GERIATRIC NUTRITION
A Comprehensive Review

Geriatric Nutrition
A Comprehensive Review

Editors

John E. Morley, M.B., B.Ch.
Dammert Professor of Gerontology and Director
Division of Geriatric Medicine
St. Louis University School of Medicine
St. Louis, Missouri and
Director, Geriatric Research,
Education and Clinical Center
St. Louis Veterans Administration Medical Center
St. Louis, Missouri

Zvi Glick, Ph.D.
Associate Director
Geriatric Research, Education and Clinical Center
Veterans Administration Medical Center
Sepulveda, California, and
Professor of Medicine
University of California School of Medicine
Los Angeles, California

Laurence Z. Rubenstein, M.D.
Director
Geriatric Research, Education and Clinical Center
Veterans Administration Medical Center
Sepulveda, California
Associate Professor of Medicine
University of California School of Medicine
Los Angeles, California

Raven Press   New York

1995 · 2nd Ed / 167.00 · 0781701694

Raven Press, Ltd., 1185 Avenue of the Americas, New York, New York 10036

Library of Congress Cataloging-in-Publication Data

Geriatric nutrition : a comprehensive review / editors, John E.
  Morley, Zvi Glick, Laurence Z. Rubenstein.
        p.   cm.
  Includes bibliographical references.
  ISBN 0-88167-610-1
  1. Nutrition disorders in old age.   2. Aged—Nutrition.
I. Morley, John E.   II. Glick, Zvi.   III. Rubenstein, Laurence Z.
  [DNLM: 1. Aging—physiology.   2. Nutrition—in old age.   QU 145
G369]
RC620.6.G47   1990
618.97'639—dc20
DNLM/DLC
for Library of Congress   90-8010
                                                                    CIP

9 8 7 6 5 4 3 2 1

Preface

With the graying of the industrialized world, it has become imperative that we explore the methods by which we can decrease morbidity associated with the aging process. Nutritional intervention is an intrinsically attractive approach to the compression of morbidity. This comprehensive text explores the realities and fallacies associated with the role of nutrition in the aging process and the effects of age-associated diseases on nutrients. Each chapter attempts to demonstrate specifically the distinctions in nutrient requirements and metabolism in the old (age 70 and over) compared to the general population.

We believe that this book has brought together the expertise of some of the most outstanding individuals presently involved in research on the unique nutritional problems of the older individual. As with all multi-authored texts, there are some areas in which the experts hold different opinions. In these cases, only time will eventually sort out the truth. Overall, however, there is consensus among the different authors; all have stressed that the nutritional needs and management of the older individual differ substantially from that which is appropriate for middle-aged and younger persons.

The editors of this volume found that reading the different chapters greatly enhanced their own knowledge of geriatric nutrition. We trust that this book will prove equally useful to the interdisciplinary team members who bear the responsibility of caring for the frail elderly and who are responsible for the nutritional education of the healthy elderly. This book should be especially appealing to nutrition educators, dietitians, geriatricians, and gerontologists. We expect that our readers will find this book to be useful and as enjoyable reading.

John E. Morley
Zvi Glick
Laurence Z. Rubenstein

Acknowledgments

The editors would like to acknowledge their debt to the Sepulveda VA Medical Center's Geriatric Research, Education and Clinical Center (GRECC). This project developed out of the animated discussions at two conferences on "Nutrition and the Elderly" that were sponsored by the Sepulveda GRECC.

Contents

NUTRITION AND AGING

1. An Overview of Aging-Demographics, Epidemiology, and Health Services 1
   Laurence Z. Rubenstein

2. Molecular Theories of Aging 11
   Arshag D. Mooradian

3. Nutrition and Longevity 19
   Edward J. Masoro

4. Energy Balance 27
   Zvi Glick

5. Nutritional Requirements of the Elderly 41
   Wayne R. Bidlack

6. Nutritional Assessment of the Elderly 73
   Emma J. Lewis and Stacey J. Bell

7. The Role of Nutrition in the Prevention of Age-Associated Diseases 89
   John E. Morley

NUTRITIONAL DEFICIENCIES

8. Anorexia of Aging and Protein-Energy Malnutrition 105
   Andrew J. Silver

9. Vitamin Disorders in the Elderly 117
   Larry E. Johnson

10. Calcium, Vitamin D, and Osteopenia in the Elderly 149
    Arnold S. Brickman

11. Zinc Metabolism in the Elderly 161
    Craig J. McClain and Mary A. Stuart

12. Other Trace Elements 171
    John E. Morley

13. Nutritional Anemias in the Elderly 183
    David A. Lipschitz

14. Water Metabolism 193
    Laurel A. Pfeil, Paul R. Katz, and Paul J. Davis

SYSTEMS MALFUNCTION AND NUTRITION

15. Modulation of Age-Associated Immune Dysfunction by
    Nutritional Intervention 203
    S. Jill James, Steven C. Castle, and
    Takashi Makinodan

16. The Oral Cavity and Nutrition 225
    Michael Kaurich

17. Gastrointestinal Function and Aging 231
    Robert M. Russell

18. The Effect of Age on the Liver.............................. 239
    David H. Van Thiel and Judith S. Gavaler

19. Nutrition and Diabetes Mellitus in the Elderly 259
    Fran E. Kaiser and Mark J. Rosenthal

20. Nutrition and Cardiovascular Disease 269
    Roslyn B. Alfin-Slater and David Kritchevsky

21. Nutritional Interventions as Antihypertensive Therapy
    in the Elderly... 281
    Dalila B. Corry and Michael L. Tuck

22. Obesity 293
    John E. Morley and Zvi Glick

23. Cancer and Malnutrition 307
    David Heber

24. Cardiac Cachexia 315
    Martin J. Gorbien

SPECIAL TOPICS IN GERIATRIC NUTRITION

25. Epidemiology of Malnutrition in Nursing Homes 325
    Daniel Rudman, Vasu D. Arora, Axel G. Feller,
    Hoskote S. Nagraj, Parde Y. Lalitha, and
    Norma P. Caindec

26. Nutrition Management in Nursing Homes 333
     Ann M. Coulston

27. Nutritional Support for Elderly Patients.................... 343
     Dennis H. Sullivan

28. Pressure Sores and Nutrition 363
     Bruce A. Ferrell and Dan Osterweil

29. Drug-Food/Food-Drug Interactions 371
     Christine Hamilton Smith

30. Nutrition Misinformation: Health Fraud and the Elderly
     Population–Creation of Food Fads for Profit 397
     Wayne R. Bidlack

31. Nutrition and Behavior 419
     Allen S. Levine

32. Memory Enhancement in Mice with Chronic Menhaden
     Oil Administration.. 435
     *James F. Flood, Ernesto N. Hernandez, and
     John E. Morley*

33. Zinc Status and Impotence.................................... 441
     *Charles J. Billington, Rex B. Shafer,
     Phillip A. Krezowski, Allen S. Levine, and
     John E. Morley*

34. Exercise and Muscle Strength 447
     *R.A. Wiswell, S. Victoria Jaque, and
     M. Hamilton-Wessler*

35. Interdisciplinary Teams for the Solution of
     Nutritional Problems... 457
     Kenneth D. Cole and Freddie A. Jones

36. Choices About Food and Water: The Emerging Ethical
     and Legal Standard of Care 471
     Steven H. Miles and Gregory P. Gramelspacher

     Subject Index... 481

Contributors

Roslyn B. Alfin-Slater, Ph.D.
Professor of Nutrition
UCLA School of Public Health
Los Angeles, California 90024

Vasu D. Arora, M.D.
Department of Medicine
The Medical College of Wisconsin,
*   and Medical Service*
VA Medical Center
Milwaukee, Wisconsin 53295

Stacey J. Bell, M.S., R.D.
Nutrition Support Service
Nutrition/Metabolism Laboratory
New England Deaconess Hospital
Boston, Massachusetts 02215

Wayne R. Bidlack, Ph.D.
Associate Professor of Nutrition
Department of Pharmacology and
*   Nutrition*
University of Southern California
School of Medicine
Los Angeles, California 90033

Charles J. Billington, M.D.
Department of Food Science and
*   Nutrition*
University of Minnesota, and
*   Neuroendocrine Research*
*   Laboratory*
Section of Endocrinology and
*   Metabolism*
Medical Service
Minneapolis, VA Medical Center
Minneapolis, Minnesota 55455

Arnold S. Brickman, M.D.
Professor of Medicine
UCLA School of Medicine and
*   Chief, Mineral Metabolism*
*   Section*
Medical Service
VA Medical Center
Sepulveda, California 91343

Norma P. Caindec, M.S., R.D.
Department of Medicine
The Medical College of Wisconsin,
*   and Medical Service*
VA Medical Center
Milwaukee, Wisconsin 53295

Steven C. Castle, M.D.
Department of Medicine
UCLA School of Medicine, and
*   Geriatric Research, Education*
*   and Clinical Center*
Wadsworth VA Medical Center
Los Angeles, California 90073

Kenneth D. Cole, Ph.D.
Clinical Associate Professor
Department of Psychology
University of Southern California
*   and Program Director,*
*   Interdisciplinary Team Training*
*   in Geriatrics*
VA Medical Center
Sepulveda, California 91343

Dalila B. Corry, M.D.
VA Medical Center
Sepulveda, California 91343

Ann M. Coulston, M.S., R.D.
Research Dietician
General Clinical Research Center
Stanford University Hospital
Stanford, California 94305

Paul J. Davis, M.D.
Professor and Vice-Chairman,
  Department of Medicine; Head,
  Endocrinology Division,
  Department of Medicine
State University of New York
  (SUNY) at Buffalo and VA
  Medical Center
Buffalo, New York 14215

Axel G. Feller, M.D.
Department of Medicine
The Medical College of Wisconsin,
  and Medical Service
VA Medical Center
Milwaukee, Wisconsin 53295

Bruce A. Ferrell, M.D.
Geriatric Fellow, Multicampus
  Division of Geriatric Medicine
UCLA School of Medicine, and
  Jewish Homes for the Aging of
  Greater Los Angeles
Reseda, California 91335

James F. Flood, Ph.D.
Department of Psychiatry and
  Biobehavioral Science
UCLA School of Medicine; and
  Geriatric Research, Education
  and Clinical Center
VA Medical Center
Sepulveda, California 91343
Current Address:
Research Service
VA Medical Center
951 No. Grand Blvd.
St. Louis, Missouri 63106

Judith S. Gavaler, Ph.D.
Division of Gastroenterology
University of Pittsburgh School of
  Medicine
Pittsburgh, Pennsylvania 15261

Zvi Glick, Ph.D.
Professor of Medicine
UCLA School of Medicine, and
  Associate Director, Geriatric
  Research, Education and
  Clinical Center
VA Medical Center
Sepulveda, California 91343

Martin J. Gorbien, M.D.
Geriatric Fellow, Multicampus
Division of Geriatric Medicine
UCLA School of Medicine
  and VA Medical Center
Sepulveda, California 91343
Current Address:
The Cleveland Clinic Foundation
Section of Geriatric Medicine
One Clinic Center
9500 Euclid Avenue
Cleveland, Ohio 44195

Gregory P. Gramelspacher, M.D.
Fellow, Center for Clinical
  Medical Ethics
University of Chicago
Chicago, Illinois 60637

M. Hamilton-Wessler, M.S.
Department of Exercise Sciences
University of Southern California
Los Angeles, California 90089

David Heber, M.D., Ph.D.
Professor of Medicine and Chief,
  Division of Clinical Nutrition
Department of Medicine
UCLA School of Medicine
Los Angeles, California 90024

Ernesto N. Hernandez
Aging Research Laboratory
VA Medical Center
Sepulveda, California 91343

S. Jill James, Ph.D.
Department of Medicine
UCLA School of Medicine, and
  Geriatric Research, Education
  and Clinical Center
Wadsworth VA Medical Center
Los Angeles, California 90073
Current Address:
National Center for Toxicological
  Research
Division of Comparative
  Toxicology
365 North Country Road 3
Jefferson, Arkansas 72079

S. Victoria Jaque, M.S.
Department of Exercise Sciences
University of Southern California
Los Angeles, California 90089

Larry E. Johnson, M.D., Ph.D.
Geriatric Fellow, Multicampus
Division of Geriatric Medicine
UCLA School of Medicine
  and VA Medical Center
Sepulveda, California 91343
Current Address:
Department of Family Medicine
  (582)
University of Cincinnati Medical
  Center
Cincinnati, Ohio 45267

Freddie A. Jones, R.D.
Chief, Clinical Dietetics Section
Dietetics Service
VA Medical Center
Sepulveda, California 91343

Fran E. Kaiser, M.D.
Assistant Professor of Medicine
UCLA School of Medicine and
  Medical Director, HBHC
  Program
VA Medical Center
Sepulveda, California 91343
Current Address:
St. Louis University
School of Medicine
1402 S. Grand, Room M-239
St. Louis, Missouri 63104

Paul R. Katz, M.D.
Assistant Professor of Medicine,
  Geriatrics Division
Department of Medicine
School of Medicine
State University of New York at
  Buffalo, and VA Medical Center
Buffalo, New York 14215

Michael Kaurich, D.D.S.
Assistant Professor of Hospital
  Dentistry
UCLA School of Dentistry
Director, Dental Geriatric
  Fellowship Program
VA Medical Center
Sepulveda, California 91343

Phillip A. Krezowski, M.D.
Neuroendocrine Research
  Laboratory Section of
  Endocrinology and Metabolism
Department of Medicine
Minneapolis, VA Medical Center
Minneapolis, Minnesota 55455

David Kritchevsky, Ph.D.
Associate Director
Wistar Institute
3601 Spruce Street
Philadelphia, Pennsylvania 19104

Parde Y. Lalitha, M.D.
Department of Medicine
The Medical College of Wisconsin
  and Medical Service
VA Medical Center
Milwaukee, Wisconsin 53295

Allen S. Levine, Ph.D.
Professor of Nutrition and Surgery
Department of Medicine, Surgery,
  Psychiatry, and Food Science
  and Nutrition
University of Minnesota, and
  Neuroendocrine Research
  Laboratory
VA Medical Center
Minneapolis/St. Paul,
  Minnesota 55417

Emma J. Lewis, R.D.
Nutrition Support Service
Nutrition/Metabolism Laboratory
New England Deaconess Hospital
Boston, Massachusetts 02215

David A. Lipschitz, M.D.
Professor of Medicine
University of Arkansas School of
  Medicine, and Chief,
  Hematology and Oncology
  Division and Director, Geriatric
  Research, Education and
  Clinical Center
VA Medical Center
Little Rock, Arkansas 72206

Takashi Makinodan, Ph.D.
Professor of Medicine
UCLA School of Medicine, and
  Director, Geriatric Research,
  Education and Clinical Center
Wadsworth VA Medical Center
Los Angeles, California 90073

Edward J. Masoro, Ph.D.
Professor of Physiology and
  Chairman, Department of
  Physiology
The University of Texas Health
  Science Center
San Antonio, Texas 78284

Craig J. McLain, M.D.
Professor of Medicine
Director, Division of Digestive
  Diseases and Nutrition
University of Kentucky, and VA
  Medical Center
Lexington, Kentucky 40536

Steven H. Miles, M.D.
Associate Director, Center
  for Clinical Medical Ethics
University of Chicago Hospitals
Chicago, Illinois 60637

Arshag D. Mooradian, M.D.
Associate Professor of Medicine
Director of Gerontologic Research
Division of Restorative Medicine,
  Department of Medicine
University of Arizona College of
  Medicine
Tucson, Arizona 85719

John E. Morley, M.B., B.Ch.
Dammert Professor of
  Gerontology and Director
Division of Geriatric Medicine
St. Louis University School of
  Medicine
St. Louis, Missouri 63104 and
  Director, Geriatric Research
  Education and Clinical Center
St. Louis VA Medical Center
St. Louis, Missouri 63125

Hoskote S. Nagraj, M.D.
Department of Medicine
The Medical College of Wisconsin,
and Medical Service
VA Medical Center
Milwaukee, Wisconsin 53295

Dan Osterweil, M.D.
Assistant Professor of Medicine
UCLA School of Medicine
Medical Director, Grancell Village
Jewish Homes for the Aging
Reseda, California 91335

Laurel A. Pfeil, M.D.
Fellow, Endocrinology Division
Department of Medicine, School
of Medicine
State University of New York at
Buffalo and VA Medical Center
Buffalo, New York 14215

Mark J. Rosenthal, M.D.
Assistant Professor of Medicine
UCLA School of Medicine, and
Geriatric Research, Education
and Clinical Center
VA Medical Center
Sepulveda, California 91343

Laurence Z. Rubenstein, M.D.
Associate Professor of Medicine
UCLA School of Medicine, and
Clinical Director, Geriatric
Research, Education and
Clinical Center
VA Medical Center
Sepulveda, California 91343

Daniel Rudman, M.D.
Professor of Medicine
University of Wisconsin, and
Medical Service
VA Medical Center
Milwaukee, Wisconsin 53295

Robert M. Russell, M.D.
Professor of Medicine and
Nutrition and Director of
Human Studies
Human Nutrition Research Center
on Aging at Tufts University
Boston, Massachusetts 02111

Rex B. Shafer, M.D.
Department of Food Science and
Nutrition
University of Minnesota, and
Neuroendocrine Research
Laboratory
Section of Endocrinology and
Metabolism
Department of Medicine
Minneapolis VA Medical Center
Minneapolis, Minnesota 55455

Andrew J. Silver, M.D.
Assistant Professor of Medicine
UCLA School of Medicine
Staff Physician, Geriatric
Research
Education and Clinical Center
VA Medical Center
Sepulveda, California 91343
Current Address:
St. Louis University
School of Medicine
1402 S. Grand, Room M-239
St. Louis, Missouri 63104

**Christine Hamilton Smith, Ph.D.,
R.D.**
Professor, Division of Food
Science, Nutrition and Dietetics
Department of Home Economics
California State University,
Northridge
Northridge, California 91330

Mary A. Stuart, Ph.D., R.D.
Department of Nutrition and Food
Science
University of Kentucky Medical
Center
Lexington, Kentucky 40536

Dennis H. Sullivan, M.D.
Assistant Professor of Geriatrics
University of Arkansas School of
Medicine
Little Rock, Arkansas 72206

Michael L. Tuck, M.D.
Professor of Medicine
UCLA School of Medicine, and
Director, Division of
Endocrinology
Medical Service
VA Medical Center
Sepulveda, California 91343

David H. Van Thiel, M.D.
Associate Professor of Medicine,
and Chief, Department of
Gastroenterology
University of Pittsburgh
Pittsburgh, Pennsylvania 15261

Robert A. Wiswell, Ph.D.
Associate Professor of Medicine,
and Chairman, Department of
Physical Education
University of Southern California
Los Angeles, California 90089

Introduction

The book provides a systematic and comprehensive coverage of the field of geriatric nutrition. Emphasis is placed on how age-associated changes in physiology and function influence nutritional status, and how nutrition may influence aging and age associated morbidity. The book is divided into four sections.

The first section, "Nutrition and Aging," sets the stage for a more detailed exploration of aging-nutrient interactions in subsequent sections. The first chapter explores the changing demographics of an aging society and the effects of aging on functional status. The next two chapters examine the effects (both demonstrated and postulated) of nutritional manipulation on the aging process. The factors associated with the change in energy balance with advancing age are explored in Chapter 4. In Chapter 5, Dr. Bidlack provides a comprehensive assessment of the available knowledge of the nutrient requirements of older individuals. He particularly stresses that many of the commonly held beliefs concerning nutrient requirements for adults do not appear appropriate as we age. The next chapter describes the techniques used for nutritional assessment and stresses the need to use appropriate values for older individuals. In the final chapter of this section, the putative role of nutritional factors in primary, secondary, and tertiary prevention of age-associated diseases is discussed. In addition, the role of assistive devices in preventing the development of malnutrition in older individuals is emphasized.

The second section, "Nutritional Deficiencies," begins with a chapter discussing the pathogenesis of the increasingly recognized syndrome of anorexia associated with aging. In Chapter 9, Dr. Johnson explores the effects of vitamin deficiency and how the aging process and associated diseases can place some individuals at risk for vitamin deficiency. The potential toxicities of megavitamin use are explored. In Chapter 10, the well-recognized role of calcium and vitamin D in the development of age-related osteopenia is discussed. The unique effects of zinc deficiency in older individuals and the putative role of zinc in the therapy of age-related macular degeneration are covered in Chapter 11. The subsequent chapter deals with the emerging knowledge of the effects of aging on other trace minerals and discusses the available evidence for a role of selenium deficiency in the pathogenesis of certain cancers. In Chapter 13, Dr. Lipschitz points out the ability of nutritional factors to produce anemia in older individuals. Chapter 14 discusses the most essential and most forgotten of nutrients—water. The elderly often live in a water desert and the situation is aggravated by the presence of age-related hypodipsia.

In the third section, "Systems Malfunction and Nutrition," the interaction of disease, nutrition, and the aging process is explored. Chapter 15 discusses the alterations in immune function with aging and the role of nutrition in these changes. The oral cavity represents the portal of entry of nutrients into the body, and as discussed in Chapter 16, age-related changes in it can result in profound effects on nutrient status. In Chapter 17, Dr. Russell explores the changes in gastrointestinal function with aging and how they may impinge on nutrient availability. The next chapter discusses the interactions of nutrients and the liver. Chapter 19 examines the dietary needs of older patients with diabetes mellitus and the effects of diabetes on micronutrients. The role of nutrition in the pathogenesis and management of heart disease and hypertension is set out in Chapters 20 and 21. Obesity is a health hazard at any age. The etiology, effects, and management of late-life obesity are discussed in Chapter 22. In the final chapter in this section, Hippocrates' description of "the flesh being consumed and becoming water" is revisited as Dr. Heber and Dr. Gorbien explore the interactions of nutrition with cancer, and the pathogenesis of cardiac cachexia and its relevance to the elderly.

The section, "Special Topics in Geriatric Nutrition," begins with two chapters on the unique nutritional problems of residents in long-term care facilities. Dr. Sullivan in Chapter 27 provides an in depth look at the methods and problems associated with parenteral and enteral feeding of the elderly. The role of nutritional factors in the pathogenesis of decubitus ulcers is covered in Chapter 28. Older individuals often receive multiple medications. These medications can modify nutrient bioavailability, and equally, nutrients can alter drug absorption and metabolism. This complex topic is handled in depth in Chapter 29. Elderly people spend billions of dollars on over-the-counter health products each year, some of which are not only ineffective but may also cause harm. The controversial area of health fraud and misinformation is covered in Chapter 30. Next, Dr. Levine in Chapter 31 explores the emerging area of how nutrition may alter behavior and its implications for older individuals. A brief chapter by Dr. Flood and his colleagues alerts us to the fact that, in animals, fish oils may enhance memory retention, suggesting that there may be some truth in the old adage that "fish is brain food." Chapter 33 shows a relationship of zinc deficiency in older patients to hypogonadism and impotence. The beneficial role of exercise in the elderly is discussed in Chapter 34. The use of the interdisciplinary team approach to manage nutritional problems in the elderly is explored in Chapter 35. Finally, the ethical and legal problems associated with feeding the elderly are analyzed in the last chapter.

John E. Morley
Zvi Glick
Laurence Z. Rubenstein

GERIATRIC NUTRITION
A Comprehensive Review

Geriatric Nutrition, edited by John E. Morley,
Zvi Glick, Laurence Z. Rubenstein.
Raven Press, Ltd., New York © 1990.

1

An Overview of Aging—Demographics, Epidemiology, and Health Services

Laurence Z. Rubenstein

*Geriatric Research, Education and Clinical Center, VA Medical Center, Sepulveda,
California 91343 and Department of Medicine, UCLA School of Medicine,
Los Angeles, California 90024*

Issues in geriatric nutrition are inextricably linked to broader issues facing the growing older population. This chapter sets the stage for this volume's detailed discussion of geriatric nutrition by providing a brief overview of some of these broader issues facing older America. These issues include the demographics of aging, the epidemiology of morbidity and mortality among older Americans, the prevalence of conditions associated with nutritional problems, and the use of both general health care services and health care programs designed specifically for the special needs of older people.

DEMOGRAPHICS

In this century the older population has progressively grown and continues to do so. People aged 65 years and over represented 4% of the United States population in 1900, 9% in 1960, 11% in 1980, and 13% in 1990 and will represent between 17% and 19% by 2020, depending on which projections are used (Fig. 1). These increases are due to several factors, including immigration patterns, reductions in infant mortality, and actual increases in life expectancy for adults. The reduction in infant mortality, largely a result of improved public health and socioeconomic conditions, has had more impact on the average life expectancy from birth than any other factor. Yet, during the last few decades substantial gains have been achieved in life expectancy for older adults too, largely the result of improvements in health care and preventive practices, including nutritional patterns. The average 65-year-old man or woman in 1920 could expect to live about 12 more years; by 2000 this expectation will be about 16 years for men and 21 years for women (1).

As a result of this substantial sex differential in life expectancy, elderly females in 1980 outnumbered males by about 1.5 to 1 (2). These gender

1

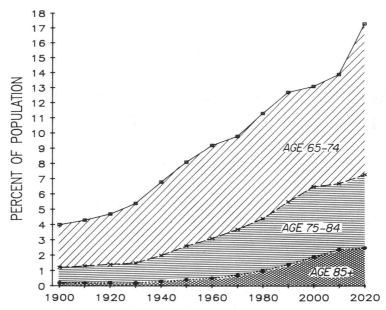

FIG. 1. Growth of the elderly segment of the U.S. population, actual and projected, 1900–2020. (From Rabin and Stockton, ref. 1.)

trends are most pronounced among the population aged 85 years and older (the "oldest old") among whom the ratio of females to males is 2.3 to 1. Moreover, because women usually marry men somewhat older than themselves, elderly women are much more likely to be widowed (52% versus 14% for women and men over age 65, respectively) (3) and to be living alone (39% versus 14%) (1).

The "oldest old" segment is growing more rapidly than any other segment of the elderly population. By the year 2000 it is projected that persons 85 years and older will comprise 15% of the elderly population (1). Clearly, this increase in the "oldest old" segment of the population is closely linked to improved health care and preventive practices.

Increases in the aged population are certainly not unique to the United States, but are occurring in developed nations worldwide. In fact, several nations had higher proportions of persons over age 65 in 1980, notably Sweden (16%), East Germany (16%), Austria (15.5%), West Germany (15%), Great Britain (15%), Switzerland (15%), Norway (15%), France (14%), and Denmark (14%) (4). In contrast, developing nations of the world have long had very small proportions of elderly persons, generally under 5%, due to their high birthrates and shorter life expectancies. In fact, some epidemiologists have proposed that a convenient definition of "developed" countries would be those in which the proportion of the population aged 65 or older is 10% or higher. However, even in developing nations, dramatic increases in the elderly populations are expected in light of recent trends of declining fertility and infant mortality rates. It is projected that, by the turn of the century, 61% of the world's elderly population will be living in developing nations (5).

There is considerable debate as to whether the increase in average life expectancy for Americans has been tapering off as it approaches a theoretical maximum life span for humans or whether average life expectancy is continuing to lengthen without a clearly defined maximum (6–8). This debate should be clarified considerably in the next decade.

Another active debate is whether the average quality of life has improved, stayed the same, or deteriorated as average life expectancy has increased, particularly during the additional years of life just before death (6–8). Two forces are at work in determining this "average quality of life." Although improvements in health status and quality of life are clearly occurring among many persons achieving old age, these are offset by the prolongation of life of disabled persons who would not have survived in previous decades. Thus, mean health and functional status among elderly people do not appear to be changing dramatically. Again, the next few years should provide data to better clarify which force—improved health status or prolongation of disability—will predominate.

The health status of the elderly population is extremely variable. Clearly, although many older people remain in good health, the oldest population segment continues to be the most susceptible to disease and disability, and the prevalence of most chronic illnesses continually increases throughout life. Although only 5% of the over-65 population live in a nursing home, 6.8% of the over-75 population and 21.6% of the over-85 population live in nursing homes (1). Over 25% of older Americans will spend some time in a nursing home before they die. Furthermore, it is estimated that, for every elderly person living in an institutional setting, there are one to three other similarly disabled persons living in the community (9).

EPIDEMIOLOGY

Causes of Death

Since the turn of the century the leading causes of death for the older population have dramatically shifted from acute infectious diseases to chronic diseases (Table 1). Currently, heart disease, cancer, and cerebrovascular disease account for 75% of all deaths for both men and women aged 65 years and older. Although mortality rates from these conditions increase markedly with age, the past two decades have witnessed a gradual decline in death rates at all ages from ischemic heart disease and cardiovascular disease. Between 1979 and 1984, death rates for ischemic heart disease decreased by 12% for men 65 years and older and 6% for women. During the

TABLE 1. *Changing causes of death: ten leading causes of death in 1900 and 1980*

1900		1980	
Cause	Rate[a]	Cause	Rate[a]
Influenza and pneumonia	210	Heart disease	205
Tuberculosis	199	Cancer	134
Heart disease	167	Accidents	43
Stroke	134	Stroke	41
Diarrhea and related diseases	134	Influenza and pneumonia	13
Cancer	81	Cirrhosis/chronic liver disease	13
Accidents	76	Suicide	12
Diabetes	13	Homicide	11
Suicide	11	Diabetes	10
Homicide	1	Tuberculosis	0.5
All other causes	775	All other causes	110
All causes	1779	All causes	594

From Detels and Breslow, ref. 10.
[a]Age-adjusted death rates per 100,000 people.

same period, death rates for cerebrovascular disease showed a 20% reduction for men and a 15% reduction for women (4). These reductions can be attributed to advances in medical treatment of these conditions; improved control of such risk factors as diet, hypertension, and smoking; and still unexplained trends and factors (10).

In contrast, the mortality rates for cancer have shown a steady increase since 1950, primarily because of the increased incidence of lung cancer, the leading cause of cancer deaths for men aged 65 to 84. For men 85 years and older, prostate cancer is the most common cause of cancer deaths. Breast cancer causes the most cancer deaths among women 65–74, but in women 75 years and older, colon cancer causes the most cancer deaths.

Infections, especially influenza and pneumonia, are still a major cause of mortality for frail older persons: 81% of these deaths occur among persons 65 years and older (11). Vaccination programs for influenza and pneumococcal disease have probably been effective in reducing the number of pulmonary deaths.

Accidents are another major cause of mortality, with falls being the leading cause of these accidental deaths. Although older persons have a lower accident rate than younger persons (probably due to lower risk-taking behavior), they have a much higher case fatality rate, most likely because of their increased fragility.

It must be kept in mind that all these trends in causes of death are based upon death certificate information, which has inevitable inaccuracies. For example, sudden or unwitnessed deaths are currently usually attributed to cardiovascular causes, often without careful assessment. Deaths from dementia and its complications are greatly underreported because the terminal event is usually reported as infection or cardiovascular disease. Because most older persons have a multitude of medical problems as they approach death, it is often virtually impossible to determine the single cause of mortality.

Morbidity

Old age is characterized by an accumulation of chronic conditions and diseases. Eighty-five percent of the noninstitutionalized elderly population have at least one definable chronic medical condition, with women having higher prevalence rates than men. Arthritis, hypertension, hearing loss, and heart disease account for 60% of these conditions (1). The prevalences of heart disease, hypertension, and hearing and visual impairments are 50 to 100% higher among persons 65 years and older than among persons aged 45 to 64 years (1). Furthermore, the tendency for older persons to have multiple chronic conditions makes them more susceptible than younger persons to disease-related, as well as treatment-related, complications and disability.

Interestingly, the annual incidence of reported acute illnesses (eg, upper respiratory infections, influenza) is actually lower for persons aged 65 years and older than for persons aged 55 to 64 years (39/100 persons versus 51/100) (4). This lower incidence is perhaps related to greater isolation among older people from reservoirs of infection, higher rates of postexposure immunity, or simply a survival phenomenon ("survival of the fittest"). However, the rates of disability and restricted activity days related to acute illness are higher for older than for younger persons (2).

Just as the prevalence of most chronic disease increases with age, so does the prevalence of definable disability. Common chronic conditions causing major activity limitations are heart disease (24% of the population aged 65 years and older are disabled by heart disease), arthritis (23%), orthopedic problems (10%), and visual impairment (10%) (3). Approximately 45% of older persons have some limitation of activity due to a chronic condition (3). Between the ages of 65 to 74, about a quarter of older persons are limited or unable to perform a major activity (defined as the ability to work or keep house), and this percentage increases to 47% of persons 85 years and older (4).

The ability to perform self-care tasks or activities of daily living (ADLs) (ie, feeding, bathing, dressing, toileting) and activities related to household management, termed instrumental activities of daily living (IADLs) (ie, shopping, cooking, cleaning, money management), is frequently used to measure functional disability. Data from a survey of Medicare enrollees in 1982 found that 19% of noninstitutionalized older persons report limitations in performing ADLs or IADLs (1). The prevalence of functional impairment increases with age from 13% among persons aged 65 to 69 to 35% among those aged 85 years and older (1). Among functionally impaired elderly living in the community, 44% report two or more limitations in ADLs and over three-quarters report two or more IADL limitations. The rates of functional disability are even higher among institutionalized elderly persons. Over 80% of institutionalized residents need assistance with one or more ADL, and 23% are dependent in all ADLs (1).

Yet, despite these high prevalences of chronic diseases and disabilities in old age, the majority of older persons rate their overall health as being good or excellent. Health status surveys have found that only about a third of older white persons and half of older black persons consider themselves to be in fair or poor health (4).

Prevalence of Nutritional Risk Factors

Several factors common among older adults have been shown to increase the risk of malnutrition (Table 2). Their prevalences in the elderly population range between 2 and 69%. The ability to purchase and prepare food is essential to ensuring proper nutrition. Poverty, social isolation, and functional impairments can have a significant impact on an older person's nutritional intake. In 1985, approximately 15% of the elderly U.S. population had an income below the poverty line, and another 29% were considered economi-

TABLE 2. *Prevalence of risk factors for malnutrition in the population aged 65 years and older*

	Proportion of population affected				
	Total Population ≥ 65	High-risk groups			
Risk factors		Women ≥ 65	"Old-old" ≥ 85	Minority aged	Nursing home residents
Social factors					
Poverty	15	16	19	26–32	NA
Isolation (% living alone)	30	39	30	NA	NA
Psychological factors					
Depression	10–25	NA	NA	NA	NA
Dementia	10–20	NA	30–50	NA	65
Alcoholism	5–15	NA	NA	NA	NA
Bereavement (% widowed)	35	52	70	45	62
Physical factors					
Impaired mobility	8	9	18	13	69
Functional impairment					
Self-feeding	2	2	4	NA	38
Preparing meals	7	9	26	NA	NA
Shopping	11	14	37	NA	NA
Severe visual deficit	8	NA	NA	NA	26
Poor dentition	16	NA	NA	NA	NA
Difficulty chewing	35	NA	NA	NA	NA

From refs. 1, 4, 12–18.
NA, data not available or not applicable.

cally vulnerable. The highest rates of poverty are among women (16% versus 9% among men) and minorities (32% versus 11% among whites) (12). In addition to being limited in the ability to purchase food, elderly persons living in poverty may have inadequate food preparation and storage facilities or may have limited access to transportation for shopping or attending community meal programs. Social isolation often accompanies poverty. Although it is difficult to estimate the prevalence of social isolation, the 30% of older people who live alone, specifically those who are frail or impaired, are certainly at risk for decreased nutritional intake.

Functional impairments that are associated with malnutrition are the inability to self-feed, shop for food, and prepare meals. Although only 2% of older people living in the community are unable to feed themselves when food is placed in front of them, over a third of institutionalized residents require feeding assistance (1). The percentage of all persons 65 years and older who report difficulty with shopping and preparing meals is 11% and 7%, respectively. For persons 85 years and older these prevalences increase to 37% and 26%, respectively (1).

Psychological conditions, such as depression, dementia, and alcoholism, and such emotional stresses as bereavement also can significantly influence an older person's nutritional intake. Anorexia is a common symptom of depression, and it is estimated that about 10% of the noninstitutionalized elderly population suffers from depressive symptoms and about 5% are clinically depressed (13). Bereavement, a common experience especially for older women (over two-thirds of elderly females 75 years and older are widowed), also can produce both a physical loss of appetite and a disinterest in eating caused by the loss of socialization at meals or the loss of a caregiver to prepare meals. Alcoholism is another well-known risk factor for malnutrition. Based on community surveys it is estimated that the overall prevalence of alcoholism among the population 65 years and older is 5 to 15% (14), with elderly men having a higher prevalence rate than elderly women (15). Older persons at high risk for alcohol abuse are retired white men who are widowed, live alone without a good support system, and are in failing health.

Persons with dementia are at risk for malnutrition because they often forget to eat, cannot make proper judgments about the type of foods to eat, or become too impaired to obtain food or feed themselves. In the United States, it is estimated that 10 to 20% of the elderly population have some form of dementia, and the prevalence increases from 5% at age 65 to 30 to 50% among persons 85 years and older (16). Over two-thirds of institutionalized elderly persons have dementia (13).

Physical impairments, such as impaired mobility, blindness, and poor dentition, are also important risk factors for malnutrition. Although only 2% of the noninstitutionalized elderly population as a whole are bedridden, 8% of older persons have difficulty getting around in their homes, and the prevalence of mobility impairment increases to about 18% for persons 85 years and older (1). In contrast, over two-thirds of institutionalized elderly persons are nonambulatory or ambulate only with assistance (4). Severe visual impairments affect about 8% of older persons and can impede self-feeding and food preparation (17). Poor dentition can also cause inadequate nutritional intake. As chewing becomes difficult, older persons often choose soft foods that are high in sugars and carbohydrates over fresh vegetables and meats. Half of all older persons are edentulous, about 16% have inadequate dentures, and over a third report difficulty with chewing food (3).

Use of Health Care Services

The older population uses a disproportionate amount of health care services. Thirty percent of the annual U.S. health care expenditures are used to provide services for the 12% of the population who are 65 years and older (4). The total health care expenditures for those aged 65 years and older increased from $8.8 billion in 1965 to $119.9 billion in 1984 (1), and hospital and nursing home costs account for 66% of these expenditures.

The older population averages more physician visits per year and has higher rates of hospitalization and longer hospital stays than the rest of the population (eg, persons 65 years and older have an average length of stay of 11 days compared to 5.3 days for persons aged 15 to 44 years (3). These rates increase with advancing age, as the group 85 years and older has the highest rates within the elderly population (1). Although these utilization rates reflect the increased prevalence of disease and disability associated with aging, they certainly do not indicate that all, or even most, older persons are receiving appropriate levels of health care. Studies have documented that physicians spend less time with older than with younger patients (19,20) and diagnose a smaller proportion of older patients' medical problems (21). Older persons receive fewer preventive health services (mammography, Pap smears, immunizations) (22–25) and rehabilitation services (21,26) and more often receive less or inappropriate treatment (27,28) than younger persons. There is documented overutilization of drugs (21,29,30) hospitals (31), and nursing homes (32) by the older population.

The development of specialized geriatric assessment and treatment programs has been one response to the need to improve the process and outcomes of care for elderly persons. These programs use a multidimensional— usually interdisciplinary—approach to evaluate an elderly individual's medical, psychosocial, and functional capabilities and problems with the intention of arriving at a comprehensive plan for therapy and long-term follow-up. Four major types of geriatric assessment programs have been described in the literature (33): hospital assessment units, hospital consultation teams, outpatient programs, and home visit programs. The most dramatic successes have been demonstrated by hospital geriatric assessment units and home visit programs. Controlled trials of such programs have documented that patients benefit significantly in several ways, including improved diagnostic accuracy, reductions in prescribed medications, greater access to rehabilitation services, improvements in functional status and mental status, reductions in hospital and nursing home utilization rates, lower health care costs, and improved survival (34–36).

Data from these innovative programs indicate that elderly patients benefit from specialized multidimensional services that address functional and psychosocial, as well as medical, aspects of health. Although the effect of these programs on nutritional status has not been examined, these programs can clearly reduce nutritional risk factors, and it is likely that nutritional status will therefore improve.

REFERENCES

1. Rabin DL, Stockton P. *Long-term care for the elderly. A factbook*. New York: Oxford University Press, 1987.
2. Fredman L, Haynes SG. In: Phillips HT, Gaylord SA, eds. *Aging and public health*. New York: Springer Publishing, 1985;1–41.
3. Lowenstein SR, Schrier RW. In: Schrier RW, ed. *Clinical internal medicine in the aged*. Philadelphia: WB Saunders, 1982;1–23.
4. National Center for Health Statistics. *Health statistics on older persons, United States, 1986. Vital and Health Statistics*, series 3, no. 25. Washington, DC: US Government Printing Office, 1987. (DHHS Publ. No. (PHS)87-1409).
5. Shuman T. *Roy Swed Acad Sci* 1984;13:175–181.
6. Myers GC, Manton KG. *Gerontologist* 1984;24:346–353.
7. Fries JH. *Gerontologist* 1984;24:354–359.
8. Manton KG. *J Gerontol* 1988;43:5153–5161.
9. Kane RL, Ouslander JH, Abrass IB. *Essentials of clinical geriatrics*. New York: McGraw-Hill, 1984.
10. Detels R, Breslow L. In: Holland WW, Detels R, Knox G, eds. *Oxford textbook of public health*, vol. 1. Oxford: Oxford University Press, 1986;20–32.
11. Fedson DS. In: Ham RJ, ed. *Geriatric medicine annual*. Oradell: Medical Economics, 1986;62–78.
12. Villers Foundation. *On the other side of easy street: Myths and facts about the economics of old age*. Washington: Villers Foundation, 1987.
13. Gurland BJ, Cross PS. *Psychiatr Clin North Am* 1982;5:11–26.
14. Barry PP. *Clin Rep Aging* 1987;1:6–12.
15. Atkinson RM, Kofoed LL. In: Cassel CK, Walsh JR, eds. *Geriatric medicine*, vol. 2. New York: Springer-Verlag, 1984;219–235.
16. Cohen D, Eisdorfer C. In: Calkins E, Davis PJ, Ford AB, eds. *The practice of geriatrics*. Philadelphia: WB Saunders, 1986;194–205.
17. McKinney PJ, Rubenstein LZ. *Geriatr Med Today* 1988;7:43–50.
18. Longino CF. *Gerontologist* 1988;28:515–523.
19. Keeler EB, Solomon DH, Beck JC, Mendenhall RC, Kane RL. *Med Care* 1982;20:1101–1108.
20. Radecki SE, Kane RL, Solomon DH, Mendenhall RC, Beck JC. *J Am Geriatr Soc* 1988;6:713–718.
21. Rubenstein LZ, Josephson KR, Wieland GD, et al. *Clin Geriatr Med* 1987;3:131–143.
22. Brown JT, Hulka BS. *J Gen Intern Med* 1988;3:126–131.
23. Weintraub NT, Violi E, Freedman ML. *J Am Geriatr Soc* 1987;35:870–875.
24. Setia U, Serventi I, Lorenz P. *J Am Geriatr Soc* 1985;33:856–858.
25. Weiss BP, Strassburg MA, Feeley JC. *Am J Pub Health* 1983;73:802–804.
26. Herman JM, Culpepper L, Franks P. *J Am Geriatr Soc* 1984;32:421–426.

27. Greenfield S, Blanco DM, Elashoff RM, Ganz PA. *JAMA* 1987;257:2766–2770.
28. Rabins P, Lucas MJ, Teitelbaum M, Reynolds MS, Folstein M. *J Am Geriatr Soc* 1983;31:581–585.
29. Jahnigen D, Hannon C, Laxson L, LaForce FM. *J Am Geriatr Soc* 1982;30:387–390.
30. Thompson JF, McGhan WF, Ruffalo RL, Cohen DA, Adamcik B, Segal JL. *J Am Geriatr Soc* 1984;32:154–159.
31. Pawlson GL. *J Am Geriatr Soc* 1988;36:202–208.
32. Greene VL, Monahan DJ. *Am J Pub Health* 1981;71:1036–1039.
33. Rubenstein LZ. *Clin Geriatr Med* 1987;3:1–15.
34. Rubenstein LZ, Josephson KR, Wieland GD, English PA, Sayre JA, Kane RL: *N Engl J Med* 1984;311:1664–1670.
35. Hendriksen C, Lund E, Stromgard E. *Br Med J* 1984;289:1522–1524.
36. Vetter NH, Jones DA, Victor CR. *Br Med J* 1984;288:369–372.

Geriatric Nutrition, edited by John E. Morley,
Zvi Glick, Laurence Z. Rubenstein.
Raven Press, Ltd., New York © 1990.

2

Molecular Theories of Aging

Arshag D. Mooradian

Division of Restorative Medicine, Department of Medicine, University of Arizona College of Medicine, Tucson, Arizona 85719

The quest for the determinants of the aging process and the search for the "Fountain of Youth" are as old as the history of mankind. Over the years, the emphasis of this search has been on formulating theories and speculations, rather than recording experimental findings. As a result, there has been a rapid proliferation of theories and very little supportive data (1,2). Over the last 30 years, however, there has been an exponential growth both in scientific tools and in interest in gerontology that has resulted in elucidation of fundamental processes of the aging cell. In this chapter, after a brief description of various theories of aging (Table 1), the recent developments in understanding of the molecular basis of aging are reviewed.

POPULATION-BASED THEORIES OF AGING

This set of theories can be grouped into two types. Type I population-based theories are based on the generalized rate of living theory, which assumes that the primary determinant of aging is the rate of development. The life span of different species is correlated with various indicators of development or rate of living, such as the metabolic rate of the species, brain weight or body weight, and the age at sexual maturation (3,4). It is suggested that the total energy spent over the life span—the so-called life span-energy potential—is constant for all species. Because caloric intake modulates energy expenditure (as discussed in subsequent chapters), it is apparent that the phenomenon of the prolongation of the life span secondary to relative caloric restriction supports this set of theories.

Type II population-based theories, the collagen theories of aging, postulate that aging is the result of collagen cross-linking in various tissues (5). These theories are now in disfavor because various animal species with different life span potentials have similar collagen composition. It is notewor-

TABLE 1. *Theories of aging*

Population-based theories
Type I: rate of living theory
Type II: collagen theories
Organ-system-based theories
Role of immune or endocrine system
"Pacemaker" of senescence
Cellular-based theories
Somatic mutation theory
Orgel's error catastrophe theory
Free radical theory
DNA or DNA-binding protein alterations

From Hart and Tuturo, ref. 13.

thy, however, that collagen cross-linking has been suggested to be an important biologic mechanism of premature aging of some tissue in diabetes (6,7).

ORGAN-SYSTEM BASED THEORIES OF AGING

These theories attribute the aging of an organism to deterioration in certain organ systems, particularly the endocrine and the immune systems. The rejuvenating effects of sex hormones have been suspected since 1889 when Brown-Sequard injected himself with a testicular extract and reported a feeling of rejuvenation (8). Although a variety of hormonal changes occur with aging (9), none has been causally linked to the aging process. Relevant to these theories is the hypothesis that there is a "pacemaker" of aging, possibly in the central nervous system, that initiates senescence. Although a variety of biologic rhythms are regulated by pacemakers, so far none has been linked to aging.

The role of the immune system in aging has been studied extensively. Failure of the immune system is a common event preceding death. However, restoration of impaired immune functions in aging animals does not significantly prolong their life span (10). It is more likely that deterioration in immune system function is a secondary phenomenon in the aging process.

CELLULAR-BASED THEORIES OF AGING

Recent experimental findings are totally in support of cellular-based theories of aging. The history of these theories as a group dates back to 1891 when Weismann suggested the "wear and tear" theory, which attributes senescence to the wearing down of somatic cells (11). This notion was reinforced by the work of Hayflick and Moorhead (12), who demonstrated that diploid cells in culture have a limited potential to divide. The finite lifetime of cultured fibroblasts correlates with the life span of different species and, more interestingly, with the age of the donor. Fibroblasts obtained from older individuals tend to undergo fewer doublings *in vitro* than fibroblasts from a younger individual (13).

The cellular-based theories can be further subdivided into four groups. The first two groups—somatic mutation theory and error catastrophy theory of Orgel—are interrelated. Most of the experimental data do not support the error catastrophy theory. Intrinsic to this theory are two assumptions. One is the notion of the positive feedback effect of errors, which assumes that the error frequency increases with time. Second, it is assumed that the error frequency reaches a threshold level that will usher in the onset of cellular senescence and death. The first assumption has been challenged experimentally. Although there are methodologic uncertainties in measuring error frequency and despite the controversial reports, it appears that the frequency of cellular errors does not increase with age (14,15). In addition, induction of cellular errors by supplying inappropriate amino acids does not result in cellular senescence.

The free radical theory of aging is still a highly popular theory (16). A variety of free radicals can be generated during normal cellular metabolism. These include superoxide, hydroxyl, lipid peroxy, purine, and pyrimidine radicals. The source of these radicals is usually normal mitochondrial respiration or antioxidation of biomolecules, such as the flavins, hydroxyquinines, and catecholamines. Environmental pollutants or radiation damage further enhances free radical generation. Free radicals damage a variety of biologic systems through either a scission reaction, such as DNA cleavage, or addition reactions, such as covalent bond formation and generation of novel biochemically active radicals. In addition, they cause cross-linking reactions that result in membrane damage and accumulation of lipofuscin. However, the studies by Harman (16) demonstrating the extension of life span in mice treated with antioxidants could not be confirmed in subsequent studies (17,18). The earlier encouraging findings could have been due to the beneficial effect of relative food restriction that was inadvertently imposed on the animals given the antioxidants. Of interest is that supplementary Vitamin E, an antioxidant, reduced the age-related accumulation of cardiac lipofuscin without altering the life span of the animals (17,18).

The cellular-based theories have one common denominator, namely the faulty protein-synthesizing machinery of the cell. Aging is associated with alterations at each phase of protein synthesis. Changes in protein synthesis, mRNA processing, and changes in DNA structure and function are reviewed separately.

Age-Related Changes in Protein Synthesis

Protein synthesis, whether measured *in vivo* or in cell-free systems, is decreased with aging (19). This reduction has been demonstrated in different species and in different strains of rats. Although the effect in some tissues is less than in others, most tissues examined show an age-related decline in protein synthesis. It is estimated that up to 70% of protein synthesis can be reduced in aged animals. This reduction is counterbalanced by a proportionate reduction in the protein degradation rate. Thus, the total protein content per cell remains stable throughout the life span. The reduction in protein synthesis therefore can be considered a secondary adaptive response to reduced protein degradation. The opposite interpretation—reduced protein degradation is secondary to reduced synthesis—is equally plausible. It is noteworthy that the synthesis of specific proteins may either decrease, increase, or remain unaltered.

To determine which step in mRNA translation accounts for the age-related reduction in protein synthesis, various biochemical processes involved in protein synthesis have been evaluated in *Drosophila melanogaster* (Table 2) (20–22). In aged animals the amino acylation of transfer RNA (t-RNA) may be decreased by 20%. This modest reduction cannot account for the 70% decrease in protein synthesis with aging. Similarly, it appears that peptide chain initiation is at most reduced only modestly. There is some decrease in ribosome aggregation to mRNA, and metheonyl-t-RNA binding to 40 S or 80 S initiation complexes may decrease by 12 to 20%. However, the major reduction appears to be in peptide chain elongation. Thus, binding of aminoacyl t-RNA to ribosomes is reduced by 70% and peptide bond formation

TABLE 2. *Effect of aging on genomic expression*[a]

Decreased total protein synthesis and degradation while protein content per cell remains stable and specific proteins may increase or decrease
  Decreased amino acylation of t-RNA
  Peptide chain initiation
    Decreased ribosome aggregation to mRNA
    Decreased methionyl t-RNA binding by 12–20%
  Peptide chain elongation
    Decreased binding of amino acyl t-RNA to ribosomes
    Decreased peptide bond formation
    Translocation unaltered
  Peptide chain termination unaltered
Decreased total RNA transcription and degradation rates
  Decreased RNA polymerase II activity and unaltered polymerase I and III activities
  Decreased mRNA translocation from the nucleus to cytoplasm
  Decreased polyadenylation and splicing efficiency
  Increased or decreased mRNA transcription rates, depending on specific mRNA activity
Altered chromatin structure and function
  Increased thermal stability
  Decreased template activity
  Changes in DNA-binding proteins
  May be decreased histone acetylation
  May be decreased methylation of some genes

[a]Some of these changes have not been reproduced by all investigators.

is 40% lower while translocation steps are not altered significantly. Similarly, the termination step of the translational process as measured by the release of ribosome-bound N-formyl methionine is not altered in aged animals (22).

Thus, alterations in peptide chain elongation are responsible for the age-related reduction in protein synthesis. However, the age-related alterations in the synthesis of certain proteins are modulated at a pretranslational level.

Age-Related Changes in RNA Synthesis

The studies on the age-related changes in RNA synthesis are flawed by inherent methodologic uncertainties. The measurements of RNA synthesis in the intact cells are complicated by the possible age-related differences in the intracellular pool of nucleotides. This problem is eliminated in studies using isolated nuclei where the intranuclear pool of nucleotides is similar to that in the incubation buffer. However, isolating the nuclei has the disadvantage of disrupting the normal nuclear-cytoplasmic relationship. Because of such methodologic difficulties, the literature on age-related changes in RNA synthesis is replete with controversial reports.

The overall evidence suggests, however, that total RNA synthesis is reduced in various tissues examined in different aged animals. Of interest is that fibroblasts obtained from the foreskin of older people synthesize less RNA than fibroblasts from younger individuals (23). This reduction in the RNA synthesis rate is also counterbalanced by a reduction in the overall RNA degradation rate such that, at steady state conditions, the RNA content per cell does not significantly change with aging. However, the steady state level of specific mRNAs may be altered (24). The changes in the mRNA levels are usually secondary to age-related alterations in the mRNA transcription rate.

Aging is also associated with significant changes in RNA processing. An area of recent interest is the effect of aging on mRNA translocation from the nucleus to the cytoplasm. This is an energy-dependent process that appears to be reduced in aged animals (25). In addition, the efficiency of post-transcriptional processing, such as polyadenylation and splicing, is also reduced with aging (25).

It is not clear which of the changes in specific mRNA levels are the result of aging and which are secondary to an age-related change in nutritional or hormonal milieu. Aged rats consume less calories, and many specific mRNAs are modulated by the nutritional status of the animal (26,27). The changes in mRNA transcription rate may be caused by an alteration in the intrinsic capacity of the gene to be transcribed or may be secondary to alterations in transcription factors. The latter possibility has not yet been studied in the aging animals. However, there is ample evidence that aging alters the structure and function of various genes.

Age-Related Changes in Chromatin

It is generally agreed that aging is associated with significant alterations in chromatin structure. Many believe that these changes are the primary determinants of senescence (28,29). However, the precise nature of these changes is still controversial. Whereas some reports have emphasized the importance of single- or double-strand DNA breaks, others have failed to confirm these findings (28). Moreover, the urinary excretion of oxidation byproducts of DNA, such as thymine glycol or hydroxy guanosine, tends to decrease with aging. It is not known whether the plasma production rate of these compounds is also reduced with aging. There are some age-related alterations in histone acetylation that may alter the initiation of gene transcription. The age-related changes in nucleosomal length remain controversial, but it appears that they are modest at most.

The most reproducible alteration in chromatin structure is the increase in thermal stability in the aging animal (30). The melting point of chromatin from older animals is higher than that in the younger group. In aged animals, the chromatin at least in neuronal cells is also more resistant to digestion by micrococcal nuclease (31). We have also found a similar indigestibility of chromatin by alkali solutions containing high concentrations of urea (32,33). The overall evidence suggests that aging is associated with reduced digestibility of chromatin. This property in white blood cells can be a potentially useful biomarker of aging (32). Most of these changes are probably the result of alterations in DNA protein interactions as age-related changes in the thermal stability of chromatin disappear when chromatin is partially deproteinized (30).

Aging is also associated with significant changes in chromatin function. A variety of techniques have been used in the past to study the effect of aging on gene expression. The overall transcribability of chromatin is reduced with aging, which also has been attributed to changes in DNA binding proteins (30). Strehler et al. (34,35) found a decreased DNA ability to hybridize with r RNA with increasing age in postmitotic tissues (brain, heart, and skeletal muscles), but not in tissues with mitosis potential (liver, spleen, and kidney), suggesting that age-related alterations in gene expression may depend on the regenerative capacity of the tissue (7). More recent studies have focused on the gene specificity of age-related alterations in protein synthesis. The albumin mRNA content of liver is higher in aged rats than in young animals, whereas the p-450 b mRNA decreases with age (24). There appears to be an age-related derepression of viral- and globin-related mRNA in the brain and liver (36), and the expression of tyrosine hydroxylase is also increased (37). These findings suggest that some degree of "leaky" expression of genes is likely to occur in aged animals. For certain genes, this phenomenon has been attributed to an age-related decrease in methylation status (38).

CONCLUSION

Despite the controversy in the literature, it is clear that aging is associated with significant changes in gene expression. It is not known, however, whether these changes are epiphenomena or have some pathogenetic significance. It is likely that some of the reported changes are not related to tissue aging, but rather are secondary to an age-related change in the nutritional or hormonal milieu. Future research should focus on identifying changes that are specific to aging.

REFERENCES

1. Hart RW, Turturo A. *Rev Biol Res Aging* 1983;1:5–17.
2. Mooradian AD. In: *Manual of intensive course in geriatric medicine.* Los Angeles: UCLA, 1988;29–33.
3. Cutler RG. In: Cutler RG, ed. *Interdisciplinary topics in gerontology,* vol. 9. New York, Karger, 1976;83–133.
4. Sacher G. In: Cutler RD, ed. *Interdisciplinary topics in gerontology, vol. 9.* New York: Karger, 1976;69–82.
5. Bornstein P. *Mech Aging Dev* 1974;5:305–314.
6. Cerami A. *J Am Geriatr Soc* 1985;33:626–634.
7. Mooradian AD. *J Am Geriatr Soc* 1988;36:831–839.
8. Brown-Sequard CE. *Compt Rendu Soc Biol* 1889;41:415–422.
9. Mooradian AD, Morley JE, Korenman SG. *Disease-a-Month* 1988;34:398–461.
10. Hirokawa K, Sato K, Makinodan T. *Clin Immunol Immunopathol* 1982;22:297–304.
11. Weismann A. In: Poulton EB, Schonland S, Shipley AE, eds. *Essays on heredity and kindred biological problems,* 2nd ed. Oxford Clarendon Press, 1981;1–92.
12. Hayflick L, Moorhead PS. *Exp Cell Res* 1961;25:585–621.
13. Hayflick L. In: Finch CE, Hayflick L, eds. *Handbook of the biology of aging.* New York: Van Nostrand Reinhold, 1976;159–188.
14. Bozcuk AN. *Exp Gerontol* 1976;11:103–112.
15. Hoffman GW. *J Mol Biol* 1974;86:349–362.
16. Harman D. *Proc Natl Acad Sci USA* 1981;78:7124–7128.
17. Blackett AD, Hall, DA. *Gerontology* 1981;27:133–139.
18. Blackett AD, Hall DA. *Age Aging* 1981;10:191–195.
19. Richardson A, Birchenall-Sparks MC. *Rev Biol Res Aging* 1983;1:255–273.
20. Webster GC, Webster SL. *Exp Gerontol* 1981;16:487–494.
21. Webster GC, Webster SL, Landis WA. *Mech Aging Dev* 1981;16:71–79.
22. Webster GC, Webster SL. *Mech Aging Dev* 1982;18:369–378.
23. Chen JJ, Brot N, Weissbach H. *Mech Aging Dev* 1980;13:285–295.
24. Richardson A, Rutherford MS, Birchenall-Sparks MC, Robert MS, Wu WT, Cheung HT. In: Sohal RS, Birnbaum LS, Cutler RG, eds. *Molecular biology of aging. Gene stability and gene expression.* New York: Raven Press, 1980;229.
25. Muller WEG, Agutter PS, Bernd A, Bachmann M, Schroder HC. In: Bergener M, Ermini M, Stahelin HB, eds. *The 1984 Sandoz lectures in gerontology thresholds in aging.* London: Academic Press, 1985;21–57.
26. Mooradian AD, Mariash CN. *Diabetes* 1987;36:938–943.
27. Mooradian AD. *Ann Intern Med* 1988;109:890–904.
28. Gensler HL, Bernstein H. *Q Rev Biol* 1981;56:279–303.
29. Kirkwood TBL. *Mutation Res* 1988;7–13.
30. Berdyshev GD, Zhelabovskaya SM. *Exp Gerontol* 1972;7:321–330.
31. Berkowitz EM, Sanborn AC, Vaughan DW. *J Neurochem* 1983;41:516–523.

32. Hartnell JM, Morley JE, Mooradian AD. *J Gerontol Biol Sci* 1989;44:B125–B130.
33. Hartnell JM, Storrie MD, Mooradian AD. *Mutation Res* 1989;212:187–192.
34. Strehler BL, Chang M-P, Johnson LK. *Mech Aging Dev* 1979;11:371–378.
35. Strehler BL, Chang M-P. *Mech Aging Dev* 1979;11:379–382.
36. Ono T, Cutler RG. *Proc Natl Acad Sci USA* 1978;75:4431–4435.
37. Wareham KA, Lyon MF, Glenister PH, Williams ED. *Nature* 1987;327:725–727.
38. Wilson VL, Jones PA. *Science* 1983;220:1055–1057.

Geriatric Nutrition, edited by John E. Morley,
Zvi Glick, Laurence Z. Rubenstein.
Raven Press, Ltd., New York © 1990.

3

Nutrition and Longevity

Edward J. Masoro

Department of Physiology, The University of Texas Health
Science Center, San Antonio, Texas 78284

Longevity, which is defined as the length or duration of life, is a widely used parameter in gerontologic research. There are several ways of measuring and expressing longevity, and each provides different insights and information.

MEASUREMENT AND EXPRESSION OF LONGEVITY

Life expectancy is the most commonly used mode of expressing longevity. Indeed, it is almost the sole way in which longevity is discussed by the popular media. Life expectancy is defined as the mean length of life remaining for a population of a given age, eg, for Americans 50 years of age in the year 1989. When calculated from birth, life expectancy is the mean length of life measured or projected for a population born during a particular period of time, eg, for female American babies born in a given calendar year.

The life span of the species (often called the life span or the maximum life span) is defined as the length of life of the longest-lived members of a population. It is a characteristic that is peculiar for each species (1), eg, the life span of humans is about 115 years, for elephants about 70, and for house mice about 3 years. Life span is a parameter of great use to gerontologists.

Survival curves are a highly informative way to express longevity data. Kirkwood and Holliday (2) used the four theoretical survival curves shown in Fig. 1 to describe the use and meaning of survival curves. The vertical axis of the graph represents the percent of a population chosen for study that is alive, and the horizontal axis expresses the age of the population. Curve *a* is an exponential decay curve that indicates that the death rate per unit of population (eg, number of deaths per month per 100,000 individuals) does not change with age. Such a survival curve has yet to be observed for a mammalian species. Rather, all survival curves reported so far are shifted to the right of curve *a*. Curve *b* is typical of those reported for mammalian populations of small size (eg, mice and rats) living in the wild; that is without

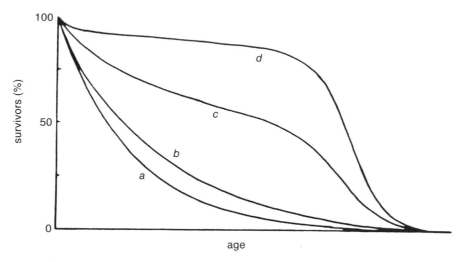

FIG. 1. Four theoretical survival curves. (From Kirkwood and Holliday, ref. 2.)

protection from environmental hazard. With protection from such environmental hazards as predators, extremes in environmental temperature, and pathogenic micro-organisms, the survival curve is shifted further to the right, becoming, with increasing protection, increasingly rectangular in shape (curves *c* and *d*). The rectangularization of the survival curve is the graphic expression of the fact that mortality is becoming increasingly associated with old age as protection from premature death increases.

RELATION OF LONGEVITY TO AGING AND TO DISEASE

Gompertz reported in 1824 that the rate and probability of death of humans increase exponentially with increasing age (3). Subsequently, similar relationships between age and death rate have been described for many animal species (4). It is generally recognized therefore that aging plays an important role in mortality and thus longevity.

This relationship is expressed quantitatively by the *age-specific death rate*, which is defined as the number of individuals who have died during an age interval (eg, between 50 and 51 years of age) in relation to the number of individuals who were alive during that age interval. In mature mammals, the age-specific death rate doubles over regular age increments, eg, in mice at 220-day increments in age, in beagle dogs at 812-day increments, and in American women based on 1969 data at 3100-day increments.

Although the aging processes clearly play an important role in longevity, disease is also a major factor. This is particularly evident when considering the changes in life expectancy that have occurred in the developed nations during this century. For example, life expectancy from birth in the United States increased from about 47 years in 1900 to 73 years in 1980 (5). Much of this increase in life expectancy occurred before 1950 and was primarily related to a reduction in the death of children from infectious diseases. Thus, this marked increase in longevity (ie, life expectancy) has little to do with the aging processes, but rather results from the effects of sanitation engineering, immunization, and, to a much lesser extent, of antibiotics on the occurrence of premature death.

The increase in life expectancy in the United States since 1960 appears to be primarily the result of factors that influence chronic degenerative diseases, such as cardiovascular disease and cancer. Because the relationship of such diseases to the aging processes remains to be defined (6), it is not clear to what extent changes in the aging processes may have been involved in these recent increases in life expectancy in the developed nations. Unfortunately, currently available information does not permit an informed choice to be made between the following possibilities: (a) the degenerative disease and aging share the same time frame, but are related in no other way; (b) the degenerative disease process is promoted by the aging processes; and (c) the degenerative disease process is part of the aging processes. Future research should make it possible to choose between these possibilities for each degenerative disease.

The life span of a species is believed by gerontologists to reflect the aging processes of the species. For example, gerontologists use the life span of a species as an index of the rate of aging for a species (7); that is, the rate of aging is believed to be related inversely to the life span of the species. This view is likely to be valid if the true life span of a species were being measured; however, in practice, it is only an apparent life span that is being determined, which could very well be influenced by disease or less than optimal environmental conditions. Nevertheless, the findings of Kohn (8) and Maeda et al. (9) indicate that the longest-lived human and rats in their respective studies may have longevities close to those of the true life span. Kohn (8) found that people who died at ages in excess of 90 years appear to be remarkably free of disease processes; this finding led him to propose that senescence is the basic cause of such deaths. Maeda et al. (9) found that with rats in environments and on dietary programs that enabled them to live long lives, death could occur in the absence of sufficient pathologic lesions.

NUTRITION, DISEASE, AND LIFE EXPECTANCY

If nutrition can prevent, delay, or retard disease processes, it should increase life expectancy. Indeed, there is evidence from both human and animal model research that nutrition can influence disease processes and thereby increase life expectancy.

Food restriction of rats markedly slows the age-associated progression of nephropathy (9) and greatly increases life expectancy (10). Brenner et al. (11) suggested that this action of food restriction is due to the reduced dietary intake of protein. This view has been challenged by Tapp et al. (12) who feel that it is the reduction of caloric intake, rather than protein intake, that is responsible. In agreement with Brenner et al., the findings from studies carried out in our laboratory show that protein restriction in the absence of caloric restriction slows the age-associated progression of nephropathy (9) and, by so doing, increases life expectancy (13). Moreover, our studies (14) show that the nature of the dietary protein is also an important factor. Rats fed a diet in which casein is the protein source exhibit a greater progression of nephropathy and a shorter life expectancy than rats fed a diet in which soy protein is the protein source. Nevertheless, in accord with the view of Tapp et al., caloric restriction was found to be more effective than protein restriction in slowing the age-associated progression of nephropathy in rats (9); however, the marked increase in life expectancy in these calorically restricted rats is primarily the result of slowing the primary aging processes, rather than the retardation of the nephropathy (9,13,15,16). Our findings on the influence of dietary calories and protein on nephropathy are summarized in Table 1.

An increase in glomerular sclerosis also occurs with age in humans (17). However, its rate of progression is usually not rapid enough to result in kidney failure unless during an earlier part of the life span the kidney suffered a loss in the number of functioning nephrons because of an acute disease or other insult (11). If an acquired acute insult did cause an abrupt reduction in the number of functioning nephrons, the age-associated progression of glomerular sclerosis can often result in renal failure long after the acquired insult is no longer active. Clearly, retarding the progression of this renal lesion should result in an increase in life expectancy. Based on the views of Brenner et al., restricting the dietary protein of these patients is currently being done (18). If the nephropathy occurring spontaneously with age in rats is relevant to the human condition, this emphasis on restricting dietary protein

TABLE 1. *Influence of dietary calories and protein on nephropathy in male Fischer 344 Rats*

Diet	Rats with severe renal lesion at time of spontaneous death (%)
Standard diet (21% casein) *ad lib*	68
Protein-restricted diet (12.6% casein), but no caloric restriction	36
Soy protein (21%) diet *ad lib*	27
No restriction of casein but 40% restriction of calories	8
40% restriction of casein and calories	1

From Maeda et al., ref 9.; Masoro et al., ref. 16.; and Iwasaki et al., ref. 14.

as a treatment should be re-evaluated. Caloric restriction may be more effective than protein restriction and may also avoid the risk of malnutrition inherent in the use of low-protein diets.

Coronary heart disease is age-associated and is a major contributor to human morbidity and mortality (19). Almost 50% of the deaths of people over 65 years of age are associated with coronary heart disease. Clearly, if nutrition can retard this disease process (ie, coronary atherogenesis), life expectancy should be increased. It is believed by many that dietary changes (20) involving a reduction in the consumption of cholesterol and an increase in the ratio of dietary polyunsaturated to saturated (P/S) fatty acids are at least in part responsible for the recent decrease in the occurrence of coronary heart disease in the American population. In addition, the recent societal emphasis on reducing body fat content in part by decreasing caloric intake results in the lowering of blood pressure (21) and of serum low-density lipoprotein cholesterol (22), both of which probably reduce the risk of coronary heart disease. Thus, many feel that the increase in life expectancy of Americans observed during the past 10 years or so is at least in part the result of alterations in the American diet.

It has been shown with mouse models that nutritional manipulations markedly increase the life expectancy of mice prone to autoimmune diseases (23). For example, restricting the caloric intake of the (NZB X NZW) F_1 mouse more than doubles the life expectancy, which appears to be the result of retarding the development of autoimmunity and renal disease (24). Food restriction was also found to more than double the life expectancy of the MLR/Mp-lpr/lpr mouse by inhibiting autoimmunity and lymphoproliferative disease (25).

Several other disease processes that influence life expectancy are believed to be influenced by nutrition. Examples are dietary calcium and osteoporosis (26), overnutrition and Type II diabetes (27), and dietary sodium and hypertension (28).

NUTRITION AND THE LIFE SPAN OF THE SPECIES

The only manipulation that has been reproducibly found to increase the life span of a mammalian species is that of food restriction in rodent species (29). Survival curves shown in Fig. 2 from a study of Yu et al. (30) with male Fischer 344 rats are typical of the kind of effects that food restriction has on rodent longevity. In that study, 115 rats were fed *ad libitum* throughout life, and another 115 rats were restricted to 60% of the *ad libitum* intake from 6 weeks of age on. When the last of the *ad libitum* fed rats died, approximately 70% of the food-restricted rats were still living; that is, food restriction resulted in a marked increase in the life span of this rat strain. This action of food restriction has been noted in experiments that have used widely differ-

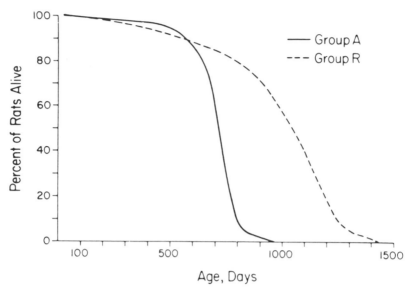

FIG. 2. Survival curves of populations of male Fischer 344 Rats. Group A (n = 115) were fed *ad libitum*. Group R (n = 115) were restricted to 60% of the *ad libitum* intake from 6 weeks of age on. (From Yu et al., ref. 30.)

ent methods of restricting food intake and many different strains and stocks of rats and mice (10).

In addition to increasing life span, food restriction retards a broad range of age-associated physiologic changes; moreover it either delays or prevents most age-associated diseases (31). From this spectrum of findings, the conclusion has been drawn that food restriction extends the life span by retarding the primary aging processes. Moreover, available evidence points to caloric restriction, rather than that of a specific nutrient, as being primarily responsible for the life span extension (31).

The current research emphasis is on the mechanisms by which caloric restriction retards the aging processes. The hypotheses that it retards the aging processes by delaying growth and development or by reducing fat content have been ruled out by recent research (31). Also, the widely held concept of Sacher (4) that food restriction retards the aging processes by decreasing the metabolic rate is not supported by metabolic measurements carried out under the usual living conditions (32). There is growing evidence that food restriction may influence the aging processes by protecting the animal from free radical damage (33–35) and from glycation reactions (36). Also, recent findings indicate that food restriction may produce its antiaging action by modulating age-related changes in gene expression (37,38). Determining the mechanisms by which food restriction retards the aging processes should yield two benefits. First, it should provide insights on the basic nature of the primary aging processes, and second, it should yield a valuable data base for the development of effective interventions of human aging.

REFERENCES

1. Kirkwood TBL. In: Finch CE, Schneider EL, eds. *Handbook of the biology of aging,* 2nd ed. New York: Van Nostrand Reinhold, 1985;27–44.
2. Kirkwood TBL, Holliday R. *Proc Roy Soc London* 1979;B205:531–546.
3. Kohn RR. *Principles of mammalian aging,* 2nd ed. Englewood Cliffs, NJ: Prentice Hall, 1978.
4. Sacher GA. In: Finch CE, Hayflick L, eds. *Handbook of the biology of aging.* New York: Van Nostrand Reinhold, 1977;582–638.
5. Fries JF, Crapo LM. San Francisco: W.H. Freeman & Co., 1981.
6. Brody JA, Schneider EL. *J Chron Dis* 1986;39:871–876.
7. Masoro EJ. *Arch Intern Med* 1987;147:166–169.
8. Kohn RR. *JAMA* 1982;247:2793–2797.
9. Maeda H, Gleiser CA, Masoro EJ, Murata I, McMahan CA, Yu BP. *J Gerontol* 1985;40:671–688.
10. Weindruch R. *J Am Geriatr Soc* 1985;33:125–132.
11. Brenner BM, Meyer TW, Hostetter TH. *N Engl J Med* 1982;307:652–657.
12. Tapp DC, Wortham WG, Addison JF, Hammonds DN, Barnes JL, Venkatachalam MA. *Lab Invest* 1989;60:184–195.
13. Yu BP, Masoro EJ, McMahan CA. *J Gerontol* 1985;40:657–670.
14. Iwasaki I, Gleiser CA, Masoro EJ, McMahan CA, Seo E, Yu BP. *J Gerontol Biol Sci* 1988;43:B5–12.
15. Iwasaki I, Gleiser CA, Masoro EJ, McMahan CA, Seo E, Yu BP. *J Gerontol Biol Sci* 1988;43:B13–21.
16. Masoro EJ, Iwasaki K, Gleiser CA, McMahan CA, Seo E, Yu BP. *Am J Clin Nutr* 1989;49:1217–1227.
17. Kaplan C, Pasternack B, Shah H, Gallo G. *Am J Pathol* 1975;80:227–234.
18. Mitch WE. *Annu Rev Med* 1984;35:249–264.
19. McGandy RB. In: Hutchison MC, Munro HN, eds. *Nutrition and aging.* Orlando, FL: Academic Press, 1986;263–275.
20. Goor R, Hosking JD, Dennis BH, Graves KL, Waldman GT, Haynes SG. *Am J Clin Nutr* 1985;41:299–311.
21. Kaplan NM. *Ann Intern Med* 1985;102:359–373.
22. Wolf RN, Grundy SM. *Arteriosclerosis* 1983;3:160–169.
23. Fernandes G. *Pharmacol Rev* 1984;36:1235–1295.
24. Fernandes G, Friend PS, Good RA, Yunis EJ. *Proc Natl Acad Sci USA* 1978;75:1500–1504.
25. Kubos C, Day NK, Good RA. *Proc Natl Acad Sci USA* 1984;81:583A–583C.
26. Osteoporosis Consensus Conference. *JAMA* 1984;252:799–802.
27. Silverberg AB. In: Armbrecht HJ, Prendergast JM, Coe KM, eds. *Nutritional intervention in the aging process.* New York, Springer-Verlag, 1984;191–208.
28. Laragh JH, Pecker MS. *Ann Intern Med* 1983;98:735–743.
29. Kalu DN, Masoro EJ. *Gerodontics* 1986;1:121–126.
30. Yu BP, Masoro EJ, Murata I, Bertrand HA, Lynd FT. *J Gerontol* 1982;37:130–141.
31. Masoro EJ. *J Gerontol Biol Sci* 1988;43:B59–64.
32. McCarter R, Masoro EJ, Yu BP. *Am J Physiol* 1985;248:E488–490.
33. Chipalkatti S, De AK, Aijar AN. *J Nutr* 1983;113:944–950.
34. Koizumi A, Weindruch R, Walford RL. *J Nutr* 1987;117:361–367.
35. Laganiere S, Yu BP. *Biochem Biophys Res Comms* 1987;145:1185–1191.
36. Masoro EJ, Katz MS, McMahan CA. *J Gerontol Biol Sci* 1989;44:B20–22.
37. Kalu DN, Herbert DC, Hardin RR, Yu BP, Kaplan G, Jacobs JW. *J Gerontol Biol Sci* 1988;43:B125–131.
38. Richardson A, Butler JA, Rutherford MS, Sensei I, Gu M, Fernandes G, Chiang W. *J Biol Chem* 1987;262:12821–12825.

Geriatric Nutrition, edited by John E. Morley,
Zvi Glick, Laurence Z. Rubenstein.
Raven Press, Ltd., New York © 1990.

4

Energy Balance

Zvi Glick

*Geriatric Research Education and Clinical Center, VA Medical Center, Sepulveda,
California 91343 and Department of Medicine, University of California,
School of Medicine, Los Angeles, California 90024*

In developed countries, such as the United States, a deficiency in a single vitamin or mineral is rare, but energy and protein deficiency is common, especially in the elderly population (1–3). How much energy we eat is determined by a complex mechanism involving central and peripheral components that is usually geared toward maintaining a caloric balance or retaining energy, especially during growth spurts and pregnancy. This mechanism monitors energy needs so that when energy expenditure is raised by an increased metabolic rate or by physical activity, food intake is also increased (4). In addition to food intake, there is also a control mechanism of energy expenditure, governed by the autonomic nervous system. The metabolic rate decreases during energy deprivation and increases during energy surfeit (5).

A malfunctioning control mechanism of either food intake or energy output will lead to abnormal changes in body weight: cachexia at the one end of the spectrum and obesity at the other end of the energy balance equation. Each of these conditions is associated with increased risk of mortality and morbidity. In this chapter the influence of aging on energy balance is described.

AGE-ASSOCIATED CHANGES IN ENERGY BALANCE

Though the cutoff point is not clearly defined and has great interindividual variability, age-related changes in the energy balance status of adults appear to be divided into two distinct, nonsymmetric phases. The first phase is typically associated with a positive energy balance and an increase in weight and adiposity, with more than 20% of the U.S. adult population being overweight (6). This phase usually occurs between the ages of 20 and 65 years of age (6). The second phase, usually beginning after the age of 65 to 70, is

27

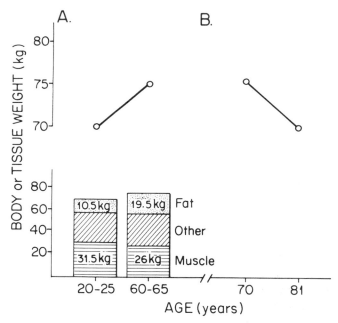

FIG. 1. Age-associated changes in weight and composition. **A:** Between 20 and 65 years. (From Shepard, ref. 46, with permission.) **B:** Between 70 and 81 years (From Steen, ref. 8, with permission.) Body composition changes past the age 70 were not included because of the small number of subjects studied longitudinally. Lean body mass and body fat tend to be reduced past the age of 70.

associated with a loss of weight, including lean body mass and apparently adipose mass as well (7–9) (Fig. 1), and with a high prevalence of malnutrition (1–3). Recent data indicate that, depending on economic status and race, some 16 to 36% of Americans over 60 years of age consume less than 1,000 kcal/day (3). Interestingly, with advancing age above 60, the mortality risk of being underweight becomes greater, whereas being mildly overweight is associated with the least mortality (10).

Understanding the age related changes in energy balance requires a separate discussion of its two components: energy output and intake.

ENERGY OUTPUT—CONTROL AND AGE-RELATED CHANGES

Until recently, energy balance was thought to be regulated chiefly by control of food intake (11). Energy expenditure was considered to be an independent variable, and weight abnormalities were seen as a result of a defective control mechanism for food intake. The first evidence for autonomic control over energy expenditure was obtained in experimental animals only about 10 years ago (12,13).

Energy expenditure may be divided into the following components: (a) basal metabolic rate (BMR), (b) the thermic effect of meals (TEM), (c) physical activity, and (d) adaptive thermogenesis.

Basal Metabolic Rate

The basal metabolic rate reflects the energy cost of maintaining normal body functions, including cardiopulmonary work, muscle tone, activity of the involuntary muscles in the gastrointestinal tract, and the chemical work necessary for normal homeostasis. BMR is determined in a postabsorptive state (12–14 hours after the last meal), at a neutral environmental temperature, and at complete rest, both physical (while lying down) and mental. The BMR is about 1,400–1,600 kcal/day or 60 to 65% of the total energy expenditure in a moderately active person (5). It originates primarily from and therefore, is highly correlated with lean body mass: men, having a greater lean body mass, have a higher BMR than women. The resting metabolic rate (RMR) refers to a value that is obtained postabsorptively at rest, but under operational experimental conditions.

The metabolic origins of BMR, especially the quantitative contribution of its individual components, are not clearly established. On the basis of our knowledge of the rate and the metabolic cost of protein synthesis, protein turnover is thought to constitute about 15 to 25% of the BMR (14,15). Should protein breakdown require energy, as has been proposed recently (16,17), the contribution of protein turnover to BMR may be even higher. The energy cost of the "sodium pump," which is needed to keep sodium extracellular and potassium intracellular against their concentration gradients, is estimated at more than 20%, with some estimates as high as 40% (18,19). The energy cost of other "futile" cycles in the metabolism of carbohydrate and fat has been estimated at less than 5% (20). The energy costs of the other components of BMR—the maintenance of muscle tone and the activity of involuntary muscles—have not been determined experimentally.

The BMR is governed by thyroid hormones through a mechanism that is not understood fully. These hormones stimulate activity of the sodium pump (21), as well as protein turnover (22), the latter both through enhancement of protein breakdown via lysosomal proteinases (22) and through stimulation of protein synthesis in conjunction with other anabolic hormones. Triiodothyronine (T_3) stimulates release of both insulin (23) and growth hormone (24). T_3 is also required for sympathetic nervous system activation (25), which can in turn stimulate the metabolic rate as described below. Thus, in addition to its direct effect, T_3 can influence the metabolic rate by enhancing sympathetic activity (25). Conversely, sympathetic activity plays an important role in facilitating the conversion of T_4 to T_3 in tissues (26,27) and influencing the metabolic rate through T_3 production, as well as its direct effect at a cellular level.

During food deprivation, the BMR is reduced by 20% or more (5,28). This reduction is caused by the associated loss in lean body mass and adaptive metabolic changes, including a decrease in T_3 and sympathetic activity (29,30). The obverse takes place during chronic overfeeding (5).

With advanced age there is a gradual 10 to 20% decline in the BMR (31,32), which may be accompanied by a reduced serum T_3 (33) and a reduced responsiveness to norepinephrine (34,35). This decline also parallels the loss of muscle mass (Fig. 1). The metabolic origins of the age-dependent compositional changes have not been clearly identified. The activity of growth hormone and testosterone, which promote lean tissue growth, is reduced with aging; this reduction may contribute to the shift in balance from lean to adipose tissue. A decreased trophic effect of the autonomic nervous system on muscle and a decreased capacity for muscle fiber regeneration have also been implicated (36).

Of the known biochemical contributors to the BMR, only protein turnover is consistently reduced with aging (37). Based on the limited data available, there is no clear age-associated change in activity of the sodium pump (38). Simat et al. (39) found that although there was no change in erythrocyte $Na+K+$ ATPase activity with age in men, women did demonstrate a decline in this activity with advancing age.

Thermic Effect of Meals (TEM)

The thermic effect of feeding is the increment in energy expenditure that is observed upon eating and that lasts for several hours thereafter. The total energy of this thermic effect amounts to about 5 to 10% of the energy intake. It has an "obligatory" and an "adaptive" component.

The *obligatory* component reflects the metabolic cost of converting the ingested macronutrients into body protein, fat, and glycogen. The heat produced in the process is a by-product of these metabolic conversions. TEM is minimal (3 to 5%) after a fat meal, where it reflects the energy for reesterification of glycerol in the intestine and adipose tissue. TEM is maximal (25 to 30%) after a protein meal, reflecting the cost of protein synthesis from the absorbed amino acids (40).

In the *adaptive* component, heat appears to be the primary end product. In rodents this heat is produced primarily in the brown adipose tissue where substrate oxidation is uncoupled from phosphorylation (41). The adaptive component of the TEM is mediated by norepinephrine through a dense sympathetic innervation of brown fat. It is abolished by the beta blocker propranolol, and in the rat the adaptive component amounts to no more than 25% of the total TEM (41). A norepinephrine-mediated adaptive component of TEM has also been demonstrated in man (5), but the tissues of origin are not known.

The thermic responses to a glucose (42) and to a protein meal (43) are decreased with advancing age. One would not expect an effect of aging on the obligatory component of the TEM, but based on a reduced capacity for adaptive thermogenesis observed in old rodents (44, but see 45) a reduced adaptive component of TEM in the elderly is feasible.

Physical Activity

Physical activity is an important determinant of energy balance status. Muscle mass is increased and adiposity is decreased with physical training (46). Such training has a much greater influence in reducing adiposity in overweight young subjects than in normal-weight subjects. Physical training also improves the energy balance status of very thin subjects (47). The amount of energy spent in physical activity varies greatly, with very highly active individuals expending in excess of 2,000 kcal, and those moderately active expending 700–800 kcal, or about 30% of their total energy expenditure (5,48). In young subjects as physical activity increases there is a compensatory rise in spontaneous food intake, but data from animals suggest that older subjects do not adequately compensate intake for an increased expenditure, displaying a negative balance (49).

Aging is associated with a decline in physical working capacity (VO_2max), amounting to about 10% per decade between the ages 25 and 65 (46). A decline in physical working capacity means that a greater effort is necessary to carry out the same physical tasks. This will tend to cause a reduction in spontaneous physical activity, which will result in a further decline in the capacity for work. This trend toward a reduction in activity with aging is exacerbated by age-related diseases, such as cardiovascular and musculoskeletal diseases, osteopenia, obesity, and others (46). A vicious cycle is created, which tends to limit physical activity and to reduce the physical working capacity. It is important to note that the elderly do retain the capacity to enjoy the benefits of physical training and that physical training can correct some age-related deterioration in physical working capacity by as much as 50% (50). In old rodents physical training improves the tolerance to cold (51). Should this hold true for humans, it will constitute an additional important benefit for the physically active elderly.

Diet-Induced Thermogenesis

Diet-induced thermogenesis (DIT) refers to the phenomenon whereby excess caloric intake can be dissipated as heat. Although it was hypothesized in the beginning of this century, the first clear evidence for the existence of DIT was only obtained some 10 years ago in experimental animals (12).

Chronically overfed rats accrued only a fraction of the excess energy intake while the rest was dissipated as heat. Clearly, a component of this heat originated from the additional metabolic costs incurred in depositing excess calories as fat (obligatory component), but the major portion of DIT originated in the metabolically active brown adipose tissue (BAT) (52). The counterpart to this finding is that the development of obesity in animal models is usually associated with a reduced DIT caused by a brown fat malfunction (53).

Recent data suggest that DIT observed during chronic overfeeding, and the thermic effect of single meals (TEM), may reflect the same phenomenon and that DIT is the summation of the TEMs during chronic overfeeding (41). The adaptive component of the TEMs is considerably greater in the overfed than in the normal fed state (41,52).

Due to the small amount of BAT in man (12,13), the ability to dissipate a large amount of excess caloric intake by adaptive thermogenesis is apparently limited and difficult to clearly demonstrate (54). DIT in elderly persons has not been studied, but in rats the capacity for DIT (and for cold induced thermogenesis) declines with age to about 10 to 20% of the level in younger animals (44, but see 45). A decline in the capacity for adaptive thermogenesis is compatible with an earlier finding that tissue norepinephrine turnover is reduced in aging rats (55).

ENERGY INTAKE—CONTROL AND AGE-RELATED CHANGES

The control of energy intake involves complex anatomic, autonomic, hormonal, and metabolic mechanisms that are only partially understood. Although we can identify some of the changes that are associated with aging, the significance of each of these changes for feeding behavior is not certain. With age, there is a gradual decline in food intake that corresponds to the decline in energy expenditure caused by a decrease in metabolic rate and physical activity (31). During the early decades of adult life, the total energy balance is positive and, in the United States, is associated with a high prevalence of overweight and obesity (6). With advancing age, anorexia of aging becomes more common as food intake falls short of expenditure and a negative energy balance ensues. In the United States, one out of every five to six individuals aged 60 years or older, and above the poverty level consumes less than 1,000 kcal/day (3).

Central Mechanisms

Anatomic and Autonomic Centers

The central control mechanism of feeding is a complex network of interconnected brain structures (56). The most studied anatomic sites are the

TABLE 1. *Age-related changes that may reduce energy intake and output*

ENERGY INTAKE
  Hypothalamic control
    Opioid feeding drive ↓
  Senses
    Sensory stimuli ↓
  Peripheral mechanism
    Insulinemia ↑
    CCK suppression of intake ↑
  Others
    Poverty ↑
    Mobility ↓
    Depression ↑
    Psychosocial problems ↑
    Dementia ↑
    Oral hygiene and dentition ↓
ENERGY EXPENDITURE
  Basal metabolic rate
    Protein turnover rate ↓
    Na-K ATPase ?
  Physical activity ↓
  Thermic effect of meals ↓
  Diet-induced thermogenesis ↓

↓, decrease; ↑, increase; ?, unknown.

ventromedial nucleus (VMH), the paraventricular nucleus (PVN), and the lateral area (LH) of the hypothalamus. Ablation of the VMH or PVN leads to hyperphagia and obesity and ablation of the LH to a suppression of feeding. Stimulation of these sites electrically or chemically by neuroreceptor agonists causes effects opposite to those brought about by ablation (57). In the past, the VMH and LH have been perceived as "centers" for satiety and hunger, respectively (the dual-center hypothesis). These centers were thought to integrate signals from the periphery reflecting the nutritional status with feeding behavior, producing a hunger drive (LH) in energy deficit and satiety (VMH) after energy replenishment.

Concepts regarding central control of feeding must now accommodate a series of additional findings. Lesions in many sites other than the VMH and LH can exert major effects on feeding. These sites are located in the hypothalamus, as well as in other brain structures (56). Severing neuronal fiber tracts that leave the VMH and LH intact can still have major effects on feeding, emphasizing the importance of neuronal pathway systems in the control of feeding (58). In addition to its proposed role in the control of feeding, the hypothalamus is also a prime activator of the autonomic nervous system. The VMH activates the sympathetic branch and exerts an inhibitory effect on the parasympathetic branch of the autonomic nervous system (58). Accordingly, VMH lesions stimulate parasympathetic (vagal) activity, hyperinsulinemia, and lipogenesis, whereas LH lesions stimulate sympathetic activity and lipolysis. It follows that feeding in the VMH-lesioned animal may not result from destruction of a "satiety center," but it may be induced indirectly by hyperinsulinemia and depletion of circulating substrates (58). Conversely, aphagia following LH lesions may result from sympathetic hyperactivity that mobilizes fat and glycogen stores and reduce the feeding drive through "autocannibalism" and not necessarily through destruction of the "appetite center." The relative importance of a "feeding center" imbalance versus an "autonomic" imbalance in the development of obesity, or in other energy balance abnormalities is not clear. It may depend on the type of obesity, the type of diet offered, and other factors (59).

In rodents, the effect of VMH lesions on food intake and the development of obesity varies with age. In very young rodents, VMH lesions have no effect on feeding, but in mature (58) and aged (58a) rodents the effect is very large. Conversely, it is not clear to what extent the age-associated shifts in energy balance—positive in early aging and with a negative trend in old age—reflect autonomic inbalances. Existing data suggest that activity of both the parasympathetic and the sympathetic branches is reduced in the elderly (60), but the proportionate reductions as pertaining to regulation of energy balance are not clear.

Neurochemical Mechanisms

The central control mechanism of feeding responds to cues from the periphery reflecting the nutritional state, as well as to sensual stimulation. The proposed signals reflecting the nutritional state, that trigger a feeding response include the rate of glucose utilization in the VMH, the level of energy stored, the thermic effect of feeding, and fullness of the stomach (4). Whatever effect a peripheral stimulus has on feeding, whether transmitted in the form of a metabolite, a hormone, or by a sensory input, is encoded into the neurotransmitter system in the brain to elicit a feeding behavior in response to the specific neurotransmitter signal. These neurotransmitters include monoamines and neuropeptides.

Monoamines

Norepinephrine, dopamine, and serotonin all play important roles in affecting feeding behavior (61). Direct injection of norepinephrine into the VMH or PVN will stimulate feeding, whereas its administration into the LH will inhibit feeding. This effect of norepinephrine is mediated through alpha -adrenergic receptors in the VMH and through beta- receptors in the LH (57,61). Brain tissue from aged rats has an impaired capacity for synthesis and regulation of alpha- and beta-adrenergic receptors. However, this impairment was demonstrated only in the cortex and cerebellum (62) and was not studied in the hypothalamus or in other sites known to play a role in feeding behavior.

Effects of serotonin and dopamine on feeding also appear to depend on the type of receptors involved, with a decrease in feeding induced by a serotonin 1_B receptor agonist in the PVN and an increase in feeding induced by a serotonin 1_A agonist (63). However, the effects of aging on either the serotonin or the dopamine feeding system have not been studied.

Neuropeptides

Several peptide neurotransmitters have been found in recent years in the mammalian brain. These include cholecystokinin (CCK), bombesin, substance P, neurotensin, opioids, neuropeptide Y, and others (64). A number of these peptides were shown to decrease feeding after central administration. However, a reduced food intake need not imply that these neuropeptides play a physiologic role in modulating feeding behavior, as their effect may be noxious or secondary to other nonspecific behavioral effects. Administration of either opioid peptides or neuropeptide Y (64) is reported to stimulate feeding, suggesting a physiologic role for these neuropeptides. Moreover, the opioid antagonist naloxone suppresses food intake (64).

It was recently reported that older rats respond less to opioid agonists or antagonists than younger rats (65). Older rats also have a lower concentration of opioid peptides in the hypothalamus (66). Aging is thus associated with a decreased opiate-based feeding drive, but the relative importance of this factor in the anorexia of aging is not clear. The orexigenic effect of NPY is not age dependent (67).

Peripheral Mechanism

Senses

Clearly, the extent of sensual pleasure that we derive from food influences food intake (4). We may be driven to eat appealing foods in a satiated state (a dessert is a typical example) or reject an unappealing food in a state of hunger. These sensual factors are important in experimental animals, as well as in humans, as offering animals a variety of appealing foods stimulates their appetite and causes obesity (4).

With aging there is a decreased acuity to taste (68) in association with a significant atrophy of the taste buds. Perhaps more important is the reduction in the ability to detect odors and to identify the foods eaten (68). Vision is also usually impaired, which may reduce feeding through lack of visual stimulation.

Stomach and Small Intestine

Placing nutrient solutions or even nonnutritive bulk in the stomach or in the intestine (4,69) cause a short latency suppression of feeding in hungry animals, suggesting that there is a gastrointestinal (GI) component to the control mechanism of feeding. This component could be mediated by afferent nerves from stretch, osmotic, or possibly nutrient receptors in the GI tract, or it may be mediated by GI hormones.

It is not clear whether any of the age-related changes in the gastrointestinal tract (70) may contribute to the observed changes in feeding behavior (CCK is perhaps an exception; see below).

Liver and Adipose Tissue

Involvement of the liver in the control of feeding is implicated largely by the correlation between hepatic glucose and glycogen metabolism, and feeding behavior. It has been proposed that glycogen and glucose breakdown products in the liver, which occur with feeding, cause changes in the membrane potential of the hepatocytes, which are relayed via vagal afferents to the hypothalamus to induce satiety (71).

A role for adipose tissue in controlling feeding has been hypothesized based on the constancy of body weight and its defense against changes: Weight loss is followed by hyperphagia, and a gain is followed by aphagia (72). Fat cell size and adipose tissue metabolites have been proposed to serve as mediators in monitoring adiposity status in the "lipostatic" control of feeding (73). Interactions of aging with adipose and liver tissues and their possible consequences on feeding behavior are not known.

Peripheral Hormones

Growth Hormone

Administration of growth hormone to experimental animals stimulates food intake and the growth of lean, but not adipose tissue (74). A similar effect has been reported in man (75). It is not clear to what extent small changes in growth hormone activity, within the normal range, influence food intake nor whether the reduction in growth hormone activity, which is often observed in the elderly, contributes to their anorexia.

Insulin

Daily single injections of insulin stimulate food intake and produce obesity (4). Moreover, the hyperphagia and obesity that develop after placement of lesions in the VMH are associated with a vagally mediated insulin hypersecretion induced by the lesions (58). The stimulatory effect of insulin on food intake is thought to result from its antilipolytic action, which decreases the availability of endogenous substrate to the tissues and perhaps to specific glucose-sensitive hypothalamic sites. In contrast to single injections of insulin, a continuous administration of insulin was reported to suppress feeding (4), perhaps by a direct effect in the brain. The contribution of age-associated insulin resistance, hyperinsulinemia, and hyperglycemia to the anorexia of aging is not known.

Glucocorticoids

The stimulatory effect on food intake of norepinephrine administered into the PVN of the hypothalamus is absent in adrenalectomized rats; it is restored with corticosterone (76). Also, peak hormone concentration in the blood is observed before the onset of feeding (77). However, corticosterone administered into normal rats has little or no effect on food intake (78). These data suggest that glucocorticoids play an important "permissive" role in the central control mechanism of feeding. In both animals and humans, glucocorticoid hyperactivity is associated with a redistribution of body energy stores toward increased adiposity and decreased lean body mass (79). In humans this is known as Cushing's syndrome, which is rather rare in the elderly.

Thyroid Hormones

Thyroid hormones stimulate food intake (80), but this effect appears to be secondary to a stimulated metabolic rate and a compensatory replenishment of the greater energy losses. In the elderly hyperthyroid patient, the rise in metabolic rate is less compensated for by a corresponding rise in food intake than in the young hyperthyroid patient. Anorexia may occur in as many as 30% of the hyperthyroid elderly.

Gonadal Steroids

Estrogen suppresses food intake; its site of action is thought to be in the VMH (81). Food intake is decreased during days of estrus (high estrogen) and increased during diestrus (low estrogen) (82). Castration of the female rat results in overeating and obesity (83). Testosterone, in contrast, increases food intake and lean tissue growth, and decreases body fat (84).

Gastrointestinal Hormones

Peripheral injections of a variety of gastrointestinal hormones (and other peptides) into rats reduce food intake. These peptides include cholecysto-kinin (CCK), bombesin, gastrin-releasing peptide, glucagon, somatostatin, substance P, and neurotensin (66). However, the physiologic significance of these hormones in producing normal satiety is not clear (69,85). Higher than normal serum levels of CCK were observed in elderly men, perhaps contrib-uting to their anorexia (3). Morley and Silver (3) reported an increased ability of pharmacologically administered CCK-8 to decrease feeding in older than in younger mice.

Confounding Problems

Poverty, poor dentition, social isolation, depression, dementia, and im-paired mobility all influence food intake adversely (3) and contribute to the undernutrition observed among the elderly (see chapter 8). Table 1 summa-rizes the age associated changes in energy balance.

REFERENCES

1. Abraham S, Carroll MD, Dresser CM, et al. *Dietary intake of persons 1–74 years of age in the United States. Advance data from Vital and Health Statistics of the National Center for Health Statistics* no. 6. Rockville, MD: Health Resources Administration, 1977.
2. Pinchofsky-Devin GD, Kaminiski MV. *J Am Geriatr Soc* 1986;34:435–440.
3. Morley JE, Silver AJ. *Neurobiol Aging* 1988;9:9–16.
4. LeMagnen J. *Physiol Rev* 1983;63:314–386.
5. Woo R, Daniels-Kush R, Horton ES. *Ann Rev Nutr* 1985;5:411–433.
6. Van Italie TB. *Ann Intern Med* 1985;103:983–988.
7. Kannel WB, Gordon T, Castelli WP. *Am J Clin Nutr* 1979;23:1238–1245.
8. Steen B. *Nutr Rev* 1988;46:45–51.
9. Shimokata H, Tobin JD, Muller DC, Elahi D, Coon PJ, Andres R. *J Gerontol* 1989;44:M66–M73.
10. Andres R. In: Andres R, Bierman EL, Hazzard WR, eds. *Principles of geriatric medi-cine*. New York: McGraw-Hill, 1985;311–318.
11. Smith GP. In: Brobeck JR, ed. *Best and Taylor's physiological basis of medical practice*, 10th ed. Baltimore: Williams & Wilkins, 1979;3–12.
12. Rothwell NJ, Stock MJ. *Nature* 1979;281:31–35.
13. Himms-Hagen J. *Ann Rev Nutr* 1985;5:69–94.
14. Waterlow JC, Garlick PJ, Millward DJ. *Protein turnover in mammalian tissues and in the whole body*. New York: North Holland/Elsevier, 1978.
15. Reeds PJ, Fuller MF, Nicholson BA. In: Garrow JS, Halliday D, eds. *Substrate and energy metabolism*. London: John Libbey, 1985;46–57.
16. Desautels M, Goldberg AL. *Proc Natl Acad Sci* 1982;79:1869–1873.
17. Waxman L, Goldberg AL. *Science* 1986;232:500–503.
18. Keynes RD. In: Bolis L, Maddrell HP, Schmidt-Nielsen K, eds. *Comparative physiol-ogy-functional aspects of structural materials*. Amsterdam: North-Holland Publishing Co., 1975;155–159.
19. Milligan LP, McBride BW. *J Nutr* 1985;115:1374–1382.
20. Himms-Hagen J. *Ann Rev Physiol* 1976;38:315–351.

21. Guernsey DL, Edelman IS. In: Oppenheimer JH, Samuels HH, eds. *Molecular basis of thyroid hormone action.* New York: Academic Press, 1983;293–324.
22. Millward DJ. In: Garrow JW, Halliday D, eds. *Substrate and energy metabolism in man.* London: John Libbey, 1985;135–144.
23. Mariash CN, Oppenheimer JH. In: Oppenheimer JH, Samuels HH, eds. *Molecular basis of thyroid hormone action.* New York: Academic Press, 1983;265–292.
24. Towle HC. In: Oppenheimer JH, Samuels HH, eds. *Molecular basis of thyroid hormone action.* New York: Academic Press, 1983;179–212.
25. Rothwell NJ, Saville ME, Stock MJ. *Am J Physiol* 1982;243:R339–R346.
26. Wiersinga WM, Touber JL. *J Clin Endocrinol Metab* 1977;45:293–298.
27. Wiersinga WM, Modderman P, Touber JL. *Horn Metab Res* 1980;12:346–347.
28. Garrow JS. *Energy balance and obesity in man,* 2nd ed. New York: North Holland/Elsevier, 1978.
29. Glick Z, Wu SY, Lupien J, Reggio R, Bray GA, Fisher DA. *Am J Physiol* 1985;249:E519–E524.
30. Glick Z, Raum WJ. *Am J Physiol* 1986;251:R13–R17.
31. Lipson LG, Bray GA. In: Chen LH, ed. *Nutritional aspects of aging,* vol 1. Cleveland: CRC Press, 1986;161–171.
32. Chernoff R, Lipschitz DA. In: Shills M, Young V, eds. *Modern nutrition in health and disease,* 7th ed. Philadelphia: Lea and Febiger, 1988;982–1000.
33. Robuschi G, Safran M, Braverman LE, et al. *Endocrinol Rev* 1987;8:142–153.
34. West CD, Volicer L, Vaughn DW. In: Ambrecht HJ, Prendergrast JM, Coe RM, eds. *Nutrition intervention in the aging process.* New York: Springer-Verlag, 1984;111–137.
35. Scarpace PJ, Mooradian AD, Morley JE. *J Gerontol* 1988;43:B65–B70.
36. Evans WJ. In: Hutchinson ML, Munro HN, eds. *Nutrition and aging.* New York: Academic Press, 1986;179–191.
37. Young VR. In: Ambrecht HJ, Prendergast JM, Coe RM, eds. *Nutritional intervention in the aging process.* New York: Springer-Verlag, 1984;27–47.
38. Guernsey DL, Koebbe M, Thomas JE, Myerly TK, Zmolek D. *Mech Aging Dev* 1986;33:283–293.
39. Simat BM, Morley JE, From AHL, Briggs JE, Kaiser FE, Levine AS, Ahmed K. *Am J Clin Nutr* 1984;40:339–345.
40. Flatt JP. In: Bray GA, ed. *Recent advances in obesity research. Proceedings of the 2nd International Congress on Obesity.* London: Newman Publishing, 1978;211–228.
41. Glick Z. *J Obes Weight Regul* 1987;6:170–178.
42. Golay A, Schutz Y, Broquet C, et al. *J Am Geriatr Soc* 1986;31:144–148.
43. Fukagawa NK, Bandini LG, Lim PH, Young JB. *Fed Proc* 1989;3:A934.
44. Horan MA, Little RA, Rothwell NJ, Stock MJ. *Exp Gerontol* 1988;23:455–461.
45. McDonald RB, Stern JS, Horwitz BA. *Exp Gerontol* 1987;22:409–420.
46. Shepard JW. In: Armbrecht HJ, Prendergast JM, Coe RM, eds. *Nutritional intervention in the aging process.* New York: Springer-Verlag, 1984;315–331.
47. Glick Z, Kaufman NA. *Med Sci Sports* 1976;8:109–112.
48. Davidson S, Passmore R, Brock JF, Truswell AS. *Human nutrition and dietetics,* 6th ed. London: Churchill Livingstone, 1975.
49. Mazzeo RS, Horvath SM. *Am J Clin Nutr* 1986;44:732–738.
50. Hagberg JM. *Fed Proc* 1987;46:1830–1833.
51. McDonald RB, Hurwitz BA, Stern JS. *Am J Physiol* 1988;254:R908–R916.
52. Rothwell NJ, Stock MJ. *Pflugers Arch* 1981;389:237–242.
53. Himms-Hagen J. *J Obes Weight Regul* 1987;6:179–199.
54. Norgan NG, Durnin JVGA. *Am J Clin Nutr* 1980;33:978–988.
55. Rappaport EB, Young JB, Landsberg L. *J Gerontol* 1979;36:152–157.
56. Krahn DD, Morley JE, Levine AS. In: Beumont PJV, Burrows GD, Casper RC, eds. *Handbook of eating disorders. Part 1: Anorexia and bulimia nervosa.* New York: Elsevier, 1987;23–43.
57. Leibowitz SF. *Physiol Behav* 1975;14:743–754.
58. Bray GA. *Int J Obes* 1984;8(suppl 1):119–137.
58a. Lazaris JA, Goldberg RS, Kozlov MP. *Endocrinologia Experimentalis* 1985;19:67–76.
59. Bray GA. *Nutr Rev* 1987;45:33–43.
60. Pfeifer MA, Wenberg CR, Cook D, Best JD, Reeman A, Halter JB. *Am J Med* 1983;249–258.

61. Leibowitz SF. *Fed Proc* 1986;45:1396–1403.
62. Greenberg LH. *Fed Proc* 1986;45:55–59.
63. Morley JE, Bundell JE. *Biol Psych* 1988;23:53–78.
64. Morley JE. *Endocrinol Rev* 1987;8:256–287.
65. Gosnell BA, Levine AS, Morley JE. *Life Sci* 1983;32:2793–2799.
66. Morley JE, Levine AS, Yim GK, Lowy MT. *Neurosci Biobehav Rev* 1983;7:281–305.
67. Morley JE, Hernandez EN, Flood JF. *Am J Physiol* 1987;253:R516–R522.
68. Morley JE. *Am J Med* 1986;81:679–695.
69. Glick Z. *Am J Physiol* 1979;5:R142–R146.
70. Almy TP. In: Andres R, Bierman EL, Hazzard WR, eds. *Principles of geriatric medicine*. New York: McGraw-Hill, 1985;297–310.
71. Scharrer E, Langhans W. *Int J Vitam Nutr Res* 1988;58:249–261.
72. Kennedy GC. *Proc Res Soc* 1953—40:578–592.
73. Glick Z. *Nutr Behav* 1984;2:65–75.
74. York DA, Bray GA. *Endocrinology* 1972;90:885–894.
75. Bray GA. In: Saunders WB, ed. *Major problems in internal medicine*, vol 9. Philadelphia, WB Saunders, 1976.
76. Leibowitz SF, Roland CR, Hor L, Squillari V. *Physiol Behav* 1984;32:857–864.
77. Dalman MF. *Am J Physiol* 1984;246:R1–R12.
78. Freedman MR, Castunguay TW, Stern JS. *Am J Physiol* 1985;249:R584–R594.
79. Hollifield G. *Am J Clin Nutr* 1968;21:1471–1474.
80. Donhoffer SZ, Vonotzky J. *Am J Physiol* 1947;150:334–339.
81. Wade GH, Zucker I. *J Compr Physiol Psychol* 1978;72:328–336.
82. Wade GH, Zucker I. *J Compr Physiol Psychol* 1970;70:213–220.
83. Bray GA. *Brain Res Bull* 1985;14:505–510.
84. Numez AA, Grundman M. *Pharmacol Biochem Behav* 1982;16:933–936.
85. Billington CJ, Levine AS, Morley JE. *Am J Physiol* 1983;245:R920–R929.

Geriatric Nutrition, edited by John E. Morley,
Zvi Glick, Laurence Z. Rubenstein.
Raven Press, Ltd., New York © 1990.

5

Nutritional Requirements of the Elderly

Wayne R. Bidlack

*Department of Pharmacology and Nutrition, University of Southern California
School of Medicine, Los Angeles, California 90033*

About 27 million people, 12% of the population, are 65 years of age or older (1). Those over 85 years of age are the most rapidly growing segment. As the "Baby Boomers" reach retirement age in the next 20 to 30 years, the number of elderly will dramatically increase again. By the year 2050, there will be more than 1 million people in the United States over the age of 100.

Only two to three million elderly individuals require extensive long-term care, but yet the elderly account for 30% of all health care and medical expenses (2). The number of older individuals requiring health care doubles for each decade over the age of 65 years.

Poor nutritional status may contribute to the declining health of the elderly and thereby increase their health care costs. Several national surveys, including the USDA Food Consumption Survey (3), and the National Health and Nutrition Examination Surveys (NHANES) I and II (4,5), report the nutritional status of the elderly to be at risk. The dietary intakes of many aged people do not satisfy the recommended level of calories; of riboflavin, vitamins B_6, A, and C; and of calcium. A variety of factors contribute to the nutritional problems of the elderly (6), including low economic status and inadequate food consumption (5,7), physiologic decline (8,9), a multitude of disease processes (10,11), and the therapeutic regimens prescribed to cure or treat those ills (12–14). Increased nutrient needs should be determined as early as possible to prevent tissue breakdown and maintain organ function (15,16).

Data are limited regarding both the nutritional needs of the elderly and the effects of aging on nutritional requirements.

Between 1984 and 1989, the publication of the Recommended Dietary Allowances (RDAs) was delayed due to a conflict between the RDA committee and the National Academy of Sciences. Before the RDAs were published, members of the RDA committee wrote summary articles discussing their views on many of the nutrients (17–21). Following appointment of a new RDA committee, the 1989 RDAs have now been published (23a). Relying on national demographic data that included relatively small numbers of elderly, both groups concluded that the nutritional needs of the elderly do not differ from younger adults.

Most data are culled to reflect healthy elderly. When reported for institutionalized or hospitalized elderly data are often criticized for not being representative (22). It is essential to identify the nutritional needs of the elderly independent of their health status.

RECOMMENDED DIETARY ALLOWANCES

The RDA values were established to evaluate the nutritional status of groups and of the population, rather than of individuals (23,24). The recommendations are intended to provide for individual variations among most normal healthy persons living in the United States under usual environmental stresses. They are not designed to meet the nutritional requirements of the ill.

None of the RDAs have specifically examined the nutritional needs of the elderly (23,23a). Instead they have simply classified recommendations for everyone 51+ years of age or older in the same group (Table 1). Estimated

TABLE 1. *Recommended dietary allowances, 1989*

Nutrients	Males 51+ years	Females 51+ years
Energy (kcal)	2300	1900
Protein (g)	63	50
Vitamins		
Vitamin A (mcg RE)	1000	800
Vitamin D (mcg)	5	5
Vitamin E (mg α-TE)	10	8
Vitamin K (mcg)	80	65
Vitamin C (mg)	60	60
Thiamin (mg)	1.2	1.0
Riboflavin (mg)	1.4	1.2
Niacin (mg NE)	15	13
Vitamin B6 (mg)	2.0	1.6
Folacin (mcg)	200	200
Vitamin B12 (mcg)	2.0	2.0
Minerals		
Calcium (mg)	800	800
Phosphorous (mg)	800	800
Magnesium (mg)	350	280
Iron (mg)	10	10
Zinc (mg)	15	12
Iodine (mcg)	150	150
Selenium (mcg)	70	55

Recommended Dietary Allowances, 10th ed. Washington, DC: National Academy of Sciences, 1989.

TABLE 2. *Estimated safe and adequate daily intakes of selected vitamins and minerals for adults*

Nutrient		Amount Recommended[a]
Biotin		30–100 mcg
Pantothenic acid		4–7 mg
Copper		1.5–3.0 mg
Manganese		2.0–5.0 mg
Fluoride		1.5–4.0 mg
Chromium		0.05–0.2 mg
Molybdenum		0.075–0.25 mg
Sodium	500[b] mg	2400 mg
Potassium	1600–2000[b] mg	3500 mg
Chloride	750[b] mg	3500 mg

[a]Nutrients listed here are presented as ranges, since insufficient evidence exists on which to base allowance recommendations.
[b]Minimum requirements.
Recommended Dietary Allowances, 10th ed. Washington, DC: National Academy of Sciences, 1989.

safe and adequate (ESA) daily intakes of nutrients for the elderly are summarized in Table 2 (6). The ESA are provided as ranges of nutrient intake because there is less information available on which to base these recommendations (23).

The elderly have an increased incidence of conditions that may compromise their health. The extent to which these problems affect the nutritional status of each individual should be considered, and generalizations about nutritional requirements of the elderly must be evaluated with care.

CALORIES

The current RDA now lists energy requirements for people aged 51 and older (Table 1). The male energy allowance was decreased 20% and the female energy allowance was decreased 15% compared to the younger adult population (23a). These recommendations differ from the 1980 RDAs which included a specific category for people aged 51 to 75 years. However, the calculations are based on data presented by the Food and Agriculture Organization/World Health Organization (FAO/WHO) (25). However, the generalized use of caloric estimates is not reasonable for the elderly (6) because it ignores the individual's activity level and the role it plays in calorie balance.

The resting metabolic rate (RMR) has been determined to decrease by 15 to 20% over the life span (26). With advanced age, the amount of energy expended for work and exercise decreases as well (8), resulting in a loss of muscle mass. Thus, the decrease in RMR results primarily from a loss in lean body tissue (27).

From the results of the NHANES I and II studies, body weight increases until the individual reaches middle age and decreases in older age. More of the poor elderly are overweight (40–100% greater), with white women and black men being the most overweight (28). The distinction between overweight and obesity is made relative to the body mass index of the young (20- to 29-year-olds), being the 85th and 95th percentile, respectively.

Increasing stores of body fat are responsible for the initial increase in weight, but a decrease in lean body mass, predominantly muscle, contributes to the reversal of the weight gain with age. A decrease in body potassium stores is also seen with increased age, indicating a decrease in body cell mass and protein content (29). This interpretation has been supported by experiments using hydrostatic weighing and those measuring total body water (see Chapter 14). These experiments have indicated that the percent body fat increases from 15 to 26% in men and from 27 to 38% in women between young adulthood and old age (30).

An individual may maintain body weight, but still have decreased lean tissue (muscle) mass. Although excess calories are stored as fat, the decreased use of muscle results in a slow atrophy of the tissue. A number of studies have indicated that an exercise regimen, even if not strenuous, can maintain body weight and body composition of the elderly (31,32).

If obesity develops, the elderly individual should decrease the intake of foods high in dietary fat. Fat calories are the most dense (9 kcal/g) and can be replaced with complex carbohydrate foods, which have fewer calories (4 kcal/g) and greater nutrient density. In periods of decreased caloric intake, however, the nutrient density of the food selected must remain high because other nutrient needs remain the same and may even be increased (26,33).

If the elderly individual has heart disease, hyperlipidemia, hypertension, diabetes, arthritis, or gout, then being overweight by 20 pounds or more becomes a specific health problem. Obesity worsens these conditions and actually increases morbidity and mortality. The maintenance of desirable (ideal) body weight is recommended as the first line of therapy.

PROTEIN

In the absence of liver or kidney disease, dietary intake of protein at 12 to 15% of total calories is well tolerated. At the current RDA of 0.8 g of protein/kg/day and with a diet of 2,300 kcal/day for men and 1,900 kcal/day for women, this amount of protein would account for about 10% of the total calories. In general, the elderly consume greater than 15% of their calories as protein (34). Because the caloric intake may be low, the actual amount of protein should be determined, rather than relying on the simple percentage of calories. Although the average need for protein may not differ with advancing age, at least some elderly have difficulty maintaining nitrogen balance when consuming the RDA for protein (21,35–37).

In 1978, Cheng and coworkers (38) used a wheat-soy-milk protein mixture to evaluate nitrogen balance in seven healthy elderly men aged 60–70 years. With an intake of 0.8 g of protein/kg of body weight, three of the elderly remained in negative nitrogen balance. Although Zanni et al. (39) reported that nitrogen balance was achieved in a similar experiment using egg protein to evaluate protein requirements, the six elderly men (63–77 years) in that protocol had been placed on a protein-free diet for 17 days before evaluating nitrogen balance. Thus, even though nitogen balance was achieved, the physiologic adjustment to the protein-free diet may have improved the use of protein during the experimental period. In a 30-day study, Gersovitz et al. (36) determined that a diet containing 0.9 g of egg protein/kg/day was insufficient to maintain nitrogen balance in the elderly (age 72–99). Elderly men were characterized as more efficient than elderly women in the use of egg protein to maintain nitrogen balance (35). The reason for these differences remains unknown. Munro et al. (34) reported no evidence of protein deficiency in two groups of free-living, healthy elderly aged 60 to 75 years and over 75 years. However, in both groups, the men and women had intakes of protein exceeding 1.0 g protein/kg of body weight/day.

Protein requirements increase in response to a number of physiologic stresses, including infection, bone fractures, surgery, and burns. The nitrogen loss in these situations is directly proportional to the severity of the injury. Although it is assumed that the increased requirements for protein during physiologic stress differ little from those for the younger population, actual experimental documentation is lacking. However, with the diminished efficiency of protein utilization in the elderly, the recommended increases would seem to be reasonable. The prudent dietary recommendation should ensure a minimum intake of 0.9–1.0 g protein/kg body weight/day.

CARBOHYDRATES

There is no RDA for either simple or complex carbohydrates because no individual sugar is identified as an essential nutrient. Most diets contain 45 to 50% of their daily calories as carbohydrates.

However, the current consensus favors an increase in complex carbohydrates to 55 to 60% of total calories. A dietary increase in complex carbohydrates improves the intake of many nutrients, because starchy foods also contain vitamins, minerals, and fiber. It can also decrease total calorie consumption if the carbohydrate foods replace foods higher in fat content.

Very few clinical problems are caused specifically by the consumption of carbohydrates. However, an increased incidence of hyperglycemia, adult-onset diabetes mellitus, and lactose intolerance occurs in the elderly.

Many elderly develop a deficiency of the intestinal enzyme, lactase (B-galactosidase) (35,40). Without hydrolysis, the lactase is not absorbed, but rather is metabolized by intestinal bacteria. The resultant metabolites and gas produce the symptoms of flatulence, cramping, and diarrhea, which result in the avoidance of milk and other dairy products in the diet. This avoidance is unfortunate because of the high nutrient value of milk. Rather than avoidance, a controlled restriction of dairy product consumption should be recommended. Smaller quantities of dairy products or the use of lactase-treated milk and fermented dairy products should diminish the occurrence of adverse reactions. A simple decrease of 20 to 30% in the lactose content of these products greatly reduces symptoms of lactose intolerance (41).

By middle age, the incidence and resultant mortality of glucose intolerance and adult-onset diabetes increase (42–44), to a somewhat greater extent in women than in men. In fact, a major portion of the elderly population live with diabetes—as many as 16.5% of the persons over 65 years of age and more than one-fourth of the elderly over 85 years.

Both blood glucose levels and immunoreactive insulin levels rise with age, indicating a loss in insulin receptor responsiveness (45,46). Similar differences have been observed during an oral glucose tolerance test (OGTT). Physical activity appears to improve the OGTT response (47,48), but how this may benefit the elderly has not been characterized.

The American Diabetes Association (49) has made specific recommendations regarding dietary changes. In general, these recommendations parallel closely the U.S. Dietary Guidelines (Table 3), which recommend an increase in the intake of complex carbohydrates and a decrease in fat intake to balance total calories. Whether these recommendations have a significant effect on diabetic outcome remains controversial (50,51).

TABLE 3. *Comparison of dietary recommendations provided by the U.S. Dietary Guidelines and the American Diabetes Association*

U.S. Dietary Guidelines for Americans (1985)	American Diabetes Association (1987)
1. Eat a variety of foods Fruits. Vegetables, whole-grain and enriched breads, cereals, and other grain products. Milk, cheese, yogurt, and other dairy products. Meats, poultry, fish, eggs, and dry beans and peas. 2. Maintain desireable weight: Watch caloric intake, improve nutrient density, and maintain some physical activity 3. Avoid too much fat, saturated fat and cholesterol 4. Eat foods with adequate starch and fiber 5. Avoid too much sugar. 6. Avoid too much sodium.	1. Consume enough calories to maintain desirable body weight 2. Have carbohydrate intake that is 55–60% of total daily calories consumed 3. Decrease fat intake to 30% or less (reduction of all components) of daily calories 4. Decrease cholesterol intake to 300 mg/day or less. 5. Limit salt intake. 6. Consume protein at the RDA or as needed; certain elderly may need more to maintain nitrogen balance.

USDA, USDHHS, Second Edition, 1985.

FAT

The intake of dietary fat has increased since 1907, proportionately displacing complex carbohydrates in the diet. Although recommendations have been made to replace saturated fats in the diet with polyunsaturated fats, the net result has been an increase in total fat consumption by the population as a whole.

Dietary fat intake can be limited to 30% or less of the total calories consumed without having a negative impact on nutrient balance. Interestingly, the RDA for essential fatty acids (EFA) can be provided by as little as 2 to 3% of the total caloric intake—only 9 to 10 grams of the essential fatty acids, linoleic and linolenic acid, from animal and vegetable foods. However, overrestriction of dietary fat to less than 20% of daily calorie intake may affect the quality of the diet.

During the past two decades, major efforts have been expended to prove, not just test, the "lipid hypothesis" of coronary heart disease. As a result of using high cholesterol diets to initiate atherosclerosis in animal models, conclusions were reached suggesting that regulation of serum cholesterol levels would alter plaque formation and decrease the development of atherosclerosis.

The controversy arises over relating the coronary heart disease (CHD) mortality that occurs with hypercholesterolemia to the effect of elevated serum cholesterol levels in the general population. The lipid hypothesis predicts that anyone with a high cholesterol level has an increased risk for CHD and suggests that, if the serum cholesterol level is reduced, the risk of developing heart disease will decrease (52,53). There is some support for this hypothesis, but it is far from proven and there is most certainly not a linear relationship between serum cholesterol and CHD (53,54). In fact a great body of evidence does not support serum cholesterol as a major factor in CHD.

Dietary recommendations made by the National Heart and Lung Institute (NHLI) and the American Heart Association (AHA) include a decrease in dietary cholesterol and saturated fatty acids and an increase in polyunsaturated fatty acids. However, the vast majority of studies have indicated limited success in altering serum cholesterol levels by dietary change (55,57).

The role of dietary cholesterol in setting serum cholesterol levels is complex. The body's pool of cholesterol is derived primarily from the balance of its own synthesis and clearance. Only 20% of the cholesterol turnover comes from the diet. Between 40 and 50% of dietary cholesterol is absorbed below 500 mg/day, but less efficiently at higher concentrations. Numerous studies have demonstrated that in most individuals an increase in dietary cholesterol is compensated for by a decrease in the endogenous production of cholesterol, thereby maintaining a constant plasma level of cholesterol (54,58–60). Other compensatory mechanisms include increased biliary excretion, increased catabolism to bile acids, and the accumulation of cholesterol in the bulk of the body tissues (61). Currently, there is no way to predict who is sensitive to dietary cholesterol.

In 1979, McGill (57) provided a unique evaluation of nine or more studies evaluating the impact of dietary cholesterol on serum cholesterol levels. Some of these studies were individual evaluations and of short duration. However, the following specific points were identified:

1. Young college students had serum cholesterol levels of 171 to 188 mg/dl, which were little affected by changing dietary intake from 0 to 211 mg/ 1,000 kcal of diet (the mean elevation per 100 mg cholesterol /1,000 kcal amounted to 6 to 8 mg/dl); at dietary intakes exceeding 1,000 mg/day, the increase amounted to 23 mg/dl (62).
2. Middle-aged men who changed their dietary cholesterol from 0 to 306 mg/ 1,000 kcal for over a month increased serum cholesterol by 25 mg/dl (191 to 216 mg/dl) (63).
3. Middle-aged men who changed their polyunsaturated/saturated (P/S) fat ratio and dietary cholesterol intake for more than 2 months, with a P/S ratio near 0.5–1.0 and a serum cholesterol level of about 197, decreased the cholesterol level by 9 mg/dl by increasing the P/S ratio to 2.3; the impact of decreasing dietary cholesterol from 149 mg/1,000 kcal to 43 mg/1,000 kcal was a change of 7 to 13 mg/dl for the P/S ratio of 0.5 to 1.0 (64).

More recent experiments have reported similar findings. A shift in dietary fat intake to increase polyunsaturated fats and decrease saturated fats to provide a P/S ratio of 1 has produced a variable effect on plasma cholesterol levels (65). In agreement, McNamara et al. (66) noted that a P/S ratio of 1.45–1.90 had little effect (less than 10%) on the plasma cholesterol and was also independent of dietary cholesterol levels.

As a result of public health education efforts, the average intake of cholesterol has decreased by 100 to 150 mg/day since the mid-1960s. Even so, the average serum cholesterol has remained constant at 210 to 220 mg/dl.

If dietary cholesterol is decreased by half (from 500 to 250 mg/day) and saturated fat intake is also decreased by half, the serum cholesterol would be decreased about 30 mg/dl, producing a 15% change (56). However, whether such a change in plasma cholesterol prevents atherosclerosis or coronary events in the general population has not yet been demonstrated. High serum cholesterol (>260 mg/dl) should be of concern, but a large number of short-term and long-term studies have not substantiated the claim that dietary cholesterol is the major causative factor in CHD (57).

Another interpretation of some of these data might emphasize the relationship of increasing cholesterol levels with advancing age. The incidence of coronary heart disease increases rapidly after mid-life and throughout old age, as does that of several other diseases, such as diabetes and hypertension. In a similar manner, serum cholesterol levels also rise with age, increasing almost linearly from birth to 55 or 65 years of age (4–6).

In men, the mean plasma cholesterol level rises to 250 mg/dl by the age of

55, after which it remains relatively constant. In women, the mean plasma cholesterol level remains 5 to 10% lower than in men until the age of 50. By the age of 55 years, both sexes have similar plasma cholesterol levels. However, plasma cholesterol levels continue to rise in women for another decade, leveling off at 260 mg/dl (4,5).

In the long-term Framingham study (67), follow-up of 1,045 men was carried out periodically over 20 years. About 9% of the participants developed myocardial infarction (MI), angina pectoris, or sudden death without previous clinical evidence of MI and had serum cholesterol levels between 114 to 193 mg/dl, in contrast to 31% who had serum cholesterol levels above 259 mg/dl. Similar results were observed in the Pooling Project (68), which was conducted over a 7-year period with participants between 30 to 59 years; of the first coronary events, 13% occurred in men with serum levels less than 195 mg/dl.

Bidlack and Smith (6) offer alternative interpretations to the conclusions of the Framingham Heart Study. The 1,378 non-CHD participants were determined to have a mean serum cholesterol level of about 220 ±41 mg/dl, whereas the 193 individuals who developed CHD within 16 years had a mean cholesterol level between 240 and 245 mg/dl (69,70). The distribution of serum cholesterol values for both non-CHD and CHD groups produced essentially Gaussian curves that overlapped extensively (Fig. 1a). Even though the non-CHD group had more than six times the number of subjects as the CHD group, the data were presented as percent of the population, which means that each population group was treated independently and made equal

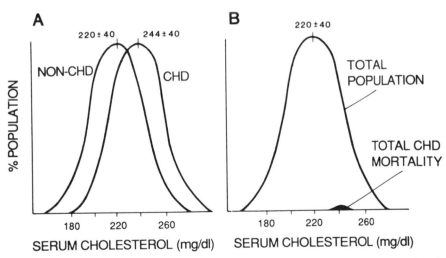

FIG. 1. Comparison of the serum cholesterol distribution in the total population and in the coronary heart disease population. **A:** Distribution relative to each population group. **B:** Distribution relative to the total population. (Modified from Bidlack and Smith, ref. 6.)

to 100 percent. This presentation makes the two groups appear equal and has been used to support the concept that CHD results from higher serum cholesterol levels. Additionally, this comparison has been used to suggest that everyone with serum cholesterol levels similar to the CHD population is developing heart disease that has not yet been detected.

However, if the distribution of CHD patients are replotted to reflect the actual CHD mortality (0.3/100) relative to the total population (Fig. 1b), several interesting observations can be made (6). First, the majority of the population have no CHD at serum cholesterol levels identified as causative for the CHD population. Second, the mortality unexpectedly does not occur at higher cholesterol levels, but at a mean of 245 mg/dl. These results would seem to be in disagreement with the lipid hypothesis and deserve further consideration.

The compounding factors that together with plasma cholesterol initiate plaque formation and increase coronary disease remain undefined. The results of the Lipid Research Coronary Prevention (LRCP) study (71,72), indicating the minimal success of diet or drug treatment, should at least bring to question the emphasis on aggressive intervention in the general population with serum cholesterol levels lower than 260 mg/dl (6). The only reports documenting a decrease in CHD mortality have been small decreases reported in studies using hypercholesterolmic patients having serum cholesterol levels in excess of 300 mg/dl.

The NIH Consensus Committee (73) made very strong recommendations to lower plasma cholesterol levels by diet and drug therapy. However, not everyone agrees with the interpretation of the data upon which these recommendations were based (6,74). Open disagreement prevents dogmatic implementation of policy, diet, and drug intervention, without thought to efficacy of the treatment, ie, decrease in serum cholesterol versus a decrease in CHD mortality.

The general public should be informed about the overall distribution of risk factors for CHD. The Pooling Project (68) identified these risks: age, sex, family history, and related genetic factors (35%), which include unidentified factors as well; obesity (5%); cigarette smoking (22%); hypertension (20%); and serum cholesterol levels (18%). Thus, the large number of interacting factors produce the high individual variance seen in most studies.

Although there has been a decrease in mortality related to coronary disease, it is highly questionable whether it is related solely to dietary changes (53,75). Therefore, physicians must consider what it means to alter the diet of the elderly before they recommend major changes in lifestyle and at the same time increase the emotional stress of their patients by inferring that failure to comply will increase their risk of dying of CHD. After all, if dietary changes reduce blood cholesterol by only 10 to 15%, major emphasis has been placed on interventions that may only alter the risk by 2 to 3% (6).

FIBER

Dietary fiber is composed of plant materials resistant to hydrolysis by the normal digestive enzymes located within the ileum of man. It comprises a variety of polysaccharides, including cellulose, hemicellulose, pectic substances, mucilages, gums, waxes, and algal polysaccharides, such as agar and carageenan (76,77).

Although dietary fiber is not a nutrient, it does benefit gastrointestinal functioning. The physical properties of fiber—its water-holding capacity, viscosity, binding, and fermentability—may affect digestion and absorption (77). Fiber is not digested in the small intestine, thereby allowing the physical properties of the polysaccharides to affect food digestion and nutrient absorption.

Dietary fiber is composed of soluble and insoluble fiber. Insoluble fibers include cellulose, hemicellulose, and lignin, a nonpolysaccharide. An important characteristic of this type of fiber is that it binds water at five to seven times its dry weight, resulting in a larger, softer stool that passes more easily through the intestine. Dietary sources of insoluble fiber include whole-grain breads and cereals, skins of fruits and vegetables, and wheat bran.

Soluble fibers include pectin, mucilages, and gums that adsorb less water, but form a gel matrix that slows the intestinal absorption of dietary substances. Food sources of these fibers include fruits, vegetables, legumes, oat bran, and gums used as thickening agents and stabilizers. Soluble fiber can be degraded and metabolized almost completely by bacteria in the large intestine, whereas insoluble fiber cannot. The resultant degradation and fermentation produce short chain fatty acids, such as acetic acid, proprionic acid, and butyric acid, which decrease the large bowel pH and may also produce flatulence. An increase in fecal mass may occur as a result of an increase in bacterial cell mass. In addition, the feces are concentrated following absorption of water in the large intestine.

One of the most frequent geriatric complaints is constipation or irregularity. The elderly average five to seven bowel movements per week, which should be satisfactory (78). However, the authors did not determine either the ease of elimination nor the quality (soft or hard) of the fecal mass. Constipation occurs when the frequency of bowel movements decreases, resulting in a prolonged transit time. Water absorption continues, producing a hard stool that is difficult to pass. Low-fiber diets aggravate this condition, and several other factors, including inadequate fluid intake and a loss of muscle tone (due to lack of exercise) with age, exacerbate this problem. Fiber adds bulk and softens the stool, providing a natural stimulation to the intestine to maintain peristalsis. Neither the specific amount of fiber nor the type of fiber that is needed has been established.

Diverticular disease can be severe enough to disable 5 to 10% of the elderly population (79). In the United States, two-thirds of the elderly have colonic diverticula. Low-fiber diets aggravate the condition in humans, and in a large majority of cases an increase in fiber intake will relieve the disorder (81,82). Thus, consumption of about 25 g/day of dietary fiber should result in a softer stool with increased bulk, enabling improved ease of elimination and one or more bowel movements each day.

Soluble fibers, including oat fiber, pectin, or guar gum, have been shown to reduce the rate of glucose absorption and diminish the blood glucose level. Apparently total glucose absorption remains constant, but the absorption occurs over the entire surface of the intestine. The slower absorption rate prevents the high increase in blood glucose levels; thus, less insulin response is required. This modulation in insulin needs is observed in normal individuals, as well as in glucose-intolerant and diabetic subjects (83,84). Legumes were demonstrated to produce a similar response and could therefore be used to modify the diet as well.

An increase in soluble fiber in the diet can decrease the plasma cholesterol levels in hypercholesterolemic patients by about 10 to 15%. The extent of this decrease does not appear to be additive with other dietary changes, such as decreased dietary fat and cholesterol.

The amount of dietary fiber intake ranges from 25 to 30 g/day. Dietary fiber content is actually three to seven times the crude fiber estimates. Thus, choosing fiber-rich foods, including whole-grain breads, cereals, fresh fruits, vegetables, and nuts, can provide the necessary health benefit for the elderly without needing fiber supplementation.

VITAMINS

Nutritional requirements for vitamins have not been established for persons over the age of 65 years (23). In addition, nutrition surveys evaluating the intake of nutrients by population groups have rarely included a representative sampling of the 75 + age group. (The existing RDAs for the 51 + years of age group are noted in Table 1.) Vitamin deficiencies may be subclinical in many elderly persons. The physiologic stress of illness may be sufficient to deplete rapidly any residual stores, placing the individual in a depleted or deficient nutritional state (16). The effects of ongoing chronic or acute disease states are not clearly identified in many of the reports.

In the large nutritional surveys, inadequate nutrient intake of the elderly was most frequently caused by limited food consumption, even though the selection of food was of high nutrient quality. The poor elderly were unable to purchase enough food to meet their needs (4,5). Data on vitamin intake accumulated from a large number of smaller investigations have varied. Specific dietary patterns that may place the individual elderly person at risk for vitamin deficiency include being finicky eaters, strict vegetarians, having an aversion to fruits and vegetables, being on rigid weight reduction diets, having a loss of appetite because of an underlying disease process, or the drug regimens being used (85).

McGandy et al. (86) examined the nutritional intake of healthy, noninstitutionalized elderly men and reported that the percentage of elderly consuming less than two-thirds of the RDA for vitamins and minerals increased dramatically in those individuals having a low calorie intake (<21.5 kcal/kg body weight). The nutrients determined to be at high risk (affecting more than 20% of the group) were vitamin A, folate, vitamin B_{12}, vitamin B_6, calcium, and zinc. In those elderly consuming more than 27.5 kcal/kg body weight, only folate and vitamin B_6 were at high risk.

In an effort to assure good health, the elderly consume large amounts of vitamin and mineral supplements. McDonald (87) summarized the use of vitamin/mineral supplements as reported in the Nationwide Food Consumption Survey (3), NHANES I and II (4,5) and other smaller surveys. A great range of intakes between 20 and 70% was noted, with the greatest consumption occurring in California, Nevada, and New Mexico (88). Numerous other studies have reported similar findings (89–92).

The elderly do not appear to be at risk for toxicity, especially when consuming multivitamin/mineral supplements formulated near the RDA levels. However, concern is warranted for ill-informed consumers who consume high doses.

Experiments comparing the nutritional status of elderly, using supplements to those not using them have suggested in most cases that the supplemented group has a higher vitamin status. However, these experiments have not assessed the direct health benefit of supplementation for individuals who otherwise do not meet their nutritional needs.

A limited number of studies have evaluated nutritional status before and after the use of vitamin supplements. Kirsch and Bidlack (16) collated these experiments and found that 0 to 56% of the elderly are deficient in one or more vitamins (Table 4). Table 5 provides a few examples of the biochemical parameters used to assess vitamin status, including enzyme activation coefficients (enzyme activity with excess coenzyme addition/initial enzyme ac-

TABLE 4. *Vitamin deficiencies in the elderly before and after supplementation*

Vitamin	Percent deficient		Reference
	Nonsupplemented	Supplemented	
Thiamine	13–40	0–6	123, 132
Riboflavin	3–42	0	113, 126, 127, 132
Niacin	0–33	0–33	16, 74, 96, 121
Pyridoxine	19–56	2–39	96, 132, 133
Folacin	14–43	0–13	107, 139, 142
Cobalamin	4–43	0–18	96, 107

From Bidlack and Smith, ref. 6.

TABLE 5. *Vitamin deficiency and efficacy of supplementation*

Elderly subjects	Deficiency criteria	No supplement deficient		Amount supplement (mg)	Supplemented deficient		Reference
		Number	%		Number	%	
		Thiamin ETK-AC					
Hospital	>1.27	153	40	25	153	0	132
Institutional	>1.20	89	16	2.5	54	2	123
Free living	>1.20	37	14	2.5	16	6	123
		Riboflavin EGR-AC					
Hospital	>1.29	153	12	10	153	0	132
Institutional	>1.20	143	8	2.5	143	0	126
Free living	>1.35	373	4	varied	373	0	113
		Pyridoxine EGOT-AC					
Hospital	>1.86	153	19	20	153	2	132
		EGPT-AC					
Institutional	>1.15	89	56	2.5	54	15	133
Free living	>1.15	37	51	1.0–5.0	16	38	133
		Folacin Serum					
Institutional	<5 ng/ml	167	24	100	160	13	96, 139
Free living	<5 ng/ml	74	15	N.S.	70	3	96, 139

ETK-AC, erythrocyte transketolase-activation coefficient; EGR-AC, erythrocyte glutathione reductase-activation coefficient; EGOT-AC, erythrocyte glutamate-oxaloacetate transaminase-activation coefficient.

tivity), and indicates the degree of efficacy of supplement use. In a recent publication with a similar experimental design to these reports, Mann et al. (93) assayed blood vitamin levels of elderly and then supplemented them either with a placebo or multivitamin supplement for 4 months. The erythrocyte glutathione reductase activation coefficient (EGR-AC) improved, plasma vitamin C increased, plasma and erythrocyte folate increased, vitamin B_{12} increased, and slight increases in plasma vitamins A and E were observed. These results indicate that increased vitamin intake can improve nutritional status.

Vitamin A

Although 42 to 65% of the elderly surveyed in NHANES I had vitamin A intakes of less than two-thirds of the RDA, only 0.3% had serum vitamin A levels low enough (less than 20 ug/dl) to be considered deficient (94). In a more limited study of healthy and wealthy retirees, Garry and coworkers (89) reported that 12% of those examined had low (<3/4 RDA) vitamin A intakes. In both reports, elderly men had higher intakes of vitamin A than elderly women. Similarly, Yearick et al. (95) and Baker et al. (96) reported little evidence of low vitamin A status based on serum levels, even though about 20% of the elderly participants consumed less than two-thirds of the RDA.

Plasma levels have not closely paralleled dietary intake in many studies. Most likely this results from the large liver storage of vitamin A and the efficiency by which these reserves maintain plasma levels independent of immediate dietary intake. Thus, a decline in plasma vitamin A would not occur until there was a severe deficiency (97). To date, no effect of age on the biochemical or physiologic parameters regulating the liver stores of vitamin A has been reported.

The dietary intake of vegetables and fruits rich in carotenoids has been associated by epidemiologic correlation with a lower incidence of some types of cancer (13,98,99). Although carotenoids can trap singlet oxygen, potentially decreasing one form of free-radical-initiated cancer, the epidemiologic relationship does not consider other dietary factors in the correlation (13,100). A diet high in vegetables and fruits would also be high in fiber and may be lower in fat and calories, which have also been associated with a decreased cancer risk (98). Thus, because it remains only a hypothesis, caution should be used in universally recommending use of beta-carotene supplements to prevent cancer.

Vitamin D

Several factors affect the vitamin D status of the elderly (101). McGandy et al. (86) reported that more than half of the elderly population consume less than two-thirds of the RDA for vitamin D. In addition, a lack of exposure to the sun decreases the production of vitamin D in the skin (102). Elderly individuals who are confined to bed at home or in an institution or live in harsh winter areas can be affected by the lack of sun exposure. There is also evidence suggesting that vitamin D absorption may be decreased with age (103,104).

Osteomalacia and osteoporosis are the major clinical problems associated with poor vitamin D status (101,105). Calcium uptake and deposition in the bone require many steps and several different metabolic forms of vitamin D. The most physiologically important vitamin D metabolite, 1,25-dihydroxy vitamin D, is formed by hydroxylation in the liver and in the kidney. There is weak evidence for an age-related decline in 25-hydroxylation of vitamin D in the liver (106) derived from reports that identified lower circulating serum levels of 25-hydroxy vitamin D (107,108). However, the evidence for an age-related decline in the 1α-hydroxylation in the kidney is stronger (109,110).

Francis et al (111) reported that treatment of osteoporotic women, with and without fractures, with 25(OH)D produced similar increases in plasma levels of 1,25(OH)D. However, calcium absorption in the osteoporotic patients did not increase to the same extent as in normal patients. These results suggest a loss of metabolic response within the mucosal cells, which may indicate a loss of receptor response or a diminished transcription either of the calcium transport protein or the calcium binding protein.

Chapuy et al. (112) reported that, when supplemental vitamin D (20 µg/dl) and calcium (1 g/day) were taken by elderly patients over a 6-month period, an increase in serum calcium and in 25(OH)D resulted, as well as a subsequent increase in parathyroid hormone. These researchers stated that adherence to this regimen eliminated signs of secondary hyperparathyroidism in the elderly as well.

Vitamin E

Although Garry et al. (113) noted that about 40% of the elderly have vitamin E intakes less than two-thirds of the RDA, Baker et al. (96) found little more than 2% of the elderly to have low serum vitamin E (<0.5 mg/dl). This Zlow incidence was similar to that noted in the younger control population and is therefore not age related.

Although Kelleher and Losowsky (114) reported that blood tocopherol levels have a tendency to increase with age into the seventh decade, other investigators have not found this relationship (115). In fact, other researchers have indicated a decline in plasma tocopherol levels that parallels the change in plasma lipoprotein levels above the age of 65 (116,117). Both the low-density lipoprotein and the high-density lipoproteins carry tocopherol in the plasma. However, unlike vitamins A and D, no specific carrier protein has been identified.

Vitamin E absorption is not altered with increasing age in humans (114). Most likely, this finding simply reflects that absorption of vitamin E occurs as part of the lipid micell required for dietary fat absorption. To date, no deficiency of vitamin E has been reported for the healthy elderly.

Vitamin K

The diverse distribution of vitamin K (phylloquinone) in green leafy vegetables ensures good dietary intake of this nutrient. In addition, the production of vitamin K (menaquinone) by gut microflora also contributes significantly to the daily intake. There are no major stores of vitamin K in the body, but the liver retains the highest reserve of the phyloquinones.

Vitamin K is well absorbed (40 to 70%) from the jejunum and ileum, but is poorly absorbed from the colon (19). In the elderly, malabsorption problems or ongoing antibiotic therapy may compromise the availability of vitamin K for absorption. In addition, the clearance rate for vitamin K is very high, with a half-life of a few hours (118).

The RDA for vitamin K is based on the amount of vitamin K needed to correct plasma prothrombin levels in subjects with little or no endogenous vitamin K synthesis. The incidence of abnormal prothrombin times does increase with age, occurring in 8% of the elderly at 60 to 70 years and in 24% of the elderly above 80 years of age (119). However, the use of prothrombin time has a marker of vitamin K status is weak because other factors may also alter clotting times.

Vitamin B_1

Thiamine intakes in the elderly vary widely. In the NHANES I study, 18 to 46% of the elderly had intakes of vitamin B_1 less than two-thirds of the RDA; race and income were the major factors in the low intake (94,120). When corrected for caloric intake, both NHANES I and II studies suggested that the intake of thiamine was above the RDA (0.5 mg/1,000 kcal).

Among noninstitutionalized healthy elderly, 3 to 25% have been determined to have low erythrocyte transketolase activation coefficient (ETK-AC), whereas based on urinary output only 0 to 15% of the elderly had low values (121–123).

Accurate quantitation of blood thiamine levels is difficult, and ETK activity has been found to decrease with age. Thus, ETK-AC is used most frequently as an indicator. As such, 3 to 15% of elderly were determined to have inadequate or deficient thiamine levels (120).

Alcoholism and low dietary intake are the major causes of vitamin B_1 deficiency in the elderly (120). Alcohol decreases thiamine absorption and its phosphorylation and may increase thiamine clearance from the cell by enhancing phosphate hydrolysis by thiamine pyrophosphate phosphatase (alkaline phosphatase) activity (120,124). The resultant alcoholic polyneuropathy and amylopia stem largely from vitamin B_1 deficiency and respond positively to thiamine supplementation, as does the Wernicke-Korsakoff syndrome.

Vitamin B_2

Low dietary intake is the cause of most of the riboflavin deficiency in the elderly. Both NHANES I and II studies found a higher incidence of deficiency among the poor and the black participants (4,5). Bowman and Rosenberg (94) reported that 36% of the elderly were reported to consume less than two-thirds of the RDA. Yet, less than 6% of noninstitutionalized wealthy elderly had intakes less than three-quarters of the RDA (113).

When the erythrocyte glutathione reductase activation coefficient (EGR-AC) was used to evaluate riboflavin status, 0 to 28% of the elderly were found to be deficient (121,125,126). The mean EGR-AC decreases with age independent of riboflavin intake.

Between 4 and 42% of the elderly have been described as biochemically deficient in riboflavin (113,127). Low intake was determined to be the major cause because all participants responded to an increase in the dietary intake of riboflavin. No experimental evidence has suggested that there is altered riboflavin absorption with age (128).

Vitamin B$_6$

Vitamin B$_6$ intakes vary widely, and food composition data are incomplete. Approximately 50 to 90% of the elderly have intakes below the 1980 RDA (128). Garry et al. (113) noted that 80% of noninstitutionalized healthy elderly had low intakes (<3/4 of the RDA), whereas Guilland et al. (129) reported that half of the elderly consumed less than 50% of the RDA. McGandy et al. (86) also noted that 48% and 62% of the elderly men and women, respectively, had a low intake of vitamin B$_6$ (<2/3 RDA) while receiving an adequate caloric intake (>27.5 kcal/kg). Eighty-five percent of those elderly consuming less than 21.5 kcal/kg each day were determined to have intakes of vitamin B$_6$ less than two-thirds of the RDA.

Caution must be used in the evaluation of B$_6$ deficiency because serum and plasma levels of pyridoxal phosphate decline with increasing age (130,131). Nevertheless, a biochemical deficiency was reported for 19 to 56% of the elderly tested (132,133). Guilland et al. (129) determined that 70% of the elderly were deficient compared to only 12% in the control population.

Kant et al. (134) reported that baseline pyridoxal phosphate (PLP) and total vitamin B$_6$ were lower, 54% and 60%, respectively, in the elderly (aged 65 to 75) than in the younger comparison group aged 25 to 35 years. In addition, about 20% of the elderly with low transaminase activation coefficient (TA-AC) activity did not return to normal values after supplementation (129,132,133). Both results may suggest an increased requirement for vitamin B$_6$ with age.

The requirements for vitamin B$_6$ appear to be in need of additional clarification. The incidence of deficiency is high, and it may not respond completely to increased intake. As noted in the review by Kirsch and Bidlack (16), 15 to 40% of the elderly were still deficient after receiving vitamin B$_6$ supplements; both plasma vitamin B$_6$ levels and enzyme activation coefficient tests were evaluated.

Niacin

The NHANES I data indicated that between 0 and 53% of the elderly had niacin intake below the 1980 RDA. Forty-three percent of the black elderly had low (less than 2/3 of the RDA) dietary intakes of niacin, primarily those having an income below the poverty level. In a population of healthy and wealthy elderly, all had dietary intakes above the RDA (89).

Using urinary excretion of N-methyl nicotinamide as a marker, 1 to 50% of the elderly were determined to have low niacin status. The oldest and sickest elderly were most affected. Currently, the urinary 2-pyridone: N-methyl nicotinamide ratio is considered to reflect niacin status best. Little additional information is available, and until improved biochemical assessment can be established little can be stated about niacin status.

Folate

Folate intakes in the elderly vary widely, although it should be recognized that food composition tables are relatively incomplete for folate. Also, the extent of altered bioavailability of folate in different foods or changes caused by food processing have not been well characterized (80).

Halstead (135) has described the physiologic processes associated with folate absorption from the intestine. Folate uptake by gut epithelium is pH dependent and reaches its maximum at pH 6.3 (136). Thus, any factor, such as gastric atrophy or antacids, that would alter intestinal pH would affect folate absorption (137). In addition, a decrease in conjugase activity would decrease the availability of monoglutamyl folate for absorption. Although, age-related changes of folyl conjugase activity have been reported, other experiments found no age-associated changes (138–140).

Garry et al. (89,141) determined that 70 to 84% of the elderly consumed less than three-fourths of the RDA for folate. Yet, only a few healthy elderly had indications of biochemical deficiency, and this incidence was not greater than among the healthy young controls. However, Vir and Love (142) and Meindock and Dvorsky (143) reported that 7.8 to 34% of the elderly had serum folate levels less than 3 ng/ml and were therefore considered to be in a deficient state.

Certain therapeutic agents as well as alcohol are known to alter folate absorption and utilization (14,144). Thus, the extent of alcohol use or the length of time that certain medications are used should be determined at the time of nutritional assessment for folate status.

Vitamin B_{12}

Garry et al. (141) indicated that 24% of the men and 39% of the women had vitamin B_{12} intakes less than three-quarters of the RDA. True dietary deficiency of vitamin B_{12} is rare, but loss of gastric instrinsic factor is more common.

Decreased absorption of vitamin B_{12} as well as decreased serum vitamin B_{12} levels, has been associated with increasing age (140,145–147). However, even though serum vitamin B_{12} levels decline with age, they appear to remain within normal limits.

A decline in serum B_{12} levels with age may result from pernicious anemia and/or B_{12} malabsorption caused by atrophic gastritis with advancing age. Up to 50% of the elderly may be afflicted with atrophic gastritis. The lack of gastric acid decreases the release of vitamin B_{12} from food protein (148). A decrease in the secretion of intrinsic factor is also apparent (149,150).

Transcobalamin II (TC II) serves as the primary plasma carrier of vitamin B_{12} (151). Newly absorbed vitamin B_{12} is bound to TC II, which delivers vitamin B_{12} to the tissues. In the elderly the number of unbound vitamin B_{12} sites on TC II increases by 25%, but the binding of vitamin B_{12} to TC II decreases more than 80%. Total serum vitamin B_{12} is 20 to 30% lower in normal elderly and 85% lower in elderly with a low intake of vitamin B_{12}. The other binding sites (TC I and TC III) are decreased by 30 to 40%. Thus, the combined decrease in absorption and the diminished serum delivery system for vitamin B_{12} may alter vitamin B_{12} status in the elderly. Perhaps, vitamin B_{12} injections could benefit those individuals who can no longer maintain their vitamin B_{12} status (152).

Vitamin C

The NHANES I and II studies indicated that the mean intakes of the entire population for vitamin C were close to the RDAs. However, the range of intake was quite extreme. Bowman and Rosenberg (94) noted that 23 to 58% of the elderly participants consumed less than 30 mg/day of vitamin C.

In a healthy and wealthy elderly population, vitamin C intake (150 mg/day) was determined to be above the mean of the population (82 mg/day), primarily because of high intakes of vitamin supplements (153). Still, 25% of the noninstitutionalized elderly show low (<0.2 mg/dl) plasma levels of vitamin C. Similar observations were made by Yearick et al. (95) and Cheng et al. (154).

An interesting experiment evaluating vitamin C needs was reported by VanderJagt et al. (155). These authors noted that plasma ascorbic acid levels were lower in elderly men than in elderly women for vitamin C intakes ranging from 30–280 mg/day. In addition, to reach and maintain a steady state level of vitamin C of 1.0 mg/dl in men, an intake of 150 mg/day was required, whereas in females only 80 mg/day produced the same effect. The difference in plasma vitamin C levels between men and women at different vitamin C intakes has also been noted by Garry et al. (153).

Such factors as smoking and physiologic stress (154,156) may alter vitamin C status and increase the need for vitamin C intake. Certain medications and pathologic alterations may further compromise the vitamin C status at the level of renal reabsorption. Again, this does not suggest a need to increase the RDA, but simply emphasizes the need to ensure that those individuals at risk have an adequate intake.

Summary

Whether the RDAs for vitamins are sufficient to meet the needs of the elderly remains to be established. The young, healthy elderly probably differ little from the younger population in terms of vitamin requirements. However, with advanced age and the increased onset of acute and chronic health problems, nutrient intake may need to be increased to maintain nutritional status. Many areas of vitamin metabolism need to be examined more carefully in the elderly.

Rather than continuing to argue about the necessity for taking vitamin supplements, it would seem more appropriate to educate the elderly about their dietary and health needs and ensure that they consume only safe levels (not more than 100% RDA) as needed as a multivitamin preparation.

MINERALS

The current edition of the RDAs provides recommended intakes for calcium, phosphorus, magnesium, iron, zinc, and iodine and suggests estimated safe and adequate daily intakes (EASDI) for six other minerals—chromium, copper, fluoride, manganese, molybdenum, and selenium (23). The EASDI category was created to provide some guidance until requirements have been established.

Currently, the two major health concerns relating to mineral intake are iron (anemia) and calcium (osteoporosis). Zinc, magnesium, and some other trace minerals may be present in less than optimal concentrations, but much more work is needed before recommendations can be made about their intake (157). Additionally, dietary sodium and its role in hypertension have stimulated concern and controversy.

Iron

There is little evidence for a high prevalence of iron deficiency in the elderly (122). According to the NHANES I and II studies, iron intake in elderly men met the RDAs, whereas in elderly women the intake was less than the RDA. Again, based on the age classification of 51 + years, the iron level for women may be set too high because at that age they are postmenopausal and are not losing iron through blood loss. The percent deficiency as measured by low transferrin saturation was only 5 to 10% in all groups in the NHANES I and II surveys (4,5). Fifteen percent of the elderly black females had low total iron-binding capacity (TIBC), and they were also identified as the group with the lowest iron intake. Thus, the RDA for iron can be assumed to be the same for elderly men and women as for adult men (158).

In ensuring an adequate iron intake, emphasis should be placed on altering the diet to include more iron-containing foods. The bioavailability of iron depends on the type of food and the form of iron in the food (159). Heme iron is absorbed much more efficiently than nonheme iron. The greatest source of heme iron is hemoglobin and myoglobin found in animal tissues. During digestion, hydrolysis of meat protein produces peptide factors that enhance iron absorption. Thus, the recent trend to avoid meat because of fat and cholesterol content may result in decreased dietary iron intake. Another nutrient, vitamin C, can also enhance iron absorption, but may diminish copper absorption.

Although hematocrit and hemoglobin are used frequently as markers to determine iron status, they should be used carefully when comparing elderly populations to younger populations (160). Many factors can affect hemoglobin levels, and changes in it may reflect the process of aging, rather than a specific biochemical deficiency (151).

When anemia is observed, the first consideration should be blood loss. Once this is ruled out, iron deficiency should be considered (161). The cause may be as simple as low dietary intake of iron, but certain illnesses, such as achlorhydria, may also interfere with iron absorption.

Calcium

A variety of foods supply calcium (162,163). The primary source, providing three-fourths of the dietary calcium, is dairy products. Other sources include meat, fish (sardines and salmon), shellfish, almonds, beans, and green leafy vegetables.

The data from the NHANES I and II studies indicate that the mean consumption of calcium by women is one-third less than the RDA from early teenage years throughout old age. The mean intake of calcium by men does not fall below the RDA until 60 to 65 years of age. However, Pao and Mickle (164) have reported that 40 to 50% of male and female elderly had intakes of calcium less than 70% of the RDA. In addition, negative calcium balance occurs frequently in the elderly, especially in patients suffering from osteoporosis.

Osteoporosis, the incidence of which increases with age, is characterized by a reduction in the quantity of bone (108,165). The osteoclasts and the osteoblasts participate actively in bone turnover and repair by constantly causing the dissolution of calcium and its redeposition. Net bone loss occurs because of an increase in calcium resorption from the bone, a decrease in bone formation, or a combination of the two processes (166).

Osteoporosis is a severe disease affecting one-fourth of postmenopausal women. After menopause, the rate of bone loss may approach 1% per year

(167). This rate of loss may be twice the normal rate and seems to occur to a greater extent in the trabecular bone, including the vertebrae and the ends of long bones. The osteoporotic process also occurs in men, but at a much slower rate. The etiology of osteoporosis is largely unknown, but numerous factors have been implicated: calcium deficiency, estrogen deficiency, inadequate vitamin D, and a lack of exercise (104,165,168–171).

Heaney et al. (172) examined the diets of 130 young women (30 to 35 years) and determined that they required 1,200 mg of calcium/day to maintain calcium balance. In 1978 Heaney and coworkers (173) further reported that postmenopausal women required 1,500 mg/day versus 1000 mg/day for premenopausal women to maintain calcium balance. Interestingly, similar results were reported by Spencer et al. (174) for men as well. These results strongly suggest that the RDA may underestimate calcium needs from mid-age through older age in both sexes.

However, the most significant time period for increased calcium need may occur in women at the immediate onset of menopause (170,175,176). In the absence of estrogen replacement, vitamin D and calcium intakes at the RDA level were not sufficient to maintain calcium balance and bone mass.

Spencer and coworkers (174) have reported improved calcium balance when the calcium intake was increased from 800 mg/day to 1,200 mg/day. Positive calcium balance was obtained using milk or calcium lactate as the calcium source. Similarly, Heaney and coworkers (169,172,173) and Nilas et al. (177) have also reported an improvement in calcium balance with increased calcium intake.

Unfortunately, the methods currently available to quantify calcium deposition in the bone matrix are still not as accurate as desired. Thus, whenever calcium balance is improved, it can only be assumed that calcium deposition in the bone has also been affected. Interestingly, in populations where dairy products are often consumed and the intake of calcium is relatively high, the incidence of osteoporosis, determined by the incidence of hip fractures, is still high. Are all osteoporotic patients in negative calcium balance? Have they had poor dietary intake of calcium over an extended period of their lives? It is important to quantify the relationship between calcium balance and osteoporosis to test further the existing hypothesis and to provide insight into alternative mechanisms.

To date, the RDA of dietary calcium should prove sufficient if consumed with no more than the RDA for vitamin D and with the support of estrogen therapy as needed in postmenopausal women (176,178). At best, however, the treatment may only be slowing calcium bone loss, rather than reversing the devastating disease process.

Long-term controlled human studies do not support the view that increased intakes of either dietary protein (179) or high phosphorus intake (180) enhances calcium loss and increases the risk for osteoporosis (181). A balanced diet still provides the most effective source of calcium and its utilization in bone maintenance.

Phosphorus

Dietary deficiency of phosphorus is very rare. However, when it occurs, hypophosphatemia can cause osteomalacia, cardiomyopathy, and pseudo-myopathy. A decrease in intracellular phosphorus can affect all energetic reactions, including muscle contraction, neurologic function, and electrolyte balance, as ATP stores are diminished (182,183).

In the elderly, the greatest risk for decreasing phosphorus absorption is posed by the frequent use of antacids, such as aluminum hydroxide, in the treatment of peptic ulcers. As stomach acid is neutralized, the aluminum chloride salt is formed. The aluminum then reacts further with phosphorus to form insoluble aluminum phosphate salts that cannot be absorbed. Thus, patients using these agents must use care in their dietary selection to prevent phosphorus depletion.

Magnesium

The mean intake of magnesium appears to be close to the RDA (163). Yet, based on a 24-hour recall and a 2-day diet record, 40 to 50% of the elderly were identified as consuming less than 70% of the RDA (164).

In the NHANES data, the serum levels of magnesium did not differ between younger and older populations. In two smaller studies, Seelig (184) reported that older subjects appeared to have decreased intestinal absorption of magnesium than younger control subjects. These studies were very difficult to do, but indicate the need for much more research in this area.

Touitou et al. (185) examined the magnesium and potassium status of a large population of elderly men and women over the age of 75. Use of erythrocyte concentrations of the cations was more accurate than the plasma concentration in estimating nutritional status for these cations. About one-fifth of this elderly population had low erythrocyte concentrations for magnesium.

Reduction in dietary intake and decreased absorption may explain the deficiencies in part. The decrease could not be attributed to any ongoing disease process or treatment. Hypomagnesemia occurs concurrently with hypokalemia, hypophosphatemia, hyponatremia, and hypocalcemia (186). Whether magnesium or potassium supplementation is beneficial to the elderly remains to be determined.

The increased intake of calcium supplements may be of concern. In animal studies, calcium may interfere with magnesium absorption, but only in large amounts. However, these relationships have not been examined in the elderly.

Increased losses of magnesium through the kidney occur in alcoholics, diabetics, and patients being treated with certain diuretics (187,188). Hypokalemia and hypocalcemia are also commonly associated with hypomagnesemia. Thus, its clinical impact can be very severe.

Sodium and Potassium

The major health concern related to dietary sodium and potassium is hypertension, which increases with age regardless of sex or race (4,5). However, men tend to have a greater incidence of hypertension than women, and black adults are more prone to hypertension than whites (5). About 18% of the U.S. population have hypertension; 95% of these have essential hypertension, whereas another 5% have elevated blood pressure as a consequence of kidney disease or diabetes (189).

The association between dietary sodium and hypertension was based initially on the epidemiologic correlations of high salt consumption by various populations and the incidence of hypertensive disease. However, it is now apparent that a variety of factors contribute to hypertensive disease (190–192). Sodium restriction only benefits 40% of hypertensive patients. Other nutritional factors include the intake of potassium, calcium, and possibly chloride and of course excess calories (obesity). It is important to identify these other mechanisms so that the majority of hypertensives can be provided appropriate therapy.

Zinc

Data on zinc levels in the elderly are very limited. Sandstead et al. (193) evaluated the zinc intake from the NHANES II data (5) and the Ten State Nutrition Survey (194). They determined that the zinc level was directly related to calorie consumption in both surveys and that intake decreased with age. The results of the NHANES study indicate dietary zinc intakes of 12.6 mg/day and 8.2 mg/day for 55- to 64-year-old men and women, respectively. These intakes decrease by more than 10% for the next decade of life.

Zinc is an integral part of 60 or more vital enzymes involved in activities ranging from digestion to the intricacies of nucleic acid metabolism and cellular replication. Thus, it is not surprising that, as zinc deficiency develops, dermatitis and gastrointestinal problems are common characteristics.

Zinc status is currently determined by plasma and erythrocyte concentrations and certain static enzyme activities. Lindeman et al. (195) determined the mean plasma zinc concentrations in a normal healthy population (aged 20 to 84 years) to be 96 ug/dl in men and 99 ug/dl in women. An inverse relationship between age and plasma zinc was described, with no change in the erythrocyte zinc concentration. However, the plasma values actually indicate a very large scatter in data points, namely 70 to 140 ug/dl in men 20 to 40 years of age and 65 to 120 ug/dl in men over age 65. A similar lack of difference was reported by Flint et al. (53) and Vir and Love (142,196). Thus, these data would suggest little difference in zinc status related to age and thus little cause for concern.

Copper

Copper is another essential mineral affected slightly by age. In 1965, Harman (197) noted a 15% increase in serum copper from 124 ug/dl to 145 ug/dl with an increase in age over 60 years. More recently, an elderly population receiving 15 mg/day of zinc and 2 to 3 mg/day of copper reported that zinc and copper balance was maintained (198).

Summary

One-third of the elderly consume magnesium, calcium, and zinc supplements, 20% consume phosphorus, and 10% use potassium supplements (88). Because minerals interact at a variety of levels, including competition for absorption, transport, and storage, such supplements may affect the uptake and utilization of other nutrients.

Thus, if the diet is limited or deficient in certain minerals, the appropriate means of correcting the problem should be to improve the quality of the diet. Only when this alternative is not effective should supplements be used and even then they should be used with care.

FLUIDS

Although fluids are very important to health, they are frequently overlooked in the diets of the elderly. Young adults require 2 to 2.5 liters/day to ensure fluid balance, based on an intake of 1 ml/kcal or 30 ml/kg body weight. It has not been determined whether this same volume is required in the elderly. Fluid intake replaces normal physiologic losses, ensures better digestion and intestinal function, and provides for renal clearance. For these reasons, the elderly should be encouraged to consume more fluids.

Perhaps the most significant reason for decreased fluid consumption is the unfortunate decrease in bladder control that is a consequence of aging. The elderly restrict their fluid intake in an effort to decrease the frequency of urination or to limit incontinence. Urinary incontinence affects 5 to 10% of the noninstitutionalized elderly population and as many as 50% of the elderly in institutions (199,200).

Although most fluid consumption occurs in association with meals or during social interactions, thirst (the conscious desire to consume fluids) still plays a very important role. Signals initiating thirst may not be as effective in the elderly (201). In fact, a longitudinal study of body composition of the same individuals from 70 to 81 years of age indicated a decrease in body water with age, especially a loss of extracellular water (202).

The consumption of alcohol and many therapeutic agents, such as diuretic agents, can increase the rate of fluid loss. Overexertion from activity or exercise can be a problem. In the elderly, nausea, constipation, elevated body temperature, hypotension, and mental confusion can be associated with dehydration (203).

With a decreased perception of changes in temperature and with decreased mobility, the elderly are at great risk during exposure to extreme heat (178,204). Indeed, two-thirds of heat stroke victims are over the age of 60 (205).

Fluid balance should be monitored whenever the elderly individual undergoes medical therapy. The presence of fever, infection, or climatic heat should provide significant reason to check and ensure proper fluid intake.

CONCLUSION

A great deal of experimental work needs to be done to establish well-defined nutritional norms for the healthy and active elderly populations at 10- to 15-year intervals of life. The lack of detailed studies in the elderly, especially for the 75 and older age groups of elderly, makes it difficult to determine their nutritional needs accurately.

In general, the healthy elderly probably differ little from other healthy adults in the population. However, there is a need to evaluate those groups at risk within the elderly population to make specific recommendations for them. Whether or not these same recommendations should then be applied uniformly to all of the elderly population remains to be determined.

Improved medical care and a quality food supply have allowed the elderly to increase their life span. Our current efforts should be directed toward improving the quality of that life.

ACKNOWLEDGMENT

This work was supported in part by a research grant provided by CAL-RECO, Inc.

REFERENCES

1. U.S. Department of Commerce. *Statistical abstract of the United States, 1983,* 103rd ed. Washington, DC: US Government Printing Office, 1980.
2. Kohrs MB. *Am J Clin Nutr* 1982;36:735–736.

3. US Department of Agriculture. *Food and nutrient intakes of individuals in one day in the United States, Spring, 1977: Nationwide Food Consumption Survey 1977–78,* preliminary report no. 2. Hyattsville, MD: U.S. Department of Agriculture, 1980.
4. Abraham S, Carroll MD, Dresser CM, Johnson CL. *Dietary intake source data, United States, 1971–1974.* Hyattsville, MD: Public Health Service, 1979. (Publ. No. (PHS) 79–1221).
5. Carroll MD, Abraham S, Dresser CM. *Dietary Intake Source Data: United States, 1976–1980, Vital and Health Statistics,* series 11, no. 231. Washington, DC: US Government Printing Office, 1983 (DHHS Publ. no. (PHS) 83–1681).
6. Bidlack WR, Smith CH. *CRC Crit Rev Food Sci Nutr* 1988;27:189–218.
7. Kingson ER, Hirshhorn BA, Cornman JM. *Ties that bind: The interdependence of generations.* Washington, DC: Seven Locks Press, 1986.
8. Watkin DM. *Am J Clin Nutr* 1982;36:750–758.
9. Watkin DM. In: Ordy JM, Harman D, Alfinslater R, eds. *Nutrition in gerontology.* New York: Raven Press, 1984;19–42.
10. Samity AH. *Med Clin North Am* 1983;67:333–344.
11. Steinberg FU. *Care of the geriatric patient.* St. Louis: CV Mosby, 1983.
12. O'Malley K, Waddington JC. *Therapeutics in the elderly.* New York: Excerpta Medica, 1985.
13. Ritenbaugh C. *Nutr Tod* 1987;22:14–19.
14. Smith CH, Bidlack WR. *J Am Dietet Assoc* 1984;84:901–914.
15. Clemens RA, Brown RC. *Food Technol* 1986;40:71–81.
16. Kirsch A, Bidlack WR. *Nutrition* 1987;3:305–314.
17. Herbert V. *Am J Clin Nutr* 1987;45:661–670.
18. Herbert V. *Am J Clin Nutr* 1987;45:671–678.
19. Olson JA. 1987 a. *Am J Clin Nutr* 1987;45:687–692.
20. Olson JA. *Am J Clin Nutr* 1987;45:704–716.
21. Olson JA, Hodges RE. *Am J Clin Nutr* 1987;45:693–703.
22. Bidlack WR, Kirsch A, Meskin M. *Food Technol* 1986;40:61–70.
23. Food and Nutrition Board. *Recommended dietary allowances,* 9th ed. Washington DC: National Academy of Sciences, 1980.
23a. Food and Nutrition Board. *Recommended dietary allowances,* 10th ed. Washington, DC: National Academy of Sciences, 1989.
24. Harper AE. *Ann Rev Nutr* 1987;7:509–537.
25. FAO/WHO. *Energy and protein requirements.* WHO technical reports, series no. 724. Geneva: World Health Organization, 1985.
26. Calloway DH, Zanni E. *Am J Clin Nutr* 1980;33:2088–2092.
27. Young VR. In: Armbrecht HJ, Prendergast JM, Coe RM, eds. *Nutritional intervention in the aging process.* New York: Springer-Verlag, 1984;27–47.
28. Van Itallie TB. *J Int Med* 1985;103:983–988.
29. Forbes GB, Reina JC. *Metabolism* 1970;19:653–663.
30. Rossman I. In: Finch CE, Hayflick L, eds. *Handbook of the biology of aging.* New York: Van Nostrand Reinhold, 1977;189–221.
31. Pollock ML, Dawson GA, Miller HS Jr, Ward A, Cooper D, Headley W, Linnerud AC, Nomier M-M. *J Am Geriatr Soc* 1976;24:97–104.
32. Shepard JW Jr. In: Ambrecht HJ, Prendergast JM, Coe RM, eds. *Nutritional intervention in the aging process.* New York: Springer-Verlag, 1984;315–331.
33. Kohrs MB. *Am J Clin Nutr* 1982;36:796–802.
34. Munro HN, McGandy RB, Hartz SC, Russell RM, Jacob RA, Otradovec CL. *Am J Clin Nutr* 1987;46:586–592.
35. Albanese AA. *Nutrition for the elderly.* New York: Alan R Liss, 1980.
36. Gersovitz M, Motil K, Munro HN, Scrimshaw NS, Young VR. *Am J Clin Nutr* 1982; 35:6–14.
37. Munro HN, Young VR. In: Exto-Smith AN, Caird FA, eds. *Metabolic and nutritional disorders in the elderly.* London: John Wright & Son, Ltd., 1980;13.
38. Cheng AHR, Gomez A, Bergan JG, Lee TC, Monckeberg F, Chichester CO. *Am J Clin Nutr* 1978;31:12–22.
39. Zanni E, Calloway DH, Zezuller AY. *J Nutr* 1979;109:513–524.
40. Sandine WE, Daly M. *J Food Protect* 1979;42:435–437.

41. Gallagher CR, Molleson AL, Caldwell JH. *Cult Dairy Prod J* 1977;10:22–24.
42. Andres R. *Med Clin North Am* 1971;55:835–846.
43. Davidson MD. *Metabolism* 1979;28:688–705.
44. DeFonzo RA. *Diab Care* 1981;4:493–501.
45. Andres R, Tobin JD. *Adv Exp Biol Med* 1975;61:239–249.
46. Pagano G, Cassader M, Diana A, Pisu E, Bozzo C, Ferrero F, Lenti G. *Metabolism* 1981;30:46–49.
47. Reitman JS, Vasquez B, Klimes I, Naguelesparan NM. *Diab Care* 1984;7:434–471.
48. Trovati M, Carta Q, Cavalot F, Vitali S, Banausi C, Lucchina PG, Fiocchi F, Emanuelli G, Lenti G. *Diab Care* 1984;7:416–420.
49. American Diabetes Association. *Diab Care* 1987;10:126–132.
50. West KM. *Ann Intern Med* 1973;79:425–434.
51. West KM. *Postgrad Med* 1976;60:209–216.
52. Ahrens EH Jr. *Ann Intern Med* 1976;85:87–93.
53. Kritchevsky D. *Nutr Int* 1986;2:290–297.
54. Samuel P, McNamara DJ, Shapiro J. *Ann Rev Med* 1983;34:179–194.
55. Hegsted DM. *Am J Clin Nutr* 1986;44:299–305.
56. Keys A. *Am J Clin Nutr* 1984;40:351–359.
57. McGill HC Jr. *Am J Clin Nutr* 1979;32:2664–2702.
58. Beynen AC, Katan MB. *Atherosclerosis* 1985;57:19–31.
59. Messinger WJ, Porosowska Y, Steele JM. *Arch Intern Med* 1950;86:189–195.
60. Oh SY, Miller LT. *Am J Clin Nutr* 1985;42:421–431.
61. McNamara DJ. *Arch Intern Med* 1982;142:1121–1124.
62. Beveridge JMR, Connell WF, Mayer GA, Haust HL. *J Nutr* 1960;71:61–65.
63. Erickson BA, Coots RH, Mattson FH, Kligman AM. *J Clin Invest* 1964;43:2017–2025.
64. National Diet-Heart Study Research Group. *Circulation* 1968;37(suppl 1):260–274.
65. Wolf RN, Grundy SM. *J Nutr* 1983;113:1521–1528.
66. McNamara DJ, Kolb R, Parker TS, Batwin H, Samuel P, Brown CD, Ahrens EH. *J Clin Invest* 1987;79:1729–1739.
67. Anderson KM, Castelli WP, Levy D. *JAMA* 1987;257:2176–2180.
68. Pooling Project Research Group. *J Chron Dis* 1978;31:201–306, 1978.
69. Castelli WP. *Am J Med* 1984;76:4–12.
70. Kannell WB, Dawber TR, Friedman GD, Glennon WE, McNamara PM. *Ann Intern Med* 1964;61:888–899.
71. Lipid Research Coronary Prevention trial investigators. *JAMA* 1984;251:351–364.
72. Lipid Research Coronary Prevention trial investorators. *JAMA* 1984;251:365–379.
73. National institutes of Health. *Lowering blood cholesterol to prevent heart disease: Consensus development conference statement.* Bethesda, MD: National Institutes of Health, 1984.
74. Kolata G. *Science* 1985;227:40–41.
75. Levy RI. *Arteriosclerosis* 1981;1:312–325.
76. Meskin MS, Bidlack WR. *Nutr Res (Sunkist)* 1987;26:1–6.
77. Schneeman BO. *Food Technol* 1986;39:104–110.
78. Milne JS, Williamson J. *Gerontol Clin* 1972;14:56–60.
79. Berman PM, Kirsner JB. In: Steinberg FU. *Care of the Geriatric Patient,* 6th ed. St. Louis: CV Mosby 1983:118–142.
80. Parks TG. *Clin Gastroenterol* 1975;4:53–59.
81. Brodribb AMM. In: Spiller GAS, Kay RM, eds. *Medical aspects of dietary fiber.* New York: Plenum Medical Books, 1980;43.
82. Hyland JMP, Taylor I. *Br J Surg* 1980;67:77–79.
83. Anderson JW, Chen WC. In: Furda I, ed. *Unconventional sources of dietary fiber.* Washington, DC: American Chemical Society, 1983;49.
84. Anderson J, Ward K. *Diab Care* 1978;1:77–82.
85. Suter PM, Russell RM. *Am J Clin Nutr* 1987;45:501–512.
86. McGandy RB, Russell RM, Hartz SC, Jacob RA, Tannenbaum S, Peters H, Sahyoun N, Otradovec CL. *Nutr Res* 1986;6:785–793.
87. McDonald JT. *Clin Nutr* 1986;5:27–33.
88. Stewart ML, McDonald JT, Levy AS, Schuckler RE, Henderson DP. *J Am Dietet Assoc* 1985;85:1585–1590.

89. Garry PJ, Goodwin JS, Hunt WC, Hopper EM, Leonard AG. *Am J Clin Nutr* 1982;36:319–331.
90. Gray GE, Paganini-Hill A, Ross R. *Am J Clin Nutr* 1983;38:122–128.
91. Hale WE, Stewart RB, Cerda JJ, Marks RG, May FE. *J Am Geriatr Soc* 1982;30:401–403.
92. Hartz SC, Blumberg J. *Clin Nutr* 1986;5:130–136.
93. Mann BA, Garry PJ, Hunt WC, Owen GM, Goodwin JS. *J Am Geriatr Soc* 1987;35:302–306.
94. Bowman BB, Rosenberg IH. *Am J Clin Nutr* 1982;35:1142–1151.
95. Yearick ES, Wang MSL, Pisasis SJ. *J Gerontol* 1980;5:663–671.
96. Baker H, Frank O, Thind I, Jaslow S, Louria O. *J Am Geriatr Soc* 1979;27:444–449.
97. Bamji MS. In: Briggs MH, ed. *Vitamins in human biology and medicine.* Boca Raton, FL: CRC Press, 1981;1–27.
98. Committee on Diet, Nutrition and Cancer. *Diet, nutrition and cancer.* Washington DC: National Academy of Sciences, 1982.
99. Ong DE, Chytil F. *Vitam Horm* 1983;40:105–144.
100. Colditz GA, Branch LG, Lipnick RJ. *Am J Clin Nutr* 1985;41:32–36.
101. Baker MR, Peacock M, Nordin BEC. *Age Aging* 1980;9:249–252.
102. Egsmose C, Lund B, Storm T, Sorensen OH. *Age Aging* 1987;16:36–40.
103. Barragry JM, France MW, Corless D, Jupta SR, Switala S, Boucher BJ, Cohen RD. *Clin Sci Mol Med* 1978;55:213–220.
104. Gallagher JC, Riggs BL, Eisman J, Hamstra A, Arnaud SB, DeLuca HF. *J Clin Invest* 1979;64:729–736.
105. Parfitt AM, Gallagher JC, Heaney RP, Johnson CC, Neer R, Whedon GD. *Am J Clin Nutr* 1982;36:1014–1031.
106. Rushton C. *Age Aging* 1978;7:91–95.
107. Baker H, Frank O, Jaslow S. *J Am Geriatr Soc* 1980;27:42–48.
108. Nordin BE, Heyburn PJ, Peacock M, Horsman A, Aaron J, Marshall D, Crilly RG. *J Clin Endocrinol Metab* 1980;9:177–205.
109. Armbrecht HJ, Prendergast JM, Coe RM. In: Armbrecht HJ, Prendergast JM, Coe RM, eds. *Nutritional intervention in the aging process.* New York: Springer-Verlag, 1984;69–83.
110. Slovik DM, Adams JS, Neer RM, Holick MF, Potts JT Jr. *N Engl J Med* 1981;305:372–374.
111. Francis RM, Peacock M, Taylor GA, Storer JH, Nordin BEC. *Clin Sci* 1984;66:103–107.
112. Chapuy M-C, Chapuy P, Meunier PJ. *Am J Clin Nutr* 1987;46:324–328.
113. Garry PJ, Goodwin JS, Hunt WC. *Am J Clin Nutr* 1982;36:902–909.
114. Kelleher J, Losowsky MS. In: DeDuve C, Hayashi O, eds. *Tocopherol, oxygen and biomembranes.* Amsterdam: Elsevier/North Holland Biomedical Press, 1978;311–327.
115. Vatassery GT, Johnson GJ, Krekowski AM. *J Am Coll Nutr* 1983;4:369–375.
116. Barnes KJ, Chen LH. *J Nutr Elderly* 1981;1:41–49.
117. Horwitt MK, Harvey CC, Dahm CJ Jr, Searey MT. *Ann NY Acad Sci* 1972;203:223–236.
118. Shearer MJ, McBurney A, Barkhan P. *Vitam Horm* 1974;32:513–542.
119. Morgan AG, Kelleher J, Walker BE, Losawsky MS, Droller H, Middleton RS. *Int J Vitam Nutr Res* 1975;45:448–462.
120. Iber FL, Blass JP, Brin M, Leevy CM. *Am J Clin Nutr* 1982;36:1067–1082.
121. Harrill I, Cervone N. *Am J Clin Nutr* 1977;30:431–441.
122. Leichter J, Angel JF, Lee M. *Can Med Assoc J* 1978;118:40–43.
123. Vir SH, Love AHG. *Int J Vitam Nutr Res* 1977;47:325–335.
124. Breen KJ, Buttigier R, Iossifidis S, Lourensz C, Wood B. *Am J Clin Nutr* 1985;42:121–126.
125. Chen LH, Fan-Chiang WL. *Int J Vitam Res* 1981;51:232–238.
126. Vir SH, Love AHG. *Int J Vitam Nutr Res* 1977;47:336–344.
127. Rutishauer IHE, Bates CJ, Paul AA, Black AE. *Br J Nutr* 1979;42:33–42.
128. Driskell JA. In: *Human vitamin B_6 requirements.* Washington, DC: National Academy of Science, 1978;252–256.

129. Guilland JC, Bereski-Reguig B, Lequeu B, Morreau D, Klepping J, Richard D. *Int J Vitam Nutr Res* 1984;54:185–193.
130. Anderson BB, Pert MB, Falford-Jones CE. *J Clin Pathol* 1970;23:232–242.
131. Rose CS, Gyorgy P, Butler M, Andres R, Norris AH, Shock NW, Tobin J, Brin M, Spiegel H. *Am J Clin Nutr* 1976;29:847–853.
132. Hoorn RKJ, Flikweert JP, Westerink D. *Clin Chim Acta* 1975;61:151–162.
133. Vir SH, Love AHG. *Int J Vitam Nutr Res* 1977;47:364–372.
134. Kant AK, Moser-Veillon PB, Reynolds RD. *Am J Clin Nutr* 1988;48:1284–1290.
135. Halstead CH. *Am J Clin Nutr* 1979;32:846–855.
136. Rosenberg IH. In: Johnson LR, ed. *Physiology of the gastrointestinal tract*. New York: Raven Press, 1981;1221–1230.
137. Russell RM, Krasinski SD, Samloff IM, Jacob RA, Hartz SC, Brovender SR. *Gastroenterology* 1986;91:1476–1482.
138. Bailey LB, Cerda JJ, Bloch BS, Busby J, Vargas L, Chandler CJ, Halstead CH. *J Nutr* 1984;114:1770–1776.
139. Baker H, Jaslow SP, Frank O. *J Am Geriatr Soc* 1978;25:218–221.
140. Elsborg L. *Acta Haematol* 1976;55:140–147.
141. Garry PJ, Goodwin JS, Hunt WC. *J Am Geriatr Soc* 1984;32:719–726.
142. Vir SC, Love AHG. *Am J Clin Nutr* 1979;32:1934–1937.
143. Meindock H, Dvorsky R. *J Am Geriatr Soc* 1970;18:317–325.
144. Roe DA. *Geriatric nutrition*. Englewood Cliffs, NJ: Prentice-Hall, 1983.
145. Cheli R, Simon L, Aste H, Ficus IA, Nicold G, Bajtai A, Puntoni R. *Endoscopy* 1980;12:105–108.
146. McEvoy AW, Fenwick HD, Boddy K, James OFW. *Age Aging* 1982;11:180–183.
147. Ardeman S, Chanarin I. *Gut* 1966;7:99–101.
148. King CE, Leibach J, Toskes PP. *Dig Dis Sci* 1979;24:397–402.
149. Doscherholmen A, Ripley D, Chang S, Silvis SE. *Scand J Gastroenterol* 1977;12:313–319.
150. Carmel R. *Ann Intern Med* 1978;88:647–649.
151. Marcus DL, Shadick N, Crantz J, Gray M, Hernandez F, Freedman ML. *J Am Geriatr Soc* 1987;35:635–638.
152. Reisenauer AM, Halstead CH. *J Nutr* 1987;117:600–602.
153. Garry PJ, Goodwin JS, Hunt WC, Gilbert BA. *Am J Clin Nutr* 1982;36:332–339.
154. Cheng L, Cohen M, Bhagavan HN. In: Watson RR, ed. *Handbook of nutrition in the aged*. Boca Raton Fl: CRC Press, 1985;157–185.
155. VanderJagt DJ, Garry PJ, Bhagavan HN. *Am J Clin Nutr* 1987;46:290–294.
156. Pelletier O. *Ann NY Acad Sci* 1975;258:156–168.
157. Nordstrom JW. *Am J Clin Nutr* 1982;36:788–795.
158. Herbert V. *Am J Clin Nutr* 1987;45:679–86.
159. Monsen ER, Hallberg L, Layrisse M, Hegsted DM, Cook JD, Mertz W, Finch CA. *Am J Clin Nutr* 1978;31:134–141.
160. Lynch SR, Finch CA, Monsen ER, Cook JD. *Am J Clin Nutr* 1982;36:1032–1045.
161. Freedman ML, Marcus DL. *Am J Med Sci* 1980;280:81–85.
162. Marston RM, Roger N. *Nat Food Rev* 1987;36:18–23.
163. Morgan KJ, Stampley GL, Zabik ME, Fischer DR. *J Am Coll Nutr* 1985;4:195–201.
164. Pao EM, Mickle SJ. *Food Technol* 1981;33:58–69, 79.
165. National Institutes of Health. *Osteoporosis. Consensus development conference statement*. Bethesda, MD: National Institutes of Health, 1984;5:1–9.
166. Riggs NL. *Endocrinol Jap* 1979;1:31–41.
167. Nordin BEC. *Drugs* 1979;18:484–492.
168. Gossard D, Haskell WL, Taylor CB, Mueller JK, Rogers F, Chandler M, Ahn DK, Miller NH, Debusk RF. *Am J Cardiol* 1986;57:446–449.
169. Heaney RP, Gallagher JC, Johnston CC, Neer R, Parfitt AM, Whedon GD. *Am J Clin Nutr* 1982;36(suppl):986–1013.
170. Kiel DP, Felson DT, Anderson JJ, Wilson PWF, Moskowitz MA. *N Engl J Med* 1987;317:1169–1174.
171. Spencer H, Kramer L. *J Nutr* 1986;116:316–319.
172. Heaney RP, Recker RR, Saville PD. *Am J Clin Nutr* 1977;30:1603–1611.

173. Heaney RP, Recker RR, Saville PD. *J Lab Clin Med* 1978;92:953–963.
174. Spencer H, Kramer L, Lesniak M, DeBartolo M, Clemontain N, Osis D. *Clin Orthop* 1984;84:270–280.
175. Riggs BL, Wahner HW, Melton LJ, Richelson LS, Judd HL, O'Fallon WM. *J Clin Invest* 1987;80:972–982.
176. Riis B, Thomsen K, Christiansen C. *N Engl J Med* 1987;316:173–177.
177. Nilas L, Christensen C, Rodbro P. *Br Med J* 1984;289:1103–1106.
178. Ettinger B, Genant HK, Cann CE. *Ann Intern Med* 1987;106:40–45.
179. Spencer H, Kramer L, DeBatolo M, Norris C, Osis D. *Am J Clin Nutr* 1983;37:924–929.
180. Spencer H, Kramer L, Osis D, Norris C. *J Nutr* 1978;108:447–457.
181. Spencer H, Karmer L, Osis D. *J Nutr* 1988;118:657–660.
182. Tolstoi LG. *US Pharmacist* 1987;April:H7–H13.
183. Tolstoi LG, Fosmire G. *Nutr Tod* 1987;22:March/April:22–28.
184. Seelig MS. *Magnesium Bull* 1981;1a:26–47.
185. Touitou Y, Godard J-P, Ferment O, Chastang C, Proust J, Bogdan A, Auzeby A, Touitou C. *Clin Chem* 1987;33:518–523.
186. Whang R, Oei TO, Aikawa JK, Watanabe A. *Arch Intern Med* 1984;144:1794–1796.
187. Flink EB. *Acta Med Scand* 1981;647(suppl):125–137.
188. Shils ME. *Medicine* 1969;48:61–85.
189. Kaplan NM. *Ann Intern Med* 1983;98:705–709.
190. Pacy PJ, Dodson PM. *Ann Nutr Metab* 1985;29:129–137.
191. Weaver CM, Evans GH. *Food Technol* 1986;39:99–101.
192. Weinberger MH, Miller JZ, Luft FC, Grim CE, Fineberg NS. *Food Technol* 1986;39:96–98.
193. Sandstead HH. In: Prasad AS, ed. *Clinical, biochemical and nutritional aspects of trace elements.* New York: Alan R Liss, 1982;83–101.
194. US Department of Health, Education and Welfare. *Ten State Survey Highlights.* Washington, DC: US Government Printing Office, 1972 (DHEW Publ. No. (HMS) 72–8134).
195. Lindeman RD, Clark ML, Colmore JP. *J Gerontol* 1971;26:358–363.
196. Flint DM, Wahlquist ML, Smith TJ, Parish AB. *J Hum Nutr* 1981;35:287–295.
197. Harman D. *J Gerontol* 1965;20:151–153.
198. Turnland J, Costa F, Margen S. *Am J Clin Nutr* 1981;34:2641–2647.
199. Williams ME, Pannill FC III. *Ann Intern Med* 1982;97:895–907.
200. Yarnell JWG, St. Leger AS. *Age Aging* 1979;8:81–85.
201. Phillips PA, Rolls BJ, Ledingham JGG, Forsling ML, Morton JJ, Crowe MJ, Wollner L. *N Engl J Med* 1984;311:753–759.
202. Steen B, Lundgren BK, Isakson B. In: Chandra RK, ed. *Nutrition immunity and illness in the elderly.* Elmsford, NY: Pergamon Press, 1985:49–52
203. Leaf A. *N Engl J Med* 1984;311:791–792.
204. Fish PD, Bennett GCJ, Millard PH. *Age Aging* 1985;14:243–245.
205. Halle A, Repasy A. *Hosp Pract* 1987;22:26–35.

Geriatric Nutrition, edited by John E. Morley,
Zvi Glick, Laurence Z. Rubenstein.
Raven Press, Ltd., New York © 1990.

6

Nutritional Assessment of the Elderly

Emma J. Lewis and Stacey J. Bell

New England Deaconess Hospital, Boston, Massachusetts 02215

As the fastest growing age group in the United States, the elderly pose a new
and increasingly important challenge to the health care profession. By the
year 2000, approximately 13% of the U.S. population will be 65 years or
older, and by 2030 this figure is expected to increase to approximately 21.2%
(1). Five percent of the elderly population presently reside in nursing homes,
and another 15% of the total population require some degree of assistance
at home (2,8). To serve this population, quality nutritional care is needed to
identify and to alert the clinical team to elderly patients at nutritional risk.
It is only through proper and continuous monitoring that a patient's nutritional status can be evaluated and deficiencies identified and resolved. Such
assessment techniques as anthropometrics, biochemical indices, and immune testing are presently well understood and easily obtainable for hospitalized and nursing home patients under 55 years. However, when assessing
the needs of older patients, the existing data may be insensitive or
inappropriate.

TYPES OF MALNUTRITION

Protein-Energy Malnutrition

The incidence of protein-energy malnutrition (PEM) in the hospitalized
patient ranges from 30 to 65% (3) and around 50% in nursing homes (4).
Among the elderly in particular, PEM may develop secondarily from chronic
disease, isolation, poverty, diminished physical or mental status, or poor
dentition prevalent among this age group. There are three types of PEM:
marasmus, hypoalbuminemia (kwashiorkor), or a mixture of both.

Marasmus

Marasmus results from an inadequate supply of calories. In this type of
starvation, skeletal muscle, fat, and glycogen are mobilized for energy

sources while visceral protein levels remain normal. In the absence of stress caused by the decrease in blood volume and body size, immune function is usually unaffected during marasmus (5). Marasmus may be detected by depressed triceps skinfold (TSF) and arm muscle circumference (AMC), weight loss, and decreased height for weight values.

Hypoalbuminemia

Hypoalbumenemia is noted by a decrease in serum albumin concentrations, reflecting the depletion of visceral protein stores. Additionally, the immune response at the cellular level (ie, IL-1 production) is decreased (5). In this type of malnutrition, however, muscle mass and weight may be normal or even above normal as a result of obesity or edema.

Mixed

The types of malnutrition previously defined may be present simultaneously, resulting in what is called a mixed marasmic state. Based on body composition changes, weight loss, laboratory indices, and anthropometrics, moderate and severe protein-calorie malnutrition can be assessed among the elderly.

CHANGES IN BODY COMPOSITION

Lean Body Mass

Decreased muscle mass or lean body mass (LBM) and an accompanying increase in body fat are the normal changes in body composition caused by aging. Using K^{40} analysis Forbes et al. have documented a 6.3% decrease in LBM per decade, averaging a total loss of 5 kg for women and 12 kg for men between the ages of 25 to 70 years (6). The accelerated decline seen in the elderly may in part be attributed to lower physical activity, poor diet, reduced body water and overall loss in cell mass (BCM), or metabolically active tissue. Basal energy expenditure, which is influenced by BCM, also decreases with age at a rate of 20% between ages 30 and 90 years (7). In old age muscle size can decrease as much as 40%. In addition, other organs shrink so that a reduction in size of as much as 9% for the kidney, 18% for the liver, and 11% for the lung can occur. These losses have profound effects on overall nutrient dynamics (8). During malnutrition, body composition changes are more drastic in the elderly because decreasing BCM is associated with increases in extracellular mass (ECM), leading to a profound diminution in metabolic and excretory capacity.

Total Body Fat

As overall lean body mass decreases, the percentage of fat increases by 2% of body weight per decade after the age of 30 (9). This can result in a total increase of between 10 to 15% during an adult's life span. In addition, the distribution of fat deposits around the trunkal area and internal organs changes with aging.

Total Body Water

The aging process is not only marked by changes in LBM and fat. Total body water also decreases with age, especially extracellular water, which explains in part the loss of total body weight. LBM in normal healthy adults is 70% water, which declines to 60% in the elderly (10). Dehydration, edema, and ascites associated with illness can, however, alter markedly these normally occurring hydrostatic weight changes, especially in the nutritionally compromised patient.

ASSESSMENT OF BODY COMPOSITION

The body compartments are conventionally divided into fat and fat-free mass and may be measured using several techniques. Data used to assess body composition within the elderly population should be obtained serially so that an assessment relating change to time can be made. The following methodologic approaches have been found useful in assessing nutritional status.

Bioelectrical Impedance

Bioelectrical impedance is a noninvasive method of determining the relative proportion of fat and lean tissue. The principle governing electrical impedance plethysomography is that lean tissue, comprised largely of water, readily conducts an applied electrical current (low resistance), whereas fat acts as an insulator and conducts little current (high resistance). In this test four electrodes placed on the hands and feet conduct a 50-kHz current at 800 microamps to determine, through a ratio of reactance to resistance, sites of hydration and changes in intra- and extracellular mass. Using regression equations based on a normal population, fat and fat-free mass can be calculated (11). The formulas deduced in this study may be applied to the elderly, providing the following limitations are kept in mind: (a) The data base for the regression analysis included few elderly and no very old persons; (b) the regression formulas were generated using data from healthy subjects, in whom the normal percentage of fat ranges between 11 and 16% for men and between 18 and 25% for women (12). These formulas do not take into account that in old age the percentage fat ranges are substantially less for men and higher for women.

Other Body Composition Techniques

Nuclear magnetic resonance (NMR), radiographic imaging, K40, and isotope dilution methods are useful in determining muscle diameter and area (6,13). Underwater weighing or densitometry gives an accurate measurement of body fat. However, all are impractical to conduct in a clinical setting and may be difficult in the geriatric population.

ANTHROPOMETRICS

Height

Height may be difficult to assess in the elderly, who tend to report the values they had in their youth. It is thus important to obtain an exact present measurement.

Hertzog et al. have calculated that height decreases in women at a rate of 0.03 cm/year until age 45 and then at 0.28 cm/year per decade thereafter (14). More recent data by Chumlea et al. indicate even greater values of height loss, with a mean value of 0.5 cm/year in a smaller sample of healthy patients (15).

The primary reason for decreased height in the elderly appears to be the shortening of the spinal column (16). Other factors contributing to altered height in the elderly include an actual bone loss of 12% in men and 25% in women (8), leading to osteoporosis (reduction in bone density) and kyphosis (curvature of the spinal column). Inactivity or non-weight-bearing exercise appears to be a risk factor.

Weight

Weight should be measured weekly while the patient is hospitalized and every few months in a nursing home to reflect dietary changes and to monitor the nutritional impact of existing disease processes. A calibrated balance scale is most accurate for ambulatory adults and a calibrated chair or bed scale for nonambulatory persons. Using the same scale helps avoid nonphysiologic errors.

The Metropolitan Life Insurance Tables of 1983 (17) based on data from a young healthy population aged 25 to 59 years are most often used today for reference height and weight. However, this table fails to include data derived from very old people.

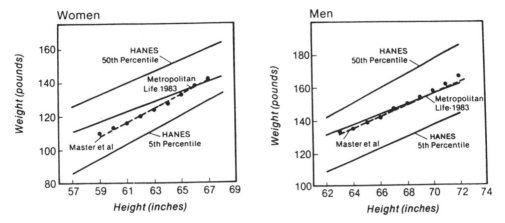

FIG. 1. The data from the NHANES survey[18], Master and associates[19], and Metropolitan Life Height/Weight Table[17] are displayed. Data from the NHANES survey and Master and associates were subjected to regression analysis, and the resulting equations were used to construct the lines. The regression equations for the NHANES data appear in Table I. For the Master and associates data, the published mean weight/height values were plotted ($\bullet$) and the line (-----) was constructed using the following equations: For women, weight (in pounds) (Y) = 4.08 × height (in inches) (X) − 132.36. For men, weight (in pounds) (Y) = 3.52 × height (in inches) (X) − 90.18. The Metropolitan Life values, when plotted directly, form the line shown.

Analysis of the 1971–74 National Health and Nutrition Examination Survey (NHANES) data (18) shows that weight appears to increase for men between 35 to 54 years and for women between 55 to 65 years. Weight stabilizes thereafter for the next 15 to 20 years and then progressively declines. In this study however, no relationship between weight/height ratios and mortality rates was examined.

Master and Lasser (19) have the most comprehensive data base from an elderly population up to 94 years. Unlike NHANES, these investigators documented a steady increase in the weight/height ratio from 84 to 94 years. However, few data exist in the oldest group, aged 90 to 94. The data for persons aged 85 to 89 years lie between the 5th and 50th percentile of these weights documented by NHANES (Fig. 1) (20). Until more reliable reference data are compiled, we suggest use of a table developed by Simpoulos (21) based on desirable weights for height obtained from mortality statistics of the Metropolitan Life Insurance Data (Table 1). These data approximate the Master and Lasser study and the 5th and 50th percentile of the NHANES data.

Weight Loss

Because of the difficulties in determining ideal body weight (IBW), weight loss may be a sensitive indication of individuals at nutritional risk. A non-

TABLE 1. *Ideal body weight (IBW) useful for elderly persons*

Height (ft/in)	Average IBW of men (lb)	Average IBW of women (lb)
4 9	—	100
4 10	—	103
4 11	—	106
5 0	—	109
5 1	117	112
5 2	120	116
5 3	123	120
5 4	126	124
5 5	129	128
5 6	133	132
5 7	138	136
5 8	142	140
5 9	146	144
5 10	150	148
5 11	155	—
6 0	159	—
6 1	164	—
6 2	169	—
6 3	174	—

From Simpoulos, ref. 21.

volitional weight loss of 10% or more, especially over a short period of time (<3 months), demonstrates malnutrition and requires further evaluation to determine the cause (8). Table 2 shows weight loss over time as a guide for monitoring malnutrition in the elderly and may be of particular value in the nursing home setting (22).

Anthropometry

Anthropometric measurements on a regular basis (yearly in a nursing home and monthly in a hospital) are an important aspect of nutritional as-

TABLE 2. *Duration of weight loss over time*

Time	Significant weight loss[a] (%)	Severe weight loss[a] (%)
One Week	1–2	>2
One month	5	>5
Three months	7.5	>7.5
Unlimited time	10–20	>20

From Clark, ref. 22.

[a]Percentage weight change = $\frac{\text{usual weight-actual weight}}{\text{usual weight}} \times 100$.

Weight loss of greater than 40% is usually associated with mortality.

sessment for elderly patients. Such measurements are simple to perform, noninvasive, and inexpensive. They are reasonably sensitive indices because they are adjusted according to the height, weight, age, and sex of a patient and compared against established standard tables developed from the NHANES.

Upper Arm Anthropometry

Triceps skinfold (TSF) thicknesses (measured by calipers) and midarm circumferences (MAC) provide estimates of body fat and skeletal muscle, respectively. Bistrian (5) has found that values on the standard NHANES tables provide a reliable estimation of body fat and nutritional status for individuals and that those between the 5th and 50th percentile correspond to moderate nutritional risk and those below the 5th percentile correspond to severe depletion. During the aging process, TSF measurements increase 14% in women and decrease 8% in men by 65 to 75 years of age (Table 4) (23). Sex differences in TSF norms for the elderly may be attributed to the distinct fat and muscle composition changes noted between sexes.

MAC is reflective of somatic protein stores (LBM) and is simply measured in centimeters using a flexible tape measure. Frisancho has reported on the most recent MAC norms for the elderly population from the NHANES data, finding that between ages 22 to 70, arm muscle circumference increases by about 6% in women and only slightly in men (Table 4) (23).

Arm muscle circumference (AMC), a better indicator of protein status, is derived by

$$\text{AMC (cm)} = \text{MAC (cm)} - \frac{[(3.14 \times \text{TSF mm})]}{10}$$

Bistrian (5) suggests calculating percent of standard (actual/standard $\times$ 100) using the 5th to 50th percentile of the NHANES data in the denominator as the limit of acceptable ranges for the elderly. Older patients who fall below 85% of standard are at nutritional risk (20).

TABLE 3. *Changes in triceps skinfold thickness (TSF)[a] and arm muscle circumference (AMC)[a] with aging*

	25.0–34.9 years	65.0–74.9 years	% change
Women			
TSF (mm)	21	24	14%
AMC (cm)	21.2	22.5	6%
Men			
TSF (mm)	12	11	8%
AMC (cm)	27.9	26.8	4%

From Frisancho, ref. 23.
[a]50th percentile values.

TABLE 4. *Creatinine height index as a function of age*

Age (years)	Number of patients	Creatinine excretion	Creatinine height index
		mg/24 hr	
17–24	10	1790 ± 52	10.2
25–34	73	1862 ± 31	10.6
35–44	122	1746 ± 24	10.0
45–54	152	1689 ± 18	9.6
55–64	94	1580 ± 22	9.0
65–74	68	1409 ± 25	8.0
75–84	29	1259 ± 45	7.2

From Driver and McAlevy, ref. 28.

Accurate AMC assessment in the elderly is questionable because axial tomography now shows that the arm is not circular and that fat distribution is uneven (24). In addition, Heymsfield et al. (25) state that only 85 to 95% of somatic protein loss may be detected by muscle mass measurements, thereby underestimating protein stores by 5 to 15%.

Unfortunately, there are limitations in assuming that TSF and AMC reflect the size of body compartments in older adults. First, one needs to assume that most body fat is subcutaneous fat and evenly distributed around the arm. Second, the data used to define standards do not include an adequate number of elderly people. Third, the accuracy of TSF and AMC measurement depends upon observer skill. Lastly, precise measurements may also be affected by such changing physiologic processes as decreased skin elasticity and compressibility and hydration status, all factors that can be influenced by age, disease, and drug therapy (22,23).

BIOCHEMICAL INDICES

Urine

Urinary Urea Nitrogen (UUN)

A 24-hour urine collection may provide a sensitive assessment of protein balance and catabolic stress. Urinary urea nitrogen (UUN) is the largest contribution of protein in the urine and is often used in the nitrogen balance equation.

$$\text{Nitrogen Balance} = \frac{[\text{Protein Intake}]}{6.25} - (\text{UUN (g)} + 4)$$

Total urinary nitrogen could be substituted, but it is more time consuming to measure and consequently more costly. UNN (g) + 4 represents nitrogen loss from the urine and to insensible losses, such as exhaled air, sweat, or feces. Clark (22) and others have found that, as age increases, the ability to concentrate urine and to excrete acid decreases. As a result, the correction factor of 4 g may overestimate true losses, and a correction factor lower than 4 g/day may be more representative for the elderly.

Urinary Creatinine

Twenty-four-hour urinary creatinine excretion may be used to reflect LBM, as 98% of total body creatinine lies within the muscle (9). From age 25 to 75 there is a decline in creatinine of 36% in women and 30% in men. Creatinine excretion decreases quickly in a malnourished or wasted state in the absence of renal failure because of the reduction in muscle mass. Additionally, such factors as low meat consumption that are prevalent among the elderly may cause a further depreciation in creatinine muscle concentration (26).

The Creatinine height index (CHI) as reported by Blackburn et al. (27) compares the value of urinary creatinine with that of a standard based on ideal excretion for a person of the same height. Predicted urinary creatinine is 18 mg/kg IBW for women and 23 mg/kg IBW for men.

$$CHI = \frac{\text{Actual urinary creatinine (mg)}}{\text{predicted urinary creatinine (mg)}} \times 100\%$$

Driver and McAlevy (28) have incorporated an age and renal function factor into the CHI equation to create a more sensitive index for the elderly (Table 4). From this information, it was found that CHI decreases normally about 18% between the ages of 20 and 70 years, reflecting the overall changing body composition in elderly persons.

Blood Parameters

Serial measurements, such as blood urea nitrogen (BUN), creatinine, hemoglobin, hematocrit, serum, iron and total iron-binding capacity, sodium, potassium, albumin, prealbumin, and cholesterol are useful to monitor the impact of nutritional therapy and in targeting those at risk of malnutrition. Abnormalities of anemia, hypoalbuminemia, hypotransferrinemia, lymphocytopenia, and immunosuppressed states indicate undernutrition, whereas serum BUN, creatinine, sodium, and potassium may be used to analyze disturbances in fluid, electrolyte, and acid-base homeostasis.

Albumin

Serum albumin concentration is an indication of visceral protein stores, which although slightly decreased by the aging process, have been found to

TABLE 5. *Serum standards for nutritional assessment*

	% of Deficit		
	Mild	Moderate	Severe
Albumin (g/dl)	3.5–3.2	3.2–2.8	<2.8
Transferrin (mg/dl)	200–180	180–160	<160
TLC (no./mm^3)	1800–1500	1500–900	<900

From Clark, ref. 22.

be the most sensitive marker of malnutrition. Assessment of serum albumin concentration is rendered insensitive in the presence of severe edema and anorexia (29). In normal healthy subjects, albumin concentrations lie between 4.1–5.5 g/dl. In ambulatory subjects values below 4.0 g/dl should be considered suspect. With recumbency, extracellular fluid is redistributed, lowering serum albumin levels by 0.5 g/dl.

Greenbalt (30) found average mean serum albumin concentration to be 3.97 g/dl in hospital patients under 40 years of age, decreasing to 3.58 gm/dl for those over 80 years. The lower levels noted in the elderly population may be attributed to a decreased rate of protein synthesis and increased breakdown. Despite a half-life of 21 days, albumin should be monitored weekly in the hospital, but in an extended care facility it can be checked once every 6 months. Transferrin, because of its smaller plasma pool and shorter half-life, responds more rapidly to dietary supplementation. Therefore, it may be a better monitoring tool to assess rapid changes that characterize unstable metabolic situations (29). Iron stores increase with age, and serum transferrin decreases concomitantly. Such findings may result in some elderly subjects being inappropriately termed malnourished. Percentage of transferrin saturation (TIBC) may be more predictive of those at risk (16,21).

Stratification of serum values of albumin and transferrin into mild, moderate, and severe malnutrition is depicted in Table 5 (22).

Hematologic Tests

Hematologic tests are also useful for the nutritional assessment of the elderly. Both hemoglobin (Hgb) and hematocrit (Hct) levels decline in the free-living elderly, suggesting the need for a downward adjustment of standards to prevent the misdiagnosis of anemia (3). In a study by Burns et al. (3), hemoglobin was normal or decreased by 20 to 30% in free-living elderly. Mitchell and Lipschitz (32) found that hemoglobin values below 12 g/dl for men and 10 g/dl for women distinguished healthy elderly from these malnourished individuals.

Immune System Parameters

Because of the diminished activity of their immune system, the elderly respond poorly to infection. Poor nutrition, pre-existing organ impairment, and the stresses of sepsis and surgery cause this group of patients to exhibit a high vulnerability to infection, which adversely affects tissue growth, wound healing, and cell-mediated immune responsiveness.

Immune status may be monitored by total lymphocyte count (TLC) and other more specific immune tests, which include acute phase proteins, complements, monokines, immunogammaglobulin levels, and helper suppressor cells.

Total Lymphocyte Count

As a simple assessment of immune competency the TLC is easily obtained from a complete blood count and differential. Levels of white blood cells found in the lymph tissues do not change significantly with aging, but are markedly suppressed in states of malnourishment and elevated during stress and sepsis (27). The following formula can be used to obtain TLC in the elderly:

$$TLC = \frac{\% \text{ Lymphocytes} \times WBC}{100}$$

Values below 1,500 mm³ (Table 5) may indicate marked immunosuppression. Unfortunately, TLC is insensitive in the presence of a bacterial infection, which increases the TLC count even in the presence of malnutrition.

Delayed Hypersensitivity Skin Testing

Certain white blood cells, the B cells responsible for the production of immunoglobulins, appear to decrease naturally with age and even more acutely during malnutrition (32). Delayed hypersensitivity skin test antigens measure patients' ability to mount an immune response. Anergy is often associated with hypoalbuminemia.

Immunity and Stress

Both increased levels of white blood cells (WBC) and the presence of sepsis are good indicators of monokine activation. Lipschitz et al. (32) have

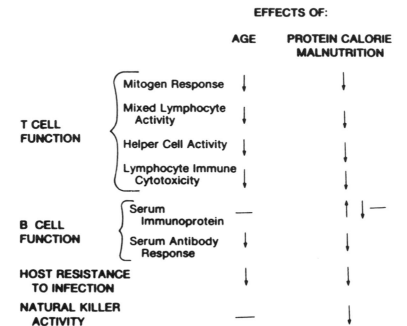

FIG. 2. A comparison of the effects of age or protein-calorie malnutrition on lymphocyte function. (From Adler, ref. 34, with permission of Ross Laboratories.)

shown a marked impairment in the ability to mount a neutrophil response in the malnourished elderly. Interleukin-1 (IL-1) and tumor necrosis factor (TNF) are released from monocytes and macrophages during infection or injury, but these may have diminished functional capacity during a malnourished state (32). Organ impairment, common among the elderly, may also adversely affect these cells' ability to mount a response to injury.

Nutrition plays an important role in the host defense system. Chandra et al. (33) showed a marked recovery from anergy upon refeeding elderly subjects, thus indicating the delicate interrelationship between nutrition and immune response.

Figure 2 exhibits the dual effect of aging and protein-calorie malnutrition on lymphocyte function and host defense systems. The ability of B cells to produce antibodies for a variety of antigens and the TLC both decrease in malnutrition, yet appear unaffected by aging alone.

Whether abnormal laboratory values in the elderly are consequences of disease states or the natural aging process is presently difficult to evaluate. However, by obtaining a well-rounded biochemical profile, nutritional status may be clearly determined and protein malnutrition diagnosed.

Prognostic Power

Measurement of the serum albumin concentration has been found to be one of the best single predictors of morbidity and mortality among the aged (31,35). Reinhardt et al. (36) studied 509 men with an average of 59 years and found that those with serum albumin concentrations greater than 3.5 g/dl had a mortality of 1.7%, those with levels less than 3.4 g/dl had a 25% mortality rate, and levels less than 2.0 g/dl resulted in a 62% mortality rate.

Rudman et al. (37) later found a relationship between mortality and decreased serum albumin concentrations in undernourished, elderly male patients residing in a long-term care facility. There was a death rate of 50% when albumin fell below 3.5 g/dl and only 11% when it remained above 4.0 g/dl. Finally, Harvey and colleagues (38) found in a group of critically ill elderly patients that a serum albumin below 2.2 g/dl was associated with a greater than 75% probability of sepsis and dying in the hospital.

A low TLC is often associated with decreased serum albumin values, yet when considered alone, TLC is a poor prognostic indicator. Seltzer et al. (39) studied albumin and TLC in 500 consecutive hospital admissions and noted a 7.6% incidence of abnormal albumin and 30.2% incidence of abnormal TLC. Abnormal TLC was associated with an increase in deaths (fourfold), and abnormal albumin was related to both increased death (sixfold) and complications. In combination, abnormal TLC and albumin resulted in an eightfold increase in complication rate with a ninefold increase in mortality.

Elderly patients with cholesterol levels below 156 mg/dl have a death rate of 67 to 80%, whereas those with values above 150 mg/dl have only a 1.9% to 9% death rate (40). Obviously, this is surprising in light of current thinking about reducing cholesterol levels and health. However, conventional thinking is not always applicable as aging occurs.

The Prognostic Nutritional Index (PNI) developed by Buzby et al. (41) and the Hospital Prognostic Index of Harvey et al. (38) may be easily applied in the clinical setting to predict the degree of postoperative complications and risk of mortality. Each index incorporates common nutritional assessment indices and predicts outcome by regression analysis. Although PNI accounts for only 17% of the information needed to predict who will develop a complication, it is useful in monitoring nutritional status and predicting hospital outcome (41).

SUMMARY

When assessing the nutritional status of the elderly it is important to define the etiologic factors involved. By doing so the assessment approach can be streamlined so that maximum information can be obtained for the optimum care of the patient. Nutritional assessments based on subjective and objective data are only valuable if continued monitoring occurs; this should be planned at frequent intervals in acute states and lesser intervals in chronic illness.

Despite the lack of age-specific standards for the elderly, nutritional assessment techniques available today are helpful tools for evaluating the changes in body composition and organ function associated with the aging process. From the viewpoint of assessment it is now possible to define and quantitate nutritional deficiencies and assess the nutritional risks facing this population during periods of stress.

REFERENCES

1. Bureau of the Census. *Projections of the population of the United States: 1983 to 2080.* Washington, DC: U.S. Government Printing Office, 1984.
2. Sullivan D, Chernoff R, Lipschitz DA. *Nutr Clin Pract* 1987;6–12.
3. Burns R, Nichols L, Calkins E, Blackwell S, Pragay D. *J Am Geriatr Soc* 1986;34: 781–786.
4. Pinchcofsky-Devin GD, Kaminski MV. *J Am Coll Nutr* 1987;6:109–112.
5. Bistrian BR. *Am J Clin Nutr* 1980;33:2211–2214.
6. Forbes GB, Reina JC. *Metabolism* 1970;19:653–663.
7. Keys A, Taylor HL, Grande F. *Metabolism* 1973;22:579–587.
8. Colucci RA, Bell SJ, Blackburn GL. *Compr Ther* 1987;13:20–28.
9. Walser M. *JPEN* 1987;11:73S–78S.
10. Steen B. *Nutr Rev* 1988;46:45–51.
11. Shizgal HM. Presentation at the ASPEN 13th Clinical Conference. Miami, FL 1989; 175–177.
12. Whitney EN, Nunnelley Hamilton EM. *Understanding nutrition,* 2nd ed. New York: West Publishing Company, 1981.
13. Cohn SH, Vartsky D, Yasumura S, Sawitsky A, Zanzi I, Vaswari A, Ellis KJ. *Am J Physiol* 1980;239:E524–530.
14. Hertzog KP, Gain SM, Hempy HO. *Am J Phys Anthropol* 1969;31:111–115.
15. Chumlea WC, Garry PJ, Hunt WC, Rhyne RL. *Hum Biol* 1988;60:917–925.
16. Chernoff R, et al. *Geriatr Med Tod* 1984;3:129–141.
17. Metropolitan Life Insurance Co: *1983 Metropolitan height and weight tables. 1979 Build Study.* Society of Actuaries and Association of Life Insurance Medical Directors of America, 1983. *Food Nutrition and Diet Therapy,* 7th ed. Philadelphia: WB Saunders, 1984;963.
18. National Center for Health Statistics. *Weight by height and age of adults 18–74 years. Vital and Health Statistics,* series 11, no. 208. Washington, DC: U.S. Government Printing Office, 1974;(PH5)79-1656.
19. Master AM, Lasser RP. *JAMA* 1960;114:658–662.
20. Clark NG, Bistrian BR. *Geriatr Med Tod* 1984;3:45–59.
21. Simpoulos AP. *J Am Dietet Assoc* 1985;85:419–422.
22. Clark NG. *Clin Consult Nutr Supp* 1982;2:5–8.
23. Frisancho AR. *Am J Clin Nutr* 1981;34:2540–2545.
24. Heymsfield SB, Olafson RP, Kutner MH, Nixon DW. *Am J Clin Nutr* 1979;32:693–702.
25. Heymsfield SB, Stevens V, Noel R, McManus S, Smith J, Nixon D. *Am J Clin Nutr* 1982;36:131–142.
26. Rowe JW, Andres R, Tobin FD, Norris AH, Shock NW. *J Gerontol* 1976;31:155–163.
27. Blackburn GL, Bistrian BR, Maini BS, Schlamm HT, Smith MF. *JPEN* 1977;1:11–22.
28. Driver AG, McAlevy MT. *Am J Clin Nutr* 1980;33:2057(letter).
29. Tayek JA. *Nutr Clin Pract* 1988;3:219–221.
30. Greenblatt D. *J Am Geriatr Soc* 1979;27:20–22.

31. Mitchell CO, Lipschitz DA. *Am J Clin Nutr* 1982;36:340–349.
32. Lipschitz DA, Mitchell CO, Thompson C. *Am J Hematol* 1981;11:47–54.
33. Chandra RK, Joshi P, Au B, et al. *Nutr Res* 1982;2:223–232.
34. Adler WH. In: *Assessing the nutritional status of the elderly state of the art, Report of the Third Roundtable on Medical Issues.* Columus, OH: Ross Laboratory, 1982;42.
35. Agarwal N, Acevedo F, Leighton LS, Cayten CG, Pitchumoni CS. *Am J Clin Nutr* 1988;48:1173–1178.
36. Reinhardt GF, Myscofski JW, Wilkens DB, et al. *JPEN* 1980;4:357–359.
37. Rudman D, Feller AG, Nagraj HS, Jackson DL, Rudman DW, Mattson DE. *JPEN* 1987;11:360–363.
38. Harvey DB, Maldawer LL, Bistrian BR, Blackburn GL. *Am J Clin Nutr* 1981;34:2013–2022.
39. Seltzer MH, Bashidas JA, Cooper DM. *JPEN* 1979;3:157–159.
40. Rudman D, Mattson DE, Nagrajet HS, Caindec N, Rudman IW, Jackson DL. *J Am Geriatr Soc* 1987;35:496–502.
41. Buzby GP, Mullen JL, Mathews DC, Hobbs CL, and Rosato EF. *Am J Surg* 1980;139:160–167.

Geriatric Nutrition, edited by John E. Morley,
Zvi Glick, Laurence Z. Rubenstein.
Raven Press, Ltd., New York © 1990.

7

The Role of Nutrition in the Prevention of Age-Associated Diseases

John E. Morley

*Geriatric Research Education and Clinical Center VA Medical Center, Sepulveda,
California 91343 and Department of Medicine, UCLA School of Medicine,
Los Angeles, California 90024*

Disease prevention can be divided into primary, secondary, and tertiary prevention. Primary prevention occurs when steps are taken before the disease has developed to prevent its occurrence, eg, the use of influenza vaccine to prevent influenza epidemics or the institution of good sanitary practices in food handling to prevent food poisoning. Secondary prevention is the early detection of a disease that may remain occult for a period of time before manifesting itself. In secondary prevention can also be included the aggressive early treatment of a disease, eg, treating influenza with amantidine to ameliorate the development of serious complications. Under tertiary prevention is included the rehabilitation process, such as when an elderly patient is admitted to a geriatric evaluation unit for a period of physical therapy and nutritional support before being discharged home.

Nutritional interventions can clearly be applied at the primary, secondary, and tertiary levels of disease prevention. However, in developing an understanding of the role of nutrition in the prevention of age-associated diseases, it is important to realize that these interventions are unlikely to make major changes in life expectancy. In the United States since the beginning of this century, life expectancy has risen from 45 to 75 years. In the 10 years from 1976 to 1986, overall life expectancy for men and women increased by approximately 2 years. In those over the age of 65 years, life expectancy for men increased by 1 year, whereas that for women increased only one half-year. These figures suggest that we are closing in on the upper limit of life expectancy, making it harder for preventive interventions to have a major impact on life extension.

For these reasons, it becomes increasingly important to measure the impact of nutritional intervention programs on morbidity. Small changes in morbidity can have a major impact on the quality of life. For example, as shown in Fig. 1, the world record for the 1-mile run has improved by 1%

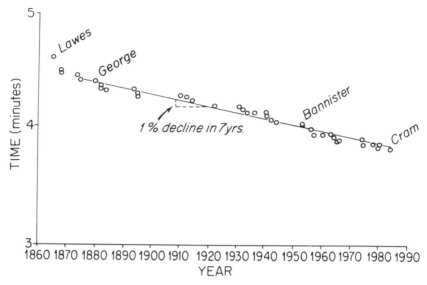

FIG. 1. Pictorial representation of the world record for the 1-mile run. (From Morley et al., ref. 37, with permission.)

every 7 years. In real terms, this means a 1% improvement in an international-class athlete would put him or her 7 years ahead of their fellow competitors. This would almost certainly guarantee an Olympic gold medal, or in the case of a professional football player, could represent the difference between being a millionaire or a street person! The impact on quality of life of a 95-year-old who does not fracture a hip when falling because of nutritional (calcium and vitamin D) and exercise interventions is immeasurable. An intervention that prevented the development of a nonfatal stroke would likewise have a major effect in compressing morbidity and improving quality of life.

Thus, it is reasonable to explore the available evidence that nutritional intervention can modulate either life expectancy or morbidity. The focus of this chapter is on the effect of nutritional manipulation in late life; that is, in humans over the age of 70 years. It should be stressed that there is no nutritional manipulation that comes close to abstaining from cigarette smoking in its power to ameliorate disease. Thus, it makes no sense to accede to requests for a dietary change in patients who persist in smoking.

PRIMARY PREVENTION

Nutrition and Hypertension

Hypertension is an extremely common problem in older individuals, with the National Health and Nutrition Examination Survey (NHANES) finding that 44% of whites and 60% of blacks aged 65 to 74 years have a blood pressure in excess of 160/95 mm Hg (1). Both the Framingham Study and the Chicago Stroke Study have shown that untreated hypertension in older individuals is strongly associated with an increased risk of stroke and cardiovascular disorders (2). Thus, nutritional interventions that would lower the prevalence of hypertension in older individuals could have a major impact on the health status of this group.

In younger patients, being overweight has been linked to hypertension, and with age there is an increase in body fat. Malnourished patients in nursing homes often display a marked amelioration of pre-existing hypertension. These findings suggest that excess weight could contribute to hypertension in older individuals. Unfortunately, the relationship between weight and blood pressure seen in younger subjects has not been substantiated in older subjects (3).

Epidemiologic studies have long suggested a relationship between hypertension and salt intake. Luft et al. (4) suggested that 25 to 30% of individuals over 40 years of age may display sodium-sensitive blood pressure responses. It has been suggested that older individuals (mean age, 85 years) are especially sensitive to the effects of a high-salt diet on blood pressure (5). This increased sensitivity may be secondary to the reduced rate of urinary sodium excretion in older individuals. It would appear prudent to suggest that most elderly should avoid adding table salt to their food and should not use excessive salt for cooking. Some drinking water is particularly high in salt; tap water should not exceed 20 mg of sodium per liter. When the sodium content of tap water is particularly high, consideration should be given to drinking and cooking with bottled water. However, severe sodium restriction should be avoided wherever possible in older individuals, as it can result in unpalatable food and the development of malnutrition.

Low calcium intake has been associated with increased arterial pressure (6), and high calcium intakes ameliorate hypertension in some subjects (7). Many older individuals have a suboptimal calcium intake. In view of the putative protective effects of high calcium intake on bone (*vide infra*), it seems reasonable to liberalize calcium intake to 1 to 1.5 g in subjects 50 years of age or older in the hope that it will also result in a lower blood pressure.

Overall, geriatric hypertension appears to have a relatively strong relationship to diet; a lifetime of moderate salt and caloric intake, as well as an adequate calcium intake, appears to be a prudent preventive medicine approach. Adequate studies on the effects of dietary intervention for hypertension in subjects over 70 years of age are not available. However, in view of the high cost of antihypertensive medications, careful dietary intervention in older subjects (mild salt restriction and/or added calcium intake) may represent the most prudent approach to the management of borderline elevations in blood pressure.

Osteopenia

The development of osteoporosis and subsequent fractures is a major cause of morbidity in postmenopausal Caucasian females. Clearly, the first approach to prevention in this group is the use of estrogen replacement at the time of the menopause in those subjects in whom no contraindication to estrogens is present. However, there is reasonable epidemiologic evidence linking the development of Type II (age-related) osteopenia to lifetime calcium intake (8). Studies in Hong Kong have suggested that subjects with a calcium intake below 400 mg/day are particularly at risk for the development of osteoporosis and hip fractures (9). Osteoporosis is more prevalent in subjects with lactose intolerance, which leads to poor intake of dairy products and thus calcium, and in subjects with malabsorption syndromes, again suggesting a role for dietary calcium in bone protection. For these reasons, it seems appropriate to suggest dietary calcium supplementation of the order of 1 to 1.5 g/day, dependent on pre-existing dietary intake.

The role of vitamin D deficiency in the pathogenesis of hip fractures in individuals over 70 years of age is rapidly emerging (10). A number of factors make older individuals at risk for developing vitamin D deficiency. These include decreased dietary intake, decreased sun exposure, the use of sunscreen to prevent recurrent skin cancer, and decreased conversion of 25(OH) vitamin D to 1,25(OH) vitamin D by the kidney. Studies from Israel have suggested that even elderly subjects living in high sun exposure areas can develop vitamin D deficiency (11). Elderly in institutions appear to be particularly vulnerable to developing vitamin D deficiency, which increases their chances of having a hip fracture. For this reason, all institutionalized older subjects should receive 100,000 IU of vitamin D twice per year (12). In view of the increased propensity to the development of vitamin D deficiency in older individuals, the use of a low-dose vitamin D supplement (200 to 400 IU per day) may be appropriate in most individuals over the age of 70 years. If this is given, calcium levels need to be checked regularly to avoid the development of unrecognized hypercalcemia. The final advisability of this approach awaits the outcome of long-term controlled trials.

Cholesterol

Cholesterol levels increase during life up to the age of 60 years in men and 70 years in women (13,14). After these ages, cholesterol levels tend to decrease slightly in the population, presumably in part because of the removal from the population of those at particular risk for atherosclerotic heart disease. Nevertheless, even in older subjects, epidemiologic studies have suggested that total serum cholesterol is positively related to atherosclerotic heart disease (15). Despite this relationship, Agner and Hansen (16) demonstrated an increased mortality in 70-year-old individuals with low serum cholesterol levels. In a relatively ill nursing home population, Rudman et al. (17) found that a cholesterol level below 160 mg/dl was the factor most predictive of death. It was presumed that this was because low cholesterol levels were a sensitive predictor of malnutrition in this population. More recently, in a somewhat healthier elderly female population (mean age, 82 years), Forette et al. (18) reported a J-shaped curve for mortality, with the highest relative death rates being at the lowest cholesterol levels and only small increases in death rates being seen at the very highest cholesterol levels. Yaari et al. (19) have reported a similar J-shaped curve in younger (40- to 65-year-old) males. These studies have led Oliver (20) to suggest that an increase in plasma cholesterol may play an adaptive process during aging by stabilizing the physical and chemical characteristics of the cell membrane.

It should be pointed out that even the most widely touted lipid reduction trials have failed to demonstrate a significant reduction in mortality. In fact, the Helsinki Heart (gemfibrozil) Study showed a 7% increase in mortality (21) and the MRFIT study a 2% decrease in mortality in the intervention group (22). Overall, there is no evidence that lowering cholesterol has any significant effect on total mortality.

Is it then rational to have embarked on a national campaign to lower cholesterol? McCormick and Skrabanek (23) have argued that future generations will look back at the era of population interventions to reduce coronary artery disease with disbelief and with contempt for the epidemiologic analysis that supported these political actions. Alternatively, Fries et al. (24), although accepting that cholesterol reduction is unlikely to reduce mortality, have cogently argued that, at least in some populations, reduction in cholesterol may compress morbidity by reducing morbid cardiovascular events. Thus, in the Helsinki Heart Study trial, for example, there was a 37% reduction in nonfatal coronaries (21). In addition, it is possible but not proven that such prevention may reduce medical expenditures. Thus, it would appear still reasonable to pursue cholesterol reduction vigorously in high-risk groups, such as those with a previous myocardial infarction or those subjects with a strong family history of atherosclerotic heart disease. The cholesterol level at which intervention should begin is uncertain, although values above 250 mg/dl would certainly warrant attention. For the best overall mortality target, levels of cholesterol should probably be in the range of 200 to 220 mg/dl in subjects under 65 years of age. A recent study has suggested that, even in subjects with a mean age of 82 years, a total cholesterol greater than 250 mg/dl and a high-density lipoprotein cholesterol less than < 35 mg/dl remain an indicator of subsequent coronary events (25). However, there is no evidence that routine intervention in subjects over 65 years of age has any benefit. In view of the fact that major interventions in diet in older subjects may result in malnutrition, it seems reckless to attempt to alter the cholesterol content of diets in the population over 70 years of age.

Fish and Fish Oils

Greenland Eskimos, despite their high fat intake, have a low prevalence of atherosclerosis and develop acute myocardial infarction at 10% the rate of Danes or North Americans. The difference is explained by the quality of fats ingested, with the Eskimos ingesting high quantities of omega-3 fatty acids derived mainly from seals and whales, whereas the other populations ate more saturated fats and omega-6 fatty acids.

These epidemiologic findings led to the suggestion that polyunsaturated fatty acids, such as eicosopentanoic and docoscipentanoic acid, may decrease coronary artery disease both by decreasing platelet adhesiveness and by lowering triglycerides and to a lesser extent low-density lipoprotein cholesterol (26). As these fatty acids are the predominant fat in fish, eating a high-fish diet may also prove protective against heart disease. Preliminary population studies have suggested that eating fish regularly may reduce atherosclerotic disease (27). Mortality from coronary artery disease was 50% lower among those who consumed fish than among those who did not. At present, no large population trials showing the efficacy of raw fish oils over a prolonged period of time have been published. Because of the increased bleeding tendency produced by fish oil ingestion, intake of fish oil should be avoided in older subjects. However, there would appear to be minimal risk and potentially some benefit of increasing fish consumption to three to four times per week.

Cancer

Approximately half of all the new cancers in the United States occur in individuals over the age of 65 years. Gastrointestinal, prostate, and breast cancer are responsible for over half the cancers in patients over 60 years of age. Although the cancer incidence rises with age, it begins to decrease in those 85 to 90 years of age. The concept that diet can modulate the prevalence of cancer is not a new one. In 1933, Orr (28) suggested that cancer in betel nut chewers was less prevalent in those with a high vitamin A intake. In the same year, Stocks and Karn (29) found that high intake of whole-meal bread, vegetables, and fresh milk was associated with a decrease in cancer incidence at multiple sites.

Animal studies have suggested that food restriction reduces the cancer rate (30). Further, feeding high-fat diets to animals induces breast and colon cancers. Human epidemiologic studies support the increased occurrence of carcinoma of the colon and breast in subjects on high-fat diets (31). Less certainty exists about the role of cholesterol in cancer of the colon, with some studies suggesting that cholesterol levels are predictive of carcinoma of the colon, whereas others found no association (31). Vegetarian groups, such as the Seventh Day Adventists, have a low occurrence of carcinoma of the colon, which could be related to low fat intake, the effect of meat, or, most likely, the increased fiber in the diet. Numerous animal and human studies have supported the protective effect of dietary fiber against the development of colon cancer.

Iron deficiency has been associated with hypopharyngeal cancers in women (32). Iodine deficiency predisposes to thyroid cancer (33). Aflatoxin, from *Aspergillus flavus*, is a contaminant of peanuts and cereals in some situations and has been associated with hepatoma (34). In Japan, eating bracken fern is associated with a fivefold increase in esophageal cancer (35).

Epidemiologic studies have suggested a decrease in lung cancer in subjects with high intakes and/or serum levels of beta-carotene or vitamin A (36). Vitamin A ingestion can lead to hypercalcemia by cathepsin D activation and release of parathormone. For this reason, supplementation with vitamin A is never recommended. Beta-carotene dietary supplementation is presently undergoing controlled trials.

Low selenium levels in the blood have been associated with an increase in cancer incidence (37). The combination of low selenium and low vitamin E levels seems to be highly predictive of increased risk, especially for gastrointestinal cancers (38). Countries with high selenium levels in the soil, such as Venezuela, have much lower colon carcinoma rates than do those with lower selenium levels in the soil, such as the United States. Overall, there is mounting evidence that selenium deficiency may predispose to the development of cancer (see Chapter 12).

Unfortunately, diets that protect against some cancers are associated with an increase in prevalence of cancers at other sites. For example, cereal cultures, such as those of Japan and Southeast Asia, have a high prevalence of stomach and esophageal cancer, whereas the incidence of breast, colon, and prostate cancers is decreased. Meat-eating cultures, such as the United States, show exactly the opposite cancer pattern. Table 1 summarizes some of the known dietary influences on cancer.

TABLE 1. *Potential dietary influences on cancer*

Cancer	Effects of nutrients
Lung	Decreased prevalence with increased beta-carotene, vitamin A, carrots, and green leafy vegetable intake
Esophageal	Increased rates with high bread or bracken from consumption
Stomach	Increased risk with dried salty fish consumption; decreased risk with vegetable and fruit consumption
Pancreas	Increased risk with butter, fried and grilled meat; decreased risk with raw fruits, vegetables, and Vitamin C
Colon	Increased risk with pasta, rice, and cereals; decreased risk with vegetables, fiber, selenium, and vitamin C
Hypopharyngeal	Increased risk with iron deficiency
Skin cancers	Decreased risk with selenium consumption

Exercise

There is mounting evidence that moderate exercise can prolong the life span (39). Exercise is associated with salutary effects on the cardiovascular system, bone, and muscle. The strengthening of muscle and bone may decrease the incidence of hip fracture. In addition, evidence in both animals (40) and human (41) studies suggests that exercise is associated with a decrease in cancer. Recent studies have shown that exercise produces an acute increase in natural killer (NK) cell activity, most probably secondary to the release of beta-endorphin from the pituitary gland (42). NK cells are responsible for scavenging circulating tumor cells. Thus, there is now a biochemical basis for the cancer-protective effect of moderate exercise.

The effects of exercise are discussed in detail in Chapter 35. Overall, it would seem that mild to moderate exercise can produce a myriad of beneficial effects when introduced at almost any age. In older individuals, the exercise program should be tailored to the individual's capacity. It has been suggested that the rhythmic Chinese exercise, Tai Chi, may be beneficial in patients with dementia of the Alzheimer's type.

Life Extension

Since Ponce de Leon set out from Puerto Rico in search of the fountain of youth, only to discover Florida instead (in view of the senior migration to Florida, he might be considered to have been at least partially successful in his quest!), many humans have craved a magic potion that would prolong their life span. Books and magazines on life extension have proved to be particularly successful with the lay public. Although clearly this author joins with Fries (43) in feeling that we should spend more time searching for ways to compress morbidity, nevertheless it is appropriate to review briefly dietary studies on life extension.

Numerous animal studies in many species from *Drosophila* to rodents have demonstrated that dietary restriction leads to a prolongation of life span (32). Dietary restriction seems to be most effective when calories are restricted by approximately 25%. Although present studies are controversial, no single macronutrient appears to be specifically responsible for the life span extension. The mechanism by which mild caloric deprivation enhances life span is uncertain, with theories ranging from a reduction in free radical generation or tissue glycation to a delay in thymic involution. It should be realized that such studies as these can be interpreted as demonstrating that overnutrition is not good for an animal, rather than demonstrating an effect of undernutrition *per se*.

Attempts to prove that the spartan existence increases life span led to searches for long-lived human populations. Three such populations were putatively identified—the Georgians in Russia, the Afghanistanis in the Khyber pass, and the people of Villacabamba in Ecuador. After much excitement concerning the ability of these individuals to live high quality lives on a frugal diet, it rapidly became obvious that the great ages attained by these individuals were more closely linked to their inability to count correctly, rather than to their dietary and exercise habits! The longest documented human life span is 120 years in a Japanese man. The most long-lived populations in the world are the Japanese, Scandinavians, and Americans (with Hawaii leading the states), hardly a group of people who follow a spartan nutritional existence!

One theory of aging proposes that the generation of three radicals causes tissue damage and ultimately death. If this is true, then one would expect that intake of free radical scavengers, such as selenium or vitamin E, or antioxidants would result in a prolongation of life span. Unfortunately, this question has been addressed in very few animal studies, and the paucity of data makes it impossible to make any conclusive comments on this issue. Of interest is the tendency of humans with parkinsonism who receive deprenyl along with L-dopa to live longer than those not receiving deprenyl (Knoll, personal communication). Deprenyl prevents the generation of free radicals. At present, there are no data to support megavitamin use in the hope that it will decrease free radical generation and thereby prolong life.

Overall, it would appear that at present there is no dietary fountain of youth and that the best advice is to partake of a balanced diet that maintains weight around that of the population average.

SECONDARY PREVENTION

Much of the approach to the early detection and treatment of nutritional diseases is reviewed in detail in other sections of this book. For this reason, approaches to secondary prevention are reviewed only briefly in this section. The development of classical nutrient deficiencies, such as pellagra or scurvy, is extremely rare in the older populations of developed countries. More commonly, some older individuals who are suffering from intercurrent illnesses may develop borderline deficiency states. For example, an older patient with Type II diabetes mellitus may be losing zinc in the urine. He then develops a leg ulcer and has recurrent urinary tract infections, resulting in anorexia and decreased intake. His leg ulcer heals slowly because he has now developed a zinc deficiency that impairs wound healing. Zinc replacement eventually allows the full healing of his ulcer. Many patients in nursing homes are at particular risk for the development of borderline vitamin and trace mineral deficiencies and, as such, should be carefully monitored for signs and symptoms of these deficiencies.

As pointed out in Chapter 30, numerous drugs that are commonly used in older individuals interfere with nutrient bioavailability. Diuretics can cause magnesium, potassium, and zinc deficiency. Tuberculosis therapy with isoniazid can lead to vitamin B_6 deficiency. Epileptic treatment with phenytoin or phenobarbitone can result in folate deficiency. Laxative abuse with mineral oil can result in deficiency of vitamins A, D, and K. For these reasons, it is important for older patients receiving medications to be monitored carefully for nutrient deficiencies. In addition, the older person's need for the variety of drugs he is receiving should be assessed carefully. Not only does polypharmacy increase the likelihood of drug interactions but it also increases the possibility of nutrient deficiencies. For the elderly, it is just as important that they learn to "just say no to drugs" when they are inappropriate as it is for our younger population.

Protein-energy malnutrition (PEM) is reaching endemic proportions among older Americans. In the prevention of this disease, primary prevention programs, such as meals at senior citizen centers and Meals-on-Wheels, can play an important role. In addition, the development of bereavement squads who visit an older person a week after a spouse dies and bring food with them may reduce the protein-energy malnutrition commonly associated with a spouse's death. In the long-term care setting, assuring sufficient money to prepare attractive food and hire a dietitian is the major primary prevention need.

Because the onset of PEM is often insidious, early detection is of paramount importance. Many older subjects present with a marasmic picture, with weight loss rather than hypoalbuminemia dominating the situation. Weight loss needs to be pursued vigorously in older individuals and treatable causes, such as occult depression, carefully excluded. Patients at risk for malnutrition include those who are unable to shop for themselves. In a DRG-driven world, the physician needs to be particularly aware that many older patients admitted with infection have occult malnutrition. If the patient is discharged home too quickly, he may be too weak to prepare meals, resulting in a vicious cycle of worsening malnutrition, further impairment of the immune system, and subsequent hospital readmissions for infection. It is important to realize that, in many cases, the best result that can be obtained from tube feeding is a maintenance of body weight at the level prevailing at the time of tube insertion. For this reason, if successful secondary prevention of PEM is to occur, it is necessary that tube feedings are begun earlier, rather than later, with the expectation that the tube may be removed as soon as weight stabilization occurs.

Diabetes mellitus is an extremely common disease, occurring in up to 18% of individuals over 65 years of age (44). Yet in approximately half of these individuals, the diagnosis is not made. Regular screening programs for diabetes mellitus in seniors should be undertaken using glucose or fructosamine levels. Not only does diabetes mellitus cause retinopathy, neuropathy, and nephropathy but there is also increasing evidence that it may result in premature aging and accelerated atherosclerosis.

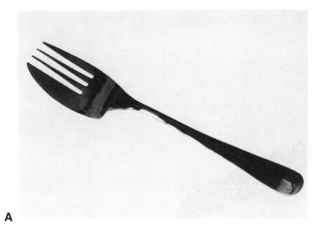

A

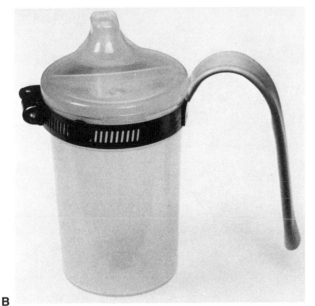

B

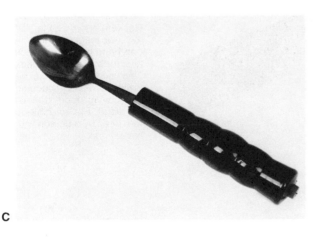

C

FIG. 2. Examples of utensils used to improve food intake in handicapped elderly. **A:** Side-cutter fork with sharpened edge, which allows cutting and eating with one hand. **B:** Flow-restricted cup in a cup holder. Cup can be used with or without a straw. Spout is large enough for thick soups. **C:** Weighted spoon for use by patients with Parkinson's disease or other tremors. (*Figure continues.*)

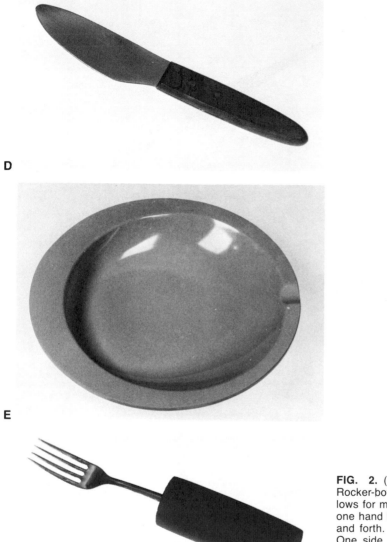

D

E

F

FIG. 2. (continued). **D:** Rocker-bottom knife allows for meat cutting with one hand by rocking back and forth. **E:** Scoop dish. One side is elevated, allowing for easier scooping by moving food against the edge. **F:** Soft built-up fork used by a person with limited grip.

TERTIARY PREVENTION

Exercise therapy and aggressive nutritional therapy are the cornerstones of the ability of the frail elderly person to return to the community.

Patients with well-established PEM often require prolonged hospitalization or admission to a skilled nursing facility. Carefully designed swallowing therapy programs may be necessary to allow the patient to eat again. When the patient fails to respond to routine measures, heroic therapy, such as the use of the anabolic growth hormone, may be indicated. Restoration of the severely malnourished patient requires a maximum effort by all the members of the interdisciplinary team. The ability of handicapped or frail elderly to eat can be greatly improved by the use of specialized eating utensils that have been developed to aid patients with strokes or amputations (Fig. 2).

Where specifically indicated, strengthening exercises are usually carried out under the supervision of a physiatrist or physical therapist. However, many patients who are recovering from a prolonged illness can benefit from a nonspecific exercise program. Exercise programs should be provided for all patients in rehabilitation or geriatric evaluation wards, as well as for those in nursing homes. Special attention should be paid to strengthening leg muscles in the hope of preventing future falls.

CONCLUSION

Our knowledge concerning nutritional prevention of age-associated diseases is similar to that of the two blind men, one at the trunk and one at the tail of the elephant. We have made an excellent start to understanding the nutritional bases of some of these diseases, but the lack of a full understanding makes it difficult to be absolutely certain that any recommendation will be proven to be correct. Table 2 summarizes the potential nutritional approaches to prevention. As we embark on the exciting field of health promotion and disease prevention in older individuals, we need to be exquisitely sensitive that the programs we institute do no harm. It should be remembered that, in many healthy older individuals, the less we intervene, the more likely they are to survive.

TABLE 2. *Nutritional approaches to prevention of age-associated diseases*

Primary prevention	Secondary prevention	Tertiary prevention
Highly recommended	**Highly recommended**	**Highly recommended**
No added salt—hypertension	Screening for weight loss	Exercise
Calcium supplementation—bone and ? hypertension	Screening for diabetes mellitus	Vigorous treatment of PEM—early tube feeding
Increased fish intake—cardiovascular disease	No megavitamin use—hypercalcemia	Specialized eating utensils—PEM
Avoidance of very high-fat diets—cancer	Use of indicated drugs only—decrease drug-nutrient interactions	
Moderate exercise—cancer, cardiovascular disease, bone		
Meals at senior citizen centers		
Meals-on-Wheels—PEM		
Possibly recommended		
Weight reduction—hypertension and diabetes mellitus; uncertain value over 60 years		
Vitamin D—hip fracture		
Cholesterol reduction—cardiovascular morbidity		
Selenium supplementation in low soil selenium areas—cancer		
Uncertain value		
Cholesterol reduction—total mortality		
Beta-carotene supplementation—lung cancer		
Dietary restriction—life extension		
Free radical scavengers—life extension		

PEM, protein-energy malnutrition.

REFERENCES

1. National Center for Health Statistics. *Plan and operation of the National Health and Nutrition Examination Survey. United States 1971–1973. Vital and Health Statistics,* series 1, nos. 10a and 10b. Washington, DC: US Government Printing Office, 1973; 1–46 (DHEW Publ. No. 73-1310).
2. Tuck ML, Griffiths RF, Johnson LE, et al. *J Am Geriatr Soc* 1988;36:630–643.
3. Pan W-H, Nanas S, Dyer A, et al. *Am J Epidemiol* 1986;124:612–623.
4. Luft FC, Weinberger MH, Feinberg N, et al. *Am J Med* 1987;82(S1B):9–15.
5. Lustig G, Palmer R, Stern N, et al. *Clin Res* 1988;36:177A.
6. McCarron DA, Morris CD, Henry HJ, et al. *Science* 1984;224:1392–1398.
7. McCarron DA, Morris CD. *Ann Intern Med* 1985;103:825–831.
8. Morley JE, Gorbien MJ, Mooradian AD, et al. *J Am Geriatr Soc* 1988;36:845–859.
9. Lou E, Donnan S, Barker DJP, et al. *Br Med J* 1988;297:1441–1442.
10. Morley JE. *J Am Geriatr Soc (in press).*
11. Goldray D, Mizraki-Sasson E, Merdler C. *J Am Geriatr Soc (in press).*
12. Davies M, Maurer EB, Hahn JJ. *Age Aging* 1985;14:349–354.
13. Bates HM. *J Cardiovasc Pharmacol* 1982;4(S2):196–200.
14. Kannell WB. *J Am Geriatr Soc* 1986;34:27–36.
15. Siegel D, Kuller L, Lazarus NB. *Am J Epidemiol* 1986;126:385–399.
16. Agner E, Hansen PF. *Acta Med Scand* 1983;214:33–41.
17. Rudman D, Mattson DE, Nagraj HS, et al. *J Am Geriatr Soc* 1987;35:496–502.
18. Forette B, Tortrat D, Wolmark Y. *Lancet* 1989;1:868–870.
19. Yaari S, Goldbourt U, Even-Zohar S, et al. *Lancet* 1981;1:1011–1015.
20. Oliver MF. *Lancet* 1981;2:1090–1095.
21. Frick MH, Elo O, Haapa K, et al. *N Engl J Med* 1987;316:1237–1245.
22. Multiple Risk Factor Intervention Trial Research Group. *Am J Cardiol* 1986;58:1–13.
23. McCormick J, Skrabanek P. *Lancet* 1988;2:839–841.
24. Fries JF, Green LW, Levine S. *Lancet* 1989;1:481–483.
25. Aronow WS, Heng AH, Etienne F, et al. *J Am Geriatr Soc* 1989;37:501–506.
26. Leaf A, Weber PC. *N Engl J Med* 1987;318:549–557.
27. Kromhout D, Borschiester EB, Coulander C de L. *N Engl J Med* 1985;312:1205–1209.
28. Orr IM. *Lancet* 1933;2:575–580.
29. Stocks P. and Karn MN. *Ann Eugenics* 1933;5:237–280.
30. Fannestil DD, Burrows CM Jr. *J Gerontol* 1965;20:462–469.
31. Linn BS, Linn MS. In: Watson RW, ed. *Handbook of nutrition in the aged.* Boca Raton, FL: CRC Press, 1986;299–311.
32. Larrson L, Sandstrom G, Westling P. *Cancer Res* 1975;35:3303–3307.
33. Cowdry EV. In: Cowdry EV, ed. *Etiology and prevention of cancer in man.* New York: Appleton, 1968;277–291.
34. Linsell CA, Peers FG. In: Hialt HH, Watson JD, Winsten JA, eds. *Origin of human cancer.* New York: Cold Spring Harbor Lab, 1977;549–560.
35. Parmukcu AM, Ertusk E, Yalciner S, et al. *Cancer Res* 1978;38:1556–1561.
36. Menken MS, Comstock GW, Vuilleumes JP, et al. *N Engl J Med* 1986;315:1250–1256.
37. Morley JE, Mooradian AD, Silver AS, et al. *Ann Intern Med* 1988;109:890–904.
38. Salonen JF, Salonen R, Lappetelainen R, et al. *Br Med J* 1985;290:417–420.
39. Paffenbarger RS Jr, Hyde RT, Wing AL, et al. *N Engl J Med* 1986;314:605–613.
40. Hoffman SA, Raschkis KE, DeBias DA, et al. *Cancer Res* 1962;22:597–599.
41. Gerhardsson M, Norell SE, Kiviranta H, et al. *Am J Epidemiol* 1986;123:775–780.
42. Fiatarone MA, Morley JE, Bloom ET, et al. *J Lab Clin Med* 1988;112:544–552.
43. Fries JF. *N Engl J Med* 1980;303:130–136.
44. Morley JE, Mooradian AD, Rosenthal MJ, et al. *Am J Med* 1987;83:533–544.

Geriatric Nutrition, edited by John E. Morley,
Zvi Glick, Laurence Z. Rubenstein.
Raven Press, Ltd., New York © 1990.

8

Anorexia of Aging and Protein-Energy Malnutrition

Andrew J. Silver

*Department of Medicine, St. Louis University School of Medicine,
St. Louis, Missouri 63104*

The elderly are one segment of the population that is particularly prone to develop malnutrition. Although the exact prevalence of this problem is unknown, many elderly suffer from some form of overt or subclinical malnutrition, and many cases are being missed because of the agist view that "old people are suppose to be skinny." The purpose of this chapter is to review the numerous factors predisposing this population toward the development of protein-energy malnutrition (PEM), with emphasis on the anorexia of aging. The assessment and treatment of malnutrition are also discussed.

A useful classification for protein-energy malnutrition, which has been developed by Bistrian (1), has two main categories: marasmus and hypoalbuminemic malnutrition. Marasmus is defined as weight loss while maintaining the serum albumin within a normal range. There is also a decrease in anthropometrics (body measurements used to describe the relative leanness or obesity of an individual) and a mild depression of immune function. Hypoalbuminemic malnutrition is defined as a serum albumin less than 3.0 g/dl ("normal" is greater than or equal to 4.0 g/dl). In the majority of cases, this state arises as a response to injury or infection with the albumin acting as an acute phase reactant. Other causes include a low protein intake with less than 3% of total calories being protein in nature, a decrease in protein production by the liver, or an increased loss of protein, as for example, through urinary losses (nephrotic syndrome).

This classification can be applied to the elderly, particularly when considering the clinical setting. For example, several nutritional surveys suggest that, in the ambulatory outpatient setting, many elderly appear to present with weight loss while maintaining their serum albumin, ie, they are marasmic-like. For example, a Boston survey (2) of over 600 independent community dwellers with no chronic diseases noted the mean serum albumin to be 4.1 g/dl. In a VA outpatient survey (unpublished), 1% of the patients had serum albumin levels less than 3.0 g/dl and 2% had levels less than 3.5 g/dl, whereas 13% had a body weight less than 90% average body weight (ABW) based on Master's table (3). Patients in the institutional setting appear to present in a similar fashion with loss of weight while maintaining the serum albumin levels within an acceptable range. For example, 18% of patients had a serum albumin less than 3.5 g/dl, whereas 23% had an average body weight less than 20% and 46% were less than 10% ABW (4). Thus, in the outpatient and institutional settings, reliance on serum albumin levels to determine nutritional status may not be adequate. On the other hand, there is ample evidence in the literature to suggest that elderly in the acute hospital setting present with hypoalbuminemic malnutrition, with the decrease in serum albumin correlating with an increased hospital stay, increased number of infections, and an increase in subsequent 1-year mortality (5-7).

ANOREXIA OF AGING

The causes of protein-energy malnutrition include anorexia or loss of appetite. Idiopathic loss of appetite was first described by Morton in 1689 as nervous atrophy, and other later concepts included pituitary cachexia, nervous malnutrition, and weight phobia. The term "anorexia nervosa" was introduced by Gull in 1874 and is typically associated with a disorder affecting young women, although there have been case reports of anorexia nervosa affecting elderly people (8). In fact a recent study suggests that body image disturbances do affect a certain percentage of the older population. Utilizing the EAT-26 questionnaire, Miller et al. (unpublished) identified elderly male veterans who were underweight yet still displayed self-control around food, liked their stomach to be empty, avoided eating when hungry, and were terrified about being overweight.

More common in occurrence is age-related anorexia, which differs from anorexia nervosa in several aspects (Table 1). In anorexia of aging, both

TABLE 1. *Age-related anorexia*

	Anorexia of aging	Anorexia nervosa ("classic anorexia")
Ages involved	65 years and above	13–20 (85%)
Socioeconomic Status	All classes	Middle/upper class
Sex	Male and female	Female (95%)
Features		
Loss of appetite	+ + +	Late if at all
Predisposing stress	+ +	+ +
Body image disturbance	—	+ + +
Fear of obesity	—	+ + +
Known physical illness	+ + +	+
Weight loss	+ + +	+ + +

+, present; −, absent.

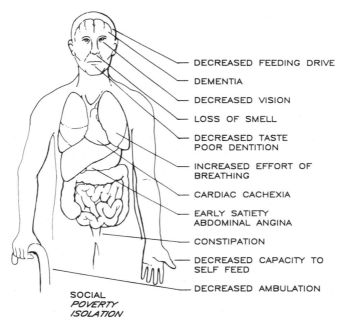

DECREASED FEEDING DRIVE

DEMENTIA

DECREASED VISION

LOSS OF SMELL

DECREASED TASTE
POOR DENTITION

INCREASED EFFORT OF
BREATHING

CARDIAC CACHEXIA

EARLY SATIETY
ABDOMINAL ANGINA

CONSTIPATION

DECREASED CAPACITY TO
SELF FEED

DECREASED AMBULATION

SOCIAL
POVERTY
ISOLATION

FIG. 1. Factors contributing to anorexia of aging.

sexes are affected, as are all socioeconomic classes. Loss of appetite is the primary symptom with minimal body image disturbance or fear of obesity. As would be expected in this population, there is frequently an accompanying physical illness.

There are numerous causes for the development of anorexia of aging with possible subsequent PEM, including social, physical, pathophysiologic, psychologic, and such miscellaneous factors as a decrease in the feeding drive and an increase in satiety (Figure 1). As in other aspects of the elderly patient, it is likely that several of these factors combine to predispose the individual towards an increased risk of developing malnutrition.

Social Factors

Social isolation is likely to contribute strongly to this increased risk. It has been estimated that 30% of older individuals live alone, and 25% need help within the neighborhood with such tasks as the procurement of food (9). Isolation at mealtimes leads to the loss of one of the symbolic meanings of food, that being warmth and sharing. Financial constraints may affect the ability of the older individual to obtain sufficient amounts of each food group to meet the recommended dietary allowances. Often, the individual's limited funds are needed for medications, or he is duped into purchasing various vitamin and mineral supplements that for the most part are unlikely to be of major benefit.

Physiologic Factors

Numerous physiologic processes that can affect appetite occur with aging. As one ages, atrophy of olfactory glomeruli increases, resulting in a decrease in smell perception (10). There is also evidence of a decrease in the number of taste buds per papilla on the tongue, as well as a possible postreceptor defect resulting in a decrease in the perception of taste (11). Both of these changes contribute to the overall decrease in the palatability or pleasant taste of food, which can reduce the desire to eat as much as in the past. Too, the basal metabolic rate of many elderly decreases because of the age-related decrease in lean body mass (12) and, more importantly, the increase in the sedentary lifestyle. For women, the recommended energy intake decreases from 2,000 cal/day at age 30 to 1,800 cal/day at age 60 to 1,600 cal/day at age 80 (13). For men the corresponding figures are from 2,700 cal/day at age 30 to 2,400 at age 60 to 2,000 at age 80 (13). Thus, physiologic processes that occur with normal aging can affect appetite and overall nutrient intake.

Pathophysiologic Factors

Pathologic processes or certain disease states occurring in older individuals can affect their appetite and subsequent intake. There may be a decreased ability to bring food from the plate to the mouth secondary to a stroke or Parkinson's disease, as well as difficulty in chewing, eg, from Parkinson's disease, temporomandibular joint pain. Certain systemic disorders can interfere with eating, including chronic obstructive pulmonary disease in which energy is expended in breathing, rather than in eating; abdominal angina in which pain accompanies eating; cancer, either from cachexia or radiation therapy; chronic constipation, which creates a sensation of fullness; or congestive heart failure, leading to cardiac cachexia (chapter 25). Finally, weight loss despite apparent adequate intake may occur because of processes that increase metabolism, such as cancer, hyperthyroidism, or pheochromocytoma.

Psychologic Factors

One segment of the elderly that may be particularly prone to malnutrition is the psychiatrically impaired, ie, those with depression or dementia. One study (14) noted that 30% of institutionalized psychogeriatric patients were malnourished, whereas another (4) found a higher prevalence of dementia and depression in nursing home patients who were less than 20% average body weight and thus at risk for malnutrition. Finally, subclinical malnutrition as detected by low serum levels of vitamin C, folic acid, riboflavin, and vitamin B_{12}, were noted in individuals who scored lower on tests of cognitive function (15).

Between 2 and 13% of older individuals experience a major depressive episode (16), and one-third note a depressed mood to some extent (17). Depressive symptoms that can interfere with nutrient intake—nausea, vomiting, and weakness—have been reported in a significant proportion of elderly men (18). Zung noted that, among North American elderly, a decreased appetite was one of the most common depressive symptoms reported (19). With depression there is decreased activity which can decrease appetite; a loss of food's symbolism of warmth and sharing; and the use of food as a weapon (20), as manifested by a subconscious death wish expressed by a refusal to eat. There may also be malabsorption secondary to laxative and enema abuse as the individual attempts to purge himself.

At least two neurotransmitters have been proposed to contribute to the anorexia of depression. Norepinephrine is a potent stimulator of feeding (21), and antidepressants that enhance its function and that of the catecholamine system as a whole have been found to increase appetite (19). Also, elevated levels of corticotropin-releasing factor, a potent inhibitor of food intake (22), have been noted in the cerebrospinal fluid of depressed patients (23).

The prevalence of dementia (16) is 2 to 3% between the ages of 65 to 79 and 20% above the age of 80. Despite a mean dietary intake of 2,059 kcal/day, Sandman et al. (24) noted malnutrition of 50% of patients studied, with a mean ideal body weight of 82%. In another study (25), it was found that patients acutely admitted to a geropsychiatry ward had low serum levels of several vitamins and minerals and thus were felt to be at increased risk for developing malnutrition.

In dementia, numerous factors can increase the risk of malnutrition, such as indifference to food, memory loss, and impairment of judgment. Changes in behavior may cause alterations in food intake, such as apraxia or "cheeking of food" (holding food in the mouth). Finally, a lack of time spent feeding institutionalized demented patients, many of whom are dependent on others for their activities of daily living, may increase the potential for anorexia and malnutrition. In one study (26), 18 minutes per day were spent feeding demented patients in a nursing home compared to 99 minutes per day when these patients were kept at home.

The potential neurotransmitter abnormalities associated with anorexia in dementia are less clear than those in depression. Norepinephrine levels have been found to be reduced in brain tissue of patients with senile dementia of the Alzheimer's type (27), as have levels of neuropeptide Y (28), another stimulant of feeding.

Miscellaneous Factors

A decrease in the central feeding drive may also contribute to the anorexia of aging and subsequent malnutrition. Various neurotransmitters have been shown to modulate feeding; inhibitors include serotonin, epinephrine, calcitonin, and cholecystokinin, whereas enhancers include norepinephrine, neuropeptide Y, and the opioid peptides (29). In fact, research suggests that opioid blockers may be used in the management of eating disorders, such as bulimia (30). In aging studies, older animals have been found to be less sensitive to the enhancement effect of opioid agonists and to the suppressive effect of opioid antagonists than younger animals (31). This decrease in the effectiveness of the opioid ingestive drive with aging may be related to the reduction in concentration of opioid receptors (28) and opioid peptides (32) in old compared with young animals, and it may help contribute to a decreased feeding drive.

Nutrient intake is also regulated by a peripheral satiety system. As food travels through the gastrointestinal tract, various gut peptides are released that appear to terminate a meal, thus increasing satiety or the sensation of fullness. These include cholecystokinin, somatostatin, glucagon, bombesin (mammalian-equivalent gastrin-releasing peptide), and calcitonin. In animals, each of these peptides has been shown to decrease feeding when given in pharmacologic doses and to act as satiety agents when given in combination at physiologic levels (33). In one study (34), of all the peptides examined, cholecystokinin significantly decreased food intake in older animals compared to younger controls. As levels of circulating cholecystokinin have been reported to be higher in older than in younger individuals (35), this peptide may well play a role in the pathogenesis of anorexia in elderly persons by inducing early satiety.

NUTRITIONAL ASSESSMENT

The purpose of nutritional assessment is the same as that for any type of assessment in geriatrics—to target those persons most likely to benefit and to provide a link between assessment and follow-up services (36). There have been many approaches to nutritional assessment in the elderly, with "at risk" patients for malnutrition being identified as those with polypharmacy, a history of depression, living alone, and recent institutionalization. The assessment usually includes a history, physical examination, laboratory evaluation, and anthropometrics or body measurements used to evaluate the relative leanness of obesity of an individual. The field of geriatric nutrition now needs to improve the provision of adequate follow-up nutritional services, including management and treatment plans.

The history is perhaps the most important aspect of the assessment, for it can help identify the various risk factors that predispose many patients toward a poor nutritional status. Important historical data include weight loss; anorexia; body image disturbances; changes in smell, taste, vision, or hearing; difficulty in chewing; presence and effectiveness of dentures; dysphagia; abdominal pain; nausea; vomiting; diarrhea; ability to ambulate; weakness; impaired wound healing; cognitive impairment; and depression. Questionnaires have been developed to help key in on important historical data (37). All medications, including over-the-counter drugs, vitamins, and minerals, should be present at the time of examination. The social history should obtain information about smoking, alcohol use, who lives with the individual, cooking facilities, distance to the grocery store, lifestyle, and income. Dietary history should include any type of restrictions, ethnic preferences, food aversions, and allergies. It remains to be seen how useful detailed intake information, such as 7-day weighing or 24-hour recall, is for the elderly.

The physical examination may provide useful clues to a potential nutritional deficit. The signs of malnutrition include older than stated age (general appearance); pallor, petechiae, erythema, hyperpigmentation, xerosis (skin); alopecia, dryness (hair); xerosis, optic neuritis (eyes); cheilosis, gingivitis, glossitis, poor dentition (mouth); surgical scars, hepatomegaly (abdomen); muscle wasting (musculoskeletal); and mental status changes, loss of vibratory sensation, decreased reflexes, peripheral neuropathy (neurologic). The most frequently missed or misused sign is peripheral edema, for which the patient is often inappropriately treated for congestive heart failure, rather than for hypoalbuminemia.

The laboratory assessment may include a serum albumin, total lymphocyte count, skin testing, and vitamin levels (as warranted). Recently, it has been suggested (38) that serum cholesterol (as in undernourished Third World children) might also be an indicator of protein-calorie malnutrition in the elderly. Although serum albumin has classically been the "gold standard" for determining nutritional status and it remains the most practical to measure in terms of ease and expense, it may not be the best indicator of early protein deficiency because of albumin's long half-life and large body pool. Other markers that reflect acute changes more accurately are transferrin, thyroxine-binding prealbumin, and retinol-binding protein.

As noted earlier, many patients appear to lose weight while maintaining their serum albumin until close to the terminal event; that is, they have a marasmic rather than a kwashiorkor-type of malnutrition. One possible explanation for this may be that what is considered within normal range for laboratory parameters in the young may not be applicable in the elderly. For example, in a nursing home study by Rudman et al. (38), there was an apparent threshold value for albumin, cholesterol, hematocrit, and hemoglobin at which the risk of death increased. These threshold values were within the conventional normal range for adults; that is, there was an annual death rate of 43.4% in patients with serum albumin levels between 3.5 to 3.99 g/dl (acceptance normal range in adults is 3.5-5.0 g/dl). Thus, there may be a need to reconsider certain laboratory parameters for the elderly.

Absolute lymphocyte count helps determine the degree of protein-calorie undernutrition because of the decreased ability of stem cells to proliferate. The measurement of delayed cutaneous hypersensitivity through skin testing may be useful as well. However, it may often be difficult to separate true malnutrition from an aging effect. Therefore, all these parameters of laboratory assessment should be used to help confirm the diagnosis, with the history and perhaps the physical examination being the primary modes of diagnosis.

The last assessment tools used in a nutritional evaluation are body measurements or anthropometrics. These were originally used to help describe the various qualitative and quantitative changes in body composition that occur with aging, including a decrease in lean body mass of 6.2% per decade (39) and an increase in total body fat, the majority of which is deposited on the trunk around the internal organs. Anthropometrics are now used to help identify patients at risk for malnutrition and include weight, height, triceps skinfold, (best applicable in older women), subscapular skinfold, and mid-arm circumference. Age-adjusted tables have been devised (40), as have measurement alternatives for bedridden patients, such as knee height or arm length (41). The Metropolitan Life Insurance weight tables should not be used because they are not age-adjusted. Rather, one may use Masters' table (3), which includes data for ages up to 94 and is based on weight ranges, rather than discrete values; thus, weights are compared and noted as average body weight as opposed to the traditional ideal body weight. Experimental anthropometric techniques (42) include compute . tomography, nuclear magnetic resonance, underwater weighing (total body fat); neutron activation and gamma analysis (total body protein); and isotope dilution and electrical impedance (total body water). Although more precise than skinfold measurements, these techniques are also more costly and more difficult to perform and are therefore not likely to gain widespread acceptance and use.

TREATMENT

The geriatric approach to treatment of protein-calorie malnutrition is summarized in Table 2. The most important aspect is to rule out potentially reversible causes. However, one need not and should not delay the implementation of therapy while waiting for the workup to be completed. Although one needs to individualize treatment, a goal of 35 kcal/kg/day (5) should be aimed for, with increased protein supplementation from 12 to 15% to 20% in patients under stress (trauma, burns, starvation).

Feeding tubes remain controversial in terms of the duration of use and type. The nasogastric tube should be used as a temporizing measure as it is

TABLE 2. *Geriatric approach to treatment of protein-calorie malnutrition*

Treat early; do not wait for the underlying etiology to be identified.
Rule out reversible cause of malnutrition, such as drug effects, hyperthyroidism,
  pheochromocytoma, abdominal angina, esophageal candidiasis.
Establish realistic goals; aim initially for 35 kcal/kg/day.
Adjust medications according to symptoms not drug levels, ie, digitalis preparations,
  theophylline, cimetidine.
Temporize use of nasogastric feeding tubes; long-term feeding may require duodenal or
  gastric tube.
Measure caloric intake at least once per week; presence of stress will require adjustment of
  protein/other nutrients.
Encourage "significant others" to participate in therapy, especially important for after
  discharge.
Never use bolus feeding because of the potential for the development of large residuals
  and subsequent aspiration.
Use a team-oriented approach, as input from all members is necessary for treatment and
  management strategies.

the type most likely to cause aspiration pneumonia and nasal necrosis. Ideally, for prolonged periods of tube feedings, duodenal feeding tubes (still placing the patient at risk for aspiration pneumonia) or endoscopically or surgically placed percutaneous gastrostomy tubes are preferred. With all of these tubes, attempts at oral feeding should continue. There are many different types of commercially available formulas for tube feedings; in general, the type chosen is usually institution-dependent. To minimize diarrhea, lactose-free isomolar formulas are recommended (43).

Tube feeding is not a benign event. To prevent the complication of aspiration pneumonia, it is necessary to elevate the head of the bed at all times and to pay close attention to the poor posture of individuals in wheelchairs. Other complications include diarrhea, gastric distention, trauma to the gastric mucosa, and wound infections (primarily associated with gastrostomy tubes). One also needs to be aware of the psychologic state of the tube-fed patient in terms of cosmetic appearance. In some elderly patients, enteral feedings are not possible, and therefore, peripheral or central hyperalimentation becomes necessary. Clearly, age alone should never be a criterion for determining whether a patient is a candidate for this type of feeding modality.

Recently, we have obtained some experience with the use of growth hormone in severely malnourished elderly subjects (Kaiser, Morley, and Silver: unpublished observations). Growth hormone therapy resulted in more rapid weight gain and increased muscle mass. This new modality may prove to be an important new therapeutic modality for the treatment of protein-energy malnutrition in older patients.

Therapy should be continued until the weight goal in the particular patient is met or until they are within 10% of ideal or average body weight. It is vitally important that postdischarge planning be carefully thought out and acted upon; otherwise it is likely that malnutrition will recur.

SUMMARY

There exist elderly individuals with body image disturbances and weight loss resembling anorexia nervosa, but a greater number suffer from true loss or decrease in appetite with subsequent weight loss and potential for the development of protein-calorie malnutrition. Of greatest importance is the fact that many of the causes of anorexia of the elderly are easily treatable. Thus, the adage that old people are supposed to be skinny or that their weight loss is due to cancer and nothing can be done about it, is an agist viewpoint.

The assessment and treatment of protein-calorie malnutrition in the elderly require a multidisciplinary approach with the setting of realistic and individually tapered goals. Ideally, early identification of at risk patients should be strived for, with emphasis on weight loss and perhaps a resetting of what is considered normal as far as laboratory parameters are concerned.

REFERENCES

1. Blackburn G, Bistrian BR, Maini BS, et al., *JPEN* 1977;1:11–22.
2. Munro HN, McGandy RB, Hartz SC, et al. *Am J Clin Nutr* 1987;46:586–592.
3. Master AM, Lasser RP, Beckman G. *JAMA* 1960;114:658–662.
4. Silver AJ, Morley JE, Strome LS, et al. *J Am Geriatr Soc* 1988;36:487–491.
5. Lipschitz DA. *Prim Care* 1982;9:531.
6. Agarwal N, Acevedo F, Cayten CG, et al. *Am J Clin Nutr* 1986;43:659.
7. Linn BS. *Am J Clin Nutr* 1984;39:66.
8. Price WA, Giamini AJ, Colella J. *J Am Geriatr Soc* 1985;33:213–215.
9. Kane RL, Ouslander JG, Abrams IB. *Essentials of clinical geriatrics*. New York: McGraw-Hill, 1984.
10. Schiffman S. *J Gerontol* 1986;41:51–57.
11. Bartoshuk LM, Rifkin B, Marks LE, et al. *J Gerontol* 1986;41:51–57.
12. Keys A, Taylor HL, Grande F. *Metabolism* 1973;22:579–5877.
13. Food and Nutrition Board, National Research Council. Recommended dietary allowances, 9th revised ed. Washington, DC: National Academy of Sciences, 1980.
14. Asplund K, Normark M, Pettersson V. *Age Aging* 1981;10:87–94.
15. Goodwin JS, Goodwin JM, Garry PJ. *JAMA* 1983;249:2917.
16. Gurland B, Gross P. *Psychiatr Clin North Am* 1982;5:11–26.
17. Gianturco D, Busse E. In: Isaacs A, Post F, eds. *Studies on geriatric psychiatry*. New York: Wiley, 1978;1–16.
18. Kivela SL, Nissin A, Tuomilehto J, et al. *Acta Psychiatr Scand* 1986;73:93–100.
19. Zung WW. *Psychosomatics* 1967;8:287–292.
20. Kaplan S, Tuckman TB. *J Nutr Elderly* 1986;5:53–58.
21. Leibowitz SF, Hammer NJ, Chang K. *Pharmacol Biochem Behav* 1983;19:945–950.
22. Morley JE, Levine AS. *Life Sci* 1982;31:1459–1464.
23. Nemeroff CB, Bissette G, Widerlov E. *Science* 1984;226:1342–1343.
24. Sandman PO, Adolfsson R, Nygren C, et al. *J Am Geriatr Soc* 1987;35:31–38.
25. Greer A, McBride DH, Shenkin A. *Br J Psychiatr* 1986;149:738–741.
26. Hu T, Huang L, Cartwright WS. *Gerontologist* 1986;26:158–163.
27. Yates CM, Ritchie IM, Simpson J. *Lancet* 1981;2:39–40.
28. Messing RB, Vasquez BJ, Spiehler VR, et al. *J Neurochem* 1981;36:784–790.
29. Morley JE. *Endocrinol Rev* 1987;8:256–287.
30. Mitchell JE, Laine DE, Morley JE, et al. *Biol Psychiatry* 1986;21:1399–1406.
31. Gosnell BA, Levine AS, Morley JE. *Life Sci* 1983;32:2793–2799.

32. Gambert SR, Garthwaite TL, Pontzer CM, et al. *Neuroendocrinology* 1980;31:252–255.
33. Hinton V, Rosofsky M, Granger J, et al. *Peptides* 1986;17:615–619.
34. Silver AJ, Flood JF, Morley JE. *Peptides* 1988;9:221–226.
35. Khalil T, Walker JP, Wiener J, et al. *Surgery* 1985;98:423–429.
36. Solomon D, et al. *J Am Geriatr Soc* 1988;36:342–348.
37. Wolinsky FD, Coe RM, Miller DK, et al. *J Health Soc Behav* 1983;24:325–333.
38. Rudman D, Feller AG. *J Am Geriatr Soc* 1989;37:173–183.
39. Munro HN. *Br Med J* 1981;37:83–88.
40. Frisancho AR. *Am J Clin Nutr* 1984;40:808–819.
41. Mitchell CO, Lipschitz DA. *JPEN* 1982;6:226.
42. Lukaski HC. *Am J Clin Nutr* 1987;46:537–556.
43. Morley JE, Silver AS, Fiatarone M, et al. *J Am Geriatr Soc* 1986;34:823–832.

Geriatric Nutrition, edited by John E. Morley,
Zvi Glick, Laurence Z. Rubenstein.
Raven Press, Ltd., New York © 1990.

9

Vitamin Disorders in the Elderly

Larry E. Johnson

*Department of Family Medicine, University of Cincinnati Medical Center,
Cincinnati, Ohio 45267*

Vitamins are defined as organic compounds that are essential for life and are required in small amounts in the diet (1). The designation of a compound as a vitamin is somewhat arbitrary. Essential fatty acids are not regarded as vitamins, whereas vitamin D may be generated endogenously by the skin after sunlight exposure and vitamin K can be synthesized by intestinal bacteria. Although a very visible minority of elderly persons supplement their diets with high or potentially toxic amounts of vitamins (2,3), insufficient vitamin intake is much more serious. Marginal or inadequate vitamin intake occurs in both fully ambulatory, community-living elderly, as well as those who are homebound, disabled, or institutionalized (4–9). Vitamin deficiencies are common in both affluent and impoverished societies.

The Ten-State Nutrition Survey (10), Nationwide Food Consumption Survey, 1977–78 (11), and the National Health and Nutrition Examination Surveys (NHANES I and II) (12,13) report that the elderly often have decreased intakes of vitamins A, B_1, B_2, B_6, and C. Other reports find vitamins D, B_{12}, and niacin to be deficient frequently in the diets of elderly persons (6,14–16). Exactly what constitutes an adequate or inadequate intake of a particular vitamin, however, remains controversial because the physiologic needs and importance of tissue stores in the elderly are not definitively known (17–19). The determination of "optimum" vitamin levels that may be associated with improved performance, rather than "adequate" levels, is also controversial. When determined on a weight basis, the recommended vitamin intake for humans is well below that of other species (1).

Suter and Russell (20), in their evaluation of the literature to determine the appropriateness of the 1980 Recommended Dietary Allowance (RDA) (Table 1) with respect to the healthy elderly, concluded that the RDA for folate and vitamin A may be too high; the RDA for vitamins B_6, B_{12}, and D may be too low, at least for certain elderly subgroups; the RDA for B_1, B_2, and C seems appropriate; and that there are conflicting data for vitamin E and insufficient data to determine the appropriateness of the RDA for vita-

TABLE 1. *Recommended dietary allowances (RDAs) for vitamin intake in the elderly (over age 51) compared with the US RDA*

	RDA		US RDA
	Men	Women	
Fat-soluble vitamins			
Vitamin A (retinol)	1,000 μg[a]	800 μg[a]	5,000 IU[d]
Vitamin D	5 μg[b]	5 μg[b]	10 μg
Vitamin E (tocopherol)	10 mg[c]	8 mg[c]	30 IU[e]
Vitamin K	80 μg	65 μg	----
Water-soluble vitamins			
Vitamin B$_1$ (thiamine)	1.2 mg	1.0 mg	1.5 mg
Vitamin B$_2$ (riboflavin)	1.4 mg	1.2 mg	1.7 mg
Vitamin B$_6$ (pyridoxine)	2.0 mg	1.6 mg	2.0 mg
Vitamin B$_{12}$ (cobalamin)	2.0 μg	2.0 μg	6.0 μg
Folic acid (folacin)	200 μg	180 μg	400 μg
Niacin	15 mg[f]	13 mg[f]	20 mg
Biotin	30–100 μg	30–100 μg	300 μg
Pantothenic acid	4–7 mg	4–7 mg	10 mg
Vitamin C (ascorbic acid)	60 mg	60 mg	60 mg

From Committee on Dietary Allowances, ref. 24, and Council on Scientific Affairs, ref. 25.
[a]As retinol equivalents (1 RE = 1 μg retinol or 6 μg beta-carotene).
[b]As cholecalciferol (5 μg cholecalciferol = 200 IU vitamin D).
[c]As alpha-tocopherol equivalents (1 α-TE = 1 mg d-α-tocopherol).
[d]3.33 IU = 1 RE.
[e]1 IU = 0.67 mg α-TE.
[f]As niacin equivalents (1 NE = 1 mg niacin = 60 mg dietary tryptophan).

mins K, niacin, biotin, and pantothenic acid. It is not known whether current intake recommendations are sufficient to protect against subclinical or atypical vitamin deficiency or even whether commonly available biochemical tests can accurately detect such deficiencies. This scientific uncertainty, combined with the relative safety of most vitamins, makes the elderly prime targets for unscrupulous nutritional supplement exploitation. Conversely, until recently the medical profession's general unconcern about vitamin disorders has made the elderly equally susceptible to nutritional neglect.

How is intake measured? There is no infallible way to determine nutritional intake in large numbers of people (21,22). Subjects who will tolerate the more detailed and intrusive evaluations become less and less representative of the population as a whole. Very few nutritional surveys have included people over 75 years of age, currently the fastest-growing segment of the population in the United States. Dietary histories and interviews, food diaries, and 24-hour recalls are subject to well-recognized inaccuracies. Biochemical measures of serum vitamin levels and urinary excretion may not correlate well either with estimates of intake or actual tissue content (19,22,23). A strong clinical suspicion, a focused physical examination, and carefully selected laboratory studies, fully understanding the limitations of each, are the best means to detect a vitamin deficiency before its florid and perhaps fatal presentation. Vitamin deficiencies in the elderly, as do many

TABLE 2. *Stages in the development of a vitamin deficiency*

Stage	Characteristics
Preliminary	Decrease in tissue stores and urinary excretion
Biochemical	Decrease in enzyme activity due to coenzyme insufficiency
Physiologic	Nonspecific symptoms: anorexia, weight loss, insomnia, lethargy, irritability, impaired psychologic function
Clinical	Exacerbated nonspecific symptoms; appearance of specific deficiency syndrome
Anatomic	Clear symptoms with pathologic tissue damage

From Brin and Bauernfeind, ref. 5.

other disorders, may present atypically or be hard to differentiate when other diseases or general malnutrition is present. The stages through which a vitamin deficiency is presumed to proceed are shown in Table 2. The goal is to prevent vitamin deficiencies or to detect them in the earliest stages before permanent tissue damage occurs.

The RDA is the sum of a minimum requirement—defined as the amount needed on the basis of the available scientific evidence to maintain health in the already healthy individual or known to prevent a nutritional deficiency— plus a calculated safety factor. The RDA are neither minimal requirements nor do they claim to represent optimal intake levels (24). The RDA for vitamins, as defined by the Food and Nutrition Board of the National Research Council and the National Academy of Sciences, are listed in Table 1. The RDA should be applied to population groups; there are many conditions that require adjustment for any specific individual (24).

The RDA includes elderly persons within the category of all persons above 51 years of age. This broad grouping may not be valid, particularly for the oldest ages. Recommended dietary intakes (RDI) are frequently proposed by various nutritional experts as modifications of the RDA as new information becomes available. In addition, the Food and Drug Administration, for purposes of labeling food supplies (eg, canned food and cereal boxes) and dietary supplements, uses a more widely distributed and simplified "US RDA" (Table 1). It is the same for all (nonpregnant) persons above age 4. The US RDA is often higher than the current 1989 RDA for elderly persons (25).

There are differences in RDAs in different countries, based not only on different interpretations of the available scientific literature but also on political and socioeconomic considerations and pressures (26). Any proposed changes in the RDA have considerable impact on agricultural patterns, food assistance programs, vitamin manufacturing, and legislation for food fortification.

The well-recognized physiologic diversity and heterogeneity in the elderly and the increased prevalence of chronic diseases and disorders that accompany aging are two arguments for modifying the current RDA (27). No one is sure to what extent acute and chronic disease affects vitamin requirements

TABLE 3. *General causes of vitamin deficiencies*

Inadequate or inappropriate intake

Poverty	Bizarre diets	Cultural idiosyncracies
Ignorance	Tube feeding	Depression
Neglect	Hyperalimentation	
Alcohol abuse	Anorexia secondary to disease or medications	

Inadequate digestion or absorption
Chronic vomiting or diarrhea
Pancreatic or biliary tract disease or obstruction
Gastric or intestinal surgery
Drug interference (antibiotics, antacids, anticonvulsants, laxatives)
Increased needs

Hypermetabolic states (infection, fever, malignancy, exercise)	
Alcohol abuse	Pregnancy/lactation
Dialysis	Smoking
Intestinal parasites	Chronic liver disease
Blind loop/bacterial overgrowth states	

Increased excretion
Proteinuria and chronic renal disease
Diuretics

nor whether supplementation will invariably alleviate clinical or subclinical disorders. Defining an RDA for older persons will likely require the identification of high-risk subgroups, such as those with achlorhydria, those who are homebound or institutionalized, or alcoholics, for special monitoring and/or supplementation (18,28).

Common causes of vitamin deficiencies in adults are listed in Table 3. As a group, the elderly are especially prone to vitamin deficiencies (4,8,20,29),

TABLE 4. *Common factors causing vitamin deficiencies in the elderly*

PHYSICAL
Decreased calorie requirements and food intake
Decreased taste sensation
Dentures: poorly fitting, painful, decreased taste and swallowing
Physical handicaps and decreased mobility
Neurologic impairment of chewing and swallowing
Memory and attention disorders
Chronic disease: COPD, congestive heart failure, coronary artery disease
Atrophic gastritis
Intestinal motility disorders
Negative reinforcers of food intake: hiatal hernia, reflux, lactose intolerance, exertional hypoxia, intestinal angina
Medications (prescription and nonprescription): digoxin, fluoxitine, laxatives, antacids, diuretics, chemotherapy, anticonvulsants
SOCIAL/PSYCHOLOGIC
Social isolation and loss of conjugate meals
Depression
Unable to drive to the market
Hidden alcoholism
"Instant bachelors" who have never learned to buy, store, or cook food
Finicky eaters
Elder abuse and neglect

and those physical and psychosocial factors that contribute to nutritional disorders in the elderly are presented in Table 4. These factors serve as warning signs identifying high-risk patients.

Each vitamin is discussed separately, with an emphasis on nutritional problems specific for elderly persons. Vitamin disorders and risk factors

TABLE 5. *Common sources for vitamins*

Vitamin	Source
Vitamin A	Preformed vitamin A: animal products (liver and liver oils, egg yolks, milk fat), supplemented dairy products and margarine. Carotenoids, especially beta-carotene (pre-vitamin A): yellow and orange pigments in fruits and vegetables (carrots, spinach, yams, squash, peaches, broccoli, turnip greens). Note: color intensity not a good predictor of carotenoid content.
Vitamin D	Fish liver oils, fatty fish (eg, swordfish, sardines, salmon, mackerel), natural and supplemented dairy products. Endogenous synthesis by sunlight exposure on skin, converting 7-dehydrocholesterol into vitamin D.
Vitamin E	Seed embryos (eg, wheat germ) vegetable oils, supplemented margarine. Alpha-tocopherol is the most active form. Natural vitamin easily lost in food processing.
Vitamin K	Green leafy vegetables (cabbage, spinach, broccoli), cauliflower, soybeans, liver. Bacterial synthesis in the intestine important.
Vitamin B_1 (thiamine)	Pork, organ meats, rice bran, soybean flour, cereal germs. Heat labile.
Vitamin B_2 (riboflavin)	Milk, organ meats, poultry, fish, enriched grains and cereals. Easily destroyed by cooking and sunlight.
Vitamin B_6 (pyridoxine)	Chicken, kidney, liver, fish, pork, eggs, whole-grain cereals, potatoes. Easily destroyed by oxidation, freezing, ultraviolet light, cooking, and milling cereal.
Vitamin B_{12}	Animal products including liver, kidney, and fish. Almost entirely absent in plant material.
Folic acid	Dry beans, liver, kidney, whole grains, wheat bran, dark green leafy vegetables, such as broccoli. Sunlight, oxidation, and cooking variably destroy folic acid.
Niacin	Organ meats, tuna, halibut, white meat of fowl, rice bran, whole wheat. Poor bioavailability from some grains, such as maize. Synthesized from tryptophan, present in many foods, in the presence of thiamine, riboflavin, pyridoxine, and biotin (60 mg tryptophan = 1 mg niacin). Small amount synthesized by intestinal bacteria.
Biotin	Egg yolk, soy flour, liver, kidney. Bioavailability varies in different foods. Some synthesis by intestinal bacteria.
Pantothenic acid	Found in most foods, especially organ meats, egg yolk, whole grain cereals, dried peas. Easily destroyed by cooking.
Vitamin C	Citrus fruits, vegetables (broccoli, brussel sprouts, collards, spinach, potatoes). Content depends upon ripeness and storage conditions. Easily lost by blanching, washing, overcooking. Little loss by freezing.

TABLE 6. *Vitamin deficiencies in the elderly*

Vitamin	Manifestation of deficiency
Vitamin A	Uncommon in the elderly: night blindness, follicular hyperkeratosis; possible increased risk of epithelial cancers, particularly associated with beta-carotene deficiency (pre-vitamin A)
Vitamin D	Common in the elderly: osteomalacia with increased bone and muscle pain, weakness, and increased risk of fractures
Vitamin E	Uncommon in the elderly: nonspecific neuralgic signs. Antioxidant role: deficiency may increase risk of cancer
Vitamin K	Iatrogenic causes common (anticoagulants and antibiotics): gastrointestinal, subcutaneous, and intracranial bleeding
Vitamin B_1	Associated with alcoholism and general malnutrition. Dry beriberi (neurologic): depression, irritability, peripheral neuropathy. Wet beriberi (cardiovascular): cardiomyopathy, edema, high output failure. Wernicke's syndrome: encephalopathy, sixth nerve palsy, ataxia
Vitamin B_2	Associated with general malnutrition: pain and inflammation of mouth, tongue, and lips; seborrheic keratosis; ocular keratitis
Vitamin B_6	Associated with general malnutrition and medications (eg, isoniazid): pain and inflammation of mouth, tongue, and lips; seborrheic keratosis; peripheral neuropathy
Vitamin B_{12}	Pernicious anemia increasingly common with age: sore mouth, megaloblastic anemia, peripheral neuropathy, dementia
Folic acid	Common in the poor or alcoholic elderly: megalobastic anemia
Niacin	Associated with general malnutrition. Pellegra: sore mouth, anorexia, gastrointestinal motility disorders; dermatitis and hyperkeratosis; nonspecific mental status changes
Biotin	Associated with general malnutrition: nonspecific gastrointestinal and neuromuscular symptoms
Pantothenic acid	Uncommon in the elderly: nonspecific neuropathy
Vitamin C	Associated with general malnutrition and smoking. Scurvy: pinpoint skin hemorrhages followed by purpura, hyperkeratosis, anemia, poor wound healing. Antioxidant role in cancer prevention remains controversial

found primarily in younger persons are not discussed. Each section summarizes each vitamin's biochemical functions, how it can be measured in the body, what factors make the elderly especially at higher risk for a particular vitamin disorder, and how hypo- and hypervitaminosis may present. Common sources for each vitamin are listed in Table 5. Table 6 summarizes the major manifestations of each of the vitamin deficiency states.

VITAMIN A—RETINOL

Function

Vitamin A regulates epithelial tissue regeneration and protects its integrity. In addition, it is involved in the production of rhodopsin in the retina, which affects dark vision adaptation. Vitamin A affects growth and reproduction in young animals and appears to have multiple effects on immune function (30).

Assessment

The preferred unit for the measurement of vitamin A is the retinol equivalent (RE) in which 1 RE = 1 μg all-trans retinol = 3.33 IU = 6 μg beta-carotene. There is a poor correlation between vitamin A intake and retinol plasma levels, except in the extreme ranges. Plasma retinol levels are frequently affected by many diseases. For example, vitamin A levels decline during infections, but usually return to normal without treatment once the infectious process ceases. Also, only 50 to 60 of the 400 to 500 existing carotenoids have known biologic activity, so serum carotenoid levels have little clinical value. There is no association between age and retinol or carotene levels (31).

Risk Factors

Hypovitaminosis A is usually caused by prolonged malnutrition, biliary obstruction and other enteropathies, chronic liver disease, or proteinuria (1,32). Deficiencies of iron, zinc, or vitamin E may also adversely affect retinol transport, storage, and utilization. Plasma levels of beta-carotene are reduced in people who smoke and perhaps in those who abuse alcohol (31,33). A number of drugs, such as mineral oil, neomycin, and cholestyramine, can interfere with vitamin A absorption (34).

Deficiency

The current RDA for vitamin A is 1,000 RE for adult men and 800 RE for women. The recommendation has been made to reduce the adult RDA to 700 RE and 600 RE in men and women, respectively (35), because of the substantial liver stores even in the very old, the increased absorption of retinol that occurs with advancing age (20), and the potential teratogenic effect of higher vitamin A doses in people of reproductive age (36).

Vitamin A deficiency primarily affects infants and children and is seldom seen in the elderly, even though intakes are often below the RDA (37). The lack of vitamin A causes normal epithelium to become inappropriately keratinized squamous epithelium. This is most acutely manifested by follicular hyperkeratosis and keratomalacia of the cornea. The follicular hyperkeratosis that is commonly found in the elderly is often caused merely by poor hygiene (34).

Vitamin A deficiency still remains among the most common causes of blindness worldwide. Gray-white plaques, known as Bitot's spots, may develop in the limbal conjunctiva as keratin debris accumulates. In addition, retinol deficiency causes impaired night vision because of the defect in rhodopsin production. It is not known how frequently these signs occur in the elderly. A much more common cause of night vision deterioration in the elderly is cataract formation. Night blindness and conjunctival changes in younger patients respond to 30,000 RE vitamin A daily for 2 to 3 weeks.

Several epidemiologic studies have suggested a correlation between retinol or carotenoid intake and cancer in humans (30,38,39). This remains controversial, and other studies have not found a strong association (40–42). It is possible that any anticancer role for carotenoids is attributable to their antioxidant properties, rather than to their conversion to retinol (20,41). Such antioxidants as the carotenoids may also protect skin from the photoaging effects of sunlight (43).

Toxicity

Side effects of beta-carotene ingestion are rare, except for carotenoidermia (44)—an orange-yellow skin discoloration that is most prominent in the palms and soles. It can be distinguished from icterus because the sclera of the eyes remains normal in carotenoidermia. Carotenoidermia is usually associated with the daily intake of more than 30 mg purified beta-carotene or equivalent (45). The lack of toxicity of carotene is due to its poor absorption from the intestine and its subsequent feedback-inhibited conversion to retinol (1). Excess intake is stored primarily in adipose tissue, rather than the liver (41). Hypothyroidism can also cause hypercarotenemia by inhibiting carotene conversion to vitamin A and by causing hyperlipidemia (44).

Hypervitaminosis A can occur both acutely and after chronic ingestion. Acute toxicity presents as headaches, drowsiness, irritability, dizziness, nausea, vomiting, and diarrhea (46). Elderly people with normal kidney and liver function may tolerate a daily dose of 50,000 RE for up to 6 months without exhibiting evidence of chronic toxicity (47), although toxicity has also been seen on daily intakes of 15,000 RE (48). Chronic toxicity may classically present as desquamation and redness of the skin and mucous membranes (of therapeutic value in topical dermatologic preparations, such as tretinoin), disturbed hair growth, loss of appetite, fatigue, irritability, thyroid suppression, cerebrospinal fluid pressure elevation producing symptoms similar to pseudotumor cerebri, and hepatosplenomegaly (1,46). Toxicity increases in the presence of renal failure or pre-existing hepatic dysfunction and decreases in the presence of excess vitamin E. Hypercalcemia and a negative calcium balance similar to that seen with hypervitaminosis D may occur, but retinol excess affects the organic bone matrix whereas vitamin D excess causes dissolution of the mineral matrix (46).

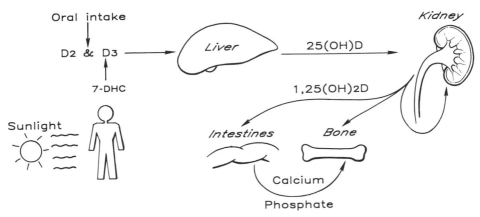

FIG. 1. Vitamin D may be ingested as ergocalciferol (D_2) or cholecalciferol (D_3) or synthesized from 7-dehydrocholesterol (7-DHC) in the skin after sun exposure. To become activated, vitamin D must undergo 25-hydroxylation in the liver (calcidiol; 25(OH)D) followed by 1-hydroxylation in the kidneys (calcitriol; $1,25(OH)_2D$). Once activated, vitamin D is free to act on bones, kidneys, and intestines to maintain calcium, phosphate, and bone homeostasis. (From Reichel et al., ref. 51.)

VITAMIN D

Function

Vitamin D enables the normal mineralization of bone, facilitates the intestinal absorption of calcium and phosphate, regulates renal reabsorption and homeostasis of amino acids and phosphate, and influences the activity of parathyroid hormone on both bone and in the kidney. Figure 1 depicts the sources of vitamin D, its conversion pathway, and its major sites of activity. Vitamin D may also be required for normal functioning of hematopoietic cells, skin, cancer cells, and for normal insulin secretion (49–51).

Assessment

Although $1,25(OH)_2D$ is the most active form, serum levels correlate poorly with clinical disease. The principal circulating metabolite of vitamin D is 25(OH)D, which currently provides the best index of body stores (52). Because of its long half-life, values of 25(OH)D usually reflect overall past intake. Changes in serum calcium, inorganic phosphate, or alkaline phosphatase are nonspecific and affected by many other diseases. Radiographic changes in osteomalacia are usually indistinguishable from those in osteoporosis, although pseudofractures are more common in osteomalacia.

Risk Factors

The current RDA for vitamin D is 200 IU (1 IU = 0.025 μg vitamin D). There is a small, age-associated decline in 25(OH)D levels, although they generally remain normal in healthy elderly persons. This is despite the fact that many elderly have an intake of vitamin D substantially below the RDA (8,20,52–54).

The capacity of the aging intestine to absorb vitamin D and calcium may decline (55). As vitamin D intake decreases with age, endogenous skin production therefore becomes more important (56). Although the concentration of 7-dehydrocholesterol decreases in the aging epidermis, with an associated decrease in the ability to synthesize vitamin D (57), the level of serum 25(OH)D in the elderly will still increase in response to sunlight exposure (58,59). The seasonal variations in vitamin D levels decrease with age as overall sun exposure also decreases, particularly in homebound and institutionalized persons (60). The long-term use of sunscreens to prevent sunlight-related skin deterioration and skin cancers may also make elderly persons prone to deficiency of vitamin D (61). Dark pigmentation of the skin is also associated with a decrease in endogenous synthesis of vitamin D.

There is little evidence for an age-related decline in liver 25-hydroxylation of vitamin D (52), but there does appear to be a marked decrease in 1-hydroxylation by the aging kidney. This reduction may be caused by a decreased responsiveness of the 1-alpha-hydroxylase enzyme to the parathyroid hormone (20), as well as an overall decline in renal function with age.

Anticonvulsant therapy (both phenytoin and phenobarbitol) decreases liver hydroxylation of vitamin D, whereas kidney hydroxylation is reduced in chronic renal failure, Wilson's disease, and during glucocorticoid therapy (1). Hepatobiliary disease, intestinal mucosal disease, partial gastrectomy, or small bowel surgery affect the absorption of all fat-soluble vitamins.

Deficiency

Vitamin D deficiency causes rickets in children and osteomalacia in adults. Bone in pure osteomalacia has normal organic matrix but decreased mineralization, resulting in soft and easily deformed bone. The resulting clinical picture is characterized by proximal bone pain, backache, difficulty rising from a chair and climbing stairs, a waddling gait, and subsequent decreased mobility because of the pain. There may be muscle tenderness and weakness, as well as anorexia and weight loss. These signs and symptoms may be difficult to recognize and are frequently attributed to "rheumatism" (62). Fractures can occur with minimal trauma. A deficiency of calcium or inorganic phosphate can cause changes identical to those seen in osteomalacia due to vitamin D deficiency.

In contrast to osteomalacia, osteoporosis is associated with a reduction in bony tissue (thinning of the bones), but the bone that remains has a normal mineral content, unlike the soft and poorly mineralized bone in osteomalacia. Osteoporosis is not caused by vitamin D deficiency, but osteoporosis and osteomalacia frequently coexist because of age-associated risk factors. Calcitriol (1,25(OH)$_2$D) does not appear to be effective in treating established postmenopausal osteoporosis (63). Osteoporosis is discussed in detail in Chapter 10.

Elderly patients who have hip fractures are frequently but not invariably found to have lower 25(OH)D levels and less sunshine exposure than control patients despite similarly low vitamin D intakes (52,64,65). In addition, vitamin D deficiency may exacerbate secondary hyperparathyroidism, which can also increase cortical bone loss (52,65).

There is considerable concern that the RDA for vitamin D is too low because of the high prevalence of osteopenia with age (66). Many other factors are also involved, such as heredity, activity level, calcium intake, and estrogen levels. It has been proposed that vitamin D deficiency can be prevented in high-risk patients (institutionalized or homebound on marginal diets) by twice yearly oral doses of 10,000 to 100,000 IU vitamin D (67,68). A daily oral vitamin D supplement of 200 to 400 IU may also suffice (62), although Parfitt et al. (52) have recommended a 600 to 800 IU total daily intake in the elderly. Sunlight exposure does increase vitamin D levels, but is often impractical for institutionalized elderly or those who live in colder environments. Patients on chronic anticonvulsant therapy and those with persistent intestinal malabsorption, chronic renal failure, or hypoparathyroidism may require higher supplementation or the use of specific substitutes, such as calcitriol, with periodic monitoring of serum and urinary calcium and vitamin D levels (51). Vitamin D therapy of 50,000 IU a day for 2 weeks followed by maintenance intake will cure osteomalacia and heal incomplete fractures in most cases (29).

Toxicity

Chronic vitamin D intake of over 25,000 to 50,000 IU a day can be extremely toxic (69). Excessive intake causes increased calcium absorption from the intestines and increased calcium mobilization from bone. The resultant hypercalcemia can cause anorexia, weakness, constipation, and soft tissue calcification of the heart (aortic stenosis), blood vessels, lungs, joints, and kidney leading to renal insufficiency. Hypervitaminosis D causes early complications in patients with renal failure, hypo- and pseudohypoparathyroidism, sarcoidosis, and accelerated atherosclerosis in the presence of hyperlipidemia (46,52).

VITAMIN E—TOCOPHEROL

Function

Vitamin E acts as an antioxidant, which may lessen the deleterious effects of free radicals. It is not known whether vitamin E intake affects cancer risk in the elderly, but it may be associated with decreased cancer risk in younger subjects (38,70). There is no evidence that topical vitamin E improves surgical scars, and it is frequently associated with minor skin reactions when applied topically in high doses (71). However, oral vitamin E may improve wound healing (71). Vitamin E may also be effective in the treatment of intermittent claudication (72).

Assessment

Vitamin E levels can be measured as serum tocopherol or by determining red blood cell (RBC) susceptibility to hemolysis. Newer functional assays for vitamin E status have been proposed recently (73). Because vitamin E circulates with HDL and LDL lipid fractions, it is now felt that vitamin E levels should be expressed relative to total serum lipids (20,74).

Risk Factors

Vitamin E deficiency can occur because of decreased intake, enteropathies (because it is linked to fat absorption and its absorption is facilitated by bile salts), or in association with lipoprotein disorders (1). Deficiency may also occur if there is a very high intake of polyunsaturated fats (1). Vitamin C and selenium help regenerate vitamin E by reducing free radicals (75).

Vitamin E blood levels do not markedly differ between old and young adults, although there is a decrease in vitamin E platelet levels with age (76). There is no relation between vitamin E: lipid ratios and age (77) nor any consistent evidence for altered vitamin E requirements with age (20).

Deficiency

The RDA for vitamin E is 10 mg for adult men and 8 mg for women. International units (IU) are still frequently used, and the activity of naturally occurring alpha-tocopherol is about 1.5 IU/mg (24). Clinical deficiency syndromes are almost exclusively restricted to premature infants, although erythrocyte hemolysis may be demonstrated *in vitro* (78). The infertility noted in animals secondary to vitamin E depletion has not been observed in man. Physical signs of deficiency are rare in adults, but may include areflexia, decreased proprioceptive and vibratory sensation, and gaze paresis

(79). Low levels of alpha-tocopherol may be associated with an increased risk of death from cancer, although they may be a consequence of the cancer, rather than its precursor (80).

Toxicity

Vitamin E is one of the most commonly supplemented vitamins in the elderly. There are minimal side effects from even very high intake up to 3,200 IU a day (81), although diarrhea or fatigue may occur. Oral vitamin E may exacerbate a coagulation disorder produced by vitamin K deficiency and potentiate oral anticoagulants (81). The effects of vitamin E on serum lipids is unclear, but there is some evidence that excessive supplementation may increase serum cholesterol in the elderly (82).

VITAMIN K

Function

Vitamin K (from the word "Koagulation") is required for the synthesis of bioactive prothrombin and factors VII, IX, and X, and proteins C and S necessary for normal coagulation. Any role for vitamin K as an antibiotic, analgesic (83), or in bone metabolism (84) is currently unclear.

Assessment

Vitamin K status is normally assessed indirectly by measuring the prothrombin time (PT).

Risk Factors

Vitamin K deficiency may occur because of (a) decreased bacterial synthesis caused by antibiotics, (b) decreased absorption because of hepatobiliary disease/obstruction, hypermotility, inflammatory bowel disease, or chronic mineral oil ingestion, or (c) decreased utilization secondary to liver disease or such anticoagulants as coumadin. Alcoholism may increase the risk of subclinical vitamin K deficiency (85). High intakes of Vitamin E may potentiate coumarin anticoagulants (81).

Deficiency

The RDA for Vitamin K is 80 μg for men and 65 μg for women (or about 1μg/kg per day). It has been suggested that this intake can be safely decreased to 35 μg for women and 45 μg for men (86). Vitamin K deficiency causes hypoprothrombinemia and an increased clotting time, which results in an increased bleeding risk into subcutaneous tissues, the gastrointestinal tract, and intracranially after minor trauma.

Toxicity

Vitamin K (phylloquinone) is usually well tolerated in adults. Because most side effects—hypotension, flushing, dyspnea, or even cardiovascular collapse—occur with intravenous administration, it should be restricted to emergency situations (46). Vitamin K may paradoxically cause a prolonged prothrombin time in patients with subclinical hepatic dysfunction (46).

VITAMIN B₁—THIAMINE

Function

Thiamine plays a role in carbohydrate metabolism as a coenzyme in the decarboxylation of pyruvate and alpha-ketoglutarate and in the pentose phosphate cycle.

Assessment

Serum and urinary thiamine, blood pyruvate, and RBC transketolase levels provide some idea of thiamine deficiency. However, aging may affect RBC transketolase activity, eliminating its value as an index of thiamine nutriture in elderly persons (87).

Risk Factors

Thiamine intake varies widely, and various studies find that 18 to 46% of elderly persons, depending upon race and income, have an intake less than two-thirds the RDA (17,88). However, when corrected for caloric intake, deficiency is less common (88).

Thiamine requirements are known to increase with increasing carbohydrate intake and in hypermetabolic states, such as hyperthyroidism, fever, and muscular activity (1). Physicians have been classically taught to include thiamine supplementation with any glucose infusions in alcoholics (who are presumed to be thiamine deficient) to avoid precipitating Wernicke's syndrome because of the increase in thiamine requirements with the sudden increase in calories. Conversely, thiamine administration may increase glucose metabolism and cause hypoglycemia.

Both alcoholism and diabetes mellitus place patients at risk for subclinical thiamine deficiency (89). Long-term hemodialysis or intravenous feedings increase risk of thiamine deficiency (24). Thiamine is destroyed by simultaneous consumption with calcium carbonate, nitrates, and sulfites (90). In addition, tea, raw fish, and shellfish consumption also are reported to destroy thiamine (1).

Deficiency

The RDA for thiamine is 1.2 mg for men and 1.0 mg for women, or 0.5 mg/1,000 kcal (minimum = 1 mg), although this may be higher than necessary (88). Vitamin B_1 deficiency can present as anorexia, constipation, depression, irritability, memory dysfunction, or a peripheral neuritis (paresthesias, muscle weakness and wasting, decreased reflexes, and diminished vibratory sensation). Beriberi (Singhalese for weakness) is the classical severe deficiency state. "Wet" beriberi refers to the presence of cardiomyopathy, high output failure, and edema. In "dry" beriberi, polyneuropathy is prominent. The typical patient has mixed signs and symptoms. Beriberi is treated by 50 mg thiamine intramuscularly for several days followed by 2.5 to 5 mg orally per day.

Wernicke's syndrome is often associated with alcoholism and presumed thiamine deficiency. It has a classic triad of signs and symptoms: (a) encephalopathy with a global confusional state (eg, apathy, lethargy) that may present rather suddenly, (b) unilateral or bilateral sixth nerve palsy and vertical or horizontal nystagmus, and (c) ataxia, with leg muscle weakness and tenderness, decreased deep tendon reflexes, foot drop, and a staggering drunken gait. Wernicke's encephalopathy may either be abated or develop into Korsakoff's syndrome once thiamine stores are renewed. Any peripheral neuropathy or gait disturbance usually requires prolonged rehabilitation.

Not all patients with Wernicke's syndrome have a demonstrable vitamin B_1 deficiency, and most patients who are thiamine deficient do not develop the syndrome. The disease may be dependent upon individual genetic variations in thiamine pyrophosphate (TPP)-dependent transketolase enzyme systems. TPP-dependent enzyme activity may also be deficient in some patients with Alzheimer's disease (91).

Toxicity

Thiamine has very low toxicity orally. Large intakes of parenteral thiamine (> 400 mg) may be accompanied by mental status changes (acute vigilance or lethargy), mild ataxia, and nausea (46). High thiamine intake may also increase riboflavin excretion.

VITAMIN B₂—RIBOFLAVIN

Function

Riboflavin is necessary for the formation of two coenzymes: flavin mononucleotide (FMN) and flavin adenine dinucleotide (FAD). These coenzymes are involved in hydrogen transport and oxidation.

Assessment

Measurement of RBC or urine riboflavin, or erythrocyte glutathione reductase is available.

Risk Factors

The current RDA for vitamin B_2 is 1.4 mg for men and 1.2 mg for women, or 0.6 mg/1,000 kcal (minimum = 1.2 mg). The NHANES I and the Ten-State Nutrition Survey found that 12 to 36% of elderly people have a riboflavin intake less than two-thirds the RDA (10,12,17). Any deficiency is almost always associated with general malnutrition and multiple B-vitamin deficiencies. There is no evidence for an age-related change in intestinal absorption, and tissue levels do not change in the healthy elderly (9). Exercise increases riboflavin requirements in younger people, but its effect in the elderly is unknown (47). Chlorpromazine increases the renal excretion of riboflavin and may place some individuals at risk for deficiency (92).

Deficiency

Signs and symptoms of vitamin B_2 deficiency include cheilosis, sore throat, angular stomatitis, a magenta hue to the tongue surface from mucosal atrophy, and seborrheic dermatitis around the nasolabial folds. Angular stomatitis is nonspecific and is more commonly related to ill-fitting dentures and drooling saliva. Eye signs are lacrimation, scleral vascularization, and superficial interstitial keratitis, often associated with conjunctivitis and photophobia.

Toxicity

High intake of riboflavin has little known toxicity.

VITAMIN B$_6$—PYRIDOXINE

Function

Vitamin B$_6$ coenzymes play an essential role in the Kreb's cycle, protein and fat metabolism, and melanin, cysteine, and porphyrin synthesis. Pyridoxine is involved in the formation of such brain metabolites as norepinephrine, epinephrine, tyramine, dopamine, 5-hydroxytryptamine, and GABA. Vitamin B$_6$ also facilitates magnesium cellular uptake.

Assessment

Serum pyridoxine levels are not useful in assessing tissue status (20). Urinary vitamin B$_6$, urinary xanthurenic acid levels after tryptophan loading, and measurement of RBC glutamic pyruvic transaminase have been used to determine vitamin B$_6$ status.

Risk Factors

The RDA for vitamin B$_6$ is 2.0 mg for men and 1.6 mg for women, or 0.016 mg/g protein. A vitamin B$_6$ intake below the RDA is common in the elderly (9,93). Pyridoxine deficiency is generally associated with general malnutrition or chronic alcoholism and a deficiency in other B-complex vitamins. However, pyridoxine metabolism or bioavailability may be specifically affected by over 40 drugs, including isoniazid, hydralazine, cycloserine, and penicillamine. The pyridoxine requirement also increases as protein intake increases. Because ingestion of estrogens increases the pyridoxine requirement, supplementation may be necessary in elderly women on estrogen replacement. There is some evidence for age-related changes in vitamin B$_6$ metabolism, but the significance of these are unknown (20).

Deficiency

As with many B-vitamin deficiencies, pyridoxine deficiency is associated with seborrheic dermatitis, cheilosis, glossitis, and angular stomatitis. Some of the drug-associated deficiencies present as a peripheral neuropathy or a pyridoxine-responsive anemia. The latter may also be seen in hemochromatosis. Pyridoxine supplementation of 30 to 50 mg a day prevents or treats the neuropathy and anemia. There is a suggestion that nausea and vomiting associated with irradiation, drug therapy, anesthesia, or travel sickness may respond to doses of pyridoxine up to 300 mg a day (1). Pyridoxine is often given prophylactically to patients on isoniazid, hydralazine, and penicillamine to prevent peripheral neuritis.

Toxicity

Vitamin B_6 intake up to 1,000 times the RDA has been tolerated without adverse side effects (94), although a sensory neuropathy and ataxia can occur at prolonged doses of 100 mg/day. Pyridoxine increases the peripheral decarboxylation of levodopa, reducing its effectiveness as a treatment for Parkinson's disease (95) and may decrease the anticonvulsant effect of phenytoin.

VITAMIN B_{12}—COBALAMIN

Function

The physiologic role of vitamin B_{12} is closely related to that of folic acid (29,96,97). It is involved in the biosynthesis of purine, pyrimidine, methionine, and choline and in the conversion of proprionate to succinate. Vitamin B_{12} also helps keep the sulfhydryl groups on enzymes in a reduced form (1).

Vitamin B_{12} is required for the isomerization of methylmalonyl CoA to succinyl CoA. When vitamin B_{12} deficiency occurs, methylmalonic acid (MMA) accumulates and urinary excretion increases. MMA excretion can be measured after giving an oral load of valine, a precursor to MMA. Urinary MMA is not affected by folate deficiency and can be used to differentiate folate from vitamin B_{12} deficiency (32). Vitamin E deficiency may also cause increased MMA excretion (32).

Assessment

Vitamin B_{12} serum levels are commonly available. Low serum B_{12} levels in the absence of folic acid or iron deficiency are felt to reflect decreased liver stores (32), although this is controversial (98). This interpretation, however, is less accurate in the presence of folate or iron deficiency. Also, liver disease tends to increase vitamin B_{12} serum levels (32). Urinary excretion of methylmalonic acid may be a more accurate method of assessing B_{12} status.

Inspection of the peripheral blood smear for macrocytosis and hypersegmented polys or the bone marrow for megaloblastosis may also help detect a vitamin B_{12} deficiency, although similar changes can occur with folate deficiency. Conversely, the hematologic abnormalities may be absent in the face of severe deficiency (99,100).

Risk Factors

Vitamin B_{12} serum level may decrease somewhat with age, but generally it remains within normal limits (20,101). Physical disability increases the risk of vitamin B_{12} deficiency (102). There does not appear to be an alteration of B_{12} absorption solely caused by aging, and it is unknown whether age influences hepatic B_{12} stores (20,28). Inadequate intake alone as a cause of vitamin B_{12} deficiency is extremely uncommon, even in pure vegetarians. The enterohepatic cycle is very important in recycling vitamin B_{12} lost in the bile, and interference with this reabsorption by pernicious anemia or small bowel disease results in more rapid depletion of vitamin stores.

Many drugs can interfere with vitamin B_{12} absorption and metabolism, including alcohol, cholestyramine, clindamycin, colchicine, and neomycin (34).

Pernicious anemia is a disease of later life, occurring in 1 to 2.5% of people over age 60. Atrophic gastritis is common, occurring in up to 50% of elderly persons. It may decrease cobalamin absorption because (a) the B_{12} vitamin cannot be extracted from meat protein without acid, (b) the bioavailability of B_{12} decreases because of bacterial overgrowth in the upper intestine when acid is not present, and (c) intrinsic factor (IF) secretion may be impaired (20). Folate and iron status also affect B_{12} levels (see Folate section). Transcobalamin II, the protein that transports vitamin B_{12} in the plasma, may also be abnormal in some elderly patients (103).

Deficiency

The RDA for vitamin B_{12} is 2 μg for both men and women. The normal presence of large liver stores of cobalamin and an effective enterohepatic circulation means that deficiency may take months or years to develop. The sequence of events in the course of vitamin B_{12} deficiency have been described in detail by Herbert (104,105). Gastrointestinal symptoms include a sore tongue and anorexia. The hematologic changes, resulting from impaired DNA synthesis, are failure of normal erythropoietic maturation with macrocytosis, megaloblastosis, and intramedullary hemolysis resulting in multilobed polys and anemia. It is important to remember that vitamin B_{12} deficiency may present solely as a nonspecific, neuropsychiatric disease in the absence of hematologic abnormalities (29,105–108). Large doses of folic acid may partially correct the hematologic abnormalities of vitamin B_{12} deficiency without affecting the course of neurologic complications. Therefore, B_{12} (and folate) levels should be determined in all older patients with intellectual impairment.

Vitamin B_{12} deficiency, but not folic acid deficiency, can be associated with subacute combined demyelination of the lateral and dorsal columns of the spinal cord. This condition is manifested by paresthesias and marked peripheral sensory loss, especially vibratory sense and proprioception, unsteady gait, foot drop, and spastic limbs with hyperactive deep tendon reflexes. The neurologic abnormalities may not be reversible with vitamin B_{12} replacement.

The Schilling test is usually part of the evaluation of the etiology of cobalamin deficiency. It helps determine whether the disorder is caused by intrinsic factor (IF) deficiency. It is now known that test results may be misinterpreted if the patient is able to absorb free oral B_{12} as given in the classic Shilling test, but remains unable to release and absorb normally ingested meat-bound B_{12} because of decreased gastric acid production (108).

Vitamin B_{12} deficiency secondary to small bowel bacterial contamination may be treated by increasing B_{12} supplementation, even if the bacterial overgrowth is resistant to antibiotic therapy (109).

Patients with pernicious anemia are usually treated with intramuscular injections of cyanocobalamin, initially daily, then weekly, and finally monthly for life. The usual maintenance dose is 100 μg once a month, although this appears higher than actually required (about 30 μg a month) for maximum hematopoiesis. A small percentage of high oral doses can be absorbed even in the absence of IF, making this an alternative method of replacement if the patient is unable to tolerate injections or visit a physician regularly. To avoid acute hypokalemia, serum potassium levels should be closely monitored during the first few days of vitamin B_{12} replacement in patients with pernicious anemia. Patients with pernicious anemia have an increased incidence of gastric and colon carcinomas.

There is often an intense feeling of well-being and increased appetite in the first few days of vitamin B_{12} replacement. It is this clinical response, seen only in patients who are truly vitamin B_{12} deficient, that has led to the undesirable practice of placebo vitamin B_{12} injections in persons without pernicious anemia or B_{12} deficiency.

Toxicity

There is little adverse effect of even large doses of oral or intramuscular vitamin B_{12}.

FOLIC ACID

Function

Folic acid, derived from the Latin word "folia" meaning leaf, is a cofactor in purine and pyrimidine synthesis, as well as in serine, methionine, glycine, and choline synthesis.

Assessment

Both serum and RBC folate levels are available, and both are fairly good reflections of tissue folate levels (32); serum folate tends to reflect recent intake, whereas RBC folate indicates folate status at the time of RBC formation because red cells take up very little folate when mature. Because serum folate levels tend to increase and RBC levels decrease in the presence of vitamin B_{12} deficiency (32), RBC folate is not useful in differentiating folate from B_{12} deficiency. In addition, in the presence of an anemia not secondary to B_{12} or folate deficiency, RBC folate increases with increasing anemia (102). In general, serum folate is probably the most cost-effective screening tool for folate deficiency.

The deoxyuridine (dU) suppression test on bone marrow cells or peripheral lymphocytes may prove useful in detecting folate deficiency in the presence of iron deficiency and in differentiating folate from vitamin B_{12} deficiency (104).

Risk Factors

Folate deficiency is common in community-dwelling as well as institutionalized elderly and is present in up to one-quarter of subjects (110). Folate levels are often reduced in those with low socioeconomic status, physical disabilities or who abuse alcohol. Methotrexate, pentamidine, trimethoprim, and triamterene are folate antagonists, and anticonvulsants (phenytoin, phenobarbitol, and primidone) and sulfasalazine inhibit folate absorption (111). Folate conjugase may decrease with age (7). Therefore, what appears to be nutritionally adequate may not supply sufficient amount of folate in some elderly. Atrophic gastritis is common in the elderly and may contribute to folate malabsorption, but it may be compensated for by increased bacterial folate synthesis due to secondary bacterial overgrowth as gastric acidity decreases (9,28). Any interference with the enterohepatic cycle or pathology of the jejunum increases the risk of folate deficiency. Vitamin B_{12} deficiency causes a secondary decrease in intracellular folic acid.

Deficiency

The RDA for folate is 200 µg for males and 180 µg for females. This RDA is much lower than the 1980 RDA of 400 µg (112,113). Nevertheless, folate deficiency is common in the poor or alcoholic elderly.

The classic study of folate deficiency in one healthy 35-year-old subject was published by Herbert in 1962 (114). The course in debilitated patients may be faster. Serum folate falls after 3 weeks on an experimentally deficient diet. Hypersegmentation of polymorphonuclear cells (polys) appears after 7 weeks of deprivation. The recognition of one six-lobed poly may be a simpler method of detecting significant hypersegmentation than other lobe index evaluations (115). The detection of a six-lobed poly may also be useful in detecting folate deficiency in patients who are iron deficient. Depleted tissue stores are seen as a low RBC folate after 17 weeks.

Macro-ovalocytes occur at 18 weeks. Normal-sized ovalocytes are non-specific, as are macrocytes. The recognition of macrocytosis, made easier by the calculation of mean corpuscular volume (MCV) by automated blood count machines, is remarkably nonsensitive, as macrocytes are found in only 59% of patients with folate deficiency (116).

Megaloblastosis occurs after 19 weeks on a folate-deficient diet. It may be masked if iron deficiency is also present. Subsequent intramedullary hemolysis causes increases in serum lactic dehydrogenase (LDH), indirect bilirubin, and transferrin saturation. The resulting anemia is usually well tolerated.

The signs and symptoms of folate deficiency are similar to those of vitamin B_{12} deficiency, except that subacute combined spinal cord degeneration does not occur with folate deficiency.

Mental status changes consistent with a dementia syndrome may occur with folate deficiency, even before the appearance of the anemia, and measurement of both vitamin B_{12} and folate levels are indicated in all elderly patients with intellectual dysfunction.

Toxicity

Folate intake is usually well tolerated in high doses with only occasional gastrointestinal disturbances. The concern with indiscriminate folate use is that it may mask the hematologic signs of pernicious anemia and yet allow the neurologic degeneration to progress and become irreversible. Folic acid and phenytoin inhibit uptake of each other, and very large doses of folic acid may precipitate convulsions in persons whose epilepsy is controlled by phenytoin (113).

NIACIN—NICOTINIC ACID

Function

Nicotinic acid and nicotinamide are converted to NAD and NADP, which are used as coenzymes with dehydrogenases in oxidation-reduction reactions in metabolism. Nicotinic acid also has clinically relevant action at pharmacologic doses. It causes vasodilation, and a trial of its use may be warranted in the therapy of migraine or peripheral vascular disease, beginning at 100 to 300 mg a day. High doses of nicotinic acid are also known to lower serum cholesterol. This effect is not seen with nicotinamide or nicotinic acid metabolites (95).

Assessment

Biochemical measurements do not accurately assess niacin status at present.

Risk Factors

Pure niacin deficiency is now rare, and deficiency normally occurs in association with general malnutrition or chronic alcoholism, except in maize-eating areas where tryptophan, a niacin precursor, is also lacking. Isoniazid, an antitubercular drug, may act as an antagonist (1). Niacin is poorly available from many cereal grains. Leucine, present in high concentrations in millet, a staple food in parts of India, is felt to increase niacin requirements by inhibiting NAD and NADP synthesis. Clinical deficiency is complicated and appears to be also related to food processing techniques and an imbalance of dietary protein, and not solely due to nicotinic acid deficiency (117). Deficiency may be caused by chronic intestinal hypermotility or be an occasional secondary manifestation of carcinoid syndrome associated with increased tryptophan catabolism.

Deficiency

The RDA for niacin is 16NE (one NE or niacin equivalent = 1 mg niacin) for men and 13 NE for women, or 6.6 NE/1,000 kcal a day (minimum = 13 NE). Sixty milligrams of tryptophan is equivalent to 1 NE of niacin. The classic deficiency state is pellegra (*pelle* = skin, *agra* = rough). Pellegra is characterized by the "three Ds": diarrhea, dermatitis, and dementia. Gastrointestinal symptoms are often the first to appear with stomatitis and a beefy red and swollen tongue. The condition eventually progresses to anorexia, nausea and vomiting, steatorrhea, and diarrhea.

The dermatitis presents as symmetric, sharply demarcated areas on sunlight-exposed skin, such as the backs of hands, forehead, and neck. These areas are dry, discolored, scaly with hyperkeratosis, and chronically inflamed with dermal edema.

Mental status changes, which may occur as a sole manifestation of niacin deficiency, include headache, lassitude, depression, failing memory, and confusion. A peripheral neuritis may occur if pellegra is complicated by a coexisting thiamine deficiency.

Toxicity

Doses of nicotinic acid above 200 mg/day are frequently associated with flushing, pruritis, altered glucose tolerance in diabetics, increased pain in peptic ulcer disease, and abnormal plasma uric acid and liver function tests (45). The side effect of flushing may often be reduced by starting at low doses, increasing slowly, taking an aspirin before the niacin, taking it with food, or using a sustained-release formula. Doses necessary to see an effect on cholesterol levels may range from 1 to 8 g/day.

BIOTIN

Function

Biotin plays a role in the formation of oxaloacetic acid and succinic acid, in purine and pyrimidine synthesis, and is a cofactor in the carboxylation of pyruvate and acetyl and proprionyl coenzyme A.

Assessment

Plasma levels of biotin are available, but have minimal clinical utility.

Risk Factors

Prolonged anticonvulsant use may be a factor in biotin deficiency. In addition, biotin may be bound and inactivated by avidin protein found in raw egg whites. Consumption of sufficient raw egg whites to cause biotin deficiency is clinically rare. Antimicrobial agents that destroy intestinal flora may decrease biotin bacterial synthesis. Failure to add biotin to parenteral nutrition formulae has caused biotin deficiency (118).

Deficiency

An official RDA for biotin is not yet established; however a daily intake of 30 to 100 μg is recommended (24). Nonspecific signs and symptoms of deficiency include glossitis, paresthesias, muscle pains, alopecia, dermatitis, nausea and anorexia.

Toxicity

High intake of biotin has no known side effects.

PANTOTHENIC ACID

Function

Pantothenic acid is used to make acetyl-coenzyme A that in turn is important in acetylation reactions, including the Kreb's cycle, and cholesterol, steroid, and porphyrin formation.

Assessment

Blood levels of pantothenic acid are available, but are rarely clinically useful.

Risk Factors

Deficiency of pantothenic acid is most likely associated with general malnutrition and alcoholism.

Deficiency

Most studies involving pantothenic acid are in animals, and their relationship to human disorders, particularly in elderly persons, is unknown. There is no RDA for pantothenic acid; it is estimated that 4 to 7 mg a day is adequate in adults (24). There is speculation that a deficiency of pantothenic acid results in nonspecific signs and symptoms, perhaps related to mild adrenal insufficiency, such as irritability, fatigue, sleep disturbances, and muscle cramps. Deficiency may be accompanied by a "burning feet" syndrome, also seen with riboflavin and niacin deficiencies, and characterized by paresthesias and circulatory disturbances in the feet. There are unproven claims for a role for pantothenic acid in the treatment of dermatitis of various kinds, postoperative ileus, and adrenal insufficiency (119).

Toxicity

Doses up to 10 g/day of calcium pantothenate have been tolerated without symptoms. Long-term toxicity in the elderly is unknown.

VITAMIN C—ASCORBIC ACID

Function

Some of the principal known functions of ascorbic acid include (a) cofactor for iron and copper absorption and metabolism; (b) free radical scavenger; (c) cofactor in the conversion of dopamine to norepinephrine; (d) stimulation of leukocyte phagocytic activity and antibody formation; (e) formation of hydroxyproline in collagen synthesis; (f) improved tissue repair and wound healing; (g) an electron donor in the metabolism of folic acid and tyrosine; (h) involvement in the synthesis of carnitine, steroids, and formation of bile acids; (i) cofactor in the conversion of tryptophan to 5-hydroxy-tryptophan; (j) and increasing maximum oxygen utilization in exercise (1,120). Ascorbic acid is known to inhibit the formation of N-nitroso compounds, which are known carcinogens, in the gastrointestinal tract (121).

Assessment

Ascorbic acid levels can be measured in the plasma, urine, platelets, or leukocytes. Measurement of levels in leukocytes (buffy coat) may be falsely low in the presence of a leukocytosis or after a myocardial infarction, surgery, or illness. An ascorbic acid tolerance test has been proposed as a better measure of vitamin C status (122).

Risk Factors

Primates, guinea pigs, and some bats are the only mammals that cannot synthesize ascorbic acid endogenously. Many elderly are at risk for decreased intake of ascorbic acid, especially those who are poor, male, living alone ("bachelor scurvy"), hospitalized, or institutionalized (123–125). Elderly men have lower vitamin C levels than elderly women when intake is identical (126), which appears to be due to decreased tubular reabsorption in men (127). There is no evidence of a decrease in intestinal absorption with age.

There is an inverse relationship between smoking and plasma ascorbic acid levels, even in light smokers (124). Smokers tend to have 20 to 50% lower vitamin C levels (26). Achlorhydria, frequently associated with gastric atrophy and pernicious anemia, reduces vitamin C absorption. Patients with rheumatoid arthritis metabolize ascorbic acid at a faster than normal rate and may require supplementation (128).

Deficiency

A grossly inadequate intake of ascorbic acid results in scurvy. Signs of scurvy appear 24 to 120 days after total vitamin C deprivation (26,124). Plasma levels may become undetectable after 40 days. The "four Hs" of scurvy (26) are (a) *h*emorrhagic signs, presenting initially as minute, perifollicular, hemorrhagic points, especially at sites of stress and trauma because of capillary fragility, followed by bleeding gums, purpura beginning on the back and the lower extremities, and bleeding into joints and muscles; (b) *h*yperkeratosis of hair follicles and coiled hairs, particularly on the outer aspects of the arms and thighs and on the abdomen; (c) *h*ypochondriasis with lassitude, weakness, and muscle pains; and (d) *h*ematologic abnormalities, with anemia exacerbated by reduced iron absorption or abnormal folate metabolism.

The daily intake of as little as 10 mg ascorbic acid prevents frank scurvy (24). However, how much ascorbic acid is sufficient to avoid other deficiency states remains controversial. The current RDA is 60 mg for both men and women over age 51; this is increased to 100 mg/day in cigarette smokers (24). Arguments have been presented that intake can be safely lowered to 40 mg and 30 mg daily in men and women, respectively, (120) or should be increased to 125 mg a day for men and 75 mg a day for women (127) or even higher (129). The controversy revolves around estimates of total body pools, importance of tissue saturation, kidney thresholds, potential toxicity, comparison with requirements recommended by other countries, the safety amount needed for reserves, and the potential role of vitamin C as an anticarcinogen. Until a consensus is reached, the clinician should ensure that his normal patients absorb at least 100 mg/day of ascorbic acid. This amount may be modified up or down if exceptional demands, such as severe malnutrition, extensive surgery, or sepsis, or potential iron toxicity (eg, hemochromatosis) are present. Smokers do require higher daily intake. Vitamin C appears necessary for transformation of cholesterol to bile acids, and it has been recommended that therapy for hyperlipidemia include an adequate ascorbic acid intake (124,129). The addition of aspirin to an ascorbic-acid-deficient diet may increase the possibility of gastric mucosal bleeding, so patients taking aspirin should also have an adequate vitamin C intake. Also, there is some indication that ascorbic acid deficiency may be involved in the pathogenesis of atherosclerosis (130).

Despite the considerable attention brought by Linus Pauling and others concerning the potential value of much higher doses of ascorbic acid, controlled scientific studies have provided little support for a role for vitamin C supplementation either in viral infection prevention (131,132), cancer prevention (133), or cancer therapy (134,135).

Toxicity

As ascorbic acid intake increases up to 90 to 150 mg/day, there is a sharp rise in plasma levels, followed by a plateau or a very gradual rise as absorption efficiency decreases and kidney tubular reabsorption is exceeded (19,136).

The most common side effect of high-dose vitamin C ingestion is occasional diarrhea. Supplementation of vitamin C averaging 300 mg/day in a healthy elderly population does not affect iron or copper levels dangerously (137). Although iron absorption improves in the presence of ascorbic acid, total body iron is not appreciably affected by long-term vitamin C use (120). However, patients who are prone to iron intoxication (eg, those with hemochromatosis, thalassemia, or sideroblastic anemia) should not take vitamin C supplements. Vitamin C also appears to stabilize ferritin intracellularly (138).

Rebound scurvy, suppression of cobalamin (B_{12}) absorption, and oxalate or urate kidney stone formation have not been proven to be important consequences of ascorbic acid use in adults. There is one report of an increased incidence of thrombotic episodes associated with use of 200 mg vitamin C in geriatric patients (139). Vitamin C decreases renal tubular reabsorption of amphetamines and tricyclic antidepressants and increases reabsorption of salicylates, but these effects are not known to be significant clinically (46). Ascorbic acid may affect the accuracy of certain laboratory tests; ingestion of over 1 g/day may reduce the accuracy of fecal and urinary occult blood tests and serum glucose measurements.

CONCLUSION

Vitamin disorders are common in the elderly. To consider the diagnosis, a high index of suspicion in the appropriate clinical setting is required (117). The presence of coexisting disease can distract the clinician from considering nutritional disorders or their prevention and mask serious nutritional deficits. Ideally, all persons should be able to obtain their vitamin intake from a nutritionally balanced diet without the need for supplements (25). Sometimes all that is required to prevent or correct a vitamin disorder is patient education about food preparation and storage or to modify vitamin-nutrient or drug-vitamin interactions. In reality, however, these steps are not always successful or sufficient in many elderly persons; nutritional intervention and appropriate supplementation may be required as well (140). To be sure, supplementation still does not exclude the possibility of continuing deficiency. In turn, patients also need instructions that vitamins are drugs and can be toxic and therefore, more is not better. In every medication history, vitamin intake must be specifically questioned because vitamin consumption is frequently forgotten. Much remains unknown about vitamin requirements in the elderly, especially regarding subclinical deficiencies. Health care professionals must establish a clear position as advocates for nutritional health and reform and monitor all of their patients closely for potential vitamin-related disorders.

REFERENCES

1. Marks J. *The vitamins: their role in medical practice.* Hingham MA: MTP Press, 1985.
2. Sobal J, Muncie Jr HL, Baker AS. *Gerontologist* 1986;26:187–191.

3. Ranno BS, Wardlaw GM, Geiger CJ. *J Am Dietet Soc* 1988;88:347–348.
4. Exton-Smith AN. *Proc Roy Soc Med* 1977;70:615–619.
5. Brin M, Bauernfeind JC. *Postgrad Med* 1978;63:155–163.
6. Baker H, Frank O, Thind IS, et al. *J Am Geriatr Soc* 1979;27:444–450.
7. Baker H, Frank O. In: Hanck A, Hornig D, eds. *Vitamins: Nutrients and therapeutic agents.* Bern, Switzerland: Hans Huber, 1985;47–59.
8. Henderson CT. *Clin Geriatr Med* 1988;4:527–547.
9. Munro HN, Suter PM, Russell RM. *Ann Rev Nutr* 1987;7:23–49.
10. US Department of Health, Education, and Welfare. *Ten-state nutrition survey 1968–1970.* Atlanta: Center for Disease Control, 1972 (DHEW Publ. No. (HSM) 72-8130 to 8134).
11. US Department of Agriculture, Science and Education Administration. *Nutrient levels in food used by households in the US, Spring, 1977. Nationwide food consumption survey, 1977–78,* preliminary report No. 3. Washington, DC: USDA, 1980.
12. National Health Statistics. *Plan and operation of the National Health and Nutrition Examination Survey, 1971–1973. Vital and health statistics,* series I, no. 10. Washington, DC: US Government Printing Office, 1975 (DHEW Publ. No. (HSM) 73-1310).
13. Public Health Service. *Plan and operation of the Second National Health and Nutrition Examination Survey, 1976–1980. Vital and health statistics,* series 1, no. 232. Washington, DC: US Government Printing Office, 1982 (DHHS Publ. No. (PHS) 81-1317).
14. Young EA. *Am J Clin Nutr* 1982;36:979–985.
15. Omdahl JL, Garry PJ, Hunsaker LA, et al. *Am J Clin Nutr* 1982;36:1125–1133.
16. Hartz SC, Otradovec CL, McGandy RB, et al. *J Am Coll Nutr* 1988;7: 119–128.
17. Bowman BB, Rosenberg IH. *Am J Clin Nutr* 1982;35:1142–1151.
18. Schneider EL, Vining EM, Hadley EC, et al. *N Engl J Med* 1986;314:157–160.
19. Garry PJ, Hunt WC. In: Hutchinson ML, Munro HN, eds. *Nutrition and aging.* Orlando, FL: Academic Press, 1986;117–136.
20. Suter PM, Russell RM. *Am J Clin Nutr* 1987;45:501–512.
21. Exton-Smith AN. *Am J Clin Nutr* 1982;35:1273–1279.
22. *The surgeon general's report on nutrition and health: 1988.* Washington, DC: US Government Printing Office, 1988; 595–627 (DHHS (PHS) No. 88-50210).
23. Sauberlich HE. In: Chen LH, ed. *Nutritional aspects of aging,* vol I. Boca Raton, FL: CRC Press, 1986;131–157.
24. Subcommittee on the Tenth Edition of the RDAs, Food and Nutrition Board, Commission on Life Sciences, National Research Council. *Recommended dietary allowances,* 10th ed. Washington, DC: National Academy Press, 1989.
25. Council on Scientific Affairs. *JAMA* 1987;257:1929–1936.
26. Gerster H. *Z Ernahrungswiss* 1987;26:125–137.
27. Rivlin RS. *Am J Clin Nutr* 1982;36:1083–1086.
28. Russell RM. In: Hutchinson ML, Munro HN, eds. *Nutrition and aging.* Orlando, FL: Academic Press, 1986;59–67.
29. Flint DM, Prinsley DM. In: Briggs MH, ed. *Vitamins in human biology and medicine.* Boca Raton, FL: CRC Press, 1981;65–79.
30. Sklan D. *Prog Food Nutr Sci* 1987;11:39–55.
31. Comstock GW, Menkes MS, Schober SE, et al. *Am J Epidemiol* 1988;127:114–123.
32. Bamji MS. In: Briggs MH, ed. *Vitamins in human biology and medicine.* Boca Raton, FL: CRC Press, 1981;1–27.
33. Stryker WS, Kaplan LA, Stein EA, et al. *Am J Epidemiol* 1988;127:283–296.
34. Watkin DM. *Handbook of nutrition, health and aging.* Park Ridge, NJ: Noyes Publications, 1983.
35. Garry PJ, Hunt WC, Bandrofchak JL, et al. *Am J Clin Nutr* 1987;46:989–994.
36. Olson JA. *Am J Clin Nutr* 1987;45:704–716.
37. Jones G. In: Chen LH, ed. *Nutritional aspects of aging,* vol I. Boca Raton, FL: CRC Press, 1986;195–212.
38. Menkes MS, Comstock GW, Vuilleumier JP, et al. *N Engl J Med* 1986;315:1250–1254.
39. Ong DE, Chytil F. *Vitam Horm* 1983;40:105–144.
40. Willett WC, Polk BF, Underwood BA, et al. *N Engl J Med* 1984;310:430–434.
41. Hennekens CH, Mayrent SL, Willett W. *Cancer* 1986;58:1837–1841.
42. Wald N. *Cancer Surv* 1987;6:635–651.

43. Gilchrest BA, Gordon PR. In: Hutchinson ML, Munro HN, eds. *Nutrition and aging.* Orlando, FL: Academic Press, 1986;35–42.
44. Vakil DV, Ayiomamitis A, Nizami N, et al. *Nutr Res* 1985;5:911–917.
45. Micozzi MS, Brown ED, Taylor PR, et al. *Am J Clin Nutr* 1988;48:1061–1064.
46. Briggs MH, Briggs M, Cumming F. In: Briggs MH, ed. *Vitamins in human biology and medicine.* Boca Raton, FL: CRC Press, 1981;187–243.
47. Roe D. *Geriatric nutrition,* 2nd ed. Englewood Cliffs, NJ: Prentice-Hall, 1987.
48. Korner WF, Vollm J. *Int J Vitam Nutr Res* 1975;45:363–372.
49. DeLuca HF, Ostrem V. *Adv Exp Med Biol* 1986;206:413–429.
50. Vitamin D and insulin secretion. *Nutr Rev* 1986;44:375–377.
51. Reichel H, Koeffler HP, Norman AW. *N Engl J Med* 1989;320:980–991.
52. Parfitt AM, Gallagher JC, Heaney RP, et al. *Am J Clin Nutr* 1982;36:1014–1031.
53. Dunnigan MG, Fraser SA, McIntosh WB, et al. *Scot Med J* 1986;31:144–149.
54. Delvin EE, Imbach A, Copti M. *Am J Clin Nutr* 1988;48:373–378.
55. Fleming BB, Barrows CH. *Exp Gerontol* 1982;17:115–120.
56. Holick MF. In: Hutchinson ML, Munro HN, eds. *Nutrition and aging.* Orlando, FL: Academic Press, 1986;45–57.
57. MacLaughlin J, Holick MF. *J Clin Invest* 1985;76:1536–1538.
58. Lore F, DiCairano G, DiPerri G. *Ann Med Interne* 1986;137:209–211.
59. Reid IR, Gallagher DJA, Bosworth J. *Age Aging* 1986;15:35–40.
60. Sem SW, Sjoen RJ, Trygg K, et al. *Compr Gerontol A* 1987;1:126–130.
61. Matsuoka LY, Wortsman J, Hanifan N, et al. *Arch Dermatol* 1988;124:1802–1804.
62. Egsmose C, Lund B, McNair P, et al. *Age Aging* 1987;16:35–40.
63. Ott SM, Chesnutt CH III. *Ann Intern Med* 1989;110:267–274.
64. Harju E, Sotaniemi E, Puranen J, et al. *Arch Orthop Trauma Surg* 1985;103:408–416.
65. Lips P, VanGinkel FC, Jongen MJM, et al. *Am J Clin Nutr* 1987;46:1005–1010.
66. Vitamin D supplementation in the elderly. *Lancet* 1987;1:306–307.
67. Davies M, Mawer EB, Hann JT, et al. *Age Aging* 1985;14:349–354.
68. Weisman Y, Schen RJ, Eisenberg Z, et al. *J Am Geriatr Soc* 1986;34:515–518.
69. Schwartzman MS, Franck WA. *Am J Med* 1987;82:224–230.
70. Knekt P, Aromaa A, Maatela J, et al. *Am J Epidemiol* 1988;127:28–41.
71. Parsa FD. *Plast Reconstr Surg* 1988;81:300–301.
72. Haeger K. *Am J Clin Nutr* 1974;27:1179–1181.
73. New functional tests of vitamin E status in humans. *Nutr Rev* 1988;46:182–184.
74. Vandewoude MFJ, Vandewoude MG. *J Am Coll Nutr* 1987;6:307–311.
75. Niki E. *Ann NY Acad Sci* 1987;498:186–199.
76. Vatassery GT, Johnson GJ, Krezowski AM. *J Am Coll Nutr* 1983;2:369–375.
77. Vatassery GT, Krezowski AM, Eckfeldt JH. *Am J Clin Nutr* 1983;37:1020–1024.
78. Horwitt MK. *Am J Clin Nutr* 1986;44:973–985.
79. Morrow MJ. *Bull Clin Neurosci* 1985;50:53–60.
80. Wald NJ, Thompson SG, Densem JW, et al. *Br J Cancer* 1987;56:69–72.
81. Bendich A, Machlin LJ. *Am J Clin Nutr* 1988;48:612–619.
82. Dahl S. *Lancet* 1974;1:465.
83. Hanck A, Weiser H. In: Hanck A, Hornig D, eds. *Vitamins: Nutrients and therapeutic agents.* Bern, Switzerland: Hans Huber, 1985;189–206.
84. Drinka PJ, Bauwens SF. *J Am Geriatr Soc* 1987;35:258–261.
85. Iber FL, Shamszad M, Miller PA, et al. *Alcohol: Clin Exp Res* 1986;10:679–681.
86. Olson JA. *Am J Clin Nutr* 1987;45:687–692.
87. Markkanen T, Heikinheimo R, Dahl M. *Acta Haematol (Basel)* 1969;42:148–153.
88. Iber FL, Blass JP, Brin M. *Am J Clin Nutr* 1982;36:1067–1082.
89. Saito N, Kimura M, Kuchiba A, et al. *J Nutr Sci Vitam* 1987;33:421–430.
90. Kutsky RJ. *Handbook of vitamins and hormones.* New York: Van Nostrand Reinhold, 1973.
91. Gibson GE, Sheu KR, Blass JP, et al. *Arch Neurol* 1988;45:836–840.
92. Pinto JT, Rivlin RS. *Drug-Nutr Interact* 1987;5:143–151.
93. Driskell JA. In: Chen LH, ed. *Nutritional aspects of aging,* vol I. Boca Raton, FL: CRC Press, 1986;227–253.
94. Bauernfeind JC, Miller ON. In: *Human vitamin B_6 requirements.* Washington, DC: National Academy of Sciences, 1978;78–110.

95. Marcus R, Coulston AM. In: Gilman AG, Goodman LS, Rall TW, et al., eds. *The pharmacological basis of therapeutics,*7th ed. New York: MacMillan, 1985;1551–1572.
96. Hillman RS. In: Gilman AG, Goodman LS, Rall TW, et al., eds. *The pharmacological basis of therapeutics,* 7th ed. New York: MacMillan, 1985;1323–1337.
97. Herbert V. *Am J Clin Nutr* 1987;45:671–678.
98. Matchar DB, Feussner JR, Watson DJ, et al. *J Am Geriatr Soc* 1986;34A:680–681.
99. Thompson WG, Babitz L, Cassino C, et al. *Am J Med* 1987;82:291–294.
100. Carmel R. *Arch Intern Med* 1988;148:1712–1714.
101. Elsborg L, Lund V, Bastrup-Madsen P. *Acta Med Scand* 1976;200:309–314.
102. Magnus EM, Bache-Wiig JE, Aanderson TR, et al. *Scand J Haematol* 1982;28:360–366.
103. Marcus DL, Shadick N, Crantz J, et al. *J Am Geriatr Soc* 1987;35:635–638.
104. Herbert V. *Lab Invest* 1985;52:3–19.
105. Herbert V. *Arch Intern Med* 1988;148:1705–1707.
106. Karnaze DS, Carmel R. *Arch Intern Med* 1987;147:429–431.
107. Lindenbaum J, Healton EB, Savage DG, et al. *N Engl J Med* 1988;318:1720–1728.
108. Carmel R, Sinow RM, Siegel ME, et al. *Arch Intern Med* 1988;148:1715–1719.
109. Chesner IM, Montgomery RD. *J Clin Gastroenterol* 1986;8:447–450.
110. Webster SGP, Leeming JT. *J Am Geriatr Soc* 1979;27:451–454.
111. Sulfasalazine inhibits folate absorption. *Nutr Rev* 1988;46:320–323.
112. Rosenberg IH, Bowman BB, Cooper BA, et al. *Am J Clin Nutr* 1982;36:1060–1066.
113. Herbert V. *Am J Clin Nutr* 1987;45:661–670.
114. Herbert V. *Trans Assoc Am Phys* 1962;75:307–320.
115. Colman N. *Clin Lab Med* 1981;1:775–796.
116. Shorvon SD, Carney MWP, Chanarin I, et al. *Br Med J* 1980;281:1036–1038.
117. Wilson JD. In: Braunwald E, Isselbacher KJ, Petersdorf PG, et al, eds. *Harrison's principles of internal medicine,* 11th ed. New York: McGraw-Hill, 1987;410–418.
118. Biotin deficiency due to total parenteral nutrition alters serum fatty acid composition. *Nutr Rev* 1989;47:121–123.
119. Fidanza A. In: Hanck A, ed. *Vitamins in medicine-recent therapeutic aspects.* Bern, Switzerland: Hans Huber, 1983;53–68.
120. Olson JA, Hodges RE. *Am J Clin Nutr* 1987;45:693–703.
121. Mirvish SS. *Cancer* 1986;58:1842–1850.
122. Neale RJ, Lim H, Turner J, et al. *Age Aging* 1988;17:35–41.
123. McClean HE, Dodds PM, Stewart AW, et al. *NZ Med J* 1976;84:345–348.
124. Cheng L, Cohen M, Bhagavan HN. In: Watson RR, ed. *CRC handbook of nutrition in the aged.* Boca Raton, FL: CRC Press, 1986;157–185.
125. Porrini M, Simonetti P, Ciapellano S, et al. *Int J Vitam Nutr Res* 1987;57:349–355.
126. VanderJagt DJ, Garry PJ, Bhagavan HN. *Am J Clin Nutr* 1987;46:290–294.
127. Garry PJ, VanderJagt DJ, Hunt WC. *Ann NY Acad Sci* 1987;498:90–99.
128. Mullen A, Wilson CWM. *Proc Nutr Soc* 1976;35:8A–9A.
129. Ginter E. In: Briggs MH, ed. *Vitamins in human biology and medicine.* Boca Raton, FL: CRC Press, 1981;95–106.
130. Ramirez J, Flowers NC. *Am J Clin Nutr* 1980;33:2079–2087.
131. Chalmers TC. *Am J Med* 1975;58:532–536.
132. Briggs M. In: Briggs MH, ed. *Recent vitamin research.* Boca Raton, FL: CRC Press, 1984;39–82.
133. Hanck A. *Prog Clin Biol Res* 1988;259:307–320.
134. Pauling L, Moertel C. *Nutr Rev* 1986;44:28–32.
135. Vitamin C and mortality. *Nutr Rev* 1987;45:77–78.
136. Spector R. In: Briggs MH, ed. *Vitamins in human biology and medicine.* Boca Raton, FL: CRC Press, 1981;137–156.
137. Jacob RA, Otradovec CL, Russell RM, et al. *Am J Clin Nutr* 1988;48:1436–1442.
138. Vitamin C stabilizes ferritin: New insights into iron-ascorbate interactions. *Nutr Rev* 1987;45:217–218.
139. Andrews CT, Wilson TS. *Lancet* 1973;2:39 (1973).
140. Kohrs MB. In: Hutchinson ML, Munro HN, eds. *Nutrition and aging.* Orlando, FL: Academic Press, 1986;139–166.

Geriatric Nutrition, edited by John E. Morley,
Zvi Glick, Laurence Z. Rubenstein.
Raven Press, Ltd., New York © 1990.

10

Calcium, Vitamin D, and Osteopenia in the Elderly

Arnold S. Brickman

*Department of Medicine, UCLA School of Medicine,
Los Angeles, California 90024 and
Mineral Metabolism Section, VA Medical Center,
Sepulveda, California 91343*

Loss of bone with aging appears to be an inevitable process. However, the rate at which bone is lost can vary and is affected by a large number of variables. These include sex, race, nutritional factors, physical activity, comorbid disease states, changes in the steady state secretion and functional activity of calcitrophic hormones, and probable age-related changes in the function of the bone cells, eg, osteoclasts, osteoblasts. Although genetic factors play a role in the development of peak bone mass, their role in determining the rate or degree of bone loss is unknown. Although considerable insight has been gained about how interactions among these variables can contribute to the dynamic processes of bone remodeling, it has remained difficult to separate effects of aging *per se* from the component of bone loss attributable to one or more of these confounding variables.

This article examines dietary calcium intake and calcium balance, and vitamin D status as they relate to development of osteopenia in the aging and the elderly.

DIETARY INTAKE OF CALCIUM

In the United States the recommended daily allowance (RDA) for calcium in adult men and women has been set at 800 mg. In reality, it has been recognized for many years that this figure is only an estimate of calcium needs because such requirements are constantly changing throughout life and there are inherent difficulties in determining the exact mineral requirements in man. Indeed, some nutritionists have suggested that the RDA for calcium should be considered as an estimate of minimum need. An RDA of 1,200 mg/day of calcium is currently recommended to meet the needs of the rapidly growing skeleton during the preadolescent and adolescent years in the majority of individuals. However, skeletal growth extends into the third and fourth decades of life, suggesting that in many young adults a higher dietary intake of calcium may be required to provide for the needs of the maturing and consolidating skeleton.

The calcium requirement of older individuals under many circumstances is also frequently increased beyond 800 mg/day. In older adults, the issue of calcium nutritional requirements is no longer focused on skeletal growth and maturation, but rather the need to ensure adequate intake to compensate for accelerated bone mineral losses, (ie, to maintain calcium balance. These mineral losses are attributable to multiple physiologic and pathologic changes that accompany aging. Conditions associated with aging or occurring more commonly in order or elderly individuals and that increase dietary calcium requirements include the menopause in females, decreased effective intestinal calcium absorption with aging, and prolonged states of negative calcium balance. This negative calcium balance may be attributable to chronic illness and periods of immobilization, decreased physical activity, reduction in muscle mass, comorbid illnesses, or treatment with medications that increase calcium losses.

Several major nutrition surveys conducted in the United States by the Public Health Service NHANES I and NHANES II (National Health and Nutrition Examination Surveys) and the Department of Agriculture (Food Consumption Surveys) have confirmed that, from childhood on, many individuals ingest diets providing substantially less than the RDA for calcium. For women, these and other surveys have shown that the median intake of calcium from the middle of the second decade of life on is well below 800 mg/day and continues to decline throughout life (1-3). Most importantly, daily median intake in many women is less than 600 mg during the years between the ages of 20 to 40 years, the period during which peak bone mass is achieved and after which a decline in bone mass begins. Although the median intake of calcium is significantly higher in men, they too show a continuing decline in dietary calcium intake with aging. In both sexes, as a consequence of substantially lower dietary intake, calcium deficiencies syndromes may occur. Thus, habitual low calcium intake has been associated with the development of hypertension, carcinoma of the colon, peridontal disease, and osteoporosis.

INCREASED CALCIUM REQUIREMENTS IN OLDER ADULTS

Menopause

In women, the onset of menopause is associated with several physiologic changes that can result in a prolonged state of negative calcium balance. In

TABLE 1. *Factors contributing to negative calcium balance in the elderly*

Inadequate dietary calcium intake
Calcium malabsorption
Nutrient-nutrient interactions
   Protein intake
   Phosphorus content
   Fiber content
Immobilization/illness
Lack of exercise
Confounding metabolic disorders
Medications

some individuals this negative calcium balance will result in the development of osteoporosis. Among the changes that occur are increased bone resorption relative to formation, increased urinary calcium losses, and decreased intestinal absorption of calcium. In this setting a dietary calcium intake at the level of the RDA is insufficient to prevent a state of negative calcium balance. Extensive metabolic balance studies performed in pre- and perimenopausal and untreated (estrogen-deficient) postmenopausal women have indicated that a daily calcium intake at or in excess of 1,000 to 1,500 mg is required to maintain a state of calcium balance (4). In some women, treatment with calcium supplements, which provide a total calcium intake at this level, can be as effective as treatment with estrogen in achieving calcium balance (5). Moreover, use of calcium supplements has been shown to reduce the dose of estrogen required to normalize calcium losses in postmenopausal women (6). Recently the RDA committee of the National Research Council (National Academy of Sciences) has recommended an RDA of 1,000 mg/day of calcium.

Immobilization, Chronic Illness, and Decreased Physical Exercise

Chronic illness (including recovery from surgery) is frequently associated with prolonged periods of absolute or relative immobilization (sustained bedrest). Numerous studies have demonstrated that under such conditions negative calcium balance and bone loss occur. Although treatment with agents that decrease bone resorption, such as calcitonin, may improve calcium balance, nutritional measures alone are unlikely to have a significant effect in restoring lost bone (7). Restoration of bone requires a combination of adequate mechanical loading of the skeleton and increased calcium intake. Thus, increased dietary calcium supplements are an important adjunct to restoring skeletal health during convaslescent period when physical activity, particularly weight-bearing activity, can occur.

A close relationship exists among exercise, muscle mass, and bone mass.

Loss of bone with aging is invariably associated with loss of muscle mass. Several studies have demonstrated that moderately enhanced physical exercise increases bone mass in older adults. Indeed, moderate exercise programs are frequently recommended as adjuncts to pharmacologic treatment of osteoporosis, including the use of oral calcium supplements.

Nutritional Factors

Phosphorus

The ratio of dietary intake of phosphorus relative to that of calcium (Ca/P) has been thought to influence the calcium balance of bone mass. Several studies in man have shown that up to threefold increases in dietary phosphorus do not decrease calcium balance (8-9). Thus, although changes in dietary intake of phosphorus produce complex changes in calcium homeostasis at the intestine, kidney, and bone, changes in the dietary Ca/P ratio do not appear to contribute to development of osteopenia in healthy adults. However, it remains possible that, in the presence of even mild renal insufficiency, which frequently occurs as a function of aging, increased dietary intake of phosphorus may be an additional factor that can contribute to the development of secondary hyperparathyroidism and hence contribute to progression of the osteopenia associated with aging.

Protein Intake

Increased dietary protein intake is associated with an increase in urinary calcium losses that is attributable both to an increase in the glomerular filtration rate and the altered renal handling of calcium (10-12). This change is not associated with an increase in intestinal calcium absorption. Thus, excessive protein intake appears to result in a state of negative calcium balance and has been implicated as a risk factor for the development of osteopenia. However, there may be individual variations in sensitivity to the calciuric effect of protein feeding. Moreover, the effect of age on this response to protein feeding in humans has not been examined.

Fiber

Ingested fiber exerts a chelating effect on calcium in the intestinal lumen. The interest in high-fiber diets as adjuncts to the management of diabetes mellitus and hypercholesterolemia has increased in recent years. It is likely that extremely high dietary intake of fiber can induce negative calcium balance and, when ingested over long periods of time, may be a risk factor for development of osteopenia.

Drugs and Dietary Manipulations that Influence Calcium Balance

A large number of medications in common use have direct and indirect effects on calcium balance and skeletal metabolism. A number of common corticosteroids, thyroid hormones, diuretics (furosenide, ethacynic acid) antacids, antibiotics, and anticonvulsant agents have profound effects on mineral homeostasis. These effects are both diverse and often complex in their interactions with nutritional factors and the metabolism and function of calcitropic hormones. A number of these agents induce excessive urinary calcium losses or impair intestinal calcium absorption. In this setting, dietary calcium requirements would need to be increased to prevent or reduce bone mineral losses.

In addition, most low-sodium diets restrict dairy production consumption. Thus, alternative sources of calcium are required to ensure adequate calcium intake.

INTERRELATIONSHIP BETWEEN CALCIUM INTAKE AND BONE MASS

Low dietary intake of calcium during the first three decades of life appears to be a major contributory factor to subsequent early development of osteoporosis. In this regard, even accepting the limitations in reliability of the diet questionnaire, most epidemiologic studies involving older subject populations have shown either no or at best a weak relationship between current dietary calcium consumption and bone mass (13-16). Earlier studies utilized metacarpal morphometry to assess cortical bone mass and found no correlation between bone mass and current calcium intake (13). A more recent study measured rates of bone loss at both a midradial site (single-photon absorptiometry) and at the lumbar spine (dual-photon absorptiometry) in a population of women without osteoporosis (17). There was no significant correlation between bone mineral density or rate of bone loss at either site and current but habitual dietary calcium intake. In a now classical study, bone mass and fracture rates were measured in a population living in two village communities in Yugoslavia with significantly different patterns of dietary calcium intake. Dietary calcium intake differed by approximately two-fold. In both men and women and independent of age, bone mass was greater and the proximal femur fracture rate lower in the community with higher calcium consumption (18). This study indicated that the major determinant of bone mass in the elderly was the peak bone mass developed during the period of skeletal mass consolidation during early adulthood. After age 40 the rates of bone loss were similar in both populations. Subsequent studies by several groups of investigators have demonstrated positive correlations between estimated habitual life long dietary calcium intake and bone density (at various predominantly cortical bone sites) in both men and women (19,20).

CALCIUM SUPPLEMENTATION AND BONE MASS

Although lifelong higher calcium intake is associated with development of a greater mature bone mass and decreased fracture rates in later life, it has not been conclusively demonstrated that supplementation of dietary calcium intake in older adults, in itself increases bone mass or reduces fracture rates. Moreover, available reports have focused on the use of calcium supplements in the management of postmenopausal osteoporosis. Investigators at the Mayo Clinic, in a study lacking randomization with a control group, found a reduction in vertebral fracture rates in subjects receiving oral calcium supplements (calcium carbonate: 1.0-1.5 g/day with or without vitamin D supplements (21). In contrast, a more recent study in Denmark found no improvement in either total body or vertebral bone mass after 2 years of calcium supplementation therapy (calcium carbonate: 2 g/day elemental calcium) in postmenopausal women. However, in this study, a tendency toward reduction in cortical bone loss (at the proximal forearm) was observed (22). It has not yet been established whether or not oral calcium supplements are as effective as enhanced dietary calcium intake in increasing bone mass. Well-designed studies are necessary to answer this question, as well as to clarify the effectiveness of calcium intake augmentation on increasing bone mass and/or reducing fracture rates in the elderly.

INTESTINAL ABSORPTION OF CALCIUM

Effective calcium absorption is determined both by the amount of calcium ingested and the efficiency of absorption. A number of studies using different techniques have demonstrated that intestinal absorption of calcium decreases with age in both men and women (23-26). It is likely that alterations in several different transport processes are involved in this decrease. Moreover, studies using different methods for measuring absorption have yielded different results with respect to the age of onset of decreased calcium absorption. Studies employing metabolic balance techniques provide information concerning net calcium absorption [calcium intake − (fecal + urine + dermal calcium loss)] and represent the summation of transport processes occurring along the entire intestine. Such studies suggest a decline in absorption beginning between the fifth and sixth decades of life (27). More sensitive double-isotope radiocalcium techniques employing a 100- to 200-mg stable calcium carrier demonstrate a steady decline in absorption after the age of 30 years (23,25,26). Single-isotope studies with a smaller calcium carrier (20 mg) have confirmed decreased absorption in the elderly (23). These results suggest that active transport of calcium is decreased. Intestinal perfusion studies with placement of the perfusion tube in the jejunum also demonstrate decreased active calcium transport in older individuals over the age of 60 years (25).

In addition to a decrease in net or fractional calcium absorption, the ability to adapt to changes in dietary calcium is blunted or absent in elderly individuals (25). In younger individuals under conditions of reduced dietary calcium intake, the fraction of calcium absorbed is increased and decreases in proportion to an increase in dietary calcium. There appears to be considerable variation in the rate at which this adaptive response occurs among individuals. This response is thought to be mediated primarily by changes in the production rate and subsequent intestinal action(s) of $1,25 (OH)_2D_3$ (calcitriol), although involvement of additional factors has not been excluded.

Several studies have shown that levels of calcitriol are decreased in older individuals. In addition, women with postmenopausal osteoporosis have lower levels of calcitriol and a greater degree of reduced calcium absorption than do nonosteoporotic individuals (26,28). Lower levels of calitriol have been attributed to a reduction in estrogen-mediated calcitriol synthesis. However, other factors may also contribute to the reduction in calcitriol levels, including a mild reduction in renal function and age-related reduced renal sensitivity to the trophic action of parathyroid hormone (PTH). Finally, there is some evidence to suggest that relative intestinal resistance to the action of calcitriol may develop in older individuals with osteoporotic syndromes.

VITAMIN D

A number of studies have demonstrated that both vitamin D nutriture and metabolism change with aging (Table 2). These changes may be central to the development of age-related osteopenia. As a generalization, two types of processes may be involved. Vitamin D deficiency can result in the malabsorption of calcium and subsequent development of secondary hyperparathyroidism and/or the development of overt osteomalacia with more profound vitamin D depletion. Alternatively, impaired calcium absorption, independent of vitamin D depletion, may contribute to the development of secondary hyperparathyroidism and subsequently to osteopenia. In this setting, relative vitamin D resistance may have some role. It is likely that both processes are part of the spectrum of development of age-related osteopenia and spinal or hip fracture syndromes.

TABLE 2. *Factors contributing to Vitamin D deficiency in the elderly*

Inadequate dietary intake
Deprivation of sunlight exposure
Decreased cutaneous formation of vitamin D
Reduced calcitriol production
Malabsorption of fat-soluble vitamins

Vitamin D Status in the Elderly

The total body store of vitamin D in an individual is determined both by dietary (exogenous sources) intake and endogenous production. The latter is determined by cutaneous production of the prohormonal metabolite, vitamin D_3 (cholecalciferol), which is subsequently metabolized to physiologically more active vitamin D analogs. Under appropriate conditions, either source can provide the total vitamin D requirements. Measurement of the plasma level of 25-hydroxyvitamin D [25(OH)D], quantitatively the major circulating metabolite, is considered the most useful index for assessment of vitamin D status of the individual. Most commercial assays report total 25(OH)D levels that include both 25(OH)D_3 and 25(OH)D_2, which is a metabolite of vitamin D_2 (ergocalciferol). Sources for these metabolites are vitamin preparations and vitamin-fortified foods, particularly dairy products. More recently, vitamin D_3 has also been used as a food additive and thus can arise from both exogenous and endogenous sources.

A number of studies have reported decreased levels of 25(OH)D (hypovitaminosis) in elderly individuals (29-33). Detailed studies have examined the multiple factors that can contribute to the age-related decline in vitamin D nutriture: (a) reduced intake of vitamin D in the elderly, (b) reduced capacity for the cutaneous production of D_3; (c) changes in intestinal absorption of vitamin D_2 (or D_3), and (d) changes in hepatic metabolism of D_2 and D_3 or the 25-hydroxymetabolites of these analogs.

Recent studies have demonstrated an age-dependent decline in epidermal concentrations of 7-dehydrocholesterol (provitamin D_3) (34). This decline is correlated with a decreased capacity to form previtamin D_3 on exposure to ultraviolet radiation. The significance of this observation must be considered in the context that many elderly individuals have decreased exposure to sunlight and frequently dress so as to allow exposure of smaller amounts of skin. In this regard, several studies have reported that institutionalized elderly patients have lower levels of 25(OH)D than do healthy ambulatory elderly subjects (30-33). In a study of elderly subjects living in New York, 25(OH)D_3 was observed to be the predominant circulating metabolite in ambulatory subjects, whereas in two-thirds of the institutionalized elderly patients subjects, 25(OH)D_2 was the predominant metabolite (33). However, both groups of subjects had levels of total 25(OH)D that, although reduced, were regarded as within the absolute normal range. The implication of such observations is that institutionalized individuals frequently have less sunlight exposure, and nutitional supplements take on greater importance in providing for their adequate vitamin D nutriture. In a large study of healthy elderly subjects living in the southwest United States, lower measured levels of 25(OH)D were observed when compared to those in younger (control) subjects. Moreover, levels of 25(OH)D showed seasonal variation, with lowest levels occurring in the winter months and highest levels during the late summer months (31). The latter observation has been made by several groups of investigators (35-36). Thus, seasonal variation as an expression of differing hours of sunlight exposure (as a function of geographic location) is an important determinant of vitamin D stores. Finally, several reports have underscored the observation that higher levels of 25(OH)D are observed in elderly subjects who are receiving supplements providing greater than 100 IU/day of vitamin D than those not receiving supplements (31,33).

It has been speculated that aging may be associated with the decreased efficiency of absorption of vitamin D. However, available published results are conflicting. One study compared plasma levels of radiolabeled vitamin D_3 after oral dosing in young and elderly individuals (38). The investigators observed significantly lower plasma levels of ^{3}H-vitamin D_3 in the elderly group, suggesting an age-related defect in its absorption. In contrast, in studies measuring plasma levels of 25(OH)D_2 after oral administration in a group of elderly individuals without evidence of malabsorption, attained levels over short time intervals did not differ from those observed in younger control subjects (33,38). The latter technique is capable of determining gross malabsorption of vitamin D, although it may not detect a subtle impairment of vitamin absorption. However, the observation in several studies that administration of small amounts of vitamin D supplements can maintain normal plasma levels of 25(OH)D in elderly individuals suggests that most elderly individuals have adequate absorption of dietary vitamin D.

In addition to the decline in plasma levels of 25(OH)D, levels of 1,25(OH)$_2$D may also decrease with aging (26,28). However, as in the case of 25(OH)D, levels of 1,25(OH)$_2$D may range from low to normal in populations of older individuals. Multiple factors are involved in the regulation of 1,25(OH)$_2$D production and appear to be involved in the reduced levels observed in the elderly. It is likely that aging-related mild to moderate reduction in renal function is a common and significant contributing factor to the fall in plasma levels of 1,25(OH)$_2$D. Other alterations include diminished PTH-mediated 1,25(OH)$_2$D secretory reserve and, in postmenopausal women, decreased estrogen-modulated 1,25(OH)$_2$D production (39).

Reduction in 1,25(OH)$_2$D production has been correlated with diminished intestinal absorption of calcium, which in turn contributes to development of secondary hyperparathyroidism. That condition is associated with increased bone resorption and is thought to constitute a major pathway for age-related bone loss. Other actions of 1,25(OH)$_2$D include interaction with PTH in modulating bone remodeling and regulation of PTH secretory activity. At the present time it is unknown if these actions of 1,25(OH)$_2$D are altered as a function of aging. Finally, a recent preliminary study has provided results in conflict with previous observations, suggesting that plasma levels of 1,25(OH)$_2$D may actually be increased with aging both because of increased production and decreased metabolic clearance (40). Increased plasma levels of 1,25(OH)$_2$D were correlated with increased levels of PTH.

However, although levels of 1,25(OH);2D were increased, intestinal absorption of calcium was unchanged, consistent with intestinal resistance to vitamin D.

Significance of Hypovitaminosis D and Deficiency in the Elderly

In individual elderly subjects, the distinction between low levels of 25(OH)D (hypovitaminosis D) and vitamin D deficiency is poorly defined. Severe and sustained vitamin D depletion with levels of 25(OH)D below 5 ng/ml is associated with development of overt metabolic bone disease, eg, osteomalacia. A state of more modest or even subtle vitamin D depletion may exist with levels of 25(OH)D between 5 and 30 ng/ml (41). Such levels are commonly observed in elderly individuals, particularly institutionalized patients or elderly individuals who have repeated episodes of hospitalizations. Low levels of 25(OH)D$_3$ in these patients have been found to be associated with malaborption of calcium. Treatment with modest doses of 25(OH)D$_3$ results in an increase in levels of 1,25(OH)$_2$D$_3$ in direct proportion to the 25(OH)D level before treatment. Subclinical osteomalacia may be present in these patients (42).

The incidence of osteomalacia in older adult or elderly populations in the United States is not known and has not been extensively studied. This information is important because the primary causes of osteomalacia in the elderly are poor nutrition and sunlight deprivation, both of which can be treated easily. The incidence of femoral neck fractures has been reported to be increased in elderly individuals with osteomalacia and/or vitamin D depletion (43-47). Most of these reports have come from Great Britain. In the United States a recent study in Boston reported that approximately 41% of 142 consecutive patients with hip fractures had low to very low levels of 25(OH)D, and approximately one-third of bone biopsies available in 39 patients were considered consistent with osteomalacia (47). An earlier study reported evidence of low-grade osteomalacia in 8 of 31 femoral head specimens from patients with hip fractures (48).

Varying degrees of severity of osteomalacia occur. In clinically overt osteomalacia, fractures may occur through sites of Looser zones (pseudofractures). In occult or subclinical osteomalacia fractures might occur as a result of mechanical weakening caused by multiple micropseudofractures; for example, a characteristic femoral subcapital fracture (48).

Because of the increased incidence of hip fracture associated with osteomalacia in the elderly, early diagnosis is important. In subclinical or occult osteomalacia, such biochemical markers as serum calcium, phosphorus, and alkaline phosphatase may be normal. Moreover, symptoms associated with vitamin D depletion, such as bone and joint pain and tenderness and/or muscle weakness, may be overlooked or attributed to degenerative arthritis and frailty in the elderly. Thus, awareness of this metabolic bone disease, which is caused primarily by nutritional deprivation of vitamin D, is probably the most important factor in its diagnosis.

REFERENCES

1. Abraham S, Carroll MD, Dresser CM, Johnson CL. *Dietary intake findings, United States 1971–1974.* Hyattsville, MD: National Center for Health Statistics, 1977 (DHEW Publ. No. (HRA) 77–1647).
2. Abraham S, Carroll MD, Desser CM, Johnson CL. *Dietary intake findings, United States 1976–1980.* Hyattsville, MD: National Center for Health Statistics, 1983. (DHHS Publ. No. (PHS) 83–1681).
3. US Department of Agriculture, Consumer Nutrition Center. *Food and nutrient intakes of individuals in 1 day in the United States, Spring 1977.* Hyattsville, MD: Nationwide Food Consumption Survey 1977–1978. (Preliminary Report no 2).
4. Heaney RP, Recker RR, Saville PD. *J Lab Clin Med* 1978;92:953–963.
5. Recker RR, Saville PD, Heaney RR. *Ann Intern Med* 1977;87:649–655.
6. Ettinger B, Genant HK, Cann CE. *Ann Intern Med* 1987;106:40–45.
7. Pezeshki C, Brooker AF, Jr. *J Bone Joint Surg* 1977;59-A:971–973.
8. Heaney RP, Recker RR. *J Lab Clin Med* 1982;99:46–55.
9. Spencer H, Kramer L, Osis D, Norris C. *J Nutr* 1978;108:7–57.
10. Margen S, Chu J-Y, Kaufman NA, Calloway DH. *Am J Clin Nutr* 1974;27:584–589.
11. Spencer H, Margen S, Costa FM. *Am J Clin Nutr* 1978;31:1028–1035.
12. Schuette SA, Zemel MD, Linkswiler HM. *J Nutr* 1980;110:305–315.
13. Garn SM. *The earlier gain and the later loss of cortical bone in nutritional perspective.* Springfield, IL: Charles C Thomas, 1970.
14. Smith RW, Frame B. *N Engl J Med* 1965;273:72–78.
15. Hurxthal LM, Vose GP. *Calcif Tissue Res* 1969;4:245–254.
16. Garn SM, Solomon MA, Friedl J. *Ecol Food Nutr* 1981;10:131–133.
17. Riggs BL, Wahner HW, Melton LJ III, et al. *J Clin Invest* 1986;77:1487–1491.
18. Matkovic V, Kostial K, Simonivoc I, et al. *Am J Clin Nutr* 1979;32:540–549.
19. Barrett-Connor E. *Calcif Tissue Int* 1989;44:303–307.
20. Haliona L, Anderson JJB. *Am J Clin Nutr* 1989;49:534–541.
21. Riggs BL, Seeman E, Hodgson SF, Taves DR, O'Fallon WM. *N Engl J Med* 1982;306:446–450.
22. Riis B, Thomsen KT, Christiansen C. *N Engl J Med* 1987;316:173–177.
23. Bullamore JR, Gallagher JC, Wilkinson R, Nordin BEC. *Lancet* 1970;2:535–537.
24. Avioli LV, McDonald JE, Lee SW. *J Clin Invest* 1965;44:1960–1967.
25. Ireland P, Fordtran JS. *J Clin Invest* 1973;52:2672–2681.
26. Gallagher JC, Riggs BL, Eisman J, Hamstra A, Arnaud SB, DeLuca HF. *J Clin Invest* 1979;64:729–736.
27. Bogdonoff MD, Shock NW, Nichols MP. *J Gerontol* 1953;8:272–288.
28. Slovik DM, Adams JS, Neer RM, Holick MF, Potts JT, Jr. *N Engl J Med* 1981;305:372–374.
29. Parfitt AM, Gallagher JC, Heaney RP, Johnston, CC, Neer R, Whedon GD. *J Clin Nutr* 1982;36:1014–1034.
30. Corless D, Boucher BJ, Beer M, Gupta SP, Cohen RD. *Lancet* 1975;1:1404–1406.
31. Omdahl JL, Garry PT, Hunsaker LA, Hunt WC, Goodwin JS. *Am J Clin Nutr* 1982;36:1125–1233.
32. Hosking DJ, Campbell GA, Kemm JR, Cotton RE, Knight ME, Berryman R, Boyd RV. *Lancet* 1983;2:1290–1292.
33. Clemens T, Zhou X-Y, Myles M, Endres D, Lindsay R. *J Clin Endocrin Metab* 1986;63:656–660.
34. MacLaughlin JA, Holick MF. *J Clin Invest* 1985;76:1536–1538.
35. Lamberg-Allardt C. *Ann Nutr Metab* 1984;28:144–150.

36. McKenna MJ, Freaney R, Meade A, Muldowney FP. *Am J Clin Nutr* 1985;41:101–109.
37. Barragry JM, France W, Corless D, Gupta SP, Switala S, Boucher BJ, Cohen RD. 1978;55:213–220.
38. Holick MF. *Clin Nutr* 1986;5:121–129.
39. Cheema C, Grant BF, Marcus R. *J Clin Invest* 1989;83:537–542.
40. Eastell R, Yergey R, Vieira N, Kumar R, Riggs BL. *Clin Res* 1989;37:448A.
41. Francis RM, Peacock M, Taylor GA, Storer JH, Nordin BEC. *Clin Sci* 1984;66:103–107.
42. Francis RM, Peacock M, Storer JH, Davies AEJ, Brown WB, Nordin BEC. *Eur J Clin Invest* 1983;13:391–396.
43. Aaron JE, Gallagher JC, Anderson J, Stasiak L, Ongton EB, Nordin BEC, Nicholson M. *Lancet* 1978;1:229–233.
44. Weisman Y, Salama R, Harell A, Edelstein S. *Br Med J* 1978;2:1196–1197.
45. Chalmers J, Conacher WDH, Gardner DL, Scott PJ. *J Bone Joint Surg* 1967;49B:403–423.
46. Jenkins, DHR, Roberts JG, Webster D, Williams EO. *J Bone Joint Surg* 1973;55B:575–580.
47. Doppelt SH, Neer RM, Daly M, Bourret L, Schiller A, Holick MF. *Orthop Trans* 1983;7:512–513.
48. Sokoloff L. *Am J Surg Patho* 1978;2:21–30.

Geriatric Nutrition, edited by John E. Morley,
Zvi Glick, Laurence Z. Rubenstein.
Raven Press, Ltd., New York © 1990.

11

Zinc Metabolism in the Elderly

Craig J. McClain* and Mary A. Stuart†

*Division of *Digestive Diseases and Nutrition, University of Kentucky Medical
Center and VA Medical Center, and †Department of Nutrition and Food Science,
University of Kentucky, Lexington, Kentucky 40536*

A combination of physiologic, social, psychologic, and economic factors affect adversely a large portion of the elderly, placing them at nutritional risk. Physiologic functions naturally decline with age, which may influence absorption and metabolism. Social and economic conditions affect dietary choices and eating patterns. The elderly have a higher incidence of chronic diseases and associated intake of medications that affect nutrient utilization. Loneliness and reluctance to eat often complicate an already fragile situation. One nutrient deficiency that frequently is observed in the elderly is zinc deficiency.

Indeed, some indicator of depressed zinc status has been observed in the elderly in the majority of studies performed. For example, plasma zinc concentrations have been reported to decrease with age both in human subjects (1) and in mice (2). Plasma zinc levels have been reported to be depressed in institutionalized patients (3), housebound elderly (4), and ambulatory healthy elderly (5). A study by Wilson and coworkers (6) revealed that only 18% of patients on a hospital geriatric ward had normal serum zinc concentrations, with no differences in patients admitted from hospital wards versus home. *In vitro* studies using rat adipocytes demonstrated impaired uptake of zinc-65 in adipocytes from elderly compared to adult control rats (7). Thus, there are considerable data from both human and animal studies to suggest depressed zinc status in the elderly.

Zinc is an essential trace element required for RNA and DNA synthesis and the function of over 200 zinc metalloenzymes (8). It plays an important role in membrane stabilization (9), and as shown by our group, zinc deficiency causes a progressive increase in membrane fluidity (10). We speculate that this increase may lead to some of the metabolic alterations seen in zinc deficiency, an example being anorexia. This chapter addresses potential clinical complications of zinc deficiency in the elderly, mechanisms for zinc deficiency in the elderly, and the possible role of zinc supplementation in the elderly.

TABLE 1. *Manifestation of zinc deficiency and response to zinc supplementation*

Manifestation	Response to supplementation	Reference
Skin lesions	−	13
Hypogonadism	NS	
Impaired vision	+	26
Anorexia, impaired taste	−	28
Impaired immune function	±	30–32
Altered mental status	NS	
Impaired wound healing	±	36, 37
Diarrhea	NS	

NS, not studied.

POTENTIAL CLINICAL IMPLICATIONS OF ALTERED ZINC METABOLISM

Zinc deficiency may present in a variety of different ways in the elderly, as noted in Table 1 and in the following section.

Skin Lesions

Acrodermatitis enteropathica (AE) is a rare hereditary disease characterized by skin lesions, alopecia, failure to thrive, diarrhea, impaired immune function with frequent infections, and in some cases ocular abnormalities (11). It is now generally accepted that the signs and symptoms of AE are caused by zinc deficiency, presumably caused by impaired intestinal absorption of zinc. The skin lesions (acrodermatitis) tend to occur around the eyes, nose, and mouth and over the buttocks and perianal regions, and sometimes in an acral distribution.

These same skin lesions also have been reported in patients receiving total parenteral nutrition and in patients with underlying diseases, such as alcoholic liver disease or Crohn's disease, who then developed zinc deficiency (12). The elderly often develop nonspecific skin lesions around body orifices and about the feet and ankles. Nursing home and bedridden patients are predisposed to decubitus ulcers. Weismann et al. (13) performed a trial of zinc supplementation in geriatric patients with hypozincemia and skin lesions that could have possibly been caused by zinc deficiency. They evaluated 585 institutionalized elderly subjects, and 26 patients with skin lesions were entered into the study. Ten of these 26 patients had depressed serum zinc concentrations and were treated with 600 mg of zinc sulfate for 4 weeks. Serum zinc concentrations more than doubled during this period, documenting patient compliance and adequate zinc absorption. However, because zinc supplementation produced no beneficial effects on the skin lesions, these investigators suggested that it is unlikely that zinc deficiency plays a major role in the nonspecific skin changes observed in the elderly.

Hypogonadism

Zinc deficiency, a well-recognized cause of hypogonadism in experimental animals, has been postulated to play a pathogenetic role in the human hypogonadism observed in some underdeveloped countries and in certain disease processes, such as regional enteritis, sickle cell disease, uremia, and chronic alcoholism (14). The hypogonadism of zinc deficiency appears to be primarily a gonadal defect (14). Compared to zinc-sufficient controls, zinc-deficient animals have reduced basal testosterone levels, markedly depressed testosterone response to human chorionic gonadotropin stimulation, and depressed weights of testes and other androgen-sensitive organs. Similarly, humans placed on a zinc-deficient diet developed decreased libido, depressed serum testosterone levels, and marked reduction in sperm counts (15). The elderly can develop problems of sexual dysfunction. A single study, reported in abstract form only (16), in middle-aged and older men demonstrated that low serum zinc levels were related to lower testosterone levels. In addition, zinc supplementation in zinc-deficient men improved potency in 50% of this group (see chapter 33).

Impaired Night Vision, Retinal Function, and Macular Degeneration

Patek and Haig (17) reported in 1939 that patients with alcoholic cirrhosis had abnormal night vision that often was corrected by vitamin A supplementation. Research by Morrison et al. (18) and McClain et al. (19) demonstrated that certain alcoholic cirrhotics also required zinc to correct their abnormalities in dark adaptation. Elegant studies by Keeling and coworkers (20) showed that alcoholic cirrhotics had abnormal electroretinography and depressed B wave amplitude correlated with leukocyte zinc concentrations. Other zinc-deficient patient populations, such as those with Crohn's disease (21) or sickle cell anemia (22), have been shown to have impaired night vision that is corrected or improves with zinc therapy.

Studies in animals also provide strong evidence for the role of zinc in normal retinal function. To investigate the role of zinc in the retina, Leure-duPree (23) treated rats with the zinc chelating agents, dithizone and 1,10-phenanthroline. Degenerative changes of the retinal pigment epithelium (RPE) and unusual osmiophilic inclusion bodies in RPE were observed. Next, Leure-duPree and McClain (24) evaluated the effect of differing durations of dietary zinc deficiency upon the ultrastructure of the rat retina. Essentially identical abnormalities were seen with dietary-induced zinc deficiency as with administration of zinc chelating agents. Osmiophilic inclusion bodies in the RPE were seen early in zinc deficiency, whereas severe disruption of the outer segments was seen later in the course of zinc deficiency. We recently had the opportunity to study the eyes of a patient who died with acrodermatitis enteropathica. This patient had severe degeneration of the RPE similar to that seen in zinc-deficient rats (25). Thus, there is strong evidence that zinc deficiency causes physiologic and possibly anatomic abnormalities in the retina.

A recent investigation by Newsome and coworkers (26) showed that zinc supplementation was helpful in preventing macular degeneration. Macular degeneration is the major cause of vision loss in the elderly in this country and thus of great clinical consequence. This was a prospective, randomized, double-masked, placebo-controlled study of the effects of zinc supplementation in 151 patients with drusen or macular degeneration. Although some eyes in the zinc-treated group lost vision, this group had significantly less vision loss than the control group at 12 and 24 months. Men had less vision loss than women for unexplained reasons. Although patients were given zinc sulfate 100 mg bid, there was no significant increase in the serum zinc level over the study period, an observation of some concern to these reviewers. Also of concern was the relatively severe vision loss in the control group, which enhanced the positive findings of the zinc therapy group. This important study requires confirmation by other laboratories. The National Institutes of Health is initiating a major multicenter study evaluating the effects of zinc therapy on macular degeneration.

Anorexia

Another major manifestation of zinc deficiency is anorexia accompanied by alterations in taste and smell. The mechanisms by which zinc deficiency produces anorexia are unclear at this time. Alterations in taste acuity, in circulating amino acid concentrations and catecholamine levels in the total brain and specific regions of the hypothalamus, and in membrane fluidity and receptor function have all been hypothesized to be related to anorexia (8).

Geriatric subjects often complain of anorexia and impaired taste sensation and have decreased food consumption. Greger (27) showed that approximately 20% of elderly institutionalized patients had impaired taste acuity; however, it did not correlate with dietary zinc intake or zinc levels. A subsequent study by this same group (28) evaluated the effects of zinc supplementation on altered taste acuity in the elderly. Forty-nine institutionalized elderly subjects were randomized to 15 mg zinc as zinc sulfate or placebo for 95 days. Hair zinc significantly increased in the zinc-supplemented patients, but there was no significant improvement in taste acuity. Thus, it appears that altered taste acuity in the elderly is generally not related to zinc status. To our knowledge, no major studies have been performed on zinc and anorexia in the elderly.

Impaired Immune Function

Zinc plays an important role in immune function in both man and experimental animals. Zinc deficiency in animals causes thymic and lymph node atrophy; decreased production of the thymic hormone, Facteur Thymique Serique; loss of cytotoxic T lymphocyte response to tumor cells; impaired response to thymus-dependent antigens; and decreased natural killer cell activity (8). Elderly patients often have impaired immune function, and the defects seen are similar to those that occur with zinc deficiency (28). Data are conflicting concerning the effects of zinc supplementation on immune function in the elderly, with initial studies, such as those by Duchateau et al. (30), showing beneficial effects. Zinc sulfate (220 mg bid for 1 month) was administered to 15 subjects over the age of 70. The zinc-treated subjects showed a significant improvement in the number of circulating T lymphocytes, cutaneous hypersensitivity, and IgG antibody response to tetanus vaccine. Zinc status was not determined in these subjects. Bogden et al. (31) reported depressed dietary intake in elderly patients, and there was a significant association between skin testing and serum zinc concentrations. However, these same investigators (32) were not able to show a beneficial effect of low-dose (15 mg/day) or high-dose (100 mg/day) zinc supplementation on immune function. However, a multivitamin-mineral preparation was given, which might have masked the beneficial effects of zinc. These subjects were healthy elderly, and possibly debilitated elderly may respond more to zinc therapy.

Whether the positive effects of zinc on immune function in the elderly reported in some studies represent a simple nutrient effect or a pharmacologic immunomodulatory effect is unclear. Further work using appropriately designed studies should help clarify the role of zinc in immune function in the elderly.

Altered Mental Status

Zinc deficiency may cause alterations in mental status. Experimentally induced zinc deficiency in humans may be associated with irritability or apathy that is reversed with zinc supplementation (8,33). Children with acrodermatitis enteropathica often have apathy or confusion that responds to zinc supplementation.

The possible effect of zinc deficiency on mental function in the elderly has received only limited attention. Stafford et al. (34) evaluated zinc status using serum and leukocyte zinc and found no significant correlation between mental impairment and zinc status. However, significant relationships were observed between mental status and plasma albumin, plasma total protein concentrations, and protein intake. To our knowledge, no study has been performed concerning the effects of zinc supplementation on mental status in the elderly.

Impaired Protein Metabolism and Impaired Wound Healing

A major manifestation of zinc deficiency in both man and animals is severe growth retardation. An early biochemical marker of zinc deficiency is decreased activity of thymidine kinase, an integral enzyme in DNA synthesis. The mechanisms for growth retardation associated with zinc deficiency are probably multifactorial and include impaired synthesis of both nucleic acids and protein, increased protein catabolism, the previously described anorexia, and impaired food utilization (35).

Because of the above-noted role of zinc in nucleic acid metabolism, the synthesis of such structural proteins as collagen, various enzymatic pathways, and polyamine metabolism, it seems logical that positive zinc balance would be important to wound healing. The clinical role of zinc in wound healing was studied initially by Pories et al. (36), who observed improved healing of pilonidal sinuses with zinc administration. Subsequent controlled studies by Hallbook and Lanner (37) demonstrated that zinc supplementation improved wound healing of venous leg ulcers in patients with decreased serum zinc concentrations. Studies in rats showed that zinc deficiency slowed healing of excised and thermal injuries, but excess zinc in the diet did not enhance wound healing (38). Thus, it appears that, when subjects are zinc deficient, zinc supplementation improves wound healing. However, if patients are zinc sufficient, providing further zinc does not accelerate wound healing.

Diarrhea

Zinc deficiency may present as severe diarrhea, and we have observed patients whose diarrhea persisted while taking nothing by mouth (8). Diarrhea also is one of the principal symptoms of acrodermatitis enteropathica. Some patients who have diarrhea with zinc deficiency have high zinc losses in their stool, which accounts for a cyclic worsening of both zinc status and diarrhea in these patients. It is important for clinicians to be aware that severe zinc deficiency may manifest as diarrhea, which may thereby improve with zinc supplementation.

POSSIBLE MECHANISMS FOR ZINC DEFICIENCY

The mechanism(s) for depressed zinc status in elderly subjects is probably multifactorial. Almost every study performed has shown that there is depressed zinc intake in elderly subjects, both those living in the community and those in continuing care nursing home situations (39). Zinc intake correlates directly with protein intake, and in the elderly, protein intake may be low because of the inadequacy of meal size and food quality. Studies of zinc absorption have reported depressed zinc levels in elderly subjects. In one study demonstrating impaired zinc absorption, however, there also appeared to be a compensatory decrease in endogenous zinc losses (40). Elderly subjects frequently take diuretics for a variety of cardiovascular reasons, and thus there is a potential for an overall increased urinary zinc loss. Also, most types of stress or inflammatory processes, such as sepsis, burns, head injury, multiple trauma, etc., cause an increase in urinary losses of zinc (41). Any one of these conditions may compromise the zinc status of an already marginal state, causing true clinical zinc deficiency.

Zinc in the plasma is bound mainly to albumin. A correlation between plasma zinc and serum albumin levels has been shown in multiple studies. It is well documented that there is a decrease in plasma albumin in elderly subjects with chronic disease. Thus, the hypozincemia seen in many elderly subjects may relate in part to depressed albumin levels (13).

Furthermore, chronic inflammatory disease states, such as decubitus ulcers, recurrent urinary tract infections, rheumatoid arthritis, and the like, may cause the release of such cytokines as interleukin-1 and tumor necrosis factor, which alter zinc metabolism (42). These cytokines depress the serum zinc level with an internal redistribution of zinc and with a large amount of plasma zinc being deposited into the liver.

In summary, a variety of mechanisms for depressed zinc status and altered zinc metabolism are operational in elderly subjects.

POTENTIAL COMPLICATIONS OF ZINC-SUPPLEMENTATION

Zinc supplementation, especially in high-dose is not without potential hazard. Regular high-dose oral zinc therapy can cause copper deficiency with subsequent anemia and neutropenia (43) because of the induction of metallothionein in the intestine, which impairs copper absorption. In addition, Chandra (44) has reported immune suppression with high-dose zinc supplementation. Thus, if zinc supplementation is to be administered, it should generally be done in low levels unless the patient is on a protocol and is being regularly monitored for adverse effects, such as copper deficiency.

CONCLUSIONS

Almost all studies in the elderly show depressed zinc intake and depressed zinc status as assessed by serum zinc levels. Health care providers need to be cognizant of the variety of potential manifestations of zinc deficiency in the elderly. However, in most situations, only one or in many cases no randomized studies of zinc supplementation have been performed in the elderly to evaluate the effect of zinc supplementation on the metabolic abnormality of interest. Further studies evaluating effects of zinc supplementation on such factors as macular degeneration, depressed T cell function, and wound healing are required. At this point, if zinc supplements are to be given, we recommend "low" doses (10 to 25 mg/day) given with meals to avoid the potential complications of zinc therapy. If higher doses are given for specific reasons, such as macular degeneration, the physician prescribing the zinc should be aware of and monitor for complications, especially for copper deficiency.

REFERENCES

1. Lindeman RD, Mervin LC, Colmore JP. *J Gerontol* 1971;26:358–363.
2. Woodward WD, Filteau SM, Allen OB. *J Gerontol* 1984;5:521–524.
3. Field HP, Whitley AJ, Srinivasan TR, Walker BE, Kelleher J. *Int J Vitam Nutr Res* 1987;57:311–317.
4. Bunker VW, Hinks LJ, Stansfield MF, Lawson MS, Clayton BE. *Am J Clin Nutr* 1987;46:353–359.
5. Bunker VW, Hinks LJ, Lawson MS, Clayton BE. *Am J Clin Nutr* 1984;40:1096–1102.
6. Wilson CWM, Myskow L. *Int J Vitam Nutr Res* 1985;55:331–336.
7. Sugarman B, Munro HN. *J Nutr* 1980;110:2317–2320.
8. McClain CJ, Kasarskis EJ, Allen JJ. *Prog Food Nutr Sci* 1985;9:185–226.
9. Bettger WJ, O'Dell BL. *Life Sci* 1981;28:1425–1438.
10. Jay M, Stuart SM, McClain CJ, Palmieri DA, Butterfield DA. *Biochimica Biophysica Acta* 1987;897:507–511.
11. Moynahan EJ, Barnes PM. *Lancet* 1973;1:676–677.
12. McClain CJ. *JPEN* 1981;5:424–429.
13. Weismann K, Wanscher B, Krakauer R. *Acta Dermatovener* 1978;58:157–161.
14. McClain CJ, Gavaler JS, Van Thiel DH. *J Lab Clin Med* 1984;6:1007–1015.
15. Abbasi AA, Prasad AS, Rabbani P, DuMouchell E. *J Lab Clin Med* 1980;96:544–550.
16. Billington CJ, Levine AS, Morley JE. *Clin Res* 1983;31:714A.
17. Patek AJ, Haig C. *J Clin Invest* 1939;18:609–616.
18. Morrison SA, Russell RM, Carney EA, Oaks IV. *Am J Nutr* 1978;31:276–281.
19. McClain CJ, Van Thiel DH, Parker S, Badzin LK, Gilbert H. *Alcohol Clin Exp Res* 1979;3:135–141.
20. Keeling PWN, O'Day J, Ruse W, Thompson RPH. *Clin Sci* 1982;62:109–111.
21. McClain CJ, Su L-C, Gilbert H, Camerson D. *Dig Dis Sci* 1983;28:85–87.
22. Warth JA, Prasad AS, Zwas F, Frank RN. *J Lab Clin Med* 1981;98:189–194.
23. Leure-duPree AE. *Invest Ophthalmol Vis Sci* 1981;21:1–9.
24. Leure-duPree AE, McClain CJ. *Invest Ophthalmol Vis Sci* 1982;23:425–434.
25. Cameron JD, McClain CJ. *Br J Ophthalmol* 1986;70:662–667.
26. Newsome DA, Swartz M, Leone NC, Elston RC, Miller E. *Arch Ophthalmol* 1988;106:192–197.

27. Greger JL. *J Gerontol* 1977;32:549–553.
28. Greger JL, Geissler AH. *Am J Clin Nutr* 1978;31:633–637.
29. Thompson JS, Wekstein DR, Rhoades JL, et al. *J Am Geriatr Soc* 1984;32:274–281.
30. Duchateau J, Delepesse G, Vrijens R, Collet H. *Am J Med* 1981;70:1001–1004.
31. Bogden JD, Oleske JM, Munves EM, et al. *Am J Clin Nutr* 1987;46:101–109.
32. Bogden JD, Oleske JM, Lavenhar MA, et al. *Am J Clin Nutr* 1988;48:655–663.
33. Henkin RI, Patten BM, Re PK, et al. *Arch Neurol* 1975;32:745–751.
34. Stafford W, Smith RG, Lewis SJ, et al. *Age Aging* 1988;17:42–48.
35. Bates J, McClain CJ. *Am J Clin Nutr* 1981;34:1655–1660.
36. Pories WJ, Henzel JH, Rob CG, Strain WH. *Ann Surg* 1967;165:432–436.
37. Hallbook T, Lanner E. *Lancet* 1972;2:780–782.
38. Sandstead HH, Lanier VC, Jr, Shephard GH, Gillespie DD. *Am J Clin Nutr* 1970; 23:514–519.
39. Thomas AJ, Bunker VW, Hinks LJ, Sodha N, Mullee MA, Clayton BE. *Br J Nutr* 1988;59:181–191.
40. Turnlund JR, Durkin N, Costa F, Margen S. *J Nutr* 1986;116:1239–1247.
41. Moser PB, Borel J, Majerus T, Anderson RA. *Nutr Res* 1985;5:253–261.
42. Goldblum SE, Cohen DA, Jay M, McClain CJ. *J Physiol* 1987;252:E27–E32.
43. Prasad AS, Brewer GJ, Schoomaker EB, Rabbani P. *JAMA* 1978;240:2166–2168.
44. Chandra RK. *JAMA* 1984;252:1443.

Geriatric Nutrition, edited by John E. Morley,
Zvi Glick, Laurence Z. Rubenstein.
Raven Press, Ltd., New York © 1990.

12

Other Trace Elements

John E. Morley

*Geriatric Research, Education and Clinical Center, VA Medical Center,
Sepulveda California, and Department of Medicine,
UCLA School of Medicine, Los Angeles, California 90024*

Trace elements play an important role in the maintenance of multiple enzyme reactions and are essential for the maintenance of tissue structure. Although much information is available on the function of trace elements, there is little available information on the effects of aging on these trace elements or the role they may play in the aging process. Table I summarizes the major functions of the trace elements and the effects of aging on them.

TRACE ELEMENTS

Arsenic

Arsenic has a biologic function in the metabolism of arginine and zinc (1). Arsenic deprivation retards growth in the presence of marginal zinc status. Arsenic also plays a role in the modulation of kidney arginase activity, alkaline phosphatase activity, and plasma levels of triglycerides, uric acid, and urea. Based on animal studies, the human arsenic requirement appears to be between 12 to 25 ug daily. The role of arsenic in human malnutrition has been extrapolated from animal studies. The effect of aging on arsenic has not been studied.

Boron

Boron appears to interact with cholecalciferol in the maintenance of bone structure (1). It also interacts with magnesium. In postmenopausal women on a low-magnesium diet, boron supplementation (3 mg/day) reduced the urinary excretion of calcium, magnesium, and phosphorus (2). Boron supplementation also resulted in an increase in serum testosterone and 17 beta-estradiol in these women. These studies have led to the perhaps premature

TABLE 1. *Functions of trace elements and the effects of aging on these trace elements*

Trace element	Function	Effect of aging
Arsenic	Urea cycle, myocardial muscle function, triglyceride synthesis	Unknown
Boron	Bone structure, mineral metabolism	Unknown
Chromium	Glucose homeostasis, lipid metabolism	Decrease
Cobalt	Vitamin B_{12}, erythropoiesis, triglyceride synthesis	No change
Copper	Cholesterol metabolism, erythropoiesis, collagen cross-linking, conversion of dopamine to norepinephrine, electron transport chain, coagulation factor V	Increase
Fluoride	Bone structure, tooth enamel	Increase after 45 years
Iodine	Thyroid hormones	Unknown
Lithium	Endocrine secretory function	Unknown
Manganese	Protein and energy metabolism, mucopolysaccharides	No change (elevated in older diabetics)
Molybdenum	Uric acid production, oxidation of sulfite to sulfate	Unknown
Nickel	RNA and DNA structure, membrane stabilization, iron absorption and metabolism, pituitary function	Unknown
Selenium	Constituent of glutathione peroxidase, T and B cell function, muscle metabolism	Decrease
Silicon	Bone structure, connective tissue structure	Decrease in aorta
Vanadium	Cholesterol synthesis, catalysis of oxidation/reduction reactions	Unknown

claim that boron supplementation may play a role in the prevention of calcium loss and bone demineralization in postmenopausal women.

Chromium

Chromium is an essential trace element that may play a role in glucose homeostasis (3). Deficiency of chromium or its biologically active form, glucose-tolerance factor (a dinicotinic acid-glutathionine complex), has been shown to result in glucose intolerance (4). The glucose tolerance factor is poorly characterized. The richest sources of it are Brewer's yeast, liver, and kidney.

Hyperglycemia, which responds to chromium replacement, has been reported to occur in patients on total parenteral nutrition (5–7). However, the role of chromium in the hyperglycemia of aging remains controversial. Skeptics totally reject its role, whereas others embrace it wholeheartedly. One well-controlled study of 16 patients 65 years of age and older found that chromium in combination with nicotinic acid caused a 15% decrease in the integrated glucose area in response to a glucose load (8).

Chromium deficiency has been associated with hypercholesterolemia in some but not all studies (3). The suggestion that chromium deficiency may play a role in atherosclerosis is not supported by the available experimental data. Chromium deficiency in humans has been associated with weight loss, atoxia, and peripheral neuropathy, as well as with hyperglycemia in patients on total parenteral nutrition.

Tissue chromium levels decline with age (9,10) and may do so more dramatically in western societies that eat refined foods that are somewhat deficient in chromium (11). The RDA for chromium is between 50 to 200 ug (12). However, Bunker et al. (13) reported that healthy volunteers ingesting 13.6 to 47.7 ug/day were able to maintain a positive chromium balance. In a study of institutionalized older individuals, the average chromium content of food offered (not eaten) was 52 ug/day (14).

Cobalt

Cobalt tissue concentrations are unchanged with age (15). Cobalt is an essential portion of the vitamin B_{12} molecule. Cobalt therapy increases hemoglobin in anemic patients on dialysis (16). However, this response may be associated with an increase in tumorigenesis. Cobalt therapy also increases triglyceride levels (17). High cobalt levels in beer have been associated with the development of a cardiomyopathy (18). Cobalt may reduce thyroid function when given in pharmacologic doses (19). Elevated cobalt levels can be found in both the blood and urine of patients with metallic hip replacements (20).

Copper

Copper is involved in iron absorption and mobilization. It acts as a catalyst in multiple enzymatic reactions, including the superoxidase dismutase reaction, the cross-linking of collagen, the lipyloxidase enzyme, the electron transport chain through cytochromic oxidase, coagulation factor V, and in the conversion of dompamine to norepinephrine. Copper deficiency is associated with hypercholesterolemia, perhaps through an increased rate of cholesterol release from the liver (21). Copper deficiency also leads to an impairment of glucose tolerance (22), and copper has been shown to act synergistically with insulin to drive the incorporation of glucose into fat cells (23). In humans, a weak association between serum copper levels and fasting blood glucose has been demonstrated (24,25). Klevay (26) suggested that atherosclerosis is related to the rate of zinc to copper levels. The evidence that copper deficiency is associated with atherosclerosis is, however, extremely weak. Copper deficiency has been associated with anemia, neutropenia, and osteoporosis (22). In addition, it may cause muscle weakness and

TABLE 2. *Possible clinical syndromes associated with copper deficiency in humans*

Anemia and neutropenia
Osteoporosis
Arterial disease
Pigmentation loss
Muscle weakness
Bleeding tendency
Cardiomyopathy versus atherosclerotic heart disease
Brain degeneration
Impaired glucose tolerance

a bleeding tendency. Symptoms of congenital copper deficiency (Menkes syndrome) include arterial disease, abnormal hair, osteoporosis, cerebellar ataxia, and other brain damage. Copper deficiency in older individuals has usually been associated with total parenteral nutrition.

Serum copper levels tend to increase with aging (27), although there is no change in leukocyte copper levels (28). Absorption of copper is similar in young and old men (29). Although older subjects ingest significantly lower amounts of copper than do younger subjects, they appear to have no problem in remaining in metabolic balance (29). In the presence of Type II diabetes mellitus, both copper and ceruplasmin levels are elevated, and this elevation is more pronounced with advancing age (22).

Overall, copper metabolism seems to be conserved with aging. The potential pathophysiologic role of copper deficiency in atherosclerosis and the hyperglycemia of aging deserves further study. The potential effects of mild copper deficiency are summarized in Table 2.

Fluoride

Fluoride plays a role in the hydroxyapatite of bone and tooth enamel. Circulating fluoride levels tend to rise after middle age because of the decrease in renal function and an increased release of fluoride from bone (30).

Fluoride has been used in the therapy of osteoporosis to reduce the fracture rate (31). However, during the early course of fluoride therapy, microfractures may occur in the lower limbs, resulting in pain in the lower extremities. Fluoride therapy can cause gastrointestinal bleeding and painful joints.

Iodine

Iodine is an integral part of the thyroid hormones. Iodine deficiency can lead to the development of goiter. There are no studies on iodine metabolism with advancing age.

Lithium

Animal studies have suggested a role for lithium as an essential trace element (1). Lithium appears to be involved in the regulation of pituitary, adrenal, and thyroid hormone secretion and water metabolism. Pharmacologic amounts of lithium used for the treatment of depression can result in hypothyroidism. Studies on lithium metabolism with aging have not been carried out.

Manganese

Manganese is essential for protein and energy metabolism and the formation of mucopolysaccharides. A deficiency of manganese can result in impaired glucose tolerance and bone abnormalities. Two studies have failed to show any effects of age on manganese concentrations (32,33). Manganese levels have been reported to be elevated in diabetic patients aged 61 to 70 years old (31,34). These elevated manganese levels may cause increased hepatic arginase activity in diabetics, resulting in increased amino acid metabolism and urea synthesis (35). The recommended daily intake of manganese ranges from 2 to 5 mg.

Molybdenum

Molybdenum deficiency has been reported in a 24-year-old patient with Crohn's disease on total parenteral nutrition (36). He had symptoms of intolerance to the TPN solution as a source of nutrients. He had high urinary levels of sulfite, thiosulfate, hypoxanthine, and xanthine and low levels of sulfate and uric acid. Biochemical and symptomatic normalization occurred with molybdenum supplementation.

Molybdenum intakes of 0.15 mg/day appear adequate to maintain molybdenum balance. Molybdenum toxicity (10 to 15 mg/day) is associated with elevated xanthine oxidase activity and uric acid levels (37). Molybdenum excess increases the urinary excretion of copper. Clinically, molybdenum toxicity presents with anorexia, weight loss, skin changes, anemia, and diarrhea. No studies on molybdenum with aging have been conducted. It has been suggested that tissue damage that occurs during postischemic injury is related to dehydrogenase-to-oxidase conversion of the molybdenum-dependent enzyme, xanthine dehydrogenase (37).

Nickel

Stabilization of RNA and DNA and membrane structure requires nickel. Nickel may also be involved in hormonal release from the pituitary. Most ingested nickel is excreted in the feces, with only small amounts being ex-creted. Grains and vegetables are the major source of nickel. Phytates in the grains appear to interfere with the absorption of nickel. No information on nickel and aging is available.

Selenium

Selenium was first recognized to be an essential trace element in 1957. The most fully characterized biochemical effect of selenium is its inclusion in the glutathione peroxidase molecule. The major physiologic role of glu-tathione peroxidase is to maintain appropriately low levels of hydrogen per-oxides within cells, thus decreasing potential free radical damage. Selenium deficiency is accompanied by a decrease in glutathione peroxidase activity and results in an increase in hepatic glutathione-S-transferase activity. Glu-tathione-S-transferase catalyzes the conjugation of electrophilic compounds and metabolites with glutathione, which is an important hepatic detoxifica-tion mechanism. Glutathione-S-transferase is also involved in the storage of heme and bilirubin. Selenium deficiency also increases liver glutathione syn-thesis, which can lead to a depletion of cysteine and impairment of protein synthesis.

Selenium has also been demonstrated to alter other drug (xenobiotic) me-tabolizing enzymes in addition to glutathione-S-transferase (38). In particu-lar, selenium deficiency is associated with a decrease in some of the isoen-zymes of cytochrome P-450. In contrast, it is also associated with an increase in UDP glucoronyl transferase activity. Thus, selenium deficiency clearly affects the ability of an individual to metabolize drugs. Because of its different effects on different enzyme systems, selenium deficiency may be associated with increased toxicity of some drugs and decreased efficiency of others.

The selenium content of food is directly dependent on the soil concentra-tion of selenium. Selenium intakes vary widely throughout the world, with intakes between 7 and 38,000 μg/day having been reported. An adequate selenium intake has been estimated at 50 μg/day, with toxic levels being estimated to occur with intakes of the order of 350 to 700 μg/day. It appears that selenium in the form of selenomethionine (the form found is wheat) results in better selenium retention than does selenate or selenite (39).

Some controversy exists concerning the effects of age on selenium levels. Circulating selenium concentrations either fall slightly (40) or remain stable with aging (41,42). Elderly residents in long-term care settings who are being tube fed have both low selenium levels and a reduction in red blood cell glutathione peroxidase levels (43,44). Selenium in hair has been found to decline from a mean of 0.76 μg/g of hair in 11- to 15-year-olds to a mean of

0.55 μg in 61- to 70-year-olds (45). Dietary intake of selenium is high in adolescents and declines to 65 μg/day in individuals over 70 years of age.

Selenium deficiency may be associated with a number of pathologic conditions (Table 3). The disease state best shown to be produced by selenium deficiency is a cardiomyopathy of children and young women (Keshan disease). Although selenium deficiency provides the necessary setting for the development of cardiomyopathy, other factors, such as viral infections, seem to play a role in the pathogenesis of this disease (46). Cardiomyopathy has also been found in some patients receiving total parenteral nutrition who are selenium deficient (47–49). Whether selenium deficiency plays a role in the pathogenesis of heart failure in some older individuals is unknown.

Patients receiving hyperalimentation have been reported to develop a syndrome of muscle weakness and/or pain and nail changes (50,51,52). This syndrome responded to selenium administration.

Selenium deficiency has been implicated in carcinogenesis. There is a lower prevalence of cancer in countries with a high-selenium concentration in the soil, such as, Venezuela. Many case-controlled prospective studies have suggested a relationship of selenium deficiency to cancer risk (53). However, not all studies have demonstrated such a correlation (54). A study from Finland suggested that a major cancer risk existed for persons with both low selenium and vitamin E levels (55). This finding is in keeping with an *in vitro* study of irradiated cells that suggested that both selenium and vitamin E act at different sites to attenuate radiation-induced damage (56). Numerous animal studies have shown that high-selenium diets can prevent the development of cancer (57). Although overall it appears that a low dietary selenium intake may lead to an increase in cancer risk, final recommendations on the preventive use of selenium should not be made until the efficacy of selenium in reducing the incidence of cancer has been demonstrated in prospective replacement trials.

Selenium deficiency increases thromboxane B_2 which causes platelet aggregation, while decreasing prostacyclin, which prevents aggregation (39).

TABLE 3. *Disease states possibly associated with selenium deficiency*

Keshan disease
Cardiomyopathy in patients on total parenteral nutrition
Muscle weakness and pain
Nail changes
T and B cell dysfunction
? cancer
?? coronary artery disease

?, uncertain association.

This gives a biochemical mechanism by which selenium deficiency could enhance the development of atherosclerotic cardiovascular disease (39). A weak correlation of low selenium levels and coronary vascular disease was reported in one study (58), but not in another (59). In the study where the association with low selenium levels was found, the major dietary source of selenium was fish, suggesting that the correlation may have been spurious and related rather to fish intake. This observation was supported by the finding that serum selenium levels correlated with the eicospentanoic acid concentrations (60).

Suppressed cellular and humoral immune function has been associated with selenium deficiency (61). In animals, selenium deficiency has been associated with impaired defense against candidiasis (61). The putative role of selenium deficiency in the immune dysfunction often found in elderly nursing home residents has not been evaluated.

Studies in children have suggested that selenium-deficient kwashiorkor patients may fail to thrive until they receive selenium supplementation (39). Again, the role of selenium supplementation in older subjects with protein-energy malnutrition has not been evaluated.

Selenium toxicity was reported in subjects in the United States who ingested an over-the-counter "health food" supplement that mistakenly contained 180 times more selenium than stated on the label (39). These subjects experienced nail changes, hair loss, and peripheral neuropathy. An early sign of selenium overexposure is the development of a garlic odor on the breath. Other toxic effects include gastrointestinal disturbances, dizziness, and sweating.

The future role of selenium in human nutrition of the elderly is uncertain. Controlled trials of selenium's effects in nutritionally depleted older individuals need to be carried out. Selenium supplementation or choosing a selenium-supplemented formula should be considered in elderly subjects being tube fed.

Silicon

Silicon is important for maintaining the structural integrity of bone and connective tissue. Silicon deficiency may play a role in the development of such degenerative diseases as osteoarthritis or atherosclerosis. The silicon content of certain animal tissues, such as the aorta, skin, and thymus, decreases with aging, whereas the content is unchanged in most tissues (19). Silicon content in the human aorta decreases with age, and this decrease is more marked in association with atherosclerosis (62). Animal studies suggest a decreased absorption of silicon with advancing age (63). Silicon levels are reduced in patients with diabetes mellitus (22). Further studies on the role of silicon with aging are indicated.

Vanadium

Vanadium deficiency in animals leads to elevated cholesterol levels (19). Data on humans are controversial, with two studies failing to show an effect of vanadium on cholesterol (64,65) and one study suggesting that vandium could lower cholesterol levels (66).

Vanadate is a potent inhibitor of $Na^+K^+ATPase$ *in vitro* and may play a role in the physiologic regulation of the sodium pump and energy metabolism (1). *In vivo* evidence for this hypothesis in presently lacking. The average daily human intake of vanadium is 2 mg. Studies on alterations in the intake or excretion of vanadium in older individuals have not been undertaken.

TRACE ELEMENT INTERACTION

The effects of each trace element are heavily dependent on one another. Thus, high intakes of zinc, cadmium, or copper interfere with the utilization and tissue storage of iron (67). Similarly, zinc supplements has been shown to cause anemia secondary to hypocupremia (68). Tetrathiomolybdate inhibits copper absorption (67). Low concentrations of dietary iron enhance the absorption not only of dietary iron but also of lead, zinc, cadmium, cobalt, and manganese (67). The potentiating effect of selenium deficiency on lipid peroxidation and thus free radical damage is enhanced in some tissues by concurrent deficiency of copper or manganese (67). The role of these trace element interactions requires intensive study in older individuals who may be on one trace element supplement, such as zinc, have a poor dietary intake, and be receiving drugs, (eg, diuretics) that cause trace element loss in the urine.

CONCLUSION

Many of these trace elements appear to be important for the maintenance of normal glucose homeostasis and lipid metabolism. Others play an important role in the maintenance of bone structure. Enzymes involved in collagen cross-linking, one of the benchmarks of aging, are often catalyzed by trace elements. Selenium deficiency may play a role in carcinogenesis, is associated with immune dysfunction, and occurs commonly in tube-fed patients. Selenium is essential for the activity of glutathionine peroxidase, which protects against free radical damage by decreasing the formation of hydroxy radicals. Little is known about the role of drugs, especially diuretics, and intercurrent illness on the development of trace mineral deficiency with advancing age. Also, the interactions of trace elements with one another—particularly in the situation where the decision is made to replace a single trace element—need further investigation. Overall, there is a need for increased study of the role of trace elements in the aging process.

REFERENCES

1. Nielsen FH. *Ann Rev Nutr* 1984;4:21–41.
2. Nielsen FH, Hunt CD, Miller LM, et al. *FASEB J* 1987;1:394–397.
3. Offenbacher EG, Pi Sunyer FX. *Ann Rev Nutr* 1988;8:543–563.
4. Schwarz K, Mertz W. *Arch Biochem Biophys* 1957;72:515–518.
5. Jeejeebhoy KN, Chu RC, Marliss EB, Greenberg R, Bruce-Robertson AS. *Am J Clin Nutr* 1977;30:531–538.
6. Freund H, Atamian S, Fischer JE. *JAMA* 1979;241:496–498.
7. Brown RO, Forloines-Lynn S, Cross RE, Heizer WD. *Dig Dis Sci* 1986;31:661–664.
8. Urberg M, Zemel MB. *Metabolism* 1987;36:896–899.
9. Shroeder HA, Balassa JJ, Tipton IH. *J Chron Dis* 1962;15:941–964.
10. Shroeder HA, Nason AP, Tipton IH. *J Chron Dis* 1970;23:123–142.
11. Pi-Sunyer FX, Offenbacher EG. In: Hegsted DM, Chichester CO, Darby WJ, McNutt KW, Stalvey RM, Stotz EH, eds. *Nutrition reviews: Present knowledge in nutrition,* 4th ed. New York: Nutrition Foundation, 1976;571–586.
12. World Health Organization: *Evaluation of certain food additives and the contaminants mercury, lead and cadmium (technical report series 505).* Geneva: World Health Organization, 1972.
13. Bunker VW, Lawson MS, Delves HT, et al. *Am J Clin Nutr* 1984;39:797–802.
14. Shaper AG, Pocock SJ, Walker M, et al. *Br Med J* 1982;284:299–302.
15. Schroeder HA, Nason AP, Tipton IH. *J Chron Dis* 1967;20:869–874.
16. Duckham JM, Lee HA. *Q J Med* 1976;45:277–282.
17. Taylor A, Marks V, Shabaan AA, et al. In: Brown S, ed. *Clinical chemistry and chemical toxicology of metal.* Amsterdam: Elsevier/North Holland, 1977;105–115.
18. Alexander CS. *Am J Med* 1972;53:395–399.
19. Udipi SA, Watson RR. In: Watson RR, ed. *Handbook of nutrition in the aged.* Boca Raton, FL: CRC Press, 1985;145–156.
20. Coleman RF, Herrington J, Scales JT. *Br Med J* 1973;1:527–528.
21. Klevay LM, Inman L, Johnson LK, et al. *Metabolism* 1984;33:1112–1118.
22. Mooradian AD, Morley JE. *Am J Clin Nutr* 1987;45:877–895.
23. Fields M, Reiser S, Smith JC Jr. *Proc Soc Exp Biol Med* 1983;173:137–139.
24. Kanabrocki EL, Case LF, Graham L, et al. *J Nucl Med* 1967;8:166–172.
25. Martin Mateo MC, Bustamante J, Gonzales Cantalapiedra MA. *Biomedicine* 1978; 29:56–58.
26. Klevay LM, *Am J Clin Nutr* 1975;28:764–774.
27. Yunice AA, Lindeman RD, Czerwinski AW, et al. *J Gerontol* 1974;29:277–281.
28. Bunker VW, Hinks LJ, Lawson MS, et al. *Am J Clin Nutr* 1984;40:1096–1102.
29. Turnlund JR, Michel MC, Keyes WR, et al. *Am J Clin Nutr* 1982;36:587–591.
30. Husdan H, Vogl R, Oreopoules D, et al. *Clin Chem* 1976;22:1884–1889.
31. Morley JE, Gorbien MJ, Mooradian AD, et al. *J Am Geriatr Soc* 1988;36:845–859.
32. Pleban PA, Pearson KH. *Clin Chem* 1979;25:1915–1918.
33. Schroeder HA, Nason AP. *J Nutr* 1974;104:167–171.
34. Lisun-Lobanova VP. *Zdravookhr Beloruss* 1966;9:49–53.
35. Hirsch-Kolb H, Kolb HJ, Greenberg DM. *J Biol Chem* 1971;246:395–401.
36. Abumrad N, Schneider AJ, Steel D, Rogers S. *Am J Clin Nutr* 1981;34:2551–2559.
37. Rajagopalan KV. *Ann Rev Nutr* 1988;8:401–427.
38. Bunk RF. *Ann Rev Nutr* 1983;3:53–70.
39. Levander OA. *Ann Rev Nutr* 1987;7:227–250.
40. Thomson CD, Rea H, Robinson MF, et al. *Proc Univ Otago Med Sch* 1977;55:18–26.
41. Lane HW, Warren DC, Taylor BJ, et al. *Proc Soc Exp Biol Med* 1983;173:87–905.
42. Miller L, Mills BJ, Blocky AJ, et al. *J Am Coll Nutr* 1983;2:331–341.
43. Feller AG, Rudman D, Erve PR, et al. *Am J Clin Nutr* 1987;45:476–483.

44. Gelbert SA, Weddnech R. *Nutr Res Suppl* 1985;1:217–223.
45. Ganapathy SN, Thimaya S. In: Watson RR, ed. *Trace elements in human health and disease,* vol 3. Boca Raton, FL: CRC Press, 1985;111–122.
46. Diplerk AT. *Am J Clin Nutr* 1987;45:1313–1322.
47. Levander OA, Burk RF. *JPEN* 1986;10:545–549.
48. Fleming CR, Lie JT, McCall JT et al. *Gastroenterology* 1982;83:689–693.
49. Johnson RA, Baker SS, Fallen JT, et al. *N Engl J Med* 1981;304:1210–1212.
50. Brown MR, Cohen MJ, Lyons JM, et al. *Am J Clin Nutr* 1986;43:549–554.
51. Kien CL, Ganther HE. *Am J Clin Nutr* 1983;37:319–328.
52. Van Rij AM, Thomson CD, McKenzie JM, et al. *Am J Clin Nutr* 1979;32:2076–2085.
53. Morley JE, Mooradian AD, Silver AJ, et al. *Ann Intern Med* 1988;109:890–904.
54. Menkes MS, Comstock GW, Vuilleumier JP, et al. *N Engl J Med* 1986;315:1250–1254.
55. Brown MR, Cohen JH, Lyons JM, et al. *Am J Clin Nutr* 1986;43:549–554.
56. Berek C, Omg A, Massa H, et al. *Proc Natl Acad Sci USA* 1986;83:1490–1494.
57. Dworkin BM, Rosenthal WS, Wormster GP, et al. *JPEN* 1986;10:105–107.
58. Virtamo J, Valkeila E, Alftham G, et al. *Am J Epidemiol* 1985;122:276–282.
59. Kok FJ, deBruijn AM, Vermeeren R, et al. *Am J Clin Nutr* 1987;45:462–468.
60. Smith DK, Teague J, McAdam PA, et al. *J Am Coll Nutr* 1986;5:243–252.
61. Watson RR, Moriguchi S, McRee B, et al. *J Leukocyte Biol* 1986;39:447–456.
62. Leoper J, Leoper J, Lemaine A. *Press Med* 1966;74:865–872.
63. Schwarz K. In: Hockstra WG, Suttie JW, Ganther HE, Mertz W, eds. *Trace element metabolism in animals,* vol 2. London: Butterworths, 1975;355–370.
64. Diamond G, Caravaca J, Berchimol A. *Am J Clin Nutr* 1963;12:49–53.
65. Hopkins LL, Mohr ME. *Fed Proc* 1974;33:1773A.
66. Curran GL, Azarnoff DL, Bolinger RE. *J Clin Invest* 1959;38:1251–1259.
67. Mills CF. *Ann Rev Nutr* 1985;5:173–193.
68. Prasad AS, Brewer GJ, Schoomaker EB, et al. *JAMA* 1978;240:2166–2168.

Geriatric Nutrition, edited by John E. Morley,
Zvi Glick, Laurence Z. Rubenstein.
Raven Press, Ltd., New York © 1990.

13

Nutritional Anemias in the Elderly

David A Lipschitz

*Geriatric Research Education and Clinical Center, VA Medical Center and
Department of Medicine, University of Arkansas for Medical Sciences,
Little Rock, Arkansas 72206*

Numerous studies have shown anemia to be very common in the elderly. There is also evidence that anemia in otherwise healthy older individuals is not due to the commonly recognized causes. A close analysis of available information suggests strongly that anemia is not a consequence of aging. There is also indirect evidence linking changes in erythropoiesis with nutritional factors. This chapter summarizes the effects of age on erythropoiesis and discusses the role of nutritional factors in the etiology.

NORMAL ERYTHROPOIESIS

The production of red cells by the marrow involves a complex interaction between hematopoietic cells, their stromal microenvironment, and a series of hormones that affect cell proliferation and differentiation (1-2). Erythroid cells are derived from a small pool of pluripotent hematopoietic stem cells that have the ability, under the appropriate conditions, to give rise to progenitor cells that are committed to erythropoietic differentiation (Fig. 1). In the case of erythropoiesis two committed progenitor cells have been identified. The more primitive precursor, which forms large colonies in cultures containing high concentrations of erythropoietin, is referred to as BFU-E (burst forming unit-erythroid). It is the immediate precursor of the CFU-E (colony forming unit-erythroid) that develops in culture at much lower concentrations of erythropoietin and after a shorter interval. The CFU-E is the immediate precursor of the proerythroblast, which is the earliest morphologically recognizable erythroid precursor. Proerythroblasts divide into more mature normoblasts that begin to produce hemoglobin in their cytoplasm. With further maturation the cell becomes smaller and its nucleus pyknotic. Finally, the nucleus is extruded, resulting in a reticulocyte that has the ability to exit the marrow and enter the circulating red cell mass.

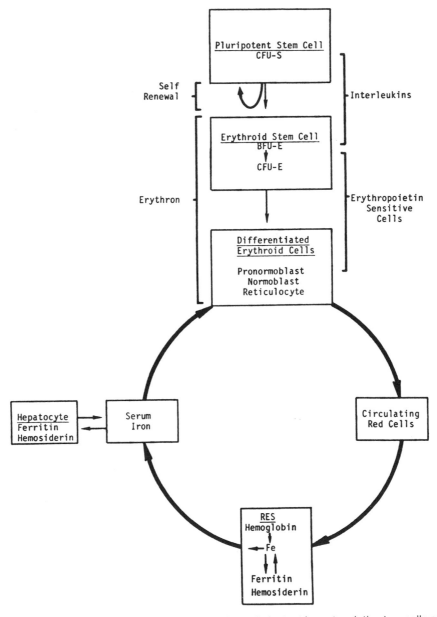

FIG. 1. The production of erythropoietic cells from pluripotent hematopoietic stem cells and committed erythroid progenitor cells. Reticulocytes enter the circulation, mature, and survive for 120 days. Senescent red cells are destroyed by the reticuloendothelial system. Iron derived from these red cells is recircuited to the bone marrow by transferrin. If body demands decrease, iron is diverted into stores. Iron is easily mobilized from stores if demands increase.

The erythron is the component of the bone marrow responsible for red cell production. The circulating red cell mass is maintained at the required level by adjusting red cell production in response to the degree of stimulation by erythropoietin. Tissue oxygen tension is the major determinant of erythropoietin production, which occurs largely in the kidney and to a lesser extent in the liver. The hormone exerts its effect on CFU-E and on proerythroblasts, resulting in increased proliferation, accelerated hemoglobin synthesis, and earlier release of reticulocytes into the peripheral blood. The hormone is not involved in the regulation of BFU-E production.

Within the circulation red cells survive for 120 days (Fig. 1). Senescent red cells are phagocytosed by reticuloendothelial cells located in the liver, spleen, and bone marrow. Within these cells the hemoglobin is broken down to its constituent amino acids, bilirubin and iron. Iron is either transferred to the cell membrane where it combines with transferrin or is stored in the cell as ferritin and hemosiderin. Iron bound to transferrin is transported back to the bone marrow where it is taken up by erythroid precursors and incorporated into heme. The recircuiting iron from senescent red cells to new red cell precursors through the reticuloendothelial system and transferrin is referred to as the iron cycle. Under normal circumstances approximately 30 mg iron passes through the plasma pool each day, the majority being derived from the breakdown of senescent red cells. Depending on marrow demands, iron is either mobilized or deposited in tissue iron stores.

Effect of Age on Normal Erythropoiesis

Because human aging is so heterogeneous, it is very difficult to determine whether a noted change in the erythropoietic system in the elderly reflects an effect of age *per se* or the numerous environmental variables that modulate erythropoiesis over time. In this regard one must rely on animal data in which chronologic aging has occurred in a constant environment.

Animal studies have generally shown that in the basal state few, if any, changes in erythropoiesis can be demonstrated (3-4). Thus, the mild anemia so frequently noted in old rodents is caused by an age-related expansion in plasma volume, rather than a decrease in red cell mass. In addition red cell life span is unaffected by aging, and the number of BFU-E, CFU-E, and differentiated cells in the bone marrow is identical in older and younger animals (Table 1).

A cardinal feature of the aging process is a reduction in reserve capacity characterized by a diminished ability to respond to increased stimulation. There is good evidence that this reduction applies to the aged erythropoietic system. Thus, the rate of return of the hematocrit to normal after phlebotomy is decreased in aged mice (3,5), and *in vivo* and *in vitro* studies have shown that erythroid cells from aged mice respond less well to stimulation than do cells from young animals (6-7).

TABLE 1. *Comparison of hematologic parameters in young and old mice housed singly or in groups*

	Young mice		Old mice	
Parameter	Single caged	Group caged	Single caged	Group caged
Hematocrit (%)	49.9 (0.4)	50.0 (0.5)	46.1 (0.7)	44.9 (0.6)[a]
BFU-E/kg ($\times 10^6$)	5.5 (0.5)	4.8 (0.4)	4.9 (0.4)	4.4 (0.2)[b]
CFU-E/kg ($\times 10^6$)	131.0 (10)	112.0 (8)	139.0 (8)	61.0 (2)[b]
Erythroid cells/kg ($\times 10^9$)	7.6 (0.5)	7.1 (0.3)	6.5 (0.6)	4.7 (0.3)[b]

From Williams et al., ref. 4.
[a]Group-housed old mice were significantly lower than the other groups ($p < .02$).
[b]Group-housed old mice were significantly lower than the other groups ($p < .01$).

Of most significance is the effect of group housing on erythropoiesis in young and old animals (4). When very old mice (42 months) are housed in groups of five animals per cage a significant alteration in bone marrow function is noted. The animals become frankly anemic, and the number of erythroid progenitor and differentiated cells in the bone marrow declines significantly (Table 1). In contrast, no change is noted if these animals are housed in individual cages. Furthermore, no change in erythropoiesis is noted if younger animals are housed in groups. The mechanism accounting for these age-related changes is unknown. Possibilities include minor infection, increased activity when strange animals are housed in groups, or increased competition for nutrients. The hematopoietic changes noted in these group-housed old mice are identical to the changes described with overcrowding. These effects are only seen, however, when young animals are housed in groups of ten per cage. These findings suggest that a minor stress that does not affect hematopoiesis in young animals causes significant abnormalities in the old. The results are of most importance to the interpretation of the changes in erythropoiesis noted with age in humans. It seems highly likely that an erythropoietic abnormality will develop more rapidly and from less of a pathologic insult in the elderly than in the young. In addition, the delineation of the etiology of anemia, for example, may be more difficult.

Prevalence of Anemia in the Elderly

It is highly likely that the erythropoietic effects of aging in humans will be similar to the changes noted in animal models. Thus, basal hematopoiesis should be unchanged. There is good evidence that bone marrow cellularity decreases in the elderly, but the functional significance of this observation is unknown (8). The major change in the hematopoietic system with age is a higher prevalence of a mild anemia. A series of epidemiologic studies from the United States, Canada, and Europe demonstrated a higher prevalence of anemia in the elderly (9-12). In women older than age 59 anemia occurs as frequently as that noted in women of child-bearing age. In men a definite increase in the prevalence of anemia is found in older age groups. Studies from Great Britain are important as they have determined the incidence of anemia in large number of subjects older than age 60 years. In both men and women, the prevalence of anemia increased significantly with each successive decade (13-14). A recent analysis of the Second National Health and Nutrition Examination Survey (NHANES 2), demonstrated a significant reduction in hemoglobin levels with advancing age in apparently healthy men and a minimal, although significant, decrease in elderly women (15). Based upon a lower normal limit of 14 g/dl, a very large percentage of elderly men were anemic. This study proposed that the reduction in hemoglobin in elderly men is a consequence of aging and suggested that age-specific reference standards for hemoglobin concentration for the elderly be adopted.

In hospitalized and institutionalized elderly the incidence of anemia is even higher. A survey of patients admitted to the Geriatric Evaluation Unit of the John L. McClellan Veterans Hospital revealed that 58% had hemoglobin values lower than 14g/dl. In the institutionalized elderly the incidence in men ranges from 30 to 50%, and for women the incidence ranges from 25 to 40%.

Etiology of Anemia in the Elderly: A Potential Role for Nutritional Factors.

Close evaluation revealed that the cause of anemia is usually not obvious in ambulatory, apparently healthy elderly (11). These subjects had evidence of mild marrow failure characterized by significant reductions in the number of bone marrow CFU-C and CFU-E and decreases in marrow-differentiated erythroid and myeloid cells (16). The elderly men and women with unexplained anemia had lower peripheral leukocyte and platelet counts. A major unanswered question is whether this unexplained anemia results from the aging process or some other related abnormality. Because animal models indicate that basal hematopoiesis is unaltered with aging and a true anemia does not occur, other causes must be considered for the anemia occurring in elderly humans. This possibility is strengthened by the recent finding that anemia is extremely rare in very affluent healthy elderly communities. In one study conducted in New Mexico, none of the elderly subjects studied was anemic or developed anemia during a 5-year follow-up (17).

Epidemiologic studies provide further clues to the etiology of the anemia in the elderly. Cross-sectional studies invariably demonstrate a higher prevalence of anemia in low socioeconomic populations (9,15). These groups also have a high prevalence of other nutritional deficiencies. We have performed a comprehensive nutritional and hematologic evaluation on a group of 73 healthy veterans living in a domiciliary facility. A high prevalence of anemia was found in this population. Multivariate analysis showed that age was the major variable affecting declines in immunologic measurements, but was not an important factor in the prevalence of anemia. In contrast, serum albumin, transferrin, and prealbumin, which assess nutritional status, appeared to be good predictors of anemia. This information provides indirect information that a nutritional variable may contribute to the unexplained anemia in these elderly populations.

If nutrition does account for the unexplained anemia seen in healthy elderly populations, mechanisms other than simple deficiencies must be considered. Based on the animal data described above (4), it is likely that significantly less stress is required to result in alterations in erythropoiesis in the elderly. Thus, a nutritional deficiency not usually severe enough to affect the hematopoietic system in younger subjects may account for the anemia in this elderly population group. Or, marginal deficiencies of one or more nutrients acting alone or in combination over prolonged periods of time may modulate or cause the anemia in the elderly. Nutrient delivery to the target organ may be affected by aging, or nutrient cell interactions may be compromised in the elderly.

The above discussion suggests that nutrition accounts for the unexplained anemia seen in the elderly. At the current time this is no more than a hypothesis that requires a great deal of further study. Other possibilities are worthy of consideration. There is some evidence that elderly subjects with anemia have higher sedimentation rates than nonanemic elderly (18). This has led to the suggestion that anemia reflects an acute or chronic disease process. On the other hand, iron-deficient erythropoiesis, which characterizes the anemia of inflammation or chronic disease, was not present. It remains likely, however, that a relatively minor inflammatory or chronic stress may result in anemia only in an elderly population.

HEMATOLOGIC MANIFESTATIONS OF PROTEIN-CALORIE MALNUTRITION (PCM) IN THE ELDERLY

A high incidence of PCM has been reported in hospitalized patients and occurs in as many as 65% of hospitalized elderly (19). The incidence is also very high in nursing homes and in other long-term care settings (20). The disorder is characterized by hypoalbuminemia and alterations in immune and hematologic function. Anemia is invariably present, the features being identical to that noted in the anemia of chronic disease or inflammation (21). In both men and women, the hemoglobin concentration ranges from 10 to 12 g/dl. The serum iron is below 60 ug/dl, and the transferrin saturation is less than 20%. In contrast to iron-deficiency anemia in which iron stores are absent, patients with PCM have increased iron stores, which are reflected in a normal to elevated serum ferritin ($<$ 60 ng/ml) and a low total iron-binding capacity (TIBC) ($<$250 ug/dl). In the elderly the immunohematopoietic sequelae of PCM tend to be more severe than in younger individuals. This may well relate to the diminished reserve capacity that we believe exists in the elderly. Table 2 demonstrates the similarities between the effects of age and PCM on immune and hematologic function. Studies in animal systems have shown that the effects of aging and protein deficiency are additive and this almost certainly applies to elderly humans.

The most appropriate definition of PCM is that it is a metabolic response to stress associated with increased requirements for calories and protein. We believe that the elderly are more susceptible to protein-energy malnutrition and develop pathology more rapidly and with less stress than do younger subjects. The stresses that cause the disorder include trauma, infection, and other acute or chronic inflammatory conditions. Considering these pathophysiologic facts, it is likely that the hematologic changes noted in these patients reflect the underlying disease and only indirectly relate to a nutritional problem.

Clinical studies have shown that the initial responses to stress that characterize PCM are beneficial and assist the patient in developing an optimal response to the underlying primary pathology. Because the acute stress is associated with severe anorexia, patients rarely if ever consume sufficient calories or protein to meet their daily needs. In young subjects inadequate nutrient intake for a period of up to 10 days usually does not affect outcome adversely. Thereafter, however, inadequate protein and caloric intake results in further lowering of the serum albumin and worsening hematologic, immune, and hepatic function, which can affect outcome adversely. In the elderly, the time before which protein-energy malnutrition exerts a negative effect is likely to be much shorter than in younger subjects. In the elderly, failure to meet nutrient needs after a period as short as 2 to 3 days can cause further lowering of the serum albumin, worsening immunohematologic function, and increased morbidity. It is essential, therefore, that the presence of PEM be appropriately diagnosed and managed in the elderly.

TABLE 2. *Comparison of hematologic and immunologic changes occurring with age and with protein-calorie malnutrition (PCM)*

	Aging	PCM
Cell-mediated immunity		
Delayed cutaneous hypersensitivity	Decreased	Decreased
T cell number	Decreased	Decreased
T suppressor cells	Increased	Increased
Blastic response to stimulation	Decreased	Decreased
Humoral immunity		
B cell number	Normal	Normal
Antibody production	Decreased	Decreased
Hematopoietic system		
Hemoglobin	Decreased	Decreased
Bone marrow precursors	Decreased	Decreased
BFU-E and CFU-E	Decreased	Decreased
Neutrophil function	Decreased	Decreased

We have studied the effects of nutritional rehabilitation on the hematologic system in elderly subjects with PEM who did not have a terminal disease (21). We confirmed previous reports that adequate nutritional support improves delayed cutaneous hypersensitivity and increases the lymphocyte count. In addition, marked improvements in the hematologic system were demonstrated. Correction of the nutritional deficits resulted in a highly significant increase in the hemoglobin concentration that was accompanied by a return of both the serum iron and the TIBC to normal (Fig. 2). Simultaneously the serum ferritin fell, presumably as a result of redistribution of iron from stores to the circulating red cell mass. In selected individuals we also demonstrated that improved nutritional status was accompanied by significant increases in the number of bone-marrow-differentiated and immature stem cells. Of interest was the observation that the delivery of adequate nutrition resulted in a prompt increase in both the serum iron and the TIBC, which occurred long before any other improvement in the clinical status.

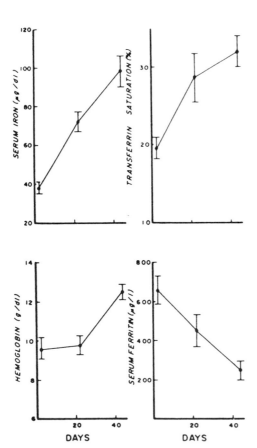

FIG. 2. Changes in hemoglobin, serum iron, transferrin saturation, and serum ferritin levels before and after nutritional repletion. The transferrin saturation is the ratio of serum iron to the TIBC expressed as a percent.

This observation provides the strongest evidence for a nutritional role in the hematopoietic alterations occurring in PEM.

The overall interpretation of the improved immunohematopoietic function in malnourished subjects is extremely difficult. Any hospitalized elderly patient with PEM has coexisting medical conditions, including infection, dehydration, and psychoneurologic changes, that also affect immune and hematologic function. Thus, the improvement seen with nutritional rehabilitation may reflect an overall improvement of the medical status of the patient.

To study this possibility more closely, we examined the effects of increased feeding on the immune and hematologic status of mildly malnourished home-based elderly (23). These individuals were underweight, had evidence of inadequate food intake, were invariably anemic, and had diminished immune function. By providing polymeric dietary supplements between meals, it was possible to increase total caloric and protein intake by 50% for a total of 16 weeks. A significant improvement in nutritional status occurred. Weight gain, increased serum albumin and transferrin, and significant increases in selected vitamins and minerals were seen. Despite this improved nutritional profile, their immune function or hematologic status remained unchanged. No anergic subject demonstrated improved delayed cutaneous hypersensitivity, T and B cell function remained abnormal, and the hemoglobin concentration did not increase.

This study and that on more severely malnourished elderly suggest that nutritional deficiencies aggravate immune and hematopoietic function in the elderly. Correction of coexisting disease and nutritional rehabilitation in the severely malnourished are associated with measurable improvements in host defense parameters. Mildly malnourished elderly individuals who have changes in immune and hematopoietic function not unlike those seen in healthy elderly do not show an improvement in their function, despite obvious improved nutritional status. A reasonable conclusion from these studies is that neither protein or calorie deprivation accounts for the immune and hematologic changes seen in the elderly.

CONCLUSIONS

There is compelling evidence that nutritional factors contribute to or account for age-related changes in the erythropoietic system. A clear relationship exists between the prevalence of anemia and socioeconomic status: the disorder being common in groups in whom poverty is prevalent and rare in the affluent elderly. In low socioeconomic populations a relationship exists between the prevalence of anemia and other nutritional deficiencies. Furthermore, nutritional deprivation reversibly aggravates hematologic changes in the elderly. If nutritional factors do contribute to the anemia seen in relatively healthy elderly, mechanisms other than simple single nutrient deficiencies must be considered. Erythropoietic reserve is diminished so that abnormalities occur with less stress in older people than in younger subjects. Thus, a minor nutritional deficit that would cause no pathology in the young may result in anemia in the elderly. Clearly, further research is required to unravel the complex nature of the interrelationship between age, nutrition, and disease in general and in erythropoiesis in particular.

REFERENCES

1. Quesenberry PJ. In: Williams WJ, Reutler E, Enslev AJ, Lichtman MA, eds. *Hematology* New York: McGraw-Hill, 1983;283.
2. Hillman RS, Finch CA. *The red cell manual,* 4th ed. Philadelphia: FA Davis, 1974.
3. Boggs DR, Patrene KD. *AM J Hematol* 1985;19:327–338.
4. Williams LH, Udupa KB, Lipschitz DA. *Exp Hematol* 198 ;14:827–832.
5. Harrison DE. *J Gerontol* 1975;30:286–291.
6. Udupa KB, Lipschitz DA. *J Lab Clin Med* 1984;103:574–580.
7. Udupa KB, Lipschitz DA. *J Lab Clin Med* 1984;103:581–587.
8. Hartsock RJ, Smith EB, Kettan CS. *Am J Clin Pathol* 1965;43:325–331.
9. US Department of Health, Education and Welfare. *Ten state nutrition survey.* Washington, DC: US Government Printing Office, 1984. (DHEW Publ. No. (HSM) 72–8132).
10. Nutrition Canada: National Survey, Ottawa, Canada, Information Canada, 1973.
11. Lipschitz DA, Mitchell CO, Thompson C. *Am J Hematol* 1981;11:47–54.
12. Timiras M-L, Brownstein H. *J Am Geriatr Soc* 1987;35:639–667.
13. Hill RD. *Practitioner* 1967;217:963–967.
14. McClellan WJ, Andrews GR, Macleod C, Caird FI. *Q J Med* 1973;52:1–13.
15. Yip R, Johnson C, Dallman PR. *Am J Clin Nutr* 1984;39:427–436.
16. Lipschitz DA, Udupa KB, Milton KY, Thompson C. *Blood* 1984;63:502–509.
17. Garry PJ, Goodwin JS, Hunt WC. *J Am Geriatr Soc* 1983;31:389–399.
18. Dallman PR, Yip R, Johnson C. *Am J Clin Nutr* 1984;39:437–445.
19. Sullivan DH, Moriarty MS, Chernoff RS, Lipschitz DA. JPEN 1989;13:249–254.
20. Rudman D, Mattson DE, Nagraj HS, et al. *J Am Geriatr Soc* 1987;35:496–502.
21. Lipschitz DA, Mitchell CO. *J Am Coll Nutr* 1982;1:17–25.
22. Lipschitz DA, Mitchell CO, Milton KY. *JPEN* 1985;9:343–347.

Geriatric Nutrition, edited by John E. Morley,
Zvi Glick, Laurence Z. Rubenstein.
Raven Press, Ltd., New York © 1990.

14

Water Metabolism

Laurel A. Pfeil, Paul R. Katz, and Paul J. Davis

*Department of Medicine, State University of New York at
Buffalo School of Medicine and Biomedical Sciences and
the Veterans Administration Medical Center, Buffalo, New York 14215*

BODY WATER

Changes in body composition that occur with normal aging in humans have been extensively described. The recent use of nuclear measurement techniques to estimate the sizes of body water compartments confirms that total body water (TBW) falls with subject age (17% decrease in women from the third to eighth decade, 11% decrease in men in the same period). This decrease primarily reflects a decline in intracellular water (ICW), as extracellular water (ECW) remains constant (1). The change in ICW is a concomitant of the age-associated fall in lean body mass (LBM), which is estimated from total body potassium (TBK) (2–4), or body cell mass (BCM). LBM and BCM are indexes of the cell mass' production and consumption of energy. (Measurement of BCM is preferred because LBM includes ECW and extracellular solids (chiefly, bone mass), in addition to BCM.) Although ICW declines over the life span, it does so symmetrically with TBK; because potassium is found almost exclusively within cells, the constancy of the TBK:ICW ratio indicates that the intracellular concentration of solute is probably unchanged with normal aging (1). Changes in body water and body cell mass as a function of age are summarized in Table 1.

The average water content of LBM is 73% (5), but in disease states this may be altered in response to changes in extracellular solute concentration. These changes may be primary alterations in extracellular water, in solute, or both or changes in intracellular solute concentration, such as the accumulation of idiogenic osmoles in uncontrolled diabetes mellitus. Thus, in assessing putatively age-associated changes in water metabolism, it is critical to exclude contributions from processes secondary to aging, such as disease states and obesity, that can affect compartments of TBW independently of aging.

TABLE 1. *Changes with normal aging in body water and other compartments*

Compartment	Alteration
Total body water (TBW)	↓
Intracellular water (ICW)	↓
Extracellular water (ECW)	None or modest ↑
Total body potassium (TBK)	↓
Extracellular solids (ECS)[a]	↓
Body cell mass (BCM)	↓
BCM + ECW + ECS (lean body mass, LBM)	↓
BCM (LBM − ECW − ECS)	↓
TBK/LBM or TBK/ICW	None

From Cohen et al., ref. 13, Fulop et al., ref. 2; and Markofsky Lesser and Markofsky, ref. 4.
[a]ECS is primarily bone mineral.

The age-related fall in ICW or the increased ratio of ECW:ICW does not promote the disorders of water metabolism that are encountered in the elderly. Rather, disease states alter more profoundly ECW:ICW relationships through altered homeostatic regulation of water excretion at the level of the kidney or through disordered thirst. Elderly subjects are more prone to disease and are therefore subjected to treatment with pharmacologic agents that alter water excretion; these factors explain the increased risk of disordered water metabolism in aged patients.

This chapter reviews the factors affecting water homeostasis as it is changed with aging. Hyperosmolar and hypoosmolar states in the elderly are also examined briefly.

RENAL FUNCTION AND WATER METABOLISM

Urine volume is determined by the osmolar clearance (C_{osm}) and free water clearance (C_{H_2O}). C_{osm} is the component of urine volume obligated by solute excretion. C_{H_2O} is that contribution to volume, positive or negative (ie, resorptive) that is independent of solute excretion. C_{H_2O} allows the elaboration of dilute or concentrated urine, according to the hydration state of the subject. A ceiling on C_{H_2O} is imposed by the glomerular filtration rate (GFR). If the GFR declines, maximum C_{H_2O} is reduced, and the ability to excrete a free water (solute-free) load is diminished. Free water loading in such a setting may result in a systematically hypo-osmolar state.

The GFR is widely acknowledged to decline as a function of age (6). In a group of 254 normal healthy subjects participating in the Baltimore Longitudinal Study of Aging (7), there was a mean decrease in creatinine clearance of 0.75 ml/min/year. Interestingly, one-third of the subjects had no measurable decrease in renal function with aging. This finding suggests that age-dependent decline in GFR is not invariable and that some of the putative age-related changes in renal function may reflect secondary aging (7). The exact contribution of occult renal disease and hyperfiltration nephropathy (8) to the decline in GFR with age has yet to be quantitated fully.

Several changes in renal anatomy have been implicated in the physiologic derangements of osmoregulation and volume regulation commonly seen in the older patient. Over a normal human life span, renal mass declines by approximately one-third, and renal blood flow falls by 50%. Accompanying these changes is a decline in proximal tubular length and volume, as well as thickening of the tubular basement membrane and mesangial proliferation (9,10).

OSMOREGULATION IN THE ELDERLY

Under normal circumstances, water balance is well maintained in the elderly through the thirst-neurohypophyseal—arginine vasopressin (AVP) or antidiuretic hormone (ADH)—renal feedback loop. Osmoreceptor-driven modulation of fluid intake and permeability of the renal collecting tubule (11) ensure a relatively constant plasma osmolality between 286 and 294 mOsm/kg H_2O. Thus, when increased fluid intake reduces plasma tonicity AVP release is suppressed, allowing for the excretion of excess water by increased C_{H_2O} and generation of dilute urine. Conversely, when fluid intake is reduced, plasma tonicity increases, which increases both thirst and ADH secretion. Water is reabsorbed in the distal renal (collecting) tubule and urine concentration increased until normal serum osmolarity is restored.

Age-related changes in hypothalamic osmoreceptor sensitivity and in end-organ (renal collecting tubule) responsiveness to AVP are well described. When combined with altered thirst sensitivity and probably a reduced ability to dilute the urine maximally, these factors can impair the older person's ability to adapt quickly to fluctuations in fluid intake. Each of these factors is addressed in the following sections.

Vasopressin Secretory Capacity

Vasopressin (AVP) secretory capacity in man is unimpaired in the course of normal aging (12–14). Secretion of AVP may, in fact, be enhanced in elderly subjects and less susceptible to pharmacologic inhibition. Basal circulating levels of AVP are increased in the elderly as well. These changes are probably secondary to decreased end-organ (renal collecting tubule) responsiveness to AVP and are not believed to contribute in the healthy elderly to the increased ECW:ICW ratio observed in the course of normal aging.

As is the case with humans, AVP secretion is unimpaired in animals during aging (15,16). Studies in rats, for example, have revealed enhanced release of ADH and sensitivity to osmotic stimuli with increasing age (17). These observations in humans and rats indicate that age-dependent decreases in urine concentrating ability cannot be attributed to limited central AVP secretory capacity.

Osmoreceptor Sensitivity

Although estimates of osmoreceptor sensitivity in healthy elderly human subjects are drawn from small numbers of subjects, it appears that sensitivity is increased. At a serum osmolality of 296 mOsm/kg H_2O, for example, elderly healthy men studied by Helderman and colleagues (12) had circulating AVP levels that were 60% higher than those in younger subjects; at a serum osmolality of 306, AVP levels were 100% increased in the elderly compared with those of younger subjects. The possibility that heightened osmoreceptor sensitivity could restrict urine diluting capacity—that is, that AVP is incompletely suppressible—is discussed in the next section.

Although AVP secretion appears to be subject more to osmoregulation than to baroreceptor regulation, under certain circumstances nonosmotic stimuli may predominate. In older patients with heart failure, for example, circulating AVP levels have been found to be elevated significantly in the face of ordinarily inhibitory levels of plasma osmolality and adequate blood pressure (18). The role played by AVP under such conditions is not well understood, although there is speculation that AVP possesses vasoconstrictive properties that may selectively augment blood flow to certain organs (19). Resetting of the osmostat in certain clinical settings as a function of age has not yet been studied.

Renal Collecting Tubule Responsiveness to AVP

Miller and Shock showed that reduced urine concentrating capacity in healthy adult men was not corrected by ADH administration (20). This observation established not only the presence of low-grade AVP resistance in the aged kidney but also that the alteration with normal aging in urine concentrating ability was not attributable to restricted central release of AVP.

The molecular basis of end-organ resistance to AVP is speculative. Age-dependent loss of the renal medullary osmotic gradient because of increased medullary blood flow may be a contributing factor. Similarly, as nephrons drop out with age, more solute must be excreted for each remaining nephron. The resultant osmotic diuresis may fix the concentrating ability. Although this hypothesis is attractive theoretically, concentrating ability does not seem to be a function of age-dependent reductions in the GFR (21,22). It has also been proposed, based on animal studies, that an age-dependent increase in central AVP release precedes collecting tubule resistance to AVP and that the latter is a consequence of downregulation of ADH receptors by high circulating levels of the hormone (17,23). Supportive evidence in man for this contention is not yet available.

Rowe and colleagues have reported that the increase in plasma AVP concentration in response to the acute assumption of the upright posture is frequently impaired in healthy elderly men and women (24). This baroreceptor-dependent response is in contrast to the heightened hypothalamic osmoreceptor sensitivity in older subjects (12). Rowe postulates that age-related changes in osmoreceptor sensitivity reflect baroreceptor modulation of osmoreceptor function, rather than a response to renal tubule resistance to AVP (25). Although applicable in the experimental setting of hypertonic saline infusion (12,26) or volume expansion, this concept of osmoreceptor/baroreceptor competition is probably not applicable to elderly subjects with normal plasma volumes who assume upright posture.

Urinary Diluting Capacity

The ability to generate dilute urine was studied by Lindeman and coworkers who reported that water loading resulted in lower U_{osm} in younger subjects than in the elderly (27). C_{H_2O} was apparently reduced in middle-aged and older subjects, with the principal change expressed by middle age. However, when free water clearance was corrected for the age-dependent decline in creatinine clearance, there was no difference in maximum C_{H_2O} between young and old men, although a significant age-associated difference did persist in women. The fact that young participants achieved lower urine osmolality than the elderly during acute water loading reflected substantial differences in the GFR (38% and 56% reductions, respectively, in middle-aged and old versus young adults) among the groups and resultant increases in solute load/residual nephron in the elderly. In a similar study of subjects with Type II diabetes mellitus of varying ages (47 to 70 years), all of whom had normal GFRs, Davis et al. found that the minimal urine osmolality generated after a water load was identical in participants younger than 60 years and those older than 60 years of age (28). These findings suggest that, in aged subjects with a relatively normal GFR, minimal urine osmolality achieved during water loading is not different from that in younger subjects. The putative increase in risk of hypo-osmolar states in elderly patients therefore should be limited to subjects with a decreased GFR (29,30). In fact, the risk even in this subpopulation is small. If minimum urine osmolality during water loading is defined as less than or equal to 100 mOsm/kg H_2O, a normal level of performance is readily achievable in elderly subjects (27,28). Extraordinary conditions of hypotonic fluid intake are required in order to induce plasma hypo-osmolarity in the setting of moderate reduction in the GFR (31). No studies have yet been reported of plasma AVP levels in healthy elderly during formal water loading to confirm that suppression of ADH is maximal.

VOLUME (SALT) REGULATION IN THE ELDERLY

Increasing age is associated with deficits in both salt conservation and excretion. Although the elderly are able to lower their urinary sodium concentrations in the face of a reduction in sodium intake, the time required to achieve sodium balance (new steady state) is markedly prolonged when compared to the young (32). Despite a somewhat delayed response in the elderly, however, older people do eventually attain sodium balance (Na intake = Na output). Indeed, after 6 days of dietary sodium restriction (33), subjects aged 60 to 70 years had weight losses similar to subjects aged 20 to 30 years.

The basis of this sluggish homeostatic adjustment is not known. Despite normal levels of renin substrate, levels of plasma renin and renin activity have been noted to decline by 30 to 50% in the elderly. The renin response to salt restriction, diuretics, and/or upright posture is also impaired in the elderly (33,34). As might be predicted, aldosterone levels in the elderly average 30 to 50% of normal values in the young. Because ACTH administration results in a normal elevation of cortisol and aldosterone in older patients, it appears that the defect in salt regulation lies in renin secretion and not in adrenal insufficiency (35).

Control over solute excretion is also dependent on atrial natriuretic peptide (ANP). Although ANP secretion is affected by age (36), it is not yet clear whether the relative contribution of ANP to volume regulation differs in the elderly.

Delayed homeostatic adjustment to altered sodium intake in older subjects prevents the rapid excretion of an acutely administered salt load. Thus, even in patients without obvious heart disease, injudicious intravenous administration of salt may cause acute volume expansion and cardiorespiratory compromise.

SYSTEMIC MODIFIERS OF WATER METABOLISM

Thirst

Alterations in thirst perception occur with normal aging. In a study comparing thirst in young versus elderly men done by Phillips et al. (37), elderly men aged 65 to 77 years old drank less than the young men after a 24-hour water deprivation, despite free access to water and higher serum sodium and plasma osmolalities. On a subjective level, the elderly men reported much less thirst overall than their younger counterparts. Miller et al. (38) reported on thirst in six stroke patients aged 68 to 91 years, all with recurrent episodes of hypernatremia. Despite apparently normal mental status, ready access to fluids and encouragement by staff, these patients did not take adequate fluids to replace volume loss and correct their serum sodium. The blunted thirst response in both normal elderly and those with central nervous system disease is an important predisposing factor to volume depletion and hypernatremia.

Access to Water

A very basic factor in water homeostasis in the elderly is impaired access to water. Acutely ill and/or stable institutionalized aged may be completely dependent on their caregivers to provide fluids in adequate and appropriate amounts. Patients with dementia or clouded sensorium may be unable to communicate their need for oral fluids, even if they can perceive and integrate the sensation of thirst. Those with severe cognitive problems who are agitated may, in fact, be physically restrained in their bed and chair. Elderly subjects are more likely than younger individuals to have visual or musculoskeletal impairments that may also hamper their ability to navigate and obtain fluids. Even relatively healthy, independent older individuals may have limited access to fluids because of environmental barriers, such as stairs, that inhibit them from freely seeking liquids and nourishment. Access to water may also be affected by incontinence, an extremely common problem in older men and women. Incontinence often prompts a self-imposed fluid restriction in hopes of decreasing the frequency and volume of urine.

CLINICAL SYNDROMES

The elderly population is at increased risk of developing derangements in salt and water metabolism largely because of the increased incidence in this population of disease states that promote aberrations in volume and tonicity or lead to use of pharmacologic agents that impair C_{H_2O}.

Hyponatremia

In all age groups, hyponatremia may present in the setting of volume contraction, euvolemia, or volume excess. The prevalence of hyponatremia in aged individuals is high, having been reported in 22.5% of patients residing in a chronic disease facility (39) and 11.3% of patients admitted to an acute geriatrics unit (30). The clinical presentation may be vague and nonspecific. In Kleinfeld's (39) study of 36 patients with hyponatremia in a chronic care facility, only 9 were symptomatic, although many had symptoms attributable to their underlying disease process. In Sunderam's study of 77 hyponatremic patients on an acute geriatric unit (30), 61% had symptoms attributable to hyponatremia, although the latter was not was diagnosed clinically. When present, symptoms include depression, lethargy, confusion, anorexia, weakness, and muscle cramps. Very low serum sodium levels or a rapid decline in sodium may be accompanied by seizures or stupor. Clinical signs that may be present in the setting of hyponatremia include altered sensorium, hypo-reflexia, pathologic reflexes, hypothermia, Cheyne-Stokes respiration, and pseudobulbar palsy (39). It is not clear which of these findings, except for altered sensorium, specifically is caused by hypo-osmolarity.

Hypoosmolarity occasionally reflects an important loss of sodium, such as hypoadrenocorticism or renal salt wasting, but usually is due to disease-related or drug-induced reduction in C_{H_2O}. The syndromes of inappropriate secretion of AVP (SIADH) caused by tumors, systemic infection, or non-tumoral central nervous system disease are states of decreased C_{H_2O} as are cirrhosis with ascites and chronic congestive heart failure.

Drug-induced hyponatremia occurs frequently in the elderly population, which is not surprising in view of the polypharmacy so commonly encoun-tered in older patients (Table 2). Diuretics, sulfonylureas, tricyclic antide-pressants, and barbiturates are notable in this regard.

Diuretics were the most common cause of hyponatremia in one study, accounting for 49 of 77 cases (30). In another study, thiazides accounted for seven cases of rapid-onset hyponatremia reported, in which six of the sub-jects were elderly (40). Hyponatremia associated with diuretics can often be distinguished from that produced by other causes by the concurrent pres-ence of hypokalemia and alkalosis. Diuretics may exert their effects by low-ering the GFR and by decreasing distal tubule delivery of hypotonic filtrate. Diuretic-induced hypokalemia may also exaggerate volume-induced ADH release (41).

Chlorpropamide is a widely used oral sulfonylurea that has antidiuretic properties in normal subjects; it may be associated with hyponatremia in up to 4% of patients (42). Interestingly, Davis et al. (43) have shown that the

TABLE 2. *Drugs associated with decreased free water clearance*

Drug	Mechanism
Vasopressin	AVP activity
Oxytocin	AVP activity
Thiazides	Decreased sodium excretion
Barbiturates	Enhanced AVP release
Carbamazepine	Enhanced AVP release
Chlorpropamide	Enhanced AVP release, enhanced renal response
Clofibrate	Enhanced AVP release
Cyclophosphamide	Renal tubular effect of cyclophosphamide metabolite
Morphine	Enhanced AVP release
Nicotine	Enhanced AVP release
Vincristine	Enhanced AVP release
Tricyclic antidepressants	Unclear
Monoamine oxidase inhibitors	Unclear
Haloperidol	Unclear
Phenothiazines	Unclear

antidiuretic effect of chlorpropamide is blunted in hyperglycemic (serum glucose concentration greater than 200 mg/dl) patients as compared to those with glucose levels less than 200 mg/dl. It appears that the persons in an antidiuretic state (eg, on chlorpropamide) improve their C_{H_2O} in the context of osmotic diuresis (hyperglycemia) and isotonic urine more than they would without the osmotic diuresis (euglycemia).

Treatment of hypo-osmolar states is reviewed extensively elsewhere (44).

Hypernatremia

Older individuals are predisposed to hypernatremia for a variety of reasons. Decreased thirst perception and decreased availability of water can limit the ability of the older individual to replace fluid losses associated with fever, vomiting, diarrhea, and/or an osmotic diuresis. Viral illnesses and febrile states are more commonly accompanied by alterations in mental status in the elderly, limiting patients' ability to replace water losses. Because of a decline in the glomerular filtration rate and the subsequent decreased ability of the aged kidney to concentrate urine, fixed urinary water loss may continue in the face of total body water deficit to the point of profound ICW loss and intracellular hypertonicity. A paucity of signs and symptoms accompany hypernatremia, although an altered sensorium and mental obtundation are not uncommon findings. Cohadon and Desbordes (45) found that older rats made hypernatremic demonstrated lethargy and ataxia while young rats appeared normal clinically.

SUMMARY

Normal aging in humans is associated with a progressive decrease in total body water (TBW), reflecting the age-dependent decline in body cell mass and intracellular water (ICW). Extracellular water (ECW) volume is unchanged over the life span. There is probably no change in intracellular solute concentration with aging. The decline in the glomerular filtration rate that accompanies aging reduces renal free water clearance C_{H_2O}; this reduction only has clinical consequences if extraordinary solute-free water intake occurs. Hypothalamic osmoregulatory control of arginine vasopressin (AVP, ADH) is heightened in the elderly, probably in response to renal collecting tubule resistance to AVP. Thus, basal circulating levels of AVP are higher in old subjects, and the AVP secretory response to increased plasma osmolality is up to twofold greater in the elderly. The thirst mechanism appears to be blunted in old subjects. These physiologic alterations in water metabolism may contribute to disorders of osmolality that occur with increased frequency in older patients; however, the major factors that promote hypo-osmolarity and hyperosmolarity in the older age group are disease states that alter water homeostasis and to which the elderly are increasingly susceptible and the increasing use in older patients of pharmacologic agents that influence water excretion.

REFERENCES

1. Cohn SH, Vaswani AN, Yasmura S, Yuen K. *J Lab Clin Med* 1985;105:305.
2. Fulop T, Worum I, Csongor J, Foris G, Leovey A. *Gerontology* 1985;31:6.
3. Cox JR, Shalaby WA. *Gerontology* 1981;27:340.
4. Lesser GT, Markofsky J. *Am J Physiol* 1979;236:215.
5. Woodward KT, Trujillo TT, Schuck RL, Anderson EC. *Nature* 1956;178:97.
6. Rowe JW, Andres R, Tobin J, et al. *J Gerontol* 1976;31:155.
7. Lindeman RD, Tobin J, Shock NW. *J Am Geriatr Soc* 1985;33:278.
8. Brenner BM, Meyer TW, Hostetter TH. *N Engl J Med* 1982;307:652.
9. Dormady EM, Offer J, Woodhouse MA. *J Pathol* 1973;109:195.
10. McLachlan MSF, Guthrie JC, Anderson CK, et al. *J Pathol* 1977;121:65.
11. Berl T, Anderson RJ, McDonald KM, Schrier RW. *Kidney Int* 1976;10:117.
12. Helderman JH, Vestal RE, Rowe JW, et al. *J Gerontol* 1978;33:39.
13. Hollenberg NK, Adams DF, Solomon HS, et al. *Circ Res* 1974;34:309.
14. Kirkland J, Lye M, Goddard C, et al. *Clin Endocrinol* 1984;20:451.
15. Fliers E, Swaab DF. *Peptides* 1983;4:165.
16. Frolkis VV, Golovchenko SF, Medved VT, et al. *Gerontology* 1982;28:290.
17. Miller M. *J Gerontol* 1987;42:3.
18. Rondeau E, deLima J, Caillens H, et al. *Mineral Electrolyte Metab* 1982;8:267.
19. Gross PA, Ketteler M, Hausmann C, Ritz E. *Kidney Int* 1987;32:567.
20. Miller JH, Shock NW. *J Gerontol* 1953;18:446.
21. Rowe JW, Shock NW, DeFronzo RA. *Nephron* 1976;17:270.
22. Lindeman RD, VanBuren HC, Raisz LG. *N Engl J Med* 1960;262:1396.
23. Handelman GE, Sayson SC. *Peptides* 1984;5:1217.
24. Rowe JW, Minaker K, Sparrow D, et al. *J Clin Endocrinol Metab* 1982;54:661.
25. Rowe JW. In: Arieff AI, DeFronzo RA, eds. *Fluid, electrolyte and acid-base disorders.* New York: Churchill Livingston, 1985;1231:1246.
26. Robertson GL, Athar S. *J Clin Endocrinol Metab* 1976;42:613.
27. Lindeman RD, Lee TD, Yiengst MJ, et al. *J Lab Clin Med* 1966;68:206.
28. Davis FB, VanSon A, Davis PJ, et al. *Exper Gerontol* 1986;21:407.
29. Lye M. *J Clin Endocrinol Metab* 1984;13:377.
30. Sunderam SG, Mankikar GD. *Age Aging* 1983;12:77.
31. Davis PJ, Davis FB. *Clin Endocrinol Metab* 1987;16:867.
32. Epstein M, Hollenberg NK. *J Lab Clin Med* 1976;87:411.
33. Weidmann P, DeMyttenaere-Bursztein S, Maxwell MH, deLima J. *Kidney Int* 1975; 8:325.
34. Crane MG, Harris JJ. *J Lab Clin Med* 1976;87:947.
35. Rowe JW. *Ann Rev Gerontol Geriatr* 1980;1:161.
36. Dlouha H, Krecek M. *Life Sci* 1985;37:2523.
37. Phillips PA, Phil D, Rolls BJ, et al. *N Engl J Med* 1984;311:753.
38. Miller PD, Krebs RA, Neal BJ, McIntyre DO. *Am J Med* 1982;73:354.
39. Kleinfeld M, Casimir M, Borra S. *J Am Geriatr Soc* 1979;27:156.
40. Ashraf N, Locksley R, Arieff AI. *Am J Med* 1981;70:1163.
41. Fichman MP, Vorherr H, Kleeman CR, Telfer N. *Ann Intern Med* 1971;75:853.
42. Weisman PN, Shenkman L, Gregerman RI. *N Engl J Med* 1971;284:65.
43. Davis FB, Boh D, Davis PJ, et al. *J Clin Pharmacol* 1982;22:97.
44. Schrier RW. *N Engl J Med* 1985;312:1121.
45. Cohadon F, Desbordes G. *Gerontology* 1986;32:46.

Geriatric Nutrition, edited by John E. Morley,
Zvi Glick, Laurence Z. Rubenstein.
Raven Press, Ltd., New York © 1990.

15

Modulation of Age-Associated Immune Dysfunction by Nutritional Intervention

S. Jill James, Steven C. Castle, and Takashi Makinodan

*Geriatric Research, Education and Clinical Center, VA Medical Center West
Los Angeles, Los Angeles, California 90073 and Department of Medicine,
UCLA School of Medicine, Los Angeles, California 90024*

Both clinical and experimental investigations have confirmed that thymus-dependent cell-mediated immunity is consistently more vulnerable to chronic nutritional imbalances than antibody-dependent humoral immunity (1). Coincidentally, those T-cell functions most sensitive to given nutritional perturbations are precisely those that have been established to decline with age in the individual (2). Moreover, the progressive T cell dysfunction with advanced age has been implicated in the etiology of many of the chronic degenerative diseases of the elderly, including arthritis, cancer, vascular injury, and autoimmune-immune complex diseases, as well as a pronounced increased susceptibility to infectious disease (3). Thus, the possible attenuating role of nutritional intervention during progressive immunosenescence is a provocative, although still relatively unexplored area of research.

This chapter begins with a review of the changes in T-cell-dependent immunologic responses that occur during senescence, as both immunologic and nutritional deficiencies interact critically in determining host resistance to disease. Recent studies documenting nutritional modulation of T-cell-mediated immunity are then evaluated, including clinical and experimental protein-calorie deprivation, dietary lipid interactions, and specific micronutrient deficiencies. Finally, directions for future research are discussed in order to determine those points proximal to effector T-cell function that are critically affected by a given nutritional intervention.

T-CELL-DEPENDENT IMMUNOLOGIC CHANGES WITH OLD AGE

A decrease in the ability to mount a T-cell-dependent primary antibody response to sheep red blood cell was first demonstrated in mice in 1962 (4). Since then, studies from various laboratories have established that other

T-cell-dependent and independent immunologic activities in various species are also vulnerable to aging (5). Three interesting results emerged from these studies:

1. Certain immunologic activities decrease with age, others show no change, and still others show an increase. The polymorphic effects of aging on immune response indices underscore the complexity of the cellular and molecular mechanisms involved in aging of the immune system.
2. T-cell-, B-cell-, and macrophage-dependent immunologic activities and macrophages are vulnerable to aging. This finding suggests that immune cells undergo quantitative and/or qualitative changes because they are vulnerable to age-related extrinsic changes in their milieu and/or intrinsic somatic changes.
3. Of the immunologically active cells, T cells are perhaps most vulnerable to aging. Because the thymus undergoes involution before the onset of age-related changes in immune functions (6), the thymus could be partly responsible for age-related T cell changes by not generating T cells and/ or synthesizing differentiation factors for intra- and postthymic precursor T cells as it undergoes involution.

Changes in the Cellular Milieu

As indicated above, alterations in immunologic activities could result from changes in the immune cells, changes in their milieu, or changes in both. Reciprocal cell transfer studies were employed in mice to determine whether the age-related changes in immunologic activities are due to intrinsic cellular changes or to extrinsic changes in the systemic milieu. Immunocompetent cells from young (Y) and old (O) mice were assessed for their ability to mount a humoral or cell-mediated immune response in an immunologically neutral environment of x-irradiated old and young synergic recipients, respectively; ie, $(Y \rightarrow O)$ and $(O \rightarrow Y)$ (7-9). The results showed that both intrinsic and extrinsic changes affect the immune response, but much of the age-related alteration can be attributed to changes in the donor cells, ie, $(Y \rightarrow Y) > (Y \rightarrow O) > (O \rightarrow Y) > (O \rightarrow O)$.

The influence of the cellular milieu could be due to an accumulation of a deleterious substance of a molecular or viral nature or a loss of an essential factor. In this regard, Antonaci et al. (10) recently detected a dissociable inhibitory factor on the surface of circulating lymphocytes of old, but not young humans.

Cellular Changes

Changes in the T-cell-dependent immune response with age can result from (a) a change in the number of T cells, (b) a shift in the enhancing and suppressive activities of regulator cells, or (c) qualitative changes in T cells. All three types of changes have been observed (5).

Quantitative Changes

In humans it was found through the use of monoclonal antibody reagents that the total number of circulating lymphocytes decreases with age by about 15%, primarily because of a decrease in the number of T cells (11–13). In mice the pattern and magnitude of change in the number of T cells were found to vary with the tissue and organ source; in general, the number does not change appreciably with age (14). Thus, cell loss does not appear to contribute significantly to the changes in T-cell-dependent immune functions with age.

Imbalance in Regulatory Cells

In recent years, subpopulations of T cells with helper and suppressor cell markers have been assessed with monoclonal antibody reagents in aging humans and mice with a greater degree of accuracy. In humans, both subpopulations decrease to about the same extent with age, and therefore, their proportion is not altered by aging (11,12). In mice, the total number and proportion of T cells with helper and suppressor cell markers are also not appreciably affected by age (15). Functionally, however, both decreases and increases in T-helper and suppressor activities of significant magnitude have been described (16–19). Investigations of the regulator monocytes/macrophages show that the suppressor activity is elevated in old humans and old mice, and this suppressor activity seems to be related to an increase in prostaglandin sensitivity and/or production with age (20,21). In regard to the immunoenhancing activity of monocytes/macrophages, it was found that the capacity of macrophages to synthesize interleukin-1, a cytokine required for proliferation and differentiation, is reduced with age in mice (22).

These results suggest that a shift in the regulatory activities of T cells and monocytes/macrophages is occurring with age in the absence of a shift in the numbers of regulatory T cells and monocytes/macrophages.

Qualitative Changes

The evidence for qualitative changes in T cells derived from metabolic, morphologic, and genetic studies is most impressive.

At the surface membrane level, both receptor and postreceptor changes have been detected, including a decrease in the number of interleukin-2 (IL-2) binding receptors (16,23,24) and in adenylate cyclase activity (25). Morphologically, swollen mitochondria containing a myelin-like structure with reduced numbers of cristae have been observed in the cytoplasm of T cells of old, but not young humans (26). Metabolically, a variety of age-related changes have been detected at the cytoplasmic level, including alteration in Ca^{2+} uptake (27) and a decrease in the levels of cyclic adenosine monophosphate (28), nicotinamide adenosine dinucleotide (29), and adenosine triphosphate (30). These morophologic and metabolic changes suggest that the ability of antigen-stimulated old T cells to generate metabolic energy may be impaired.

At the nuclear level, a variety of morphologic alterations have been observed with age, including (a) the loss of chromosomes (31); (b) a decrease in the nucleolar organizing region (32), which would indicate that a decrease in the ribosomal DNA (rDNA) content and/or the transcriptional activity of rDNA (33) may be occurring in T cells of aging individuals; and (c) an increase in the frequency of T cells with micronuclei (34), which could contribute to the inability of certain T cells of old individuals to proliferate extensively in response to antigenic or mitogenic stimulation.

Several functional changes have been detected in the nucleus of T cells of old individuals, including (a) a decrease in the ability to repair ultraviolet-light-induced damages (35,36), (b) a decrease in the level of low molecular weight DNA polymerase (37), and (c) a decrease in the activity of purine nucleotide phosphorylase, a purine salvage enzyme, the absence of which can cause an increase in the level of toxic deoxyribonucleoside (38).

Finally, an age-related increase in the proportion of T cells that can proliferate in the presence of 6-thioguanine has been observed in humans (39,40) and mice (41). The fact that these 6-thioguanine-resistant T cells possess levels of hypoxanthine guanine phosphoribosyl transferase (HGRPT) activity as low as those of HGPRT-deficient mutant cells and that they cannot grow in hypoxanthine-aminopterin-thymidine medium suggests that these metabolic changes are reflective of changes at the genomic level. The studies of individual aging mice by Inamizu et al. (41) further show that an inverse correlation exists between the frequency of 6-thioguanine-resistant T cells and the ability of T cells to produce IL-2 or proliferate in response to mitogenic stimulation. This would mean that old mice with a high frequency of HGRPT-deficient T cells tend to have a reduced T cell function, and those with a low frequency of HGRPT-deficient T cells tend to have a heightened T cell function. Of course, this does not necessarily mean that specific mutation of the HGRPT gene is responsible for the decline in T cell activities with age. However, it validates the use of 6-thioguanine-resistant T cells as cellular probes to assess the role that gene alterations play in T cell aging.

AGE-RELATED CHANGES IN THE THYMUS

The thymus is involved in four important functions:

1. The production of chemotactic factors to attract prethymic stem cells to the gland (42)

2. The induction of self-tolerance and major histocompatibility complex (MHC) restriction (43)
3. The production of factors that act on intrathymic immature T cells, influence the peripheralization of T cells, and modulate postthymic immature T cells (42,44)
4. The production of factors that modulate the neuroendocrine circuit (45)

To date, four thymic peptides with hormonal activities have been chemically defined: thymic humoral factor (46), thymopoietin (47), thymosin α_1 (48), and thymulin (49). These hormones are found in the thymic epithelial cells (50,51) and therefore are presumed to be synthesized by them. However, very little is known about what role other stromal cells (fibroblasts, macrophages, and dendritic cells) play in the differentiation and regulation of the parenchymal T cells.

The most dramatic age-related change in the anatomy of the immune system is the involution of thymus. Shortly after reaching maximum cellular mass at around sexual maturity, it starts to involute in humans (52) and mice (53). The beginning of involution coincides with the cessation of prethymic stem cell migration into the thymus as judged by parabiosis of mice of different ages (54) and with the onset of age-related decline in the T-cell-dependent antibody response (4). This suggests that thymic involution contributes to the decline in T-cell-dependent immunity with age. Evidence in support of this view is substantial. One example is that adult thymectomy of autoimmune-susceptible and autoimmune-resistant mice accelerates the decrease in T-cell-dependent humoral and cell-mediated immune responses (55), increases autoimmunity (56), and decreases longevity (57).

Immunohistologic studies by Hirokawa et al. (51) of thymic tissues from 1-day to 62-year-old humans established that thymosin α_1, a representative thymic hormone, is found in the epithelial cells of the cortical surface and the medulla and that aging affects these cells selectively in the medulla. Thus, they found that the number of thymosin-α_1-containing epithelial cells in the medulla decreases progressively beginning at sexual maturity, so that only a fraction can be detected by the third decade of life. In contrast, those cells covering the cortical surface could still be detected in adequate numbers even in the atrophic thymus of a 62-year-old individual. In regard to thymosin-α_1-containing epithelial cells, it is interesting to note that Haynes et al. (50) found that they also contain thymopoietin and the human T cell leukemia virus antigen p19.

In order to understand better the functional changes occurring in the involuting thymus, we assessed the capacity of involuting thymic grafts to generate antigen/mitogen-responsive mature T cells (58,59). Thymic lobes were grafted from donor mice ranging in age from 1 day to 33 months into either (a) thymectomized, x-irradiated, and bone-marrow reconstituted T-cell-deficient adult mice or (b) naturally athymic T-cell-deficient adult mice. Both of these mouse models are deficient in T cells but rich in B cells, macrophages, null cells, precursor stem cells, and stromal cells. At intervals for a period of 12 weeks after grafting, both groups of recipient mice were assessed for various T-cell-dependent immunologic activities; comparable results were obtained that showed that T cell activities are inversely related to the age of the donor mice (ie, the older the donor mice, the lower the T cell activity), but the degree of the inverse relationship differed with the T cell activity index. For example, it appears that the ability of thymic grafts to generate cytolytic T cells against allogeneic target cells declines rapidly starting at birth, long before the thymus reaches its maximum size. In contrast, the ability of thymic grafts to generate mitogen-sensitive T cells decreases only slightly with age, with the decline beginning at midlife, long after the start of the involution process. These results suggest that the intrathymic and postthymic immature T cells could be the major, if not the sole, progenitor source of antigen/mitogen-responsive T cells after adulthood. If so, the thymus can be looked upon as the pacemaker of aging of the T cell arm of the immune system.

To gain a more precise understanding of how the thymus is aging physiologically, a series of studies were initiated to characterize the influence of age on the stromal cells (60). Plastic-adhering stromal cells, which include epithelial cells, macrophages, dendritic cells, and fibroblasts, participate in the differentiation and proliferation of parenchymal thymocytes by producing either the differentiation factors, proliferation factors, or their modulators. Thymic adherent cells, obtained from mice ranging in age from 1 day to 20 months, were cultured for 1 month *in vitro* with weekly supernatant collection. The supernatants were then assessed for their ability to augment or inhibit the antigen/mitogen-induced proliferation of indicator thymocytes and of indicator prethymic splenic cells obtained from syngeneic nude mice. The results revealed that intrathymic but not prethymic T indicator cells are responsive to the modulating influence of the supernatant. It is therefore likely that the prethymic stem cells require a direct contact with the adherent cells in order to undergo differentiation. The results further showed that the ability of thymic adherent cells to synthesize the augmenting factor declines drastically between 2.5 and 5 months of age, which is consistent with the findings derived from histologic and thymic graft studies (58,59). Perhaps the most interesting findings in terms of homeostasis are those indicating that the thymic adherent cells can also synthesize an inhibitory factor. Thus, thymic adherent cells of newborn mice were shown to synthesize both the augmenting factor and the inhibitory factor, whereas those of young adult mice synthesize primarily the augmenting factor and those of 20-month-old mice synthesize primarily the inhibitory factor. Mixture studies of the two factors suggest that these factors can coexist and that the augmentable thymocytes are the target of the inhibitory and augmenting factors.

Further studies of the inhibitory factor showed that the inhibitory factor suppresses the proliferation of mitogen-stimulated thymocytes, but not of mitogen-stimulated T blast cells nor of crude mitogen-stimulated cytolytic T cells (61). These results would suggest that the inhibitory activity of the factor is stage-specific T cell differentiation. Ion exchange and gel filtration chromatographic analysis of the supernatant of thymic adherent cells showed that the fraction with the highest inhibitory activity was confined to the 68,000 fraction, which contains serum albumin. However, albumin itself had no inhibitory activity. Moreover, the inhibitory activity was heat resistant (75°C/30 min).

NUTRITIONAL MODULATION OF
CELL-MEDIATED IMMUNITY (CMI)

Acute or chronic nutritional imbalance, as an environmental variable, can critically modify the cell-mediated immune (CMI) response. Depending on the severity and type of nutritional deficiency, humoral immunity and nonspecific immune defense mechanisms, such as phagocytic cell function and complement synthesis, may also be affected adversely. However, the focus in this chapter is on specific nutrient interaction with CMI.

Protein-Calorie Malnutrition (PCM)

Human Studies

Human studies of PCM, whether in children of underdeveloped countries or in hospitalized adults, have confirmed a causal association between undernutrition and secondary immunodepression resulting in impaired host resistance to infection and/or physiologic stress. So consistent in this association that several studies of clinical malnutrition in medical and surgical patients have demonstrated the potential of immunologic status (eg, delayed hypersensitivity reaction) as a predictor of clinical outcome (62,63). The response to physiologic stress—infection, trauma, surgery, catabolic disease—and nutritional status are mutually interdependent variables that can interact in two directions: (a) Malnutrition can impair the response to physiologic stress via the secondary depression of lymphoid tissue, or (b) chronic physiologic stress can precipitate acute malnutrition via increased nutrient demands and catabolic losses. The pathophysiology of one exacerbates the other, leading to a negative synergistic and cyclic interaction that underlies increased morbidity and mortality.

The voluminous literature of human PCM and immune function has been extensively reviewed by Gross and Newberne (1). Consistent results and precise definitions of immunologic derangement have proven difficult to assess in field studies for several reasons: (a) Multiple and variable nutrient deficiencies often coexist, (b) immune responses are often evaluated after nutritional therapy has begun, (c) assessment is often confounded by concurrent infection, and (d) the degree of malnutrition (severe versus moderate, chronic versus acute) varies among studies. Nonetheless, the general pattern indicates that cell-mediated immunity is more profoundly affected in generalized malnutrition than is humoral immunity.

It must be emphasized that human PCM is a multifaceted complex syndrome involving multiple and variable nutrient deficiencies, not only in protein and energy but also in various vitamins and minerals. The combined deficiencies interact to impair aspects of CMI consistently at all ages, with a negative impact on host resistance as previously described.

Animal Studies

Because multiple and uncontrolled variables confound immunologic evaluation in human PCM, more recent investigation has focused on the impact of single-nutrient variables on aspects of CMI in laboratory animal models in which environmental conditions can be controlled precisely. However, extrapolation of data from animal models to human PCM should be made with caution because these univariate models are, at best, an academic approximation of a complex and multivariate condition. Nonetheless, these studies represent an important first step. Accordingly, several investigators have evaluated either protein or calorie restriction as isolated variables in an otherwise replete diet in laboratory animals. The effect of this regimen on patterns of CMI belied expectations by consistently *enhancing* T-cell-dependent responses when assessed after midlife and by significantly extending life span.

The cause of these disparate effects on CMI, depending on whether undernutrition is naturally occurring in human populations or is imposed as an isolated restriction in the laboratory, is not clear. Laboratory models of PCM are restricted to protein and/or calories, but are supplemented with control levels of micronutrients. Schloen and associates (64) have strongly implicated the importance of micronutrient deficiencies, particularly zinc, in the etiology of depressed CMI in human malnutrition.

In attempting to dissect human PCM into its component parts, most of the controlled studies in animal models try to investigate immunologic effects of either protein or calorie restriction independently. However, considerable metabolic overlap exists when proteins or calories are independently restricted. For example, caloric restriction is generally imposed by feeding the restricted group one-half the quantity of diet consumed *ad libitum* by the control group. Because most control diets contain approximately 20% protein, the restricted animals thus receive about 10% dietary protein, which approaches the level of protein (8%) imposed in studies of chronic protein deprivation. Furthermore, metabolic alterations in response to caloric insufficiency cause a decreased utilization of available protein. When calories are limiting, the carbon skeleton of amino acids is converted to glucose in the liver to meet priority energy requirements. It is likely therefore that caloric restriction is not an independent variable, but may have a component of protein deficiency as well. Conversely, dietary protein restriction, despite the isocaloric adjustment of the diet, often causes inanition, a marked reduction in food intake, as a metabolic adaptation to insufficient protein. Therefore, it is likely that a degree of caloric restriction is simultaneously imposed when protein is limiting. Such nutrient interactions are important considerations.

Caloric Restriction

In 1935, McCay et al. (65) observed that, if the growth rate in rats was retarded in a controlled manner by withholding calories, the surviving animals lived significantly longer than *ad libitum* fed controls. In the early 1960s, Ross et al. (66) confirmed and extended these observations. However, both McCay and Ross observed significant losses to infection *early in life* in the restricted groups.

The immunologic consequences of caloric restriction have been evaluated in several strains of rats and mice. Gerbase-DeLima et al. (67) imposed caloric restriction on a long-lived strain of weanling mice, using a casein-based diet (14.5 cal/21% casein) by feeding the restricted group on alternate days. Various indices of T cell function were followed throughout the life span of the animals and were observed to be *depressed* uniformly in the *early* months of restriction, which corroborated the findings of McCay (65) and Ross et al. (66). However, by midlife the pattern reversed, with enhanced activity in the restricted group compared with *ad libitum* fed controls. The relative enhancement of T cell function was associated with a significant increase in life span. However, life span extension through caloric restriction is not a universal phenomenon. Thus, Harrison and Archer (68) have recently shown that long-lived male C57BL/6J mice fed a calorically restricted diet had in fact shorter median and mean life spans than those fed the standard normal diet, ie, median life span, 591 days versus 878 days; mean life span, 593 days versus 858 days.

Delayed malnutrition and involution of thymic tissue induced by caloric deprivation have been suggested by Good et al. (69) as an important determinant of life span because the rate of thymic involution has been implicated as a major factor in immunologic aging. These investigators chose to study short-lived autoimmune-prone strains of mice (NZB, NZB/NZW) as models for immunologic diseases associated with aging in humans. They found that restricted feeding of 10 cal/day (with control levels of micronutrients) from weaning, regardless of variations in protein, carbohydrate, or fat in the diet, dramatically increased life span in these strains, delayed the onset of autoimmune manifestations, and enhanced indices of CMI. It is not clear, however, whether caloric restriction in autoimmune-prone strains affects life span by altering the tempo of a common aging process or by affecting the life-shortening disease process.

Of considerable interest, although not a focus of longevity studies, is the repeated observation of early suppression of CMI by caloric restriction during the growth period. As documented in other studies, Fernandes et al. (70) similarly observed a depressed *in vitro* response to T cell mitogen, phytohemagglutinin, and depressed response to sheep RBC injected *in vivo* during the first few months of caloric deprivation. These results suggest that the increased longevity and immunoenhancement are not univariate and appear to apply only to the surviving cohort. Nevertheless, the calorically deprived animals display increases in antigen/mitogen-responsiveness, delayed deposition of lethal autoimmune complexes, increased cytotoxicity to allogeneic tumor cells, and significant extension of life span when compared with *ad libitum* fed animals (70).

It should be recognized that, in these studies of food restriction and its effects on CMI and life span, the normal or control level of consumption is, in fact, an arbitrary definition, based on the *ad libitum* intake of caged animals that are deprived of exercise and housed in an unvarying environment. It may be argued that, under these artificial conditions, the restricted intake may be more optimal for CMI reactivity relative to the "normal" control, or alternatively that *ad libitum* feeding is an unnatural environment has a negative impact on life span and CMI.

The reference diet for caloric restriction is designed for rapid growth, maturation, and reproductive capacity. It was never intended to promote longevity, and yet the implicit assumption in studies of caloric restriction is that life span is being extended from a normal or maximum. The high content of protein, fat, and simple sugars in the *ad libitum* diet undoubtedly exceeds physiologic requirements, especially as needs decline with age. Therefore, an important interpretive question is whether the reference diet is in fact *less than optimal* in terms of reflecting the genetic potential for life span in a given species. In terms of the relative immunoenhancement observed with restricted regimens, there is strong evidence that the high-fat content of the control diet may be immunosuppressive, as discussed in the next section.

Lipids and Immune Function

Immunoregulatory aspects of dietary lipid composition are inherently interesting and may have particular relevance to the aging individual in whom lipid profiles tend to increase. The immunosuppressive qualities of high dietary fat could contribute to or potentiate the natural decline in immune activity with age and conceivably exacerbate immune-related disease.

Lipids are essential for the structural and functional integrity of cell membranes. Membrane events are integrally involved in all aspects of cellular immune reactivity. Both the type and quantity of dietary lipid have been found to modulate immune activity in several ways. First, endogenous cholesterol synthesis appears to be an essential prerequisite to DNA synthesis in lymphocyte proliferative responses in order to accommodate new membrane formation (71). Thus, if cholesterol synthesis is blocked, directly or indirectly, proliferative events are abrogated proportionately. Second, the degree of saturation of fatty acids (FA) esterified to membrane lipids can be altered dramatically by the level of FA intake. The degree of unsaturation (number of double bonds) of constituent FAs perturbs the molecular configuration and fluidity of cell membranes; increased membrane fluidity has been associated with immunosuppression (72). Third, circulating lipoproteins (LP) interact with specific membrane receptors on lymphocytes and have been shown to inhibit antigen/mitogen-induced blastogenesis (73). Although the precise biochemical interactions have yet to be elucidated, it is clear that dietary lipids have dynamic immunoregulatory effects through alterations of the cellular lipid constituents and membrane-related activity.

Cholesterol

Several studies have demonstrated that nutritionally induced hypercholesterolemia is associated with impaired host resistance to both bacterial and viral infection (74). However, the apparent immunosuppressive effects of cholesterol must be re-evaluated in the light of recent evidence. Humphries (75) has demonstrated that the dietary cholesterol included in experimental hypercholestrolemic diets is often contaminated with auto-oxidative metabolites, which act as potent immunosuppressive agents by inhibiting sterol synthesis. In related studies, Heiniger (76) found that purified cholesterol, free of oxidized metabolites, was not immunosuppressive. Further, *de novo* cholesterol synthesis was shown to be an obligatory prerequisite to mitogen-stimulated DNA synthesis. Chen (71) has confirmed that endogenous cholesterol synthesis must and does precede DNA synthesis and is apparently required for new membrane synthesis. Agents that block cholesterol synthesis *in vitro* result in impaired mitogen responsiveness (77) and decreased cytotoxicity (78). Enhanced mitogenesis has been associated with increased levels of membrane cholesterol and relative reduction in membrane fluidity (79).

Studies by Broitman et al. (80) suggest that the degree of saturation of dietary polyunsaturated fatty acids (PUFA), rather than the level of serum cholesterol, correlates best with immunosuppressive activity. A tenfold greater depression in mitogen response was observed in hypercholesterolemic rats fed PUFA compared with equally hypercholesterolemic rats fed saturated fats, suggesting that serum cholesterol *per se* was not a regulatory factor.

Polyunsaturated Fatty Acids (PUFA)

High dietary intake of PUFA can alter dramatically the composition of esterified membrane lipids. The *cis* conformation of double bonds in esterified fatty acids alters the molecular configuration of cell membrane lipid and increases membrane fluidity. A reduction in the ratio of PUFA to saturated FA in the membrane or an increase in cholesterol content reduces the fluidity of the membrane. These changes have been associated with enhanced mitogen responsiveness (78) and increased cytolytic activity (77). Dynamic changes in membrane fluidity and phospholipid and cholesterol metabolism occur normally with antigen/mitogen stimulation. Membrane alterations induced by changes in FA composition may affect receptor aggregation, configuration, and availability for ligand binding, thereby affecting immune reactivity negatively (81).

Essential fatty acids [linoleic (18:2) and arachidonic (20:4)] are known precursors of prostaglandin (PG); however, dietary manipulation of PG levels by increased precursor intake has been difficult to demonstrate *in vivo*. Nonetheless, it is tempting to postulate that dietary PUFA exert an immunosuppressive effect via increased PG synthesis, especially because the availability of arachidonic acid is the rate-limiting step in PG synthesis. In support of this notion are the recent studies demonstrating that macrophage-derived PGE_2 activates suppressor cell populations (82). Increased suppressor cell activity could contribute to the immunosuppressive effects of PG precursors, particularly in older animals with an increased sensitivity to PG (21).

Lipoproteins (LP)

In addition to providing a transport mechanism for hydrophobic lipids, lipoproteins have immunoregulatory properties as well. In particular, a species of low-density lipoprotein (LDL), termed intermediate-density lipoprotein (IDL), has been shown to have specific saturable receptors on T cell membranes (72). The binding of IDL to these receptors has been shown to interrupt the sequence of membrane-related events initiated by PHA activation. The normal sequence of events after mitogenic stimulation includes an increase in Ca^{++} flux, arachidonic acid release, phospholipid turnover, and an elevation of cyclic guanidine monophosphate (GMP). Evidence presented by Harmony and Hui (72) suggests that the binding of IDL interferes with intracellular accumulation of Ca^{++}, which effectively blocks the progression of events. The quantity of IDL bound to surface receptors correlated directly with a reduction in Ca^{++} accumulation intracellularly. Furthermore, internalization of IDL was not required to depress Ca^{++} flux, and the effect was independent of the cholesterol content of the bound LP.

It is apparent that abnormalities in lipid intake can reversibly affect cell-mediated immune function. The potential for therapeutic nutritional intervention, particularly for autoimmune diseases in the elderly, is an interesting consideration. It must be emphasized, however, that immunosuppressive diets high in PUFA have also been convincingly related to cancer promotion (81).

Micronutrients and Immune Function: Zinc

Inclusive review articles have recently been published that explore the experimental evidence relating each of the micronutrients to immune function (1,73). The focus here is on the single micronutrient zinc because it is highly likely that zinc deficiency is a component of human malnutrition and may contribute significantly to secondary immunodeficiency. In addition to zinc, deficiencies in vitamin A and iron are most likely to contribute to secondary immunodeficiency in chronic moderate PCM.

Human Studies

According to a recent review by Sandstead (83), chronic moderate zinc deficiency in humans may be more prevalent than previously appreciated. Inadequate zinc status is most likely during early rapid growth, old age, and periods of physiologic stress, such as pregnancy, lactation, and catabolic illness. Alcoholism and malabsorptive states may also predispose to zinc deficiency.

There are no major storage sites for zinc in the body, so that when availability or intake is reduced, deficient symptoms are apparent within a few weeks. Because zinc content and availability are highest in meat protein and lowest in cereal-based diets, it is not surprising that concomitant zinc deficiency has been documented in children with PCM (84). Many of the clinical symptoms of PCM, including growth retardation, dermatitis, lymphoid hypoplasia, impaired wound healing, and immunodeficiency, mimic those observed in acrodermatitis enteropathica, a genetic disorder that impairs zinc absorption and results in severe deficiency. Golden et al. (84) have demonstrated that local cutaneous application of zinc ointment to children with chronic moderate PCM resulted in significant restoration of impaired delayed hypersensitivity response.

Although isolated zinc deficiency in man is rare, severe zinc deficiency has been inadvertently produced in patients maintained on total parenteral nutrition (TPN) in which the nutrient solution was insufficient in zinc (85). Lymphocytopenia, anergy, and a profound depression of PHA response was dramatically reserved when zinc was added to the TPN solution. The importance of this study is that the single variable zinc was shown to reverse immunodeficiency in otherwise well-nourished humans.

Animal Studies

A means of adaptation to severe zinc deficiency is a pronounced reduction in food consumption (inanition). Because inanition can independently depress immune function, well-designed studies must necessarily include a pair-fed control group that is fed the same quantity of food consumed by the deficient group. However, when deficiency and inanition are severe, it is questionable whether the pair-fed animals are adequately nourished. Faraji and Swendseid (86) have circumvented problems of inanition control in rats by enteral feeding via a gastric tube, so that both deficient and control animals receive an adequate quantity of the diet, which varies only in zinc content.

Severe zinc deficiency imposed during rapid growth invariably results in total weight loss and lymphoid atrophy. Thymic hypoplasia is severe, with massive depletion of cortical thymocytes. Moderate zinc deficiency, on the other hand, has been shown to impair mitogen-induced blastogenesis dramatically without reducing lymphoid or body weight (87). Severity and duration of the deficiency and age of the animal appear to be interdependent variables, which must be considered critically when interpreting the extent and type of immunologic impairment with nutritional intervention.

Fraker and associates (88) have shown that the spleen plaque-forming-cell response (PFC) to sheep red blood cells (a T-cell-dependent response) is markedly reduced in severe or moderate zinc deficiency in young adult mice. In these studies, the PFC response was expressed per spleen and thus could be misleading because spleen size is invariably reduced in zinc-deficient animals. More recently, the PFC response was re-evaluated in zinc-deficient rats, and when expressed per 10^6 spleen cells, differences between the groups were not significant (89). It would appear that total PFC capacity is reduced with severe zinc deficiency, but remaining splenocytes appear to react normally to challenge with sheep erythrocytes.

In vitro blastogenesis in response to mitogenic lectins has been shown to be depressed significantly in lymphocytes from zinc-deficient animals, despite the presence of zinc in the culture medium (90). In other studies, delayed hypersensitivity (91) and cytotoxic activity against allogeneic tumor cells (90) have been shown to be impaired with zinc deficiency.

At the subcellular level, it has not been determined whether immunodeficiency with zinc deprivation is primarily due to changes in zinc-dependent enzyme activities or to changes in cell membrane integrity or function. Enzymatic and/or membrane changes may occur singly or in combination depending on the severity, duration, and age of intervention.

It is apparent that effector cell dysfunction with zinc deficiency has been well described; however, the cellular-molecular basis for dysfunction is not well understood.

Dietary Supplementation

The most comprehensive long-term dietary supplementation study with an immunopotentiating substance was undertaken by Heidrick et al. (92). They investigated the effect of 2-mercaptoethanol on the immune system, tumor incidence, lipid peroxidation damage, and life span of long-lived mice by adding the chemical (0.25% w/w) to a nutritionally adequate diet starting when the mice were 16 weeks old. Their results showed that the animals fed the 2-mercaptoethanol diet had an elevated T cell immune response, a decrease in the accumulation of lipid peroxidation damage, a postponed onset and decreased incidence of tumor, and an increased mean and maximum life span. It is important to note that 2-mercaptoethanol preferentially enhances the T-cell-dependent immune response of old over young mice (93), and this is associated with a preferential translocation of protein kinase C from the cytosol to the membrane of mitogen-activated T cell (94), a critical step in signal transduction.

Equally encouraging are the results of studies on the immunopotentiating effectiveness of short-term supplements. Thus, Fabris et al. (95) showed that the serum level of thymulin, a thymic hormone, of old mice receiving lysine and arginine (about 0.3 g/kg body weight/day) orally for 15 days is elevated, with the elevated level being comparable to that of adult mice. This would suggest that the serum level of thymulin of old mice can be modulated upward by nutritional supplementation. The 15-day lysine-arginine regimen also enhanced the mitogenic activity of T cells, but the maximum level of enhancement attained was still below that of adult mice. More recently, Furukawa et al. (96) reported that when old mice are fed a nutritionally adequate diet containing 1.0% of reduced glutathione for 4 weeks, both their delayed-type skin hypersensitivity reaction and T cell mitogenic response are elevated. It would seem that these chemically defined supplements could be used as probes to identify the cellular and intracellular biochemical events in T cells of old individuals that are responsive. Such cells and biochemical events may reflect age-related changes that can be reversed by nutritional intervention.

By supplementing the tissue culture with zinc (10^{-4}M), Winchurch et al. (97) demonstrated that the T-cell-dependent antisheep RBC response by spleen cells of young mice could be enhanced by 30 to 40% over that of spleen cells in unsupplemented cultures. In contrast, the magnitude of enhancement of spleen cells from old mice induced by zinc was 5- to 12-fold over that of spleen cells of old mice in unsupplemented cultures. Moreover, the level of response approached that of young mice. It is interesting to note that this concentration of zinc, however, was toxic to the production of interleukin-2 by T helper cells (98). As in the case of the chemically defined supplements used in the *in vivo* studies, zinc could also be used as a probe to identify which of the cascading intracellular metabolic event(s) is first potentiated by it.

NUTRITIONAL CHANGES WITH OLD AGE

The consequences of nutritional deficiencies in early individuals in whom immunocompetence is already compromised are likely to be particularly severe in terms of resistance to disease. Several recent nutritional surveys have documented an alarming prevalence of clinical malnutrition in medical and surgical wards in this country (99). Among institutionalized elderly, malnutrition diagnosed by biochemical indices is particularly high (100). Bienia and associates (101) have assessed the prevalence and consequence of malnutrition among hospitalized elderly individuals. Clinical malnutrition was diagnosed in 61% of patients over 65 years old compared with 28% in patients under 65. A comparison between malnourished and well-nourished elderly revealed that mortality, incidence of infection, anemia, and anergy were significantly higher in the malnourished group. Of particular interest was the finding that the incidence of these abnormalities in the well-nourished elderly individuals did not differ from the incidence in the younger group, suggesting that nutritional status and not age *per se* could be the more significant variable. However, Goodwin and Garry (102) reported that they were unable to detect any association between malnutrition and depressed immunologic function in a population of 230 independently living healthy elderly men and women. This would suggest that subtle nutritional deficiency may not be a noticeable contributor to immunodeficiency in healthy elderly individuals.

Chandra (103) has recommended the use of various measures of immunocompetence as possible functional indicators of general malnutrition. This approach would have the advantage of predicting disease vulnerability, as well as early nutritional deficiencies. However, because of the age-related decline in these indices, the sensitivity would be low in assessment of the elderly and would require age-specific norms to be established.

In conclusion, when periods of nutritional vulnerability overlap with suboptimal immune function caused by senescent changes, a synergistic interaction could occur. The exaggerated susceptibility to disease emphasizes the pivotal role that nutritional status may play in modulating susceptibility to diseases. Nutritional intervention studies that aim to define the severity and duration of deficiency required to affect immunologic activity must be qualified in terms of age because the impact of a given deficiency can be expected to vary with the age-specific changes in immune responsiveness.

FUTURE RESEARCH: A MECHANISTIC APPROACH TO MODULATION OF AGE-ASSOCIATED CELL-MEDIATED IMMUNE DYSFUNCTION WITH NUTRITIONAL INTERVENTION

For the most part, past studies have been descriptive, with emphasis on the characterization of effector response as a consequence of a given nutritional intervention. Recent advances in molecular biology and cellular immunology can now be used to explore the nutritional dependence of the various stages in T-cell ontogeny from bone marrow stem cell to activated effector T cell. The derivation and interactions of T cells and B cells are schematically presented in Fig. 1.

The thymus is the major site in the differentiation, growth, and selection of T cells and appears to be particularly vulnerable to nutritional imbalance. Peripheral cell dysfunction secondary to derangement in the thymic microenvironment can now be evaluated by analyzing quantitative and qualitative changes in the purified subpopulations of mature and immature thymocytes. Alterations in thymic hormone production; in terminal deoxytransferase (TdT) activity; or in the appearance of Thy 1, L3T4, Lyt 1, Lyt 2, and other surface antigens by nutritional intervention would suggest a nutritional dependence in the thymic differentiation pathway. Regarding the

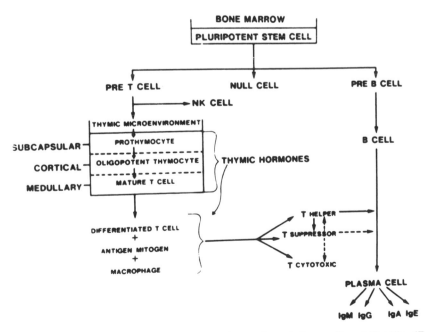

FIG. 1. Differentiation pathways and cellular interactions between T and B cells. (From James and Makinodan, ref. 105.)

modulation of thymic hormone production, Weindruch et al. (104) recently reported that they could not prevent the age-related decline in serum level of a thymic hormone, thymosin α_1, by subjecting long-lived mice to a calorically restricted diet starting at 3 weeks of age. This would suggest that the thymosin-α_1-producing thymic epithelial cells are not responding favorably to the life-extending calorically restricted diet. However, caution should be taken of such a view because we do not know whether the calorically restricted diet alters the rate of utilization of the hormone and whether nonthymic epithelial cells can also produce the hormone and, if so, how they are affected by the calorically restricted diet.

Peripheral T cell activation is initiated by the production and release of IL-1 by macrophage cells. The binding of IL-1 to splenic lymphocyte receptors appears to be an absolute requirement for the differentiation of certain T lymphocytes into cells capable of producing a second mediator, IL-2. The binding of IL-2 provides a trigger for cell proliferation in subpopulations of T helper and cytolytic cells. Nutritional dependence of the proliferative response can be assessed by analyzing the release and binding of the ILs by purified cell populations. A shift in the balance of subpopulations of T lymphocytes, specifically in T helper and suppressor cells, may underlie the nutritional modulation of CMI. In addition, age-related alterations in intracellular events after antigen/mitogen activation could be monitored, including Ca^{++} flux, protein kinase C translocation, and specific messenger RNA synthesis, which may be modified with nutritional intervention.

In summary, recent knowledge of the cellular and subcellular events that comprise the intact immune response now permits a more sophisticated approach to assessing the effects of dietary manipulation at the cellular-molecular level. It is now possible to delineate which phase in the lymphocyte differentiation pathway is most susceptible to a given dietary manipulation. The potential for therapeutic intervention by dietary modulation of immune responsiveness depends on more precise elucidation at the molecular level.

CONCLUSION

The exaggerated susceptibility of humans to disease with age, when periods of nutritional vulnerability coincide with suboptimal immune function, underscores the negative interaction between compromised nutritional status and immunocompetence. Adequate nutrition may be of pivotal importance in terms of disease prognosis, especially in the frail elderly in whom immune function has already declined.

Single-nutrient modulation has been extensively documented in animal models under controlled laboratory conditions. However, these attempts to isolate the individual components of PCM are, by definition, academic approximations that cannot approach the multivariate interactions involved in the human condition. Nonetheless, an understanding of the independent contributions of individual nutrients to immune dysfunction must necessarily precede the understanding of the integrated state.

We have reviewed some of the important studies of dietary manipulation of CMI. In these studies, severity and duration of the deficiency and the age of nutritional intervention appear to be interdependent variables, which must be considered critically when interpreting the extent and type of immunologic impairment.

Finally, we propose that future research effort can now extend beyond gross descriptive studies of T-cell-dependent functions by utilizing recent advances in cellular immunology and molecular biology. It is now technically possible to define nutrient interaction at the subcellular and molecular levels and in terms of T cell ontogeny in order to delineate those points proximal to effector cell function that are most sensitive to a given nutritional deficiency. In this regard, special emphasis should be given to the thymus, for the age-associated changes in T cells are closely linked to the involution and atrophy of the thymus.

ACKNOWLEDGMENT

This publication was funded by VA Medical Research Funds and contract RP8000-08 from the Electric Power Research Institute.

REFERENCES

1. Gross RL, Newberne PM. *Physiol Rev* 1980;60:188–302.
2. Makinodan T, Kay MMB. *Adv Immunol* 1980;48:287–330.
3. Makinodan T, Yunis E, eds. *Immunology and aging*. New York: Plenum Publishing Corp, 1977.
4. Makinodan T, Peterson WJ. *Proc Natl Acad Sci USA* 1962;48:234–238.
5. Goidl EA, ed. *Aging and the immune response*. New York: Marcel Dekker Inc, 1987.
6. Hirokawa K. In: Makinodan T, Yunis E, eds. *Immunology and aging*. New York: Plenum Publishing Corp, 1977;51–72.
7. Albright JF, Makinodan T. *J Cell Physiol* 1966;67(suppl 1):185–206.
8. Goodman SA, Makinodan T. *Clin Exp Immunol* 1975;19:533–542.
9. Price GB, Makinodan T. *J Immunol* 1972;108:403–412.
10. Antonaci S, Jirillo E, Lucivero G. *Clin Exp Immunol* 1983;52:387–392.
11. Ligthart GJ, Schuit HRE, Hijmans W. *Immunology* 1985;55:15–21.
12. Nagel JE, Chrest FJ, Pyle RS. *Immunol Comm* 1983;12:223–237.
13. O'Leary JJ, Jackola DR, Hallgren HM. *Mech Aging Dev* 1983;21:109–120.
14. Kay MMB, Mendoza J, Diven J., et al. *Mech Aging Dev* 1979;11:295–346.
15. Utsuyama M, Hirokawa K. *Mech Aging Dev* 1987;40:89–102.
16. Gillis S, Kozak R, Durante M, et al. *J Clin Invest* 1981;67:937–942.
17. Ceuppens JL, Goodwin JS. *J Immunol* 1982;126:2429–34.
18. Hallgren HM, Buckley EC III, Gilbertsen VA, et al. *J Immunol* 1973;111:1101–07.
19. Makinodan T, Albright JW, Good PI, et al. *Immunology* 1976;31:903–11.
20. Delfraissy JF, Galanaud P, Wallon C, et al. *Clin Immunol Immunopathol* 1982;24:377–85.
21. Goodwin JS, Messner RP. *J Clin Invest* 1979;64:434–439.

22. Inamizu T, Chang M-P, Makinodan T. *Immunology* 1985;55:447–455.
23. Gilman SC, Rosenberg JS, Feldman JD. *J Immunol* 1982;128:644–650.
24. Chang M-P, Makinodan T, Peterson WJ, et al. *J Immunol* 1982;129:2426–2430.
25. Abrass IB, Scarpace PJ. *J Clin Endocrinol Metab* 1982;55:1026–1028.
26. Biro J, Beregi E. *Acta Gerontol* 1979;9:235–239.
27. Kennes B, Hubert C, Brohee D, et al. *Immunology* 1981;42:119–126.
28. Tam CF, Walford RL. *Mech Aging Dev* 1978;7:309–320.
29. Chapman ML, Zaun MR, Gracy RW. *Mech Aging Dev* 1983;21:157–167.
30. Verity MA, Tam CF, Cheung MK, et al. *Mech Aging Dev* 1983;23:53–65.
31. Jacobs PA, Court Brown WM, Doll R. *Nature* 1961;191:1178–1180.
32. Buys CHCM, Osinga J, Anders GJPA. *Mech Aging Dev* 1979;11:55–75.
33. Zakharov AF, Davudov AZ, Benjush VA, et al. *Hum Genet* 1982;60:334–339.
34. Norman A, Cochrane A, Bass D, et al. *Int J Radiat Biol* 1984;46:317–321.
35. Lambert R, Ringborg U, Skoog L. *Cancer Res* 1979;39:2792–2795.
36. Niedermuller H. *Mech Aging Dev* 1982;19:259–271.
37. Barton RW, Yang WK. *Mech Aging Dev* 1975;4:123–136.
38. Scholar EM, Rashidian M, Heidrick ML. *Mech Aging Dev* 1980;12:323–329.
39. Trainor JJ, Wigmore DJ, Chrysostomou A, et al. *Mech Aging Dev* 1984;27:83–86.
40. Vijayalaxmi, Evans HJ. *Mutation Res* 1984;125:87–94.
41. Inamizu T, Kinohara N, Chang M-P, et al. *Proc Natl Acad Sci USA* 1986;83:2488–2491.
42. Pyke KW, Bach JF. *Eur J Immunol* 1979;9:317–323.
43. Zinkernagel RM, Doherty PC. *Adv Immunol* 1979;27:51–177.
44. Stutman O. *Immunol Rev* 1978;42:138–184.
45. Hall NR, Goldstein AL. In: Ader R, ed. *Psychoneuroimmunology*. New York: Academic Press, 1981;521–543.
46. Trainin N, Small M, Zipori T, et al. In: Van Bekkum DW, ed. *The biological activity of thymic hormones*. Rotterdam: Kooyker Scientific Publications, 1975;261–264.
47. Schlesinger DH, Goldstein G. *Cell* 1975;5:361–365.
48. Goldstein AL, Low TLK, McAdoo M, et al. *Proc Natl Acad Sci USA* 1977;74:725–29.
49. Dardenne M, Pleau JM, Man NK, Bach JF. *J Biol Chem* 1977;252:8040–8044.
50. Haynes BF, Robert-Guroff M, Metzgar RS, et al. *J Exp Med* 1983;157:907–920.
51. Hirokawa K, McClure JE, Goldstein AL. *Thymus* 1982;4:19–29.
52. Boyd E. *Am J Dis Child* 1932;43:1162–1214.
53. Santisteban GA. *Anat Rec* 1960;136:117–126.
54. Kay MMB. *Mech Aging Dev* 1984;28:193–218.
55. Metcalf D. *Nature* 1965;208:1336.
56. Teague PO, Yunis EJ, Rodey G, et al. *Lab Invest* 1970;22:121–130.
57. Jeejeebhoy HF. *Transplantation* 1971;12:525–526.
58. Kirokawa K, Makinodan T. *J Immunol* 1975;114:1659–1664.
59. Hirokawa K, Sato K, Makinodan T. *Clin Immunol Immunopathol* 1982;24:251–262.
60. Sato K, Chang M-P., Makinodan T. *Cell Immunol* 1984;87:273–484.
61. Kinohara N, Makinodan T. *Thymus* 1987;10:179–192.
62. Mullen JL, Gertper MH, Buzby GP, et al. *Arch Surg* 1979;114:121–125.
63. Meakins JL, Pietsch JB, Bubenick O, et al. *Ann Surg* 1977;186:241–249.
64. Schloen LH, Fernandes G, Garofalo JA, et al. *Clin Bull* 1979;9:63–75.
65. McCay CM, Crowell MF, Maynard LA. *J Nutr* 1935;10:63–79.
66. Ross MH, Lustbader E, Bras G. *Nature* 1976;262:548–553.
67. Gerbase-DeLima M, Liu RK, Cheney KE, et al. *Gerontologia* 1975;21:184–202.
68. Harrison DE, Archer JR. *Exp Gerontol* 1988;23:309–321.
69. Good RA, Fernandes G, West A. In: Singhal, Stiller, eds. *Aging and immunity*. New York: Elsevier, 1979;141–163.
70. Fernandes G, West A, Good RA. *Clin Bull* 1979;9:91–106.
71. Chen HW. *J Cell Physiol* 1979;100:147–158.
72. Harmony JAK, Hui DY. *Cancer Res* 1981;41:3799–3802.
73. Keusch GT, Wilson CS, Waksal SD. In: Gallin JI, Fauci AS, eds. *Advances in host defense mechanisms*, vol 2. New York: Raven Press, 1982;275–357.
74. Kos WL, Loria RM, Snodgrass MJ, et al. *Infect Immun* 1979;26:658–667.
75. Humphries GMK, McConnell HM. *J Immunol* 1979;122:121–126.

76. Heiniger HJ. *Cancer Res* 1981;41:3792–3794.
77. Meade CJ, Mertin J. *Adv Lipid Res* 1978;16:127–165.
78. Heiniger HJ, Brunner KT, Cerottini JC. *Proc Natl Acad Sci USA* 1978;75:5683–5687.
79. Ip SHC, Abraham J, Cooper RA. *J Immunol* 1980;124:87–93.
80. Broitman SA, Vitale JJ, Vavrousek-Jukuba E, et al. *Cancer* 1977;40:2455–2463.
81. Vitale JJ, Broitman SA. *Cancer Res* 1981;41:3706–3709.
82. Webb DR, Nowowiejski I. *Cell Immunol* 1981;63:321–328.
83. Sandstead HH. In: Prusad AS, ed. *Clinical, biochemical and nutritional aspects of trace elements.* New York: Alan R. Liss, 1982;83–101.
84. Golden MH, Harland PS, Golden BE, et al. *Lancet* 1978;1:1226–1227.
85. Allen JI, Kay NE, McClain CJ. *Ann Intern Med* 1981;95:154–157.
86. Faraji B, Swendseid ME. *J Nutr* 1983;113:447–455.
87. Gross RL, Osdin N, Fong L, et al. *Am J Clin Nutr* 1979;32:1260–1265.
88. Fraker PJ, Haas SM, Leuke RW. *J Nutr* 1977;107:1889–1895.
89. Carlomango MA, McMurray DN. *Nutr Res* 1983;3:69–78.
90. Fernandes G, Nair M, Onoe K, et al. *Proc Soc Acad Sci USA* 1979;76:457–461.
91. Fraker PJ, Zwickl CM, Leuke RW. *J Nutr* 1982;112:309–313.
92. Heidrick ML, Hendricks LC, Cook DE. *Mech Aging Dev* 1984;27:341–358.
93. Chang M-P, Tanaka JL, Stosic-Grujicic T, et al. *Int J Immunopharmacol* 1982;4:429–436.
94. Fong TC, Makinodan T. *Immunol Lett* 1989;20:149–154.
95. Fabris N, Mocchegiani E, Muzzioli M. *Int J Immunopharmacol* 1986;8:677–685.
96. Furukawa T, Meydani SN, Blumberg JB. *Mech Aging Dev* 1987;38:107–117.
97. Winchurch RA, Thomas DJ, Adler WM, et al. *J Immunol* 1984;133:569–571.
98. Winchurch RA, Togo J, Adler WM. *Clin Immunol Immunopathol* 1988;49:215–222.
99. Bistrian BR, Blackburn GL, Vitale J, et al. *JAMA* 1976;235:1567–1570.
100. Smith JL, Wickiser AA, Kuth LL. *JPEN* 4:367–370.
101. Bienia R, Ratcliff S, Barbour GL, et al. *J Am Geriatr Soc* 1982;30:433–436.
102. Goodwin JS, Garry PJ. *J Gerontol* 1988;43:M46–49.
103. Chandra RK. *Br Med Bull* 1981;37:89–94.
104. Weindruch R, Naylor PH, Goldstein AL, et al. *J Gerontol* 1988;43:B40–42.
105. James SJ, Makinodan T. In: Armbrecht HJ, Prendergast JM, Coe ER, eds. *Nutritional intervention in the aging process.* New York: Springer-Verlag; 1984:209–227.

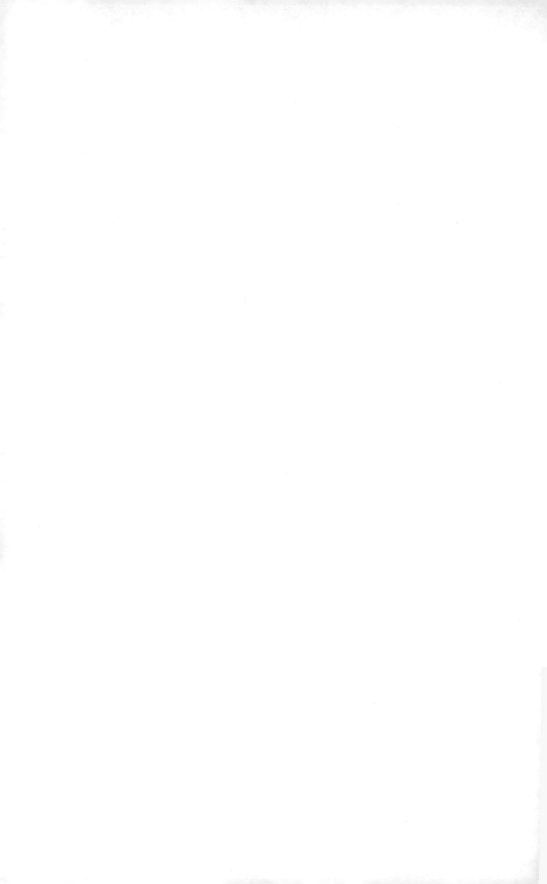

Geriatric Nutrition, edited by John E. Morley,
Zvi Glick, Laurence Z. Rubenstein.
Raven Press, Ltd., New York © 1990.

16

The Oral Cavity and Nutrition

Michael Kaurich

*UCLA School of Dentistry, and Dental Geriatric Fellowship Program,
VA Medical Center, Sepulveda, California 91343*

The condition of the oral cavity, the portal for body nourishment, can affect the nutritional status and general well-being of the elderly. Unfortunately, the importance of oral health is neglected by many elderly and by the health care system. A recent survey by the National Institute of Dental Research shows high prevalence rates of oral diseases and underutilization of dental services in the geriatric population (1). These findings are in part due to the false perception held by many elderly that age causes tooth loss, and, unlike medical care, the provision of dental services has not been extensively financed by public or private insurance.

Food ingestion is a complex activity in which the oral cavity plays a major role. Impaired oral function secondary to tooth loss can alter the sensory and psychologic aspects of eating and cause restrictions in food selection, which is determined by a complex interaction among economic, psychosocial, cultural, anatomic, and physiologic factors. Assessing the effect of poor oral health on nutrition is difficult because of the lack of definitive data and the complexity of the subject. This chapter presents the age-associated changes in the oral cavity and their nutritional relationship.

AGE-RELATED CHANGES

Many of the age-related changes in the oral cavity mirror the tissue changes seen in the body. Unfortunately, very little is known about the correlation between nutrition and normal oral aging. However, there is no doubt that poor nutrition can be a contributory factor.

The oral mucosa appears to atrophy with age. The connective tissue displays decreased elasticity and cellular regeneration, and the muscle has decreased mass and reduced tone. Nerve cells decrease in number and are characterized by calcification and fatty degeneration. Vascular tissue undergoes fibrosis and calcification. Bone formation in the maxilla and mandible is reduced (2).

Attrition or wear of the enamel surfaces of the teeth is a sign of aging that can be accelerated by an abrasive diet. Changes in enamel porosity and thickness can result in yellowing of the teeth. Recession of the gingiva, once thought to be an aging effect, is pathologically induced by poor oral hygiene.

Alveolar bone, the thin layer of bone surrounding the teeth, has decreased vascularization and cellular metabolism with age. Calcium deficiency may be an important factor in this decrease. Wical has shown a correlation between excessive alveolar bone resorption and inadequate dietary calcium intake (3). Kribb et al. have demonstrated a correlation between daily calcium intake and the bone density of the mandible (4).

Salivary glands are also affected by age. Fibrous or fatty infiltration of the glands and atrophy of secretory cells occur. However, decreased salivary secretion is not a normal corollary of aging (5). Xerostomia (dry mouth) is caused by dehydration, medication side effects, or radiation therapy.

ORAL PATHOLOGY AND NUTRITION

Caries

Many people would not expect caries, tooth decay, to be a disease of the elderly. Yet 60% of the dentate elderly have decay of the root surface of the teeth and recurrent caries, decay around existing fillings is also prevalent (1).

In order to initiate tooth decay three elements are required: bacteria, carbohydrates, and a susceptible host. The source of bacteria is plaque, a heterogeneous, sticky white film that collects on the teeth daily. Plaque consists of aerobic and anaerobic bacteria, salivary proteins, and food debris. The bacteria utilize dietary carbohydrates for their own metabolism. The acidic byproducts demineralize and destroy the hard tissues of the tooth.

A soft diet high in refined carbohydrates has been shown to increase the caries rate in children (6). A study by Papas et al. (7) indicates that this same relationship exists in older adults. Untreated caries can ultimately result in tooth loss. The functional deficits caused by this loss can alter an individual's food selection pattern (8).

Periodontitis

Periodontitis (gum disease) affects the majority of adults and is a major cause of tooth loss in the elderly. Approximately 90% of dentate elderly have some type of periodontal disease ranging from localized gingivitis to advanced periodontitis (1).

The major etiologic factor in periodontitis is plaque. If not removed daily, plaque eventually calcifies through interaction with minerals in the saliva. This calculus (tartar) acts as a tissue irritant to gingiva and alevolar bone.

A nutritional deficit has not been implicated as a direct cause of periodontitis, but nutritional intake and status can affect the quality and health of the periodontal tissues. Vitamin deficiencies, especially A, B complex, and C, can alter the tissue response to local irritants and retard repair and healing (9). The physical character of the diet also plays a role in plaque formation (10). A soft diet enhances plaque formation, whereas a hard diet has a cleansing action on the teeth and gums and provides the stimulation important in maintaining alveolar bone.

ORAL FUNCTION AND NUTRITION

Mastication

One of the most important functions of the oral cavity is mastication, the biomechanical act of comminuting food to prepare it for swallowing. Mastication also serves to induce salivation and excite taste and olfactory receptors through the liberation of gustatory and olfactory stimuli from food.

Masticatory performance or chewing ability can be quantitated by measuring the degree of pulverization that food particles undergo during chewing. For example, an individual chews a 3-g portion of peanuts or carrots until he is ready to swallow. The chewed food is expectorated and passed through a ten-mesh screen. The ratio of the volume of the food particles that pass through the ten-mesh screen divided by the total volume recovered multiplied by 100 represents the percent masticatory performance (11).

Although there is interindividual variation, the effect of missing teeth on masticatory performance is significant. Various studies have shown the strong correlation between increased tooth loss and a decline in masticatory performance (12–14). With decreased masticatory ability, alterations also take place in self-reported measures of food acceptance and consumption (8,15).

Age *per se* is not strongly correlated with masticatory performance (15). However, 42% of the overall geriatric population are completely edentulous, with higher prevalence rates with increased age and institutionalization. Kapur (16) has shown that the average masticatory performance of denture wearers is one-third that of normal dentate subjects. When the amount of effort expended to achieve a certain degree of pulverization is factored in, the chewing efficiency of a denture wearer is one-sixth of a normal dentate individual. Denture wearers also show impairments in oral sensory and motor functions and a decreased ability to discriminate among textures of food (17). They also exert three to four times less muscle activity than a dentate person to chew the same food (18).

These tooth loss changes have been postulated to alter food selection patterns. Softer, easier-to-chew foods lacking in essential nutrients are often chosen. Unfortunately, the relationship between these changes and overall nutritional status is unclear. Some investigators have found no relationship between impaired masticatory function and nutritional status (19,20). However, Gordon et al. (21), in a study of very elderly men, have shown a significant correlation between chewing problems and decreased protein and total caloric intake and increased carbohydrate intake.

Salivation

Salivation is the discharge of fluid (saliva) by the various salivary glands into the oral cavity. It has the following functions: (a) facilitating chewing and swallowing by lubricating the food, (b) dissolving and transporting gustatory stimuli released by chewing, (c) initiating the first phase of digestion through the action of amylase, (d) neutralizing acids, (e) diluting unpleasant and noxious substances, (f) flushing away food particles and other debris, and (g) lubricating and protecting the oral mucosa and teeth. Salivary production is unchanged in healthy aging adults.

Xerostomia is a marked reduction in salivation. A recent survey conducted by Berkey et al. (22) indicates that as many as one-third of the elderly have symptoms of xerostomia. Although studies have not been done on the nutritional effects of xerostomia, this condition can limit food selection and lessen the enjoyment of eating.

Gustation

Taste plays an important role in the acceptance or rejection of food. It has generally been accepted that the number of taste buds and taste activity decrease with age. However, recent studies (23,24) indicate that there is no significant loss of taste buds with age. There is a possibility that the neurophysiologic responses of the peripheral or central taste systems are impaired, but information to confirm this hypothesis is lacking. Taste detection thresholds are elevated in the elderly, but most food contains more than threshold taste amounts. These suprathreshold levels are more clinically relevant, and their detection appears to be functionally intact in healthy elderly (25,26).

A possible correlation between poor oral hygiene and taste has been reported. Improvements in oral hygiene reduced taste thresholds in some elderly individuals (27). Zinc deficiency has also been implicated in decreased taste acuity (28). However, zinc supplementation has not reversed taste abnormalities in the elderly (29).

CONCLUSION

The oral health care needs of the geriatric population are overwhelming. Tooth loss, which is the end result of poor oral health, causes a significant loss in chewing ability. Complete dentures do not restore full oral function. Impaired mastication alters the sensory and psychologic aspects of eating and causes restrictions in food selection that may induce adverse dietary changes. The effect of these changes on nutritional status are unclear. They may not be a direct cause of malnutrition, but might be a contributory factor in some elderly who have other risk factors.

REFERENCES

1. US Department of Health and Human Services. *Oral health of United States adults: National findings*. Washington, DC, US Government Printing Office, 1987 (NIH Publ. No. 87-2862).
2. Tonna EA. In: Finch CE, ed. *Handbook of the biology of aging*. New York: Van Nostrand Reinhold, 1976;470–495.
3. Wical KE. *J Prosth Dent* 1974;32:13.
4. Kribbs PJ, Smith DE, Chemut CH. *J Prosth Dent* 1983;50:719–724.
5. Baum B. *Gerodontics* 1986;2:61–64.
6. Sognnaes RF. *Am J Dis Child* 1948;75:792.
7. Papas AS, Palmer CA, McGandy RB, Hartz SC, Russell RM. *Gerodontics* 1987;3:30–37.
8. Wayler AH, Muench ME, Kapur KK, Chauncey HH. *J Gerontol* 1984;39:284–289.
9. Glickman I, ed. *Clinical periodontology*, 4th ed. Philadelphia: WB Saunders, 1974;365–382.
10. Pelzer A. *J Am Dent Assoc* 1940;27:13.
11. Yurstas A, Manly RS. *J Appl Physiol* 1950;3:45.
12. Helkimo E, Carlsson GE, Helmiko M. *Acta Odont Scand* 1978;36:33–41.
13. Wayler AH, Chauncey AH. *J Prosth Dent* 1983;49:427–433.
14. Yurkstas A. *J Prosth Dent* 1954;4:120.
15. Wayler AH, Kapur KK, Feldman RS, Chauncey HH. *J Gerontol* 1982;37:294–299.
16. Kapur KK, Soman SD. *J Prosth Dent* 1964;14:687–694.
17. Kapur KK, Collister T. In: Bosma, J, (ed). *Second symposium on oral sensation and perception*. Springfield, IL: Charles C Thomas, 1970;332–339.
18. Yurkstas AA, Curby WF. *J Prosth Dent* 1953;3:82–87.
19. Neill DJ, Philips HIB. *Br Dent J* 1970;128:581–585.
20. Baxter JC. *J Prosth Dent* 1984;51:164.
21. Gordon SR, Kelley SL, Sybyl JR, et al. *J Am Geriatr Soc* 1985;33:334–339.
22. Berkey DB, Call RL, Loupe MJ. *Gerodontics* 1985;5:213–216.
23. Miller JJ. *Anat Reconstr* 1986;216:474–482.
24. Bradley RM. *Gerodontics* 1988;4:244–248.
25. Bartoshuk LM, Riflin B, Marks LE, Bars P. *J Gerontol* 1986;41:1:51–57.
26. Bartoshuk LM. *Gerodontics* 1988;4:249–255.
27. Lanagan MJ, Yearick ES. *J Gerontol* 1976;31:413–418.
28. Sandstead HH, Hevuksen LK, Greger JL, et al. *Am J Clin Nutr* 1982;36:1046.
29. Greger JL, Geissler AH. *Am J Clin Nutr* 1978;31:633.

Geriatric Nutrition, edited by John E. Morley,
Zvi Glick, Laurence Z. Rubenstein.
Raven Press. Ltd.. New York © 1990.

17

Gastrointestinal Function and Aging

Robert M. Russell

*Human Nutrition Research Center on Aging, Tufts University,
Boston, Massachusetts 02111*

The function of the gastrointestinal (GI) tract is generally well preserved in aging (1). To date no changes in the GI tract have warranted or appear to warrant a change in the dietary requirement for any one specific nutrient. The fact that there is little change of clinical relevance in GI function with age is due to the larger reserve capacity of this multiorgan system. In addition to describing those changes that do occur with aging, this chapter examines specific disease states of the GI tract for which there is some evidence that aging affects the clinical course.

CHANGES IN THE GASTROINTESTINAL TRACT WITH AGING

Aging and the Mouth

Loss of teeth is a common finding among elderly people that (with or without ill-fitting dentures) limits dietary intake (2). Although changes in salivary secretion have been reported with advanced age, when corrected for medication use, age *per se* has no detrimental effect on stimulated parotid flow rate (3). Taste and smell detection and recognition threshholds are diminished with advancing age, particularly for sweet and salty substances (4,5). Clinical studies have yet to be carried out on the effect of age on carbohydrate and fat digestion from enzymes synthesized in the oral cavity, eg, salivary amylase, lingual lipase.

Aging and Esophageal Function

Although esophageal motility in elderly people shows a number of minor abnormalities on manometric tracings, age itself appears to produce little or no manifestations of clinical relevance with regard to disordered swallowing (6). Pathologically, there is a decrease in the number of ganglion cells and a concurrent thickening of esophageal smooth muscle in elderly compared to young people (7,8). Further, manometry has demonstrated in some studies increased tertiary contractions of a nonpropulsive nature with delayed esophageal emptying (9). Nevertheless, these test findings are of questionable relevance because there is no evidence that age alone produces dysphasia. On the other hand, dysphasia in the elderly person should be taken seriously as it could be related to benign stricture, malignant disease, or neuropathy from diabetes or stroke.

Aging and the Stomach

Gastric emptying of mixed solid-liquid meals is somewhat delayed in elderly people versus controls. For example, in one study among 25 elderly subjects, the gastric emptying time (T 1/2) of a mixed meal was 136 ± 13 minutes versus 81 ± 4 minutes in younger controls (10).

One of the most striking changes in gastric histology and function that appears to be age correlated is atrophic gastritis with hypo- or achlorhydria. From various studies among elderly people, the prevalence of atrophic gastritis ranges from 20 to 50%, depending on how the diagnosis is made and the various definitions used (11). In Boston, using pepsinogen I and II measured by radioimmunoassay (and the ratio thereof), the prevalence of atrophic gastritis among 60- to 69-year-old people was found to be 24%, among 70- to 79-year-old people 32%, and among people greater than the age of 80, 37% (12).

The physiologic consequences of atrophic gastritis include other alterations in gastric emptying and decreased intrinsic factor secretion (11). Because the pH of the stomach is higher in hypochlorhydria, gastric emptying theoretically should be quicker in this condition. However, Davies et al. (13) found just the opposite with regard to a solid meal. In a Swedish study using a liquid meal alone, patients with hypochlorhydria had a quicker gastric emptying time then did control subjects (14). Because the stomach appears to have a large reserve capacity for intrinsic factor secretion, only in the most severe cases of gastric atrophy does intrinsic factor secretion become so low as to be limiting for vitamin B_{12} absorption.

Other consequences of atrophic gastritis include increased gastric and proximal small intestinal pH and bacterial overgrowth of the proximal small intestine (11). For example, in one group of normal healthy elderly, the pH measured at the ligament of Trietz was 6.6 ± 0.1 versus 7.1 ± 0.1 in subjects with atrophic gastritis (15). This half-unit rise in pH is seemingly small, but was shown to be significant with regard to limiting the absorption of folic acid. The optimum pH for maximal active intestinal uptake of folate has been shown to be about 6.3 (16). Using a test (designed after the Shilling test) to measure folate absorption, it was shown by Russell et al. (15) that folate absorption was markedly diminished in elderly subjects with atrophic gastritis versus elderly control subjects. Further, the absorption of folic acid in the atrophic gastritis subjects could be increased by administering the oral folate along with dilute hydrochloric acid (15). Thus, the defect in absorption of the folate was overcome by the administration of acid, which lowered the pH of the proximal small intestine. Despite the malabsorption of folic acid in atrophic gastritis subjects, serum folate levels are paradoxically higher in elderly people with atrophic gastritis than in those without this condition (12). The reason for this apparent paradox appears to be the greater numbers of bacteria that reside in the proximal small intestine and that synthesize folic acid, thus making up for the absorptive defect.

Recently, atrophic gastritis has been reported to limit the bioavailability of vitamin B_{12}, but not on the basis of impaired intrinsic factor secretion (17). Vitamin B_{12} obtained from dietary sources is in a form that is bound to food proteins and peptides. The cleavage of B_{12} from food protein and peptides normally takes place in the stomach under the action of acid and pepsin. After this cleavage, vitamin B_{12} is free to bind with R binders and then migrate to the proximal small intestine where the R binders are digested under the action of pancreatic proteases. At this time, vitamin B_{12} is free to bind with its final binder, intrinsic factor, and migrate to the terminal ileum for active absorption. If the first step of this process—that is, the freeing of B_{12} from dietary protein—cannot take place because of the lack of acid pepsin digestion, then none of the rest of the sequence of events leading up to the final absorption of vitamin B_{12} in the ileum can take place.

King et al. (18) demonstrated abnormally low protein-bound vitamin B_{12} absorption tests in a group of elderly people with atrophic gastritis and achlorhydria but who had normal Schilling tests using crystalline vitamin B_{12}. Thus, the recovery of B_{12} in the urine after eating protein-bound vitamin B_{12} was abnormally low in atrophic gastritis subjects versus controls. Moreover, the feeding of protein-bound vitamin B_{12} along with oral intrinsic factor did not improve vitamin B_{12} bioavailability. However, the addition of acid or acid plus pepsin did increase the bioavailability of vitamin B_{12} in many of these patients. There is also the possibility that bacterial overgrowth in the proximal small bowel in atrophic gastritis can limit vitamin B_{12} bioavailability because various bacteria can take up or bind the vitamin.

Ferric iron absorption is known to be decreased in achlorhydria because acid normally solubilizes ferric iron (19). Various ligands, such as citrate, can maintain ferric iron solubility in a neutral or alkaline pH range, but such ligands form only at an acid pH; thus, the need for gastric acid.

There is some controversy in the literature as to how important atrophic gastritis is in limiting the bioavailability of calcium. Hydrochloric acid reacts with calcium carbonate to form soluble calcium chloride, water, and carbon dioxide. Bo-Linn et al. (20), using an intestinal washout method, were unable to demonstrate an important effect of hypochlorhydria on calcium bioavailability. However, Recker (21) did demonstrate a lowered absorbability of calcium carbonate in achlorhydric subjects versus normal subjects. When the calcium carbonate was given with a meal, however, this difference was not seen. Fiber is frequently prescribed for elderly people for relieving constipation. However, fiber-divalent cation complexes are normally disrupted in an acid millieu (22). Whether atrophic gastritis and gastric atrophy inhibit or cause a decrease in calcium bioavailability because of the inability to dissociate calcium from fiber is uncertain.

Aging and the Pancreas

In several animal studies, pancreatic secretion in terms of volume and enzyme concentration has been shown to be lower with advancing age (23). It has been harder to demonstrate this effect in humans. In one study after repeated stimulation, elderly humans showed less pancreatic enzyme output than did younger people, although after the first stimulation no differences were seen (24). Despite this relative defect in pancreatic secretion due to age, it has not been reflected by an increased prevalence of fat malabsorption with advancing age (1). For example, we have found that, in people aged 20 to 60, fecal fat on a 100-g fat diet intake is 3.3 ± 2.3 g ($N = 40$); in those aged 60 to 70, 2.5 ± 1.8 g ($N = 45$); and in those aged 70 to 91, 2.9 ± 1.9 g ($N = 50$). In one small study from Scandinavia, no difference in fecal fat output was found between elderly and younger adults when the dietary intake of fat was in the range of 85 to 90 g/day (25). However, when dietary intake of fat was elevated to an intake of 115 to 120 g/day, several of the elderly people began to malabsorb fat, whereas younger people continued to excrete only 3 to 9 g/day (25). Similarly, when dietary protein was raised to more than 1.5 g/kg/day, elderly people showed some elevation of fecal nitrogen, whereas younger adults did not (25). Whether this abnormal elevation in fecal nitrogen due to age is related to a defect in pancreatic protease secretion or intestinal digestion and/or absorption of peptides and/or amino acids is uncertain.

Aging and the Small Intestine

Human studies have shown that the small intestinal transit remains relatively stable with increasing age. However, minor differences in morphology between young adult and geriatric subjects have been described, including shorter villi in elderly subjects (26). A well-known change in the small intestine that is age related is decreased lactase of the brush border membrane, producing a higher prevalence of lactose intolerance in elderly people versus young adult controls (27). In contrast, sucrase and maltase concentrations of the human small intestinal mucosa appear to remain relatively stable over age.

A decline in the urinary excretion of D-xylose has been demonstrated to correlate directly with advancing age (1). Nevertheless, when corrected for creatinine clearance by partial regression analysis, the decline in renal function was able to account for almost all of the decline in D-xylose urinary excretion. Except in advanced aged—that is, greater than 80 years old—there does not appear to be an effect of age alone on D-xylose absorption (28). An interesting study of intestinal carbohydrate metabolism and age was carried out by Feibusch and Holt (29), who fed elderly and young adults diets of increasing carbohydrate content. Breath hydrogen was measured after each meal, and it was found that the young controls did not show abnormally elevated breath hydrogen, even at single-meal carbohydrate intakes of 200 g. However, more than 60% of the elderly subjects showed abnormal breath hydrogen excretion after eating a 200-g carbohydrate meal. This breath hydrogen rise is caused by increased bacterial metabolism of carbohydrate, either from contact within the proximal small bowel or within the colon. Thus, from these studies it is unclear whether the elevated breath hydrogen was caused by bacterial overgrowth of the small bowel or malabsorption of carbohydrate with subsequent hydrogen production by colonic bacteria.

It has recently been reported that glycocolic breath test results in elderly individuals are not significantly different from those of young adults (1). Thus, bacterial overgrowth due to atrophic gastrits may not result in bile salt deconjugation and subsequent fat malabsorption.

In a study by Hollander and Morgan (30), it was shown that the uptake of vitamin A by perfused intestinal segments of the rat increased with advancing age of the animal. It was theorized that this increase was caused by a change in thickness or character of the unstirred water layer (30). Similarly, it has been found that tolerance curves using a physiologic dose of vitamin A showed higher peak heights and areas under the curves in elderly individuals versus young adults. Because a tolerance curve is made up of both an absorptive and a clearance component, it is unclear whether these higher curves found in elderly people are in fact due to greater absorption or decreased clearance of the vitamin from the circulation. In order to clarify this, Krasinski et al. (31) fed high-fat, vitamin A rich meals to elderly and young adults and subsequently performed plasmaphoresis to obtain vitamin-A-enriched chylomicrons and chylomicron remnants. When these remnants were subsequently reinfused into the volunteers, it was found that elderly people had one-half of the clearance ability of young adults. Thus, in part, the higher tolerance curves for vitamin A appear to be due to decreased clearance capacity for chylomicron remnants in the elderly by the liver, rather than an increased absorptive ability.

Ileal absorption of vitamin B_{12} does not appear to be affected by age, although malabsorption of vitamin D has been described (32,33). It is unlikely that this is a major cause of vitamin D depletion of elderly subjects. Rather, decreased skin synthesis of vitamin D and renal synthesis of 1-25 dihydroxy vitamin D appear to be the major problems in vitamin D nutriture in aging (34).

The aged small intestine does not adapt to low calcium intakes with a higher fractional calcium absorption as does the younger intestine (35). This may be an important factor with regard to the pathogenesis of osteoporosis in the elderly. Iron absorption, except for that regarding achlorhydria, appears to remain intact with age. One study in the rat showed increased mucosal to serosal transfer of zinc with advancing age (36). However, no such studies have been carried out in humans.

Age and the Gallbladder

Although the sensitivity of gallbladder muscle to cholecystokinin (CCK) stimulation is decreased with advancing age in humans, there is an increased release of CCK after a fatty meal, thus making up for the diminished sensitivity (37).

SPECIFIC DISEASE STATES

Malignancies of the GI tract are all age related; that is, the prevalence increases with advancing age. Moreover, type B atrophic gastritis—environmental gastritis—which is commonly associated with aging, is associated with a higher prevalence of gastric cancer (38). The incidence of peptic ulcer disease is the same in the elderly as in young adults, although elderly patients with bleeding complications may fare worse and thus require therapeutic measures more quickly (39). Celiac disease should not just be considered a disease of childhood, as in a recent study approximately 10% of newly diagnosed cases of celiac disease occurred among individuals over the age of 60 (40). However, the most common cause of steatorrhea in the elderly person is not celiac disease or pancreatic disease, but rather bacterial overgrowth of the small intestine. Vascular disease of the GI tract, including ectasia, ischemia, and bleeding diverticuli, are all age related and are serious causes of morbidity and mortality among the elderly. Inflammatory bowel disease occurs less frequently among the elderly than among young adults, but the prognosis in the past has been reported to be grave in the aged person (41). However, a recent study has demonstrated a more favorable course of inflammatory bowel disease (both Crohn's disease and ulcerative colitis), in the elderly, which may be due to the more common use of maintenance drug therapy.

REFERENCES

1. Arora S, Kassarjian Z, Krasinski SD, Croffey B, Kaplan MM, Russell RM. *Gastroenterology* 1989;96:1560–1565.
2. Bowman BB, Rosenberg IH. *Hum Nutr Clin Nutr* 1983;37C:75–89.
3. Baum BJ. *J Dent Res* 1981;60:1292–1296.
4. Stevens JC, Bartoshuk LM, Cain WS. *Chem Sens* 1984;9:167–179.
5. Busse EW. *Postgrad Med* 1978;63:118–125.
6. Khan TA, Shragge BW, Crispin JS, Lind JF. *Am J Dig Dis* 1977;22:1049–1054.
7. Almy TP. *Bull NY Acad Med* 1981;57:709.
8. Eckhardt VF, Le Compte PM. *Am J Dig Dis* 1978;23:443.
9. Soergel KH, Zboralske FF, Amberg JR. *J Clin Invest* 1964;43:1472.
10. Wegener M, Borsch G, Schaffstein J, Luth I, Rickels R, Ricken D. *Digestion* 1988;39:40–46.
11. Russell RM. In: Hutchinson ML, Munro HN, eds. *Nutrition and aging.* New York: Academic Press, 1987;7:23–49.
12. Krasinski SD, Russell RM, Samloff IM, et al. *J Am Geriatr Soc* 1986;34:800–806.
13. Davies WT, Kirkpatrick JR, Owen GM, Shields R. *Scand J Gastroenterol* 1971;6:297–301.
14. Halvorsen I, Dotevall G, Walan A. *Scand J Gastroenterol* 1973;8:395–399.
15. Russell RM, Krasinski SD, Samloff IM, Jacob RA, Hartz SC, Brovender SR. *Gastroenterology* 1986;91:1476–1482.
16. Russell RM, Dhar GJ, Dutta SK, Rosenberg IH. *J Lab Clin Med* 1979;93:428–436.
17. Carmel R, Sinow RM, Siegel ME, Samloff M. *Arch Intern Med* 1988;148:1715–1719.
18. King CE, Leibach J, Toskes PP. *Dig Dis Sci* 1979;24:397–402.
19. Lockhead AC, Dagg JH. *Lancet* 1963;1:848–850.
20. Bo-Linn GW, Davis GR, Buddrus DJ, Morawski SG, Santa Ana C, Fordtran JS. *J Clin Invest* 1984;73:640–647.
21. Recker RR. *N Engl J Med* 1985;313:70–73.
22. James WPT, Branch WJ, Southgate DAT. *Lancet* 1978;1:638–639.
23. Greenberg RE, Holt PR. *Dig Dis Sci* 1986;31:970–977.
24. Bartos V, Groh J. *Gerontol Clin* 1969;11:56–62.
25. Werner I, Hambraeus L. In: Carlson LA, ed. *Nutrition in old age.* Uppsala: Almquist and Wiksell, 1972;55–60.
26. Webster SGP, Leeming JT. *Age Aging* 1975;4:168–174.
27. Welsh JD, Poley JR, Bhatia M, Stevenson DE. *Gastroenterology* 1978;75:847–855.
28. Guth PH. *Am J Dig Dis* 1968;13:565–571.
29. Feibusch JM, Holt PR. *Dig Dis Sci* 1982;27:1095–1100.
30. Hollander D, Morgan D. *Exp Gerontol* 1979;14:301–305.
31. Krasinski SD, Russell RM, Schaefer EJ. *Gastroenterology* 1987;92:1803.
32. McEvoy AW, Fenwick JD, Boddy K, James OFW. *Age Aging* 1982;11:180–183.
33. Barragry JM, France MW, Corless D, Gupta SP, Switala S, Boucher BJ, Cohen RD. *Clin Sci Mol Med* 1978;55:213–220.
34. Webb AR, Kline L, Holick MF. *J Clin Endocrinol Metab* 1988;67:373–378.
35. Ireland P, Fordtran JS. *J Clin Invest* 1973;52:2672–2681.
36. Mooradian AD, Song MK. *Mech Aging Dev* 1987;41:189–197.
37. Khalil T, Walker JP, Wiener I, Fagan CJ, Townsend CM, Greeley GH, Thompson JC. *Surgery* 1985;98:423–429.
38. Strickland RG, Mackay IR. *Dig Dis Sci* 1973;18:426–440.
39. Permutt RP, Cello JP. *Dig Dis Sci* 1982;27:1–6.
40. Price HL, Gazzard BG, Dawson AM. *Br Med J* 1977;1:1582–1584.
41. Softley A, Myren J, Clamp SE, Bouchier IAD, Watkinson G, De Dombal FT. *Scand J Gastroenterol* 1988;23(suppl 144):27–30.

Geriatric Nutrition, edited by John E. Morley,
Zvi Glick, Laurence Z. Rubenstein.
Raven Press, Ltd., New York © 1990.

18

The Effect of Age on the Liver

David H. Van Thiel and Judith S. Gavaler

*Division of Gastroenterology, University of Pittsburgh School of Medicine,
Pittsburgh, Pennsylvania 15261*

The elderly currently represent approximately 12% of the population in the United States (1). This figure is increasing rapidly and steadily. Furthermore, the elderly present a unique yet serious health care problem. For example, this segment of modern society is the most medicated and accounts for more than 25% of all prescription drugs dispensed or more than $15 million in drug costs annually (2,3). The average patient receiving Medicare reimbursement is in an acute care hospital and is the recipient of a polypharmacy regimen averaging ten different medications per day (2,3). This drug exposure results in a significantly greater incidence of adverse drug reactions in geriatric patients than in younger individuals. Moreover, there is a considerable body of clinical evidence to support an age-related decline in drug disposition capacity (3,4). This evidence is largely based on data demonstrating an increase plasma T 1/2 value for most xenobiotics. These changes in drug metabolism in the elderly can reflect changes in renal clearance, shifts in the volume of distribution due to an altered body composition, or diminished hepatic clearance or metabolism of drugs and/or their metabolites.

Individuals in their sixties are largely healthy, with only a small percentage, less than 5%, requiring long-term care. However, a considerably higher percentage of individuals in their eighties—35%—requires substantial long-term care (1). The disability of the old-old is shown by the finding that approximately 22% of this group in the United States resides in nursing homes. Yet, the fastest-growing age group in the world is that aged 85 years and above. For physicians and health care professionals, these facts have enormous consequences.

The recognition that disease rather than aging *per se* is the cause of most, if not all, disability in the elderly is crucial to the early diagnosis and prevention of many age-associated disabilities. For example, only in the last decade have physicians begun to realize that the most common cause of dementia in the latter decades of life is Alzheimer's disease. Even more important is the observation that not all individuals develop dementia as they age. Thus, the recognition of the fact that Alzheimer's disease, rather than senility *per se,* is the cause of dementia in two to three million Americans has led to a net tenfold increase in research support for this particular disease process in the last 5 years alone in the United States (5). Many other diseases are attributed to aging that may not actually be due to it *per se* and deserve similar degrees of support and research attention. A prime example is non-A non-B hepatitis, the most common cause of advanced liver disease in individuals over age 65 years of age.

Most studies of physiologic aging have been cross-sectional; that is, they involve individuals of all ages examined at a specific time (5–10). By contrast, longitudinal studies examine the same individual at different points across his life span. Frequently, cross-sectional studies are confounded by cohort and/or secular trends. Such problems do not exist in longitudinal studies. Even fewer case control studies have been performed in which appropriate controls for identified cases have been included. The latter are essential for truly determining the effects of age as opposed to disease in the elderly.

THE LIVER CELL AND THE AGING PROCESS

The life span of hepatocytes in the body is quite long. Normal hepatocytes divide only once or twice in an entire lifetime in the absence of a growth stimulus, such as a disease-induced loss of liver cells or a partial hepatectomy.

In an autopsy series Watanabe and Tanaka (11) found hepatocyte enlargement relative to nuclear size, an increase in nuclear DNA relative to nuclear size, an increasing number of binuclear cells in the liver, and an increase in the number of cells having increased ploidy with increasing age.

Onishi et al. (12), studying rats aged 70, 250, and 500 days showed that total lipid, triglyceride, and cholesterol levels increase with age in hepatocytes, whereas the phosopholipid content remains constant. Lipid levels in female animals increase with age and are almost eight times greater than at birth (13,14). The absolute level of unsaturated ground plasma in rat hepatocytes increases from 3167 μm^3 at birth to 4,054 μm^3 by 27 months of age, although the volume density of this material does not change.

David (15) has shown that the rat hepatocyte volume at birth is 5776 μm^3. It increases to about 10,000 μm^3 at 2 months of age (sexually mature animal) and stays relatively stable until 6 months of age (fully adult animal) at which time it begins to decline to a level of 7389 μm^3 by 24 to 27 months of age (senescent animal). In contrast to male rats, the volume of hepatocytes in female animals increases continuously during life to reach a limit of 17,000 μm^3 at 27 months of age. Cell volume variations between individual hepatocytes are larger in older animals because of polyploidy, with both very small and very large hepatocytes being present in increased numbers (15,16).

A net increase in cell size and a decline in cell number demonstrated by the number of nuclei per unit area are major characteristics of age-related atrophy of the liver. The presence of large nuclei with a greater DNA content with increasing age in human liver has been demonstrated. The number of large nuclei has been found to increase from 1.7% in the first decade of life to 10.3% in the third and 22.5% in the eighth decade of life (17).

In animals the percentage of binuclear forms increases from 2% in the first 2 weeks of age to 40% in animals aged 30 months and from 19% in animals aged between 3 to 4 months to 28% in animals aged 29 to 30 months (18,19).

THE LIVER AND THE AGING PROCESS

Munro and Young (20) found that the relative weight of the human liver drops from about 4% of body weight in newborn infants to 2% of body weight in aged individuals (20). Livers of aged persons between 69 to 91 years exhibited only minor histologic changes that often are interpreted as being signs of aging, but are actually not specific for aging (21).

Age-associated cell death is believed to occur in the form of apoptosis, with damaged hepatocytes disintegrating to fragments that are then phago-cytosed by surrounding macrophages without any inflammatory reaction. Aging rats of different strains exhibit spontaneous neoplastic and non-neoplastic lesions of the liver, as well as other changes that occur in parallel with neoplasia of hematopoietic tissues. These findings include a fatty change, focal cellular degeneration, and such degenerative alterations as eosinophilia, basophilia or bright areas within cells, individual cell necrosis, focal chronic hepatitis and a periportal inflammation that can be interpreted as representing nonspecific reactive hepatitis, cholangitis, bile duct prolif-eration, biliary cyst formation, sinusoidal dilatation, chronic passive conges-tion, hepatocellular atrophy, nodular regeneration, small neoplastic nodules, adenomas, and/or carcinomas (22).

HEPATOCYTE ORGANELLES AND THE AGING PROCESS

Each cell and organelle membrane appears to have its own distinct pattern of age-related alterations in biochemical and biophysical parameters. At present, it is difficult to make generalizations about membrane parameters in relationship to the aging process. It would seem reasonable to suggest, however, that structural changes should, at least in part, be responsible for some of the functional changes detected during the aging process.

In 1975, Hegner and Platt (23) reported that the fluidity of rat plasma membranes was reduced in old rats as compared to young rats. More recently, Nokubo (24) found that the fluidity of rat hepatocyte plasma membranes as assessed by steady state fluorescent polarization using the probe DPH decreases progressively with age in male rats from 2 months, whereas in female rats the fluidity of these same plasma membranes only begins to decrease after 24 months of age. Thus, in addition to age-related changes, there are sex-related changes in plasma membrane structure and possibly function. The effect of aging on the lipid composition and fluidity of hepatic mitochondrial membranes of female Fisher 344 rats has been determined by Vorbeck et al. (25). These investigators have shown a progressive age-dependent increase in the cholesterol/phospholipid molar ratio of mitochondrial membranes secondary to a progressive increase and decrease, respectively, in their cholesterol and phospholipid contents. Taken together, these findings and those of others indicate that the cholesterol/phospholipid molar ratio of hepatic mitochondrial membranes increases with aging, which in turn leads to the observed reductions in their fluidity (26–28).

In 1979, Kapitulnik et al. (27) reported an increase in rat hepatic microsomal membrane fluidity from birth to 3 months of age. More recently, Armbrecht et al. (28), using electron paramagnetic resonance techniques and the spin labels 5-nitroxide and 16-nitroxide steric acid, extended these observations to demonstrate an increase in fluidity from 3 to 27 months of age in hepatic microsomal membranes. Because the increase in membrane fluidity with age was seen with both spin labels, the data suggest that the increased fluidity extends from the surface of the membrane deep into the membrane's interior.

Studies conducted in liver of humans aged between 69 and 91 years reveal a numerical increase in the number of liver cells with large nucleoli and the numbers of nucleoli (14,16,17,29).

The rough and smooth endoplasmic reticulum and the number of free ribosomes and polysomes and their relationship to each other are important for normal hepatocyte function. The number of free ribosomes and the rough endoplasmic reticulum appear to correlate inversely (14,30). The amount of endoplasmic reticulum found in central lobular cells doubles between 1 and 10 months of age (31). It increases to 165% of its original value in the portal cells, but after 30 months of age drops to a value similar to that found in animals at 1 month of age (31). The volume density of the rough endoplasmic reticulum is 0.0470 in hepatocytes of rat liver at birth and declines to a value of 0.0311 by the age of 3 days (14,30). It then increases to 0.0545 by 6 months, only to decline again to a value of 0.498 by 27 months.

The amount of ribosomes relative to the volume of the rough endoplasmic reticulum is 44.8% at birth and declines to 35% between day 7 to 27 months of age, with a value of 21.1% being recorded at the end of 27 months (14,30). The volume density of the smooth endoplasmic reticulum is 0.0051 in newborn rats and increases to a value of 0.0226 by 21 days before it begins to decline to a value between 0.0100 to 0.0230 (14). From 6 to 18 months of age, it declines from 0.0186 to 0.0109 (58.6% in males) and 0.0411 to 0.0370 (90% in females). The need for a differential assessment of age-related changes in hepatocyte structure dependent on gender can be demonstrated in that the rough endoplasmic reticulum volume density of male rats declines from a value of 0.0545 to a value of 0.0238 (43.7%) from 6 to 18 months of age, but in females it increases from a value of 0.0336 to 0.0445 during the same time period.

The volume density of the Golgi apparatus of rat hepatocytes is 0.0170 at birth, declines to a value of 0.0150 by 1 month of age, and ranges between 0.0080 and 0.0120 at 12 months of age (14,30). The volume of this organelle is 0.0050 at 27 months. The absolute volume of the Golgi apparatus is 80.1 μm^3 at birth and 31.3 μm^3 at the end of 27 months. Values for female animals at advanced age are higher, with volumes between 92 and 139 μm^3 (14,30).

The volume density of mitochondria in aged rats is 10.48% below that found in young animals (32). Per cell mitochondrial volume for female rats are 1.036 μm^3 at 1 month of age, 868 μm^3 after 12 months, and 1.236 μm^3 after 27 months. A decline in the volume density of mitochondria with advancing age has been reported also by Tate and Herbener (33). The volume density declines from 0.283 in animals aged 8 months to 0.181 in animals between 43 and 44 months of age. The absolute mitochondrial volume per cell is 783 μm^3 at birth and reaches a value of 1,419 μm^3 at the end of 6 months of age. In female animals, the absolute mitochondrial volume increases to a level of 2,464 μm^3. The number of mitochondria in the liver of humans aged over 70 years, according to Sato and Tauchi (34), is less than that in individuals less than 50 years of age, whereas mitochondrial size is increased. The absolute number of mitochondria per hepatocyte in male rats is 204 at birth, increases to 708 at the end of 1 month, and increases further to a value of 1441 at the end of 2 months, representing an increase of 1,078% from birth (14,30). Thereafter, it declines to a level of 1516 at 27 months. The number of cristae per mitochondria increases to compensate for this decline in number. Simultaneously, the number of megamitochondria increases as aging occurs.

When one examines mitochondrial aging, it is important to bear in mind that the turnover rate of mitochondrial molecules ranges between 9 and 11 days. A half-life of 10.3 days has been calculated for the turnover of most mitochondrial proteins, lipid, and cytochrome C, whereas a half-life of 9.6 days has been derived for all other mitochondrial materials.

Protein levels are reduced in the mitochondria of old rats (35). In contrast, protease activities are increased. Impaired performance and higher fragility of mitochondria in older rats have been demonstrated and are thought to be a result of an increased level of mitochondrial neutral protease activity. The matrix protein loss recorded from mitochondria isolated from rats aged 28 months and placed in a hypo-osmotic medium is greater than that experienced by animals between 7 and 14 months. This finding suggests that an alteration in the permeability of the mitochondrial outer membrane occurs with age and is a potential cause of this increased protein loss with age (36).

The volume density of the proxisomes of rat liver is 0.021 at birth, reaches a maximum of 0.027 at 4 months of age after which it declines to a value of 0.14 at 12 months, and achieves a minimum level of 0.004 at 18 months of age (14,37,38). The absolute volume of the proxisomes per hepatocyte is 99 μm^3 at birth. It rises continuously to a value of 200 μm^3 at 6 months of age and declines thereafter to a value of 36 μm^3 at 24 months. The number of proxisomes is greater in female animals at advanced ages.

Greater numbers of enlarged lysosomes with different inclusions are found in liver cells of old rats (39). Cathepsin D activity is increased, whereas arylsulphatase B activity hardly changes with age (40). Lysosomal volume density increases by 45% between youth and old age (32). The lysosomal volume density increases from a value of 0.0054 at birth to a value of 0.0290 at 27 months of age in rats (14,30,37,41). Total lysosomal volume increases from 26 μm^3 at birth to a value of 94 μm^3 at 27 months of age. Greater values are recorded for female animals than for males with advancing age. The number of lysosomes per cell increases from 31.4 at birth to 198.3 at the end of 27 months in rats.

HEPATOCYTE DOMAINS AND THE AGING PROCESS

The three domains of the hepatocyte's plasma membrane are characterized by their unique differentiation for specialized function (14,42). The sinusoidal surface is developed as an absorbing and secreting surface. Its surface area is expanded by a factor between 1.8 and 3.7 as a result of the formation of surface microvilli. The number of microvilli per hepatocyte is 1323 at birth and increases to 5471 at 27 months. At the same time, the sinusoidal surface area increases from 689 μm^2 to 1226 μm^2 and that of the entire hepatocyte from 1900 μm^3 to 2783 μm^3.

The bile canaliculi that have been developed as a secretory site also change with age, but to a lesser extent. The bile canaliculi average 249 microvilli and have a surface area of 120.5 μm^2 at birth and 792 microvilli and a surface area of 164.1 μm^2 at 27 months of age. The extrahepatic space in rat liver increases from 11.8% of the liver volume in the first month of life to a volume of 16.2% at 6 months and 20.3% at 27 months (14,15,43–45).

LIVER CELL TURNOVER AND THE AGING PROCESS

Periportally localized hepatocytes express aerobic energy metabolism and demonstrate increased biosynthetic function as compared to intermediary zone and perivenous zone III cells (46,47). Ultrastructurally, perivenous he-

patocytes have a large number of mitochondria, peroxisomes, and lysosomes and more smooth endoplasmic reticulum than periportal cells (48,49).
DNA measurements reveal that, in adult rat liver, diploid cells prevail in the
periportal zone and that bionuclear diploid cells in this region can give rise
to mononuclear tetraploid cells. In the perivenous zone, tetraploid hepatocytes and other cells with very high ploidy predominate (50,51). The periportal zone of the hepatic lobule is thought to represent the proliferating
zone of the liver, whereas the perivenous cells are thought to represent functionally active, highly differentiated nature cells (46,52).

The nongrowth fraction of liver cells is 0.6% of the total number of cells
in young animals and increases to 21% in adults. It accounts for 70% of all
hepatocytes in senile animals. Yet even at advanced ages, 30% of all hepatocytes can proliferate if exposed to a regenerative stimulus, such as a partial
hepatectomy or injury and/or exposure to a hepatotrophic substance (53,54).

The fraction of ^{3}H-labeled thymidine taken up by hepatocytes in young
rats reaches a maximum between 20 and 27 hours after a partial hepatectomy
and is followed by a second smaller wave of DNA synthesis about 56 hours
after the partial hepatectomy. In contrast, senile rats show a much reduced
response and only a single wave of early DNA synthesis. The wave of DNA
synthesis after a partial hepatectomy in young animals starts about 18 hours
after the partial hepatectomy. Preferentially, the hepatocytes localized immediately adjacent to the portal track become labeled. At 20 hours, the wave
of DNA synthesis reaches a maximum in and about the portal area, with a
steep decline in labeling as one moves toward the hepatic vein. At 27 hours,
a high labeling index is found in all parts of lobule, except for its very central
perivenous quarter. In this area, it takes about 40 hours before the majority
of cells are labeled.

Stocker and his group (53–55) have shown that the growth fraction of rat
liver decreases with increasing age. With a 10-day continuous infusion of
tritium-labeled thymidine, a plateau of labeled cells is reached at 99.8% of
the cells with juvenile rats, at 93% of the cells with young adult animals, and
at 77% of the cells with adult senile rats at 24 to 30 months of age.

HEPATIC NONPARENCHYMAL CELLS AND THE AGING PROCESS

The parenchymal cells, the most abundant liver cell type, comprise 60%
of the total number of cells present in the liver and occupy 85% of the liver
volume (56). The nonparenchymal or sinusoidal cells consist of three different cells: the Kupffer cells, the endothelial cells, and the fat storage cells
that together account for 35% of the total liver cells but occupy only 6 to 7%
of the liver volume (56). Despite their small number and volume, they are of
primary importance for the maintenance of the structural organization and
function of the liver (57,58).

Kupffer cells are tissue macrophages that protect the animal against micro-organisms, clear foreign as well as endogenous particles, and macro-molecules from the circulation (57,59,60). These cells are primarily respon-sible for the removal of bacteria, bacterial endotoxins, colloidal substances, and cellular debris from the blood. In addition, they have the capacity to synthesize and excrete signal molecules, or cytokines, which exert profound effects on the function of other cells present in the liver and elsewhere in the body. These cytokines include pyrogens, immunomodulators, prosta-glandins, and other inflammatory mediators that modulate protein synthesis or the proliferation of both parenchymal and nonparenchymal cells. The structure of Kupffer cells is very similar to that of other tissue macrophages. They possess a ruffled membrane, and their cytoplasm contains numerous lysosomal vacules.

The endocytosis activity of Kupffer cells of rats aged 36 months is clearly less than that recorded from animals of a much younger age (61,62). The clearance capacity of the reticuloendothelium system in man also has been demonstrated to decline by about 15% between 30 and 80 years of age (63,64).

The endothelial cells that line the sinusoids of the liver are a special type of endothelial cell (57). Unlike other vacular endothelial cells, they form a porous lining without a underlining basement membrane, which facilitates direct contact between solids and small particles present in the plasma and the parenchymal and fat-storing cells that are situated beneath the endothe-lial cell lining. The endothelial cells of the liver have a remarkable capacity to take up and catabolize macromolecules, including glycosaminoglycans, glycoproteins, and lipoproteins. In addition, they can be induced to produce mediators, such as prostacylcin and other vasoactive substances.

The fat-storing cells are also located in the space of Disse in recesses between adjacent parenchymal cells. Their main function is the storage of vitamin A (65). Fat-storing cells contain large concentrations of vitamin-A-binding protein and the enzymes necessary for the metabolism of vitamin A (66). Under appropriate stimulation these cells can undergo a morphologic transformation and become myofibroblasts capable of producing collagen.

The only study available evaluating the relative numbers of various sinu-soidal cells within the liver shows that the number of Kupffer, endothelium, and fat-storing cells in rat liver is constant throughout the entire life span of the animal, with 49% of the cells being endothelial cells, 21% to 23% being Kupffer cells, and 28% to 36% being fat-storing cells (67).

The morphologic and ultrastructural changes observed in Kupffer cells during the aging process are minimal (67,68). Similarly, the ultrastructure of the endothelial cells remains fairly constant at all ages. In contrast, fat-storing cells show a clear-cut age-related change in ultrastructural morphol-ogy (65). At 3 months of age in rats, these cells contain relatively small numbers of lipid droplets; a considerable part of their cytoplasm is occupied by cell organelles, such as the Golgi system, swollen cisternae of the endoplasmic reticulum, and mitochondria. With advancing age, fat-storing cells become increasing filled with lipid droplets.

Studies evaluating the biochemistry of purified Kupffer cells, endothelium, and parenchyma have shown that different age-related changes occur in these three liver cell types. In Kupffer and endothelial cells, there are no major changes in the activity of most of the key lysosomal enzymes with increasing age (69,70). Cytochemical and biochemical studies have shown a decrease in the activity of glucose 6-phosphatase and magnesium ATPase and in glucagon-stimulated adenylcyclase activity of endothelial cells with aging. In contrast, alkaline phosphatase activity is increased in the endothelial cells of older animals. Age-related changes in the biochemical properties of fat-storing cells have not been studied in detail as of yet.

There is a significant age-related reduction in the apparent V max, the maximal uptake of colloid albumin, by Kupffer cells per milligram protein with increasing age (71,72). Because the protein count of the cells also increases with age, the percentage decrease in endocytosis with increasing age is less when the V max is expressed per 10^6 cells than it is when expressed per milligram of protein (72). The Km, which indicates the affinity of Kupffer cells for substrate, is unaffected by aging. Nonetheless, older animals appear more susceptible to endotoxin paralysis of Kupffer cells and subsequent death in response to endotoxin exposure (73,74). This effect is probably not the result of a diminished threshold dose for the toxic effect of endotoxin, because it appears that the mechanisms responsible for death in response to endotoxin is different in older animals than in younger animals (75). It appears unlikely that this increase in susceptibility to endotoxin-induced death is caused solely by a reduction in the capacity to clear endotoxin from blood because the increase in endotoxin half-life is only about 50 to 60%, whereas the lethal dose is reduced at least fourfold in older rats. Older animals probably are more sensitive to the induction by endotoxin of one or more mediators (cytokines) produced by macrophages that contribute to their adverse response to endotoxin (75).

LIVER FUNCTION AND THE AGING PROCESS

When liver volume and hepatic blood flow have been studied in healthy subjects over a wide age range, a significant inverse correlation has been found between age for both parameters (76–79). Furthermore, hepatic volume declines with increasing age even more so when the data are corrected for body weight. This reduction in liver size and hepatic blood flow with increasing age presumably accounts for the reduced drug elimination observed in the elderly.

Faulty enzyme molecules accumulate with age in cells *in vivo*. This phenomenon is associated with a 30 to 70% reduction in specific enzyme activity per unit enzyme antigen, as determined by immunotitration studies using antiserum prepared against native enzyme derived from young individuals (80). This accumulation of faulty enzyme appears to be a universal phenomenon. These faulty molecules are not the result of errors induced within the protein synthetic apparatus *per se* that is a misincorporation of amino acid residue as such errors would produce detectable alterations in the properties of the enzyme molecules under study, such as their Km or Ki values and net charge (80–83). Such changes have not been detected in extensive studies. Thus, the alterations in proteins that accumulate in cells of senescent organisms are much more likely to be posttranslational in origin. Many of these changes result in the production of inactive molecules that in younger cells would be degraded. With increasing age, the removal of these abnormal molecules becomes inadequate, however, because of an age-associated impairment in the degradation system (84,85).

The biliary bromosulfothalein (BSP) transport maximum tends to decrease with age in rats (86–88). In addition, the transport maximum for BSP conjugation with glutathione also decreases (89). The biliary excretion of intravenous injected ouabain, a neutral cardiac glycoside that is excreted efficiently into bile without any biotransformation, also declines with increasing age in both male and female animals (89–91). The V max value for the hepatic uptake of ouabain by isolated hepatocytes decreases with age from 2.98 ± 1.05 to 1.03 ± 0.39 nmol/mg/min ($p < 0.05$), whereas the Km value changes little with increasing age—31.08 ± 9.31 versus 23.47 ± 10.92 uM.

When serum enzymes of hepatic origin are assayed in blood, there are no changes in transaminase levels with age. Similarly, total and unconjugated bilirubin levels do not change with age after the newborn period. Bone alkaline phosphatase levels are increased as a consequence of growth and are increased in children relative to adults, but after age 20 to 21, no age-related changes in alkaline phosphatase activity are evident.

HEPATIC PROCESSING OF EXTRAHEPATIC LIGANDS AND THE AGING PROCESS

The two principal pathways for ligand processing have been identified in hepatocytes (92). The first is termed the transcellular pathway and uses shuttle vesicles to transport receptor-bound proteins from the sinusoidal surface to the bile cannicular membrane for exocytosis into bile. Because these vesicles are segregated from the lysosomal elements of the hepatocyte, their contents are delivered to bile intact. Immunoglobulin A (IgA) is a typical ligand transported by this pathway (93). The second pathway is termed the lysosomal or degregated pathway and involves the integradation of endocytotic vesicles with lysosomes to form multivesicular bodies. This pathway is utilized by ligands destined for degradation, such as low-density lipoproteins, lipoprotein remnants, and the desialylated glycoproteins (94,95). In general, the receptors for ligands that utilize the degradation pathway are recycled.

Fisher et al. (96) have shown that IgA rapidly binds to a nonrecyclable receptor secretory component on the sinusoidal surface of the rat hepatocytes. IgA enters bile bound to a portion of its receptor. In contrast, asialoorosomucoid is transported almost exclusively by the lysosomal pathway (94). The receptor-bound asialoorosomucoid is internalized in endocytotic vesicles that fuse to form secondary lysosomes. These secondary lysosomes become acidified and give rise to multivesicular bodies that eventually fuse with additional primary lysosomes.

A third model ligand, epidermal growth factor, has been shown to use both the transcellular and lysosomal transcellular pathway (97,98). Most of the epidermal growth factor secreted into bile is degraded, but 20% is excreted intact as immunoprecipitable epidermal growth factor (EGF). The peak secretory activity of intact EGF occurs early at 20 minutes, whereas degraded excretion peaks at approximately 40 minutes.

The biliary secretion and intracellular distribution of IgA have been compared in young and old animals (99). The biliary secretion of IgA in young rats is five times greater than that of older rats and six times greater than that of very old animals. At all age groups, the binding of IgA to rat plasma membranes demonstrates a single class of receptors, which decreases almost fourfold from 2.61×10^{12} to 0.72×10^{12} sites per mg protein between 3 months and 27 months in animals. This age-dependent reduction in the ability of the liver to take up IgA from the plasma is almost certainly due to a reduction in liver plasma membrane IgA binding capacity.

In contrast to these findings, there are no differences in the biliary secretion of asialoorosomucoid between young and old animals. This is true, despite the fact that the plasma membranes obtained from old animals have a reduced binding capacity for asialoorosomucoid. This loss of ability to remove asialoorosomucoid from plasma is offset by the recruitment of additional cells to remove the material from blood. In other words, by recruiting additional cells, the liver is able to compensate for the diminished binding capacity of individual liver cells.

The total quantity of epidermal growth factor excreted into bile decreases markedly with age (96). The biliary excretion of both intact and degraded EGF decreases to the same extent. Thus, despite an age-dependent decrease in EGF binding by approximately 50%, this reduction in binding is not sufficient to account for the total reduction in biliary excretion.

ALBUMIN SYNTHESIS AND AGING

When hepatocytes are isolated from 3-, 12-, 24-, 31-, and 36-month-old rats and examined for their capacity to synthesize albumin under optimal conditions, a significant decrease in the amount of albumin synthesized per

10^6 hepatocytes can be observed between 3 and 24 months of age (101–102). When the albumin-synthesizing capacity is expressed on the basis of cellular protein as opposed to cell number, approximately the same pattern of an age-related reduction in albumin synthesis is observed. When total protein synthesis is examined, a similar reduction is observed between the ages of 3 and 12 months. When one examines the clearance of radioactive albumin injected into animals, the T 1/2 decreases between 12 and 24 months of age and remains constant thereafter (103). The volume of distribution for albumin increases between 12 and 24 months of age, but after 24 months no additional changes occurs. Aging does not influence the transcriptional rate of albumin gene expression (104–105). The amount of albumin mRNA per mg RNA is greater at 24 and 36 months than at 3 and 12 months of age. The higher content of albumin mRNA is attributed to an increase of albumin mRNA content within the membrane-bound polyribosomal fraction. No change with age is evident in the protein synthetic activity of either the free or the membrane-bound polyribosomes.

THE MONO-OXYGENASE SYSTEM AND THE AGING PROCESS

There are no conclusive human studies of differences in hepatic mono-oxygenase activity as a function of either age or sex (106–109). The current consensus is that the data available for an age-dependent decline in hepatocellular cytochrome-P450-dependent drug metabolism in humans as compared to animals are largely circumstantial. In contrast, there exist a plethora of *in vitro* studies evaluating hepatic mono-oxygenases in inbred rodents as a function of age (4,11). These studies from a number of different laboratories have reported age-dependent reductions in noninducible enzyme activities of the hepatic mono-oxygenase system and also for some inducible mono-oxygenases (108,109). In general, such studies demonstrate a two- to fourfold reduction in the NADPH cytochrome C reductase activity, a loss of cytochrome P450 content, and a decline in the rate of ethylmorphine-N-demethylation in microsomes studied *in vitro* as a function of increasing age. The metabolism of pharmaceuticals in the liver of old male rats is considerably less than that seen in females, presumably because of a reduction of the microsomal cytochrome P450 reductase levels, as well as of NADPH cytochrome P450 reductase activity. The magnitude of the phenobarbital-inducible changes in mono-oxygenase activity is similar, regardless of the age of the animal. Thus, although the actual rate of mono-oxygenase induction may not be compromised during aging, the maximum level of induction is lower in older animals.

Concomitant qualitative fine structural studies reveal a 40 to 50% decline in the amount of hepatic smooth endoplasmic reticulum, a primary focus of the microsomal mono-oxygenases as a function of increasing age in rats

(110–111). These data have been confirmed biochemically by the finding of a parallel change in the hepatic concentration of microsomal protein with age.

Biochemical studies of hepatic microsome have demonstrated that the noninduced phenobarbital-inducible activities of the microsomal mono-oxygenase system decline, the hepatic concentration of smooth endoplasmic reticulum is reduced, the cholesterol/phospholipid ratio of microsomes increase, and the fluidity of the microsomal membrane is diminished in livers of inbred male rats as a function of increasing age (112–114). The specific activity of young adult soluble P450 reductase is twofold greater than that isolated from older animals. Furthermore, there is no change in the molecular weight, a shift to a more heat-stable form, or a decline in the immuno-titratable activity. Approximately 40 to 50% of the P450 reductase isolated from senescent microsomes, although immunoprecipitatable, is inactive catalytically.

In the Rhesus monkey, an absence of change in the cytochrome P450 content and a substantial increase in the specific activity of NADPH cytochrome C reductase within hepatic microsomes have been reported as a function of age, independent of gender (114,115).

In contrast to Class 1 mono-oxygenase enzymes, Class 2 reactions comprise a heterogeneous group of conjugations by which chemical groups derived from so-called donor substrates are coupled to acceptor substrates. The enzymes catalyzing these reactions reside in various compartments of hepatic parenchymal cells. Several of these enzymes are also present in other tissues, such as the kidney, intestine, lung, and skin. In general, Class 2 reactions result in the production of a more hydrophilic compound. A pronounced effect of gender and sex hormones has been observed for this enzyme system, with enhancement of enzyme activity, such as UDP-glucuron-oyl transferase and sulfatase activity toward bilirubin by progesterone and by testosterone (116). Acetylation rates, measured by the plasma half-life of isoniazid, show no significant or only a small increase with age (117,118). In general, Class 2 enzyme activities remain rather constant with increasing age in females and show only a slight decline with age in males.

GALLSTONE DISEASE AND THE AGING PROCESS

The putative mechanisms for gallstone development become more important with advancing age. An increase in cholesterol gallstones with increasing age is a well-established fact in many areas of the world, although the incidence and the age-related increased rate vary considerably among different ethnic groups (119). The major lipid fractions in human bile are bile acids, phospholipids, and cholesterol. Their relative molar percentages, respectively, are 70% to 75%, 20% to 25%, and 48%. In addition to lipids, bile contains proteins and biopigments. Secreted hepatic bile is concentrated three- to fivefold in the gallbladder.

In human bile, the quantitatively most important bile acids are cholic acid (30 to 40% of the bile acid pool), chenodeoxycholic acid (30 to 40% of the bile acid pool), and deoxycholic acid (20 to 30% of the bile acid pool). Bile acids are excreted into bile and conjugated either with glycine or taurine. They are reabsorbed efficiently (95% to 98%) from the intestine by an active transport process present in the distal ileum. Reabsorbed bile acids are carried in the portal blood to the liver where they are extracted efficiently from the blood and then re-excreted into bile.

The formation of bile acids in the liver is regulated homeostatically by the inflow of bile acids through the portal vein, with the rate-limiting enzyme being cholesterol 7 α-hydroxylase. Under steady state conditions, the synthesis rate of bile acids is 0.5 to 1.5 mmol/day (200 to 600 mg). Normally, the formation of cholic acid is 1.5 to 2 times that of chenodeoxycholic acid. Owing to the efficiency of the enterohepatic circulation, the bile pool circulates five to ten times per day.

Lecithin is the principal phospholipid in human bile. It generally contains a saturated fatty acid at position one and an unsaturated fatty acid at position two.

Biliary cholesterol is secreted in its nonesterified form (120). The average daily intake of cholesterol by man is about 0.5 to 1.5 mmol/day (200 to 600 mg). Between 30 to 60% of this cholesterol is absorbed from the diet. A similar amount of the cholesterol is secreted into bile daily as bile acid and cholesterol. The synthesis of cholesterol by the body, particularly the liver, is quantitatively much more important than the amount absorbed from the diet. Approximately half the cholesterol production of the body occurs in the liver.

Hepatic cholesterol synthesis is regulated by the inflow of cholesterol and possibly by the inflow of bile acids to the liver. Thirty to 50% of the daily cholesterol turnover is to bile acids.

The effect of age on biliary lipid composition was determined in a very large series of gallstone-free, healthy Scandinavians (119). Thirty percent of these healthy subjects were found to have a supersaturated bile. There were no differences between the sexes with regard to biliary lipid or bile acid composition or cholesterol saturation of hepatic bile. When biliary secretory rate studies were performed, it was evident that cholesterol secretion increased progressively with age. However, no relationship between age and bile acid or phospholipid secretion was evident. By measuring the bile acid production rate in this series of normal subjects, an inverse relationship between age and bile acid synthesis could be demonstrated to exist for both sexes. Furthermore, a negative correlation between bile acid production and biliary cholesterol saturation and between bile acid synthesis and cholesterol secretion could be demonstrated.

In male rats, it has been shown that the relative proportion of cholic acid increases and that of chenodeoxycholic acid declines with increasing age. Such a relationship has not been seen in female animals (121,122).

The key enzyme for the conversion of cholesterol into bile acids is 7 α hydroxylase. Other important enzymes for subsequent catabolism of cholesterol to bile acids are 12 α and 6 α hydroxylase, both of which are P450-dependent enzymes (123–125). P450 enzyme activity changes with age and is known to be gender dependent. In male rats, the P450 in mono-oxygenase activity declines markedly with age, whereas in females little change occurs with age.

Van der Werf et al. (126) have reported that the 7 α dehydroxylation of bile acids is enhanced in the gut of normal elderly persons. Moreover, Hellemans and coworkers (127) have reported that elderly healthy individuals have an abnormally high C14 glycocholic acid breath test, suggesting an increased deconjugation of conjugated bile acids. This increase is believed to occur as a result of an intestinal bacterial population in the small bowel. Thus, the increased production of CO_2 from the glycine component of the bile acid breath test suggests that a latent but excessive bacterial overgrowth exists in elderly individuals. This may contribute to some of the biliary lipid abnormalities found with aging. Others have not been able to replicate this finding and therefore deny its existence (128). More studies are necessary to resolve this issue.

DRUG-INDUCED LIVER DISEASE AND THE AGING PROCESS

There is an almost universal impression that adverse drug reactions are much more common in elderly subjects, and certainly hepatic adverse drug reactions are no different. Recently, Woodhouse, Mortimer, and Wiholm (129) examined all adverse hepatic drug reactions reported to the Swedish Adverse Drug Reaction Advisory Committee from 1980 to 1984. The total reported number of acute hepatic adverse drug reactions was 807, of which 239 or 29% occurred in individuals over the age of 65. In Sweden, 17% of the population is over the age of 65. Superficially therefore, there was a marked excess in the proportion of hepatic adverse drug reactions occurring in individuals over 65 years of age. By monitoring data about prescriptions, however, it was possible to show that about 30% of the prescriptions written during this period were given to individuals over age 65. By obtaining prescription data for the drugs most commonly implicated in hepatic adverse drug reactions, Woodhouse et al. (129) were able to derive a ratio (percent of reports of reactions in individuals greater than 65 years to percent of prescriptions for individuals greater than 65 years) in order to obtain a better indication whether elderly individuals are more susceptible to adverse drug reactions for individual drugs than might be expected. A high ratio would indicate an increased susceptibility in the elderly; a ratio of 1 would indicate a reduced susceptibility to a particular adverse drug reaction. For the eleven most frequently reported adverse drug reactions reported, there was no marked increase in the susceptibility (no ratio >1.5 for any of the drugs). However, there was a suggestion that a higher proportion of elderly individuals receiving nitrofuradantin might be more susceptible to an acute drug reaction as the ratio was 1.43.

SPECIFIC LIVER DISEASE AND THE AGING PROCESS

In a retrospective analysis by Potter and James (130) of all patients in whom a diagnosis of alcoholic liver disease was made, 208 patients were identified with a firmly established diagnosis of alcoholic liver disease (130). Of these, 149 presented before age 59, 49 presented for the first time between the ages of 60 and 69 years, and 12 presented over the age of 70. Thus, 57 of the 206 patients (28%) were over age 60 at initial presentation. The elderly with alcoholic liver disease tended to present with a higher proportion of symptoms suggesting severe liver disease, such as ankle swelling, jaundice, and ascites, than did younger patients. Liver histology was available on 96% of these patients, either within 3 months of their presentation or at postmortem. Elderly individuals had an increased rate of cirrhosis compared to younger alcoholic individuals.

Primary Biliary Cirrhosis

The mean age at the time of initial diagnosis for primary biliary cirrhosis (PBC) is in the mid-forties (131). Many patients are asymptomatic at the time of detection (132,133). In a large series of patients with PBC of whom 29% were greater than 65 years of age at detection, there were 12 men (10% of the total). No single sign or symptom was more common either in the younger or older individual. However, the total number of signs and symptoms recorded per patient was significantly less in the older than in the younger patients. Interestingly, there was no difference in the histology at the time of the first liver biopsy between the two groups; 40% of the younger and 37% of the older patients were found to have cirrhosis at the time of initial biopsy.

ACKNOWLEDGMENTS

This work was supported in part by NIAAA grants 04425, 06601, and 06772 and NIDDK grant 32556.

REFERENCES

1. Guralnik J, Schneider EL. In: Espenshade TJ, Stolnitz GJ, eds. *Technological prospects and population trends.* Boulder, CO: Westview Press, Inc., 1987;125–146.
2. Schmucker D. *Pharmacol Rev* 1979;30:445–456.
3. Schmucker D. *Pharmacol Rev* 1985;37:133–148.
4. Vestal R, Dawson G. In: Finch C, Schneider E, eds. *Handbook of the biology of aging.* New York: Van Nostrand Reinhold, 1985;744–819.
5. National Institute on Aging. *Annual Report 1986.* Bethesda, MD: NIH, 1987.
6. Manton KG. *J Gerontol* 1986;41:672–681.
7. Brandfonbrener M, Landowne M, Shock NW. *Circulation* 1955;12:557.
8. Rodeheffer RJ, Gerstenblith G, Becker LC, et al. *Circulation* 1984;69:203–213.
9. Rowe JW, Tobin JD, Andres RA, Norris A, Shock NW. *J Gerontol* 1976;31:155–163.
10. Lindeman RD, Tobin JD, Shock NW. *J Am Geriatr Soc* 1985;33:278–285.
11. Watanabe T, Tanaka Y. *Virchows Arch (B) Cell Pathol* 1982;39:9–20.
12. Onishi H, Tsukada S, Hayashi Y, et al. *Nature (New Biol)* 1972;239:84–86.
13. David H, Uerlings I. *Zbl Allg Pathol Pathol Anat* 1979;123:85–103.
14. David H. *Exp Pathol* 1985;(suppl 11):1:1–148.
15. David H. *Acta Biol Med Germ* 1979;38:935–952.
16. Barz H, Kunze KD, Voss K, Simon H. *Exp Pathol* 1977;14:55–64.
17. Van Zwieten MJ, Hollander CF. In: Jones TC, Mohr U, Hunt RD, eds. *Digestive system.* Berlin: Springer-Verlag, 1985;83–86.
18. Van Zwieten MJ, Hollander CF. In: Jones TC, Mohr U, Hunt RD, eds. *Digestive system.* Berlin: Springer-Verlag, 1985;86–92.
19. David H, Reinke P. In: Bianchi L, Holt P, James OFW, Butler RN, eds. *Aging in liver and gastrointestinal tract.* Boston: MTP Process LTD, 1988;143–159.
20. Munro HN, Young VR. *Postgrad Med* 1978;63:143–148.
21. Findor J, Perez V, Bruch Igartua E, Giovanetti M, Fiaravantti N. *Acta Hepatogastroenterol* 1973;20:200–204.
22. Zurcher CI, Van Zwieten MJ, Solleveld HA, Van Bezooijen CFA, Hollander CF. In: Kitani K, ed. *Liver and aging.* Amsterdam: Elsevier/North-Holland Biomedical Press, 1982;19–36.
23. Hegner D, Platt D. *Mech Aging Dev* 1975;4:191–200.
24. Nokubo M. *J Gerontol* 1985;40:409–414.
25. Vorbeck ML, Martin AP, Long JW Jr, Smith JM, Orr RR. *Arch Biochem Biophys* 1982;217:351–361.
26. Grinna LS. *Mech Aging Dev* 1977;6:197–205.
27. Kapitulnik J, Tshershedsky M, Barenholz Y. *Science* 1979;206:843–844.
28. Armbrecht HJ, Birnbaum LS, Zenser TV, Davis BB. *Exp Gerontol* 1982;17:41–48.
29. David H. *Exp Pathol* 1983;24:77–82.
30. David H. *Pathol Res Pract* 1980;166:381–399.
31. Schmucker DL, Mooney JS, Jones AL. *J Cell Biol* 1978;78:319–337.
32. Fleischer M, Meiss R, Robenek W, Themann H. *Int Arch Occup Environ Health* 1979;44:25–43. .PA
33. Tate EL, Herbener GH. *J Gerontol* 1976;31:129–133.
34. Sato T, Tauchi H. *Acta Pathol Jap* 1975;25:403–412.
35. Forbeck ML, Martin AP. *J Cell Biol* 1976;70:2,36a.
36. Spencer JA, Horton AA. *Exp Gerontol* 1978;13:227–232.
37. David H. *Acta Stereol* 1983;2:408–412.
38. David H. *Exp Pathol* 1980;18:321–328.
39. Tauchi H, Sato T. *J Gerontol* 1968;23:454–461.
40. Knook DL. In: *Fifth European symposium on basic research in gerontology.* 1977; 26:595–598.
41. David H. In: Collan Y, Romppanen T, eds. *Morphometry in morphological diagnosis.* Kuopio: Kuopio University Press, 1982;115–122.
42. David H, Reinke P. *Exp Pathol* 1987;32:193–224.
43. David H. *Gegenbaurs Morphol Jahrbuch* 1980;126:285–292.
44. David H. *Acta Histochem* (suppl XXVI):357–360.

45. Knook DL, Praaning van Dalen DP, Brouwer A. In: Kitani K, ed. *Liver and aging.* Amsterdam: Elsevier/North-Holland Biomedical Press, 1982;269–281.
46. Dubuisson L, Bedin C, Balaband C. *Falk Symp* 1986;43:161.
47. Jungermann K, Sasse D. *Trends Biochem Sci* 1978;3:198.
48. Pette D, Brandau H. *Enzymol Biol Clin* 1966;6:79–122.
49. Loud AV. *J Cell Biol* 1968;37:27–46.
50. Reith A, Schuler B, Vogell W. *Z Zellforsch* 1968;89:225–240.
51. Nadal C, Zajdela F. *Exp Cell Res* 1966;42:99–116.
52. Sulkin NM. *Am J Anat* 1943;73:107–125.
53. Rabes HM. In: Popper H, Schaffner F, eds. *Progress in liver diseases,* vol V. New York: Grune & Stratton, 1976;83–99.
54. Stocker E, Schultze B, Heine W-D, Liebscher H. *Z Zellforsch* 1972;125:306–331.
55. Stocker E. *Verh Dtsch Ges Pathol* 1975;59:78–94.
56. Heine W-D, Stocker E. *Verh Dtsch Ges Pathol* 1970;54:550–554.
57. Wisse E, Knook DL. In: Popper H, Schaffner F, eds. *Progress in liver diseases,* vol VI. New York: Grune and Stratton, 1979;153–171.
58. Kirn A, Knook DL, Wisse E, eds. *Cells of the Hepatic Sinusoid,* vol 1. Rijswijk, The Netherlands: The Kupffer Cell Foundation, 1986.
59. Benacerraf B. In Rouiller E, ed. *The Liver,* vol II. New York: Academic Press, 1964;37–62.
60. Altura BM. In: Altura BM, ed. *Advances in Microcirculation,* vol 9. Basel: Karger, 1980;252–294.
61. Popper H. In: Popper H, Schaffner F, eds. *Progress in liver disease,* vol 8. Orlando, FL: Grune & Stratton, 1986;659–683.
62. Brouwer A, Knook DL. *Mech Aging Dev* 1983;21:205–228.
63. Praaning van Dalen DP, Brouwer A, Knook DL. *Gastroenterology* 1981;81:1036–1044.
64. Praaning van Dalen DP, Knook DL. *FEBS Lett* 1982;241:229–232.
65. Hendriks HFJ, Verhoofstad WAMM, Brouwer A, De Leeuw AM, Knook DL. *Exp Cell Res* 1985;160:138–149.
66. Blaner WS, Hendriks HFJ, Brouwer A, De Leeuw AM, Knook DL, Goodman DS. *J Lipid Res* 1985;26:1241–1251.
67. DeLeeuw AM, Knook DL. In: Van Bezooijen CFA, ed. *Pharmacological, morphological and physiological aspects of liver aging.* Rijswijk, The Netherlands: Eurage, 1983;91–96.
68. Burek JD. *Pathology of aging rats.* West Palm Beach, FL: CRC Press, 1980.
69. Wilson PD, Watson R, Knook DL. *Gerontology* 1982;28:32–43.
70. Knook DL, Sleyster E. In: Kitani K, ed. *Liver and aging.* Amsterdam: Elsevier/North-Holland Biomedical Press, 1978;241–250.
71. Brouwer A, Knook DL. *Mech Aging Dev* 1983;21:205–228.
72. Brouwer A, Barelds RJ, Knook DL. *Hepatology* 1985;3:362–372.
73. Horan MA. *Endotoxin as a naturally occurring immunomodulator.* Utrecht: State University of Utrecht, 1986.
74. Brouwer A, Horan MA, Barelds RJ, Knook DL, Hollander CF. In: Van Bezooijen CFA, Miglio F, Knook DL, eds. *Liver, drugs and aging.* Rijswijk, The Netherlands: Eurage, 1986;77–82.
75. Brouwer A, Horan MA, Barelds RJ, Knook DL. *Arch Gerontol Geriatr* 1986;5:317–324.
76. Thompson EN, Williams R. *Gut* 1965;6:266–269.
77. Tauchi H, Sato T. In: Kitani K, ed. *Liver and aging.* Amsterdam: Elsevier/North-Holland Biomedical Press, 1978;3–19.
78. Firtschy P, Robotti G, Schneekloth G, Vock P. *J Clin Ultrasound* 1983;11:299–303.
79. Caesar J, Shaldon S, Chiandussi L, Guevena L, Sherlock S. *Clin Sci* 1961;21:43–57.
80. Orgel LE. *Proc Natl Acad Sci USA* 1963;49:517–520.
81. Dovrat A, Scharf Y, Eisenbach L, Gershon D. *Exp Eye Res* 1986;42:489–496.
82. Rothstein M. In: Adelman RC, Roth GS, eds. *Altered proteins in aging.* Boca Raton, FL: CRC Press, 1983;1–9.
83. Hirsch G. In: Adelman RC, Roth GS, eds. *Altered proteins in aging.* Boca Raton, FL: CRC Press, 1983;35–54.

84. Lavie L, Reznick AZ, Gershon D. *Biochem J* 1982;202:47–51.
85. Gershon D, Reznick AZ, Reiss U. In: Cherkin A, ed. *Physiology and cell biology of aging*. New York: Raven Press, 1979;21–26.
86. Kitani K, Kanai S, Miura R. In: Kitani K, ed. *Liver and aging—1978*. Amsterdam: Elsevier/North-Holland Biomedical Press, 1978;145–156.
87. Kitani K, Zurcher C, van Bezooijen CFA. *Mech Aging Dev* 1981;7:381–393.
88. Kanai S, Kitani K, Fujita S, Kitagawa H. *Arch Gerontol Geriatr* 1985;4:73–85.
89. Kanai S, Kitani K, Sato Y, Nokubo M. *Arch Gerontol Geriatr (submitted)*.
90. Sato Y, Kanai S, Kitani K. *Arch Gerontol Geriatr* 1987;6:141–152.
91. Ohta M, Kanai S, Sato Y, Kitani K. *Biochem Pharmacol* 1988;37:935–942.
92. Jones AL, Burwen SJ. *Semin Liver Dis* 1985;5:136–146.
93. Renston RH, Jones AL, Christiansen WD, Hradek GT, Underdown BJ. *Science* 1980;208:1276–1278.
94. Hubbard AL, Stukenbrok H. *J Cell Biol* 1979;83:65–81.
95. Jones AL, Hradek GT, Hornick C, Renaud G, Windler EET, Havel RJ. *J Lipid Res* 1984;25:1151–1158.
96. Fisher MM, Nagy B, Bazin H, et al. *Proc Natl Acad Sci USA* 1979;76:2008–2012.
97. Burwen SJ, Barker ME, Goldman IS, Hradek GT, Raper SE, Jones AL. *J Cell Biol* 1984;99:1259–1265.
98. St. Hilaire RJ, Hradek GT, Jones AL. *Proc Natl Acad Sci USA* 1983;80:797–801.
99. Schmucker DL, Gilbert R, Hradek GT, Jones AL, Bazin H. *Gastroenterology* 1985;88:436–443.
100. Van Bezooijen CFA, Grell T, Knook DL. *Mech Aging Dev* 1977;6:293.
101. Van Bezooijen CFA, Sakkee AN, Knook DL. *Mech Aging Dev* 1981;17:11.
102. Horbach GJMJ, Yap SH, Van Bezooijen CFA. *Biochem J* 1983;216:309.
103. Horbach GJMJ, Princen HMG, Van der Kroef M, Van Bezooijen CFA, Yap SH. *Biochem Biophys Acta* 1984;783:60.
104. Horbach GJMJ. *Albumin metabolism and aging* (thesis). Berlin: Maastricht, 1986.
105. Horbach GJMJ, Van der Boom H, Van Bezooijen CFA, Yap SH. In: Van Bezooijen CFA, Miglio F, Knook DL, eds. *Liver, drugs and aging*. Rijswijk, The Netherlands: Eurage, 1986;121.
106. Pearson M, Roberts C. *Age Aging* 1984;13:313–316.
107. Van Bezooijen CFA. *Mech Aging Dev* 1984;25:1–22.
108. Schmucker D, Wang R. *Exp Gerontol* 1980;15:321–329.
109. Schmucker D, Wang R. *Mech Aging Dev* 1981;15:189–202.
110. Schmucker D, Mooney J, Jones S. *Science* 1977;197:1005–1008.
111. Schmucker D, Mooney J, Jones A. *J Cell Biol* 1978;78:319–337.
112. Vlasuk G, Walz F. *Arch Biochem Biophys* 1982;214:248–259.
113. Schmucker D, Wang R, Vessey D, James J, Maloney A. *Mech Aging Dev* 1984;27:207–217.
114. Maloney A, Schmucker D, Vessey D, Wang R. *Hepatology* 1986;6:282–287.
115. Sutter M, Wood G, Williamson L, Strong R, Pickham K, Richardson A. *Biochem Pharmacol* 1985;34:2983–2987.
116. Muraca M, Fevery J. *Gastroenterology* 1984;87:308–313.
117. Farah F, Taylor W, Rawlins MD, James O. *Br Med J* 1977;2:155–156.
118. Gachaly B, Vas A, Hajos P, Kaldor A. *Eur J Clin Pharmacol* 1984;26:43–45.
119. Lindstrom CG. *Scand J Gastroenterol* 1977;12:341–346.
120. Angelin B. In: Calandra S, Carulli N, Salvioli G, eds. *Liver and lipid metabolism*. Amsterdam: Elsevier/North-Holland Biomedical Press, 1984;187–201.
121. Uchida K, Takeuchi N. In: Yonago H, ed. *Proceedings of the 15th Symposium on Pharmacological Activity and Mechanism*. Amsterdam: Elsevier/North Holland Biomedical Press, 1986;41–46.
122. Uchida K, Matsubara T, Ishikawa Y, Ito N. In: Kitani K, ed. *Liver and aging—1982, Liver and drugs*. Amsterdam: Elsevier/North-Holland Biomedical Press, 1982;192–211.
123. Fujita S, Uesugi T, Kitagawa H, Suzuki T, Kitani K. In: Kitani K, ed. *Liver and aging—1982, Liver and drugs*. Amsterdam: Elsevier/North-Holland Biomedical Press, 1982;55–71.

124. Kitani K. *Hepatology* 1986;6:316–319.
125. Kamataki T, Maeda K, Shimada M, Kitani K, Nagai T, Kato R. *J Pharmacol Exp Ther* 1985;233:222–228.
126. Van der Werf SDJ, Huijbregts AWM, Lanners HLM, van Berge Henegouwen GP, van Tongeren JHM. *Eur J Clin Invest* 1981;11:425–431.
127. Hellemans J, Joosten E, Ghoos Y, et al. *Age Aging* 1984;13:138–143.
128. Arora S, Kassarigian Z, Krasinski SD, Croffey B, Kaplan MM, Russell RM. *Gastroenterology* 1989;96:1560–1565.
129. Woodhouse KW, Mortimer O, Wiholm BE. In: Kitani K, ed. *Hepatic adverse drug reactions: The effect of age in liver and aging—1986.* Amsterdam: Elsevier/North-Holland Biomedical Press, 1986;75–80.
130. Potter JF, James OFW. *Gerontology* 1988;32:560–566.
131. Lehmann AB, Bassendine MF, James OFW. *Gerontology* 1985;31:186–194.
132. Christensen E, Crowe J, Doniach D, et al. *Gastroenterology* 1980;78:236–246.
133. Roll J, Boyer JL, Barry D, et al. *N Engl J Med* 1983;308:1–7.

Geriatric Nutrition, edited by John E. Morley,
Zvi Glick, Laurence Z. Rubenstein.
Raven Press, Ltd., New York © 1990.

19

Nutrition and Diabetes Mellitus in the Elderly

Fran E. Kaiser and Mark J. Rosenthal

*Geriatric Research, Education and Clinical Center, VA Medical Center,
Sepulveda, California 91343*

"What some call health, if purchased by perpetual anxiety about diet, isn't much better than tedious disease."

George Dennison Prentice
Prenticeana, 1860

Diet remains the cornerstone of the treatment of Type II diabetes mellitus, and the relationship between diet and diabetes has remained one of interest and much controversy since 1674 when Willis advocated the use of starchy and gummy, high-carbohydrate foods in diabetes. Yet, the relevance of various dietary manipulations for older adults with diabetes has received relatively little attention. This is surprising and disturbing because diabetes is very much a disease of older adults, and indeed, the prevalence of diabetes increases with advancing age. Two-thirds of all hospitalized diabetic patients are older than age 65 (1). Unfortunately, the diagnosis of diabetes is often missed in older persons. Harris et al. suggest that the prevalance of diabetes in those over age 65 is nearly 20%, and half of these cases are presently undiagnosed (2).

A much larger segment of the population has impaired glucose tolerance. Such glucose intolerance is demonstrably present in otherwise healthy older individuals. It has been widely reported that there is a 1 to 2 mg/dl increase in the 2-hour postprandial glucose level with each decade over age 50 (3). Reports of elevated glycosylated hemoglobin (4) suggest that such mild increases in glucose response to feeding are physiologically relevant. There are remarkable parallels between the toxicity of glucose and hyperglycemia upon various systems and the changes that occur with age (5). Hence, mild to modest hyperglycemia may have a profound influence on the development of age-related pathology. However, we found no age-related alteration of another glycosylated protein—fructosamine (6)—and others have failed to find age-related changes in glycosylated hemoglobin (7). The reason for

259

these discrepancies is unclear, and these findings may be related to associated factors, rather than merely to advanced age *per se*. As discussed below, nutritional considerations may have a major impact.

The significance of such changes in glucose tolerance has been supported by recent findings of impaired cognition that appears to be proportional to the degree of elevation of plasma glucose (8,9). Furthermore, glucose intolerance without overt diabetes has also been associated with a worsened prognosis after ischemic stroke (10) and an increased incidence of atherosclerotic heart disease (11).

There are therefore several strongly suggestive and important reasons for better understanding this glucose intolerance. A number of the concomitants of aging have been linked to impaired glucose tolerance, notably changes in body composition with increased adiposity and degree of activity. Clearly, nutritional factors play a role in developing adiposity, which is related to glucose intolerance and to overt diabetes (2). There may also be age-related changes in dietary preference, such as the so-called geriatric sweet tooth (12). Certain changes in dietary intake may relate not only to social factors or economic exigencies but also to alterations in taste perception. A decrease in taste acuity is found not only in diabetics but also in older people in general, and these changes are not apparently related to micronutrient deficiencies (13).

Given the potential effect of changes in dietary preference, a recent study investigated the role of dietary carbohydrates in the decreased glucose tolerance of the elderly (14). By giving a preparatory diet containing 300 g carbohydrate to a group of 50- to 80-year-old subjects for 3 days before glucose tolerance testing, 11 of the 16 glucose tolerance tests that had been abnormal when performed without dietary preparation became normal (14). Several investigators have found that older subjects consumed significantly fewer total calories and slightly less carbohydrate than younger individuals (14,15). Although insulin response was impaired in older but not in younger subjects maintained on a low-carbohydrate diet, the insulin response was adequate when subjects were fed a high-carbohydrate diet (14). The plasma glucose response to a standard oral glucose challenge appears to be impaired by caloric restriction (16), such as might pertain to the ordinary diet of many older Americans, and improves if patients ingest a high-carbohydrate diet for several days (17,18). The improvement in oral glucose tolerance has been associated with a fall in the plasma insulin response, which suggests that insulin sensitivity might also improve after ingestion of a high-carbohydrate diet, but this has yet to be confirmed (19). Despite these changes, the improvements seen are at best marginal.

Hence, dietary carbohydrate intake can partially modify some of the age-related changes in glucose tolerance, but does not entirely explain the tendency toward pancreatic failure. One major component in the development of glucose intolerance is insulin resistance, which has been well demonstrated by insulin-infusion/glucose clamp studies (20). Similar pathology has been demonstrated in aging rodents (21). Such changes occur relatively early and may be developmental, rather than sensecent. More notable in rodents than in humans is the development of pancreatic failure as indicated by deficient insulin responses (22). Although the development of pancreatic amyloidosis (amylin) has been reported to be associated with aging in man (23), rodents show enlarged multilobulated, fibrotic pancreatic islets (24). Also contributing to the glucose intolerance of aging is impairment in the second phase of insulin release, the complete physiologic significance of which has not been entirely understood. With aging in rodents, there is a 40 to 50% decrease in the short-term stimulation of insulin synthesis by glucose. The impaired short-term effects of glucose on proinsulin synthesis in pancreatic islets derived from aged rats appear to occur at a translational level (25). Furthermore, there may also be changes in the processing of insulin, resulting in increased release of relatively bioinactive products, notably proinsulin.

Dietary factors are involved in the development of pancreatic failure at least in animal models. Sucrose-fed rats were able to contend with the age-related decreased insulin release (as normalized to individual pancreatic beta cells) by expanding their pool of pancreatic beta cells (22). Sucrose *per se* did not have an adverse effect on this compensatory process. Indeed, these authors suggest that caloric restriction may prevent this pancreatic compensation. Although calorically restricted animals did not demonstrate the alterations in serum insulin levels or the pancreatic pathology exhibited by control fed rats, the islets from the restricted rats were shown to have impaired function *in vitro* (22). Food restriction has been reported to promote a sustained lowering of plasma glucose concentration. Not only does ambient glucose concentration diminish but also the percentage of glycosylated hemoglobin falls (26).

The relevance of these studies to pancreatic failure is called into question by a lack of glucose intolerance reported recently with aging in mice (27). Although the construct of pancreatic failure has generated fruitful research, the applicability to human aging is unclear at this time. Nonetheless, insulin resistance is common, has multifactorial contributions, and is of considerable relevance to the process of aging.

What are the appropriate dietary modalities for the treatment of diabetes in this very large cohort of primarily non-insulin-dependent patients? Here the applicability of most data to the geriatric population becomes even murkier because of the paucity of studies performed in the elderly. In most studies, therapeutic options are discussed, and the relevance to older patients, although tenuous, is presumed to be based on clinical experience and commonalities present in the majority of patients with diabetes. Total caloric intake must be considered carefully. Although caloric deficiency can promote glucose intolerance, excess can promote obesity. Although this can be a greater problem among younger patients with diabetes, many older diabetics are overweight, and the beneficial effects of moderate weight loss for this group have been demonstrated (28).

The involvement of other nutritional factors in the pathogenesis of diabetes among the elderly is, at best, tenous, but such factors do appear to play a significant role in the morbidity of diabetes among older people. Studies have long suggested a role for micronutrients either in the development of diabetes or its complications, and this literature has been recently and extensively reviewed (29). Although provocative, the clinical import remains to be documented definitively. Older people in general appear to be at particular risk for micronutrient deficiency (30). Diabetes compounds this risk by increasing glycosuria, which increases the urinary loss of zinc (31). Most notable is the role of zinc in potentially ameliorating the immunodeficiency that develops with aging (32). Unfortunately, recent controlled studies have failed to validate initial suppositions (33), and the benefits from zinc supplementation remain to be resolved. Both an animal and a human study have reported benefits of zinc replacement on immune function in patients with diabetes mellitus with zinc depletion as measured by T cell response to phytohemagglutin (34,35). Zinc clearly has other important roles as well. Because older diabetics are particularly prone to macrovascular disease, the role of zinc in wound healing is critical (36). Zinc supplementation has been shown to accelerate the rate of healing leg ulcers in zinc-deficient elderly patients (37). Zinc deficiency may also play a role in the cardiomyopathy associated with diabetes by altering myocardial adenylate cyclase activity (38). However, it does not appear that zinc deficiency can fully explain the decreased taste acuity that develops in older adults with diabetes (35).

Other micronutrients may be involved in the pathogenesis of diabetes. Manganese deficiency results in decreased pancreatic insulin synthesis and enhanced degradation in rats (39). In several studies, chromium has been suggested to play a role in the occurrence of diabetes. A combination of chromium and nicotinic acid improves glucose tolerance in healthy elderly volunteers, whereas either agent alone was ineffective in ameliorating hyperglycemia (36).

CALORIES AND DIET

The maintenance of ideal body weight is obviously desirable for all patients with diabetes. In obese subjects, weight loss can result in improved insulin sensitivity, diminished hyperglycemia, and decreased cholesterol, triglycerides, and blood pressure (40,41). Although the vast majority of type II diabetics are overweight (approximately 80%), it is important to recognize that some elderly are at risk for malnutrition and in fact need a diet to maintain or increase weight and improve nutrition. Weight tables, such as the

TABLE 1. *Dietary recommendations of the American Diabetes Association*

Carbohydrate:	55–60% of the total caloric intake
Protein:	12–20% of the total caloric intake
Fat:	< 30% of the total caloric intake
	< 300 mg/dl cholesterol
	Saturated and polyunsaturated fat < 10% of the total caloric intake
	(2–40 g/day)

Master table (42), should be used to assess body weight as they are more age appropriate.

There are many unresolved issues around weight reduction, such as altering body fat distribution (a high waist/hip ratio being a good predictor of cardiovascular disease and mortality (43) and altering dietary composition to conform to American Diabetes Association (ADA) recommendations (Table 1).

Although moderate to severe caloric restriction in younger and middle-aged Type II diabetics can result in weight loss in the short term, these benefits tend to be short lived (44,45). The effects of such diets have not been extensively evaluated in the elderly.

Recently, Grundy and coworkers (46) compared the effects of a high-carbohydrate, low-fat diet (60% carbohydrate, 25% fat) to a high-monounsaturated-fat diet (50% fat, 35% carbohydrate). Plasma glucose, triglyceride, and very low-density lipoprotein (VLDL) cholesterol levels fell on the high-fat diet. This finding may alter some of the current thinking regarding the ADA diet.

For many elderly people, the effort of changing the intake habits of a lifetime; the use of a complicated (at least to physicians) exchange list of foods; the alterations of dentition, taste, and smell; the economics and mobility required to purchase food; and the mistaken notion that "special food" is required may all conspire to result in dietary noncompliance, which then results in worsening of hyperglycemia, hyperlipidemia, and hypertension (Fig. 1). Furthermore, in a study of diabetic nursing home residents, no detrimental effects of a regular nondiabetic diet were seen when weight, fasting glucose, glycosylated hemoglobin, plasma triglyceride, and cholesterol were measured (47). This short-term study (16 weeks in total) may provide an impetus to examine the long-range effects of a diet that provides more choice for an individual.

Optimizing caloric intake to appropriate levels and following the dietary choices of the individual should remain a goal for all diabetes diets. Aerobic conditioning exercises—walking, swimming, "low impact" types of exercise—should be an adjunct to any dietary program. Insulin sensitivity has been enhanced by physical exercise (48).

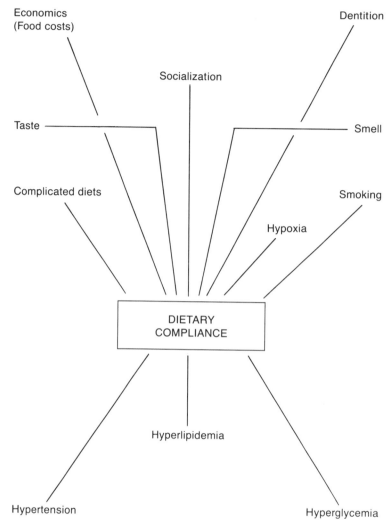

FIG. 1. The cascade of some factors that limit dietary compliance and their results.

Carbohydrates

The ADA recommendation is for 55 to 60% of total calories to be made up of complex carbohydrate and fiber. The pendulum of carbohydrate recommendations has swung from high carbohydrate and fiber in 1500 b.c. (Papyrus Ebers), to John Rollo's low-carbohydrate, high-protein diet of the 1790s, to everything in between, and finally back to the recommendations of 1,500 b.c. Although high-carbohydrate and fiber diets improve glycemic control, the type of carbohydrate to be utilized in the diet remains far from settled. The only rule that appears to be generally agreed upon is the avoidance of simple sugars, which are thought to be absorbed more rapidly, thereby promoting a greater degree of hyperglycemia than isocaloric amounts of starch (49).

The role of various carbohydrates in producing a glucose response has been quantified in the "glycemic index," which is calculated by taking the postprandial blood glucose area of a test food divided by the postprandial blood glucose area of a reference food (glucose or white bread) times 100. However, the use of the glycemic index can be problematic, as differences between various dried legumes (beans), vegetables, spaghetti, and different grains and rice can be shown (50,51). There are even glycemic index differences among differing varieties of some potatoes (eg, Idaho versus Michigan (49)), or when a food is prepared in different ways (whole rice versus rice flour). The difficulty in interpreting the various studies using the glycemic index is due to a lack of standardization of methods, such as single versus mixed meal composition, and variations in the response of a single individual. Too, there are a lack of long-term data on the benefits of eating foods with a lower glycemic index.

Glucose, fructose, sucrose, and potato and wheat starch have been compared in a more physiologically relevant manner through as meal tolerance testing. The fructose meal produced a lower (but not statistically different) increment in glucose concentration (52). Interestingly, sucrose did not cause a greater postprandial rise in glucose than other isocaloric amounts of other carbohydrates (52). Yet, the acceptance of sucrose in the diet is not universal (53), as concern regarding its effect on glucose and lipids remains. As with the glycemic index, the studies analyzing sucrose effects are also not standardized, with different dietary composition utilized (different fats/fiber content, etc.), thus making comparisons among studies difficult.

Fructose, a natural sugar, is 15 to 80% sweeter than sucrose. Fructose, which is absorbed more slowly from the GI tract than other sugars, may be metabolized without insulin, and appears to result in a slower rise in glucose postprandially (54,55). Long-term effects have not been studied, but in *in vitro* studies, fructose resulted in more rapid nonenzymatic glucosylation of protein than other sugars (56).

Sorbitol and mannitol are equicaloric to glucose, but their use can result in diarrhea and flatulence. At present few data exist regarding their long-term use in diabetic diets.

Artificial sweeteners (aspartame and saccharin) are both used extensively in the United States. Aspartame use appears to be safe, but long-term studies of this substance are needed (57). Saccharin, a coal tar derivative, has been implicated as a carcinogen in animals, although the AMA Council on Scientific Affairs found no solid evidence to link saccharin to an increased risk of bladder cancer in humans. Despite consideration of a ban by the U.S. Congress, saccharin remains on the market.

Dietary fiber (foods that are not digested or absorbed) and its role in diabetes have been reviewed extensively (58,59). Water-insoluble fiber (lignin, cellulose, etc.) causes bulky stools and more rapid intestinal transit time, whereas soluble fiber reduces blood glucose and slows gastric emptying. Therefore, soluble fiber should be recommended. It can be found in oat bran, peas, legumes, apples, and oranges.

Alpha-glucosidase inhibitors, such as acarbose and BAYm 1099, that inhibit intestinal disaccharidase, sucrase, glucoamylase, and maltase and thus result in a lower postprandial glucose may play a future role in the management of diabetes (60,61). Their side effects, however, mitigate against their use in those individuals who are not prepared to tolerate diarrhea, flatulence, and abdominal discomfort.

Fats

The shift in the American diet to a lower fat content and greater use of polyunsaturated and monounsaturated fats is in line with the recommended guidelines of the ADA. Yet, it has recently been shown that even a high-fat diet, if mostly monounsaturated fats, may be as beneficial as a low-fat diet (46) and polyunsaturated fats may promote carcinogenesis (62)! Water-soluble fiber can also be effective in lowering lipid levels, although the mechanisms underlying this effect are not completely known.

Omega-3 fatty acids (fish oils), a class of highly polyunsaturated fatty acids that lower triglyceride and cholesterol concentrations, can result in worsening of glycemic control in Type II diabetes (63) and therefore should be used with care.

Inhibitors of intestinal lipid transport, such as blockers of chylomicron formation and transport, may play a future role in dietary therapy for obesity (64). However, malabsorption of fat-soluble nutrients (fat-soluble vitamins), diarrhea, and flatulence are side effects that limit the clinical benefits offered. The use of fat substitutes might prove more popular, such as sucrose polyesters (which are undigested) but taste similar to fat, or such substances as heat-coagulated proteins that are microparticulated. Butter flavors, such as those composed of maltodextrin, are low calorie, nonfat, impart a strong butter flavor to foods, and are commercially available.

Protein

A high protein intake increases renal blood flow and the glomerular filtration rate (GFR) and may accelerate glomerulosclerosis. Dietary protein has come under additional scrutiny because patients with diabetic renal disease have shown improvement in renal function with protein restriction (65). This fact takes on additional significance as proteinuria itself confers a high rate of mortality in Type II diabetes (66).

Some diabetics, in attempting to lower carbohydrate and fat in their diets, have a relatively high protein intake. A protein intake of 0.8 g/kg body weight should result in no loss of nitrogen balance and may be beneficial in maintaining kidney function (67).

Clearly, there are as many divergent opinions about diabetic diets and their role in glycemic control as there are data supporting each of these opinions. One can only logically argue for diets appropriate in calories, nutritional composition, and palatability that can fit into an elderly patient's eating habits.

REFERENCES

1. Harrower AD. *Br J Clin Pract* 1980;34:131–133.
2. Harris MK, Hadden WCF, Knowler WC, Bennett PH. *Diabetes* 1987;36:523–534.
3. Reaven GM, Reaven EP. *J Am Geriatr Soc* 1985;33:286–290.
4. Fink FI, Koltermann OG, Olefsky JM. *J Gerontol* 1984;39:273–278.
5. Oimomi M, Maeda Y, Hata F, et al. *J Gerontol* 1988;43:B98–B101.
6. Negoro H, Morley J, Rosenthal MJ. *Am J Med* 1988;85:360–364.
7. Kabadi UM. *Diab Care* 1988;11:429–433.
8. Perlmuter LC, Hakami MK, Hodgson-Harrington C, et al. *Am J Med* 1984;77:1043–1048.
9. Mooradian AD, Perryman K, Fitten J, Kavonian GD, Morley JE. *Arch Intern Med* 1988;148:2369–2372.
10. Pulsinelli WS, Levy DE, Sigsbee B, Schere P, Plum F. *Am J Med* 1983;74:540–544.
11. Jarrett RJ, McCartney P, Keen H. *Diabetologia* 1982;22:79–84.
12. Stein EM, Stein S, Linn MW. *J Am Geriatr Soc* 1985;33:687–692.
13. Abbasi AA. *Geriatrics* 1981;36:73–78.
14. Chen M, Halter JB, Porte D. *J Am Geriatr Soc* 1987;35:417–424.
15. O'Hanlon J, Kohrs MB. *Am J Clin Nutr* 1978;31:1257–1263.
16. Anderson JW, Herman RH. *Am J Clin Nutr* 1972;25:41–46.
17. Anderson JW, Herman RH, Zakim D. *Am J Clin Nutr* 1973;26:600–607.
18. Brunzell JD, Lerner RL, Hazzard WR. *N Engl J Med* 1971;284:521.
19. Reaven GM, Coulston AM, Marcus RA. *Med Clin North Am* 1979;63:927–943.
20. Rosenthal M, Doberne L, Greenfield M, Widstrom A, Reaven GM. *J Am Geriatr Soc* 1982;30:562–567.
21. Narimiya M, Azhar S, Dolkas CB, et al. *Am J Physiol* 1984;246:E397–404.
22. Reaven E, Curry D, Moore J, Reaven GM. *J Clin Invest* 1983;71:345–350.
23. Clark A, Lewis CE, Willis AC. *Lancet* 1987;1:59–62.
24. Reaven EP, Reaven GM. *J Clin Invest* 1981;68:75–84.
25. Wang SY, Rowe JW. *Endocrinology* 1988;123:1008–1013.
26. Masoro EJ, Katz MS, McMahan CA. *J Gerontol* 1989;44:B20–22.
27. Leiter EH, Premdas F, Harrison DE, Lipson LG. *FASEB J* 1988;2:2807–2811.
28. Reaven GM. *J Am Geriatr Soc* 1985;33:93–96.
29. Mooradian AD, Morley JE. *Am J Clin Nutr* 1987;45:877–895.
30. Morley JE. *Am J Med* 1986;81:679–695.
31. Kinlaw WB, Levine AS, Morley JE, Silvis SE, McClain CJ. *Am J Med* 1983;75:273–277.
32. Duchateau J, Delepesse G, Vrijens R, Varcake P. *Am J Med* 1981;70:1001–1007.
33. Bogden JD, Oleske JM, Lavenhar MA, et al. *Am J Clin Nutr* 1988;48:655–661.
34. Mooradian AD, Norman DC, Morley JE. *Diabetologia* 1988;31:703–707.
35. Niewoehner CB, Allen JI, Boosalis M, et al. *Am J Med* 1986;81:63–69.
36. Morley JE, Mooradian AD, Rosenthal MJ, Kaiser FE. *Am J Med* 1987;83:533–544.
37. Hallbrook T, Lanner E. *Lancet* 1972;2:780–782.
38. Mooradian AD, Morley JE, Scarpace PJ. *Acta Endocrinol* 1988;119:174–180.
39. Balky DL, Curry DL, Keen CL, Hurley LS. *Endocrinology* 1985;116:1734–1740.

40. Zimmerman J, Kaufmann N, Fainaru M, et al. *Arteriosclerosis* 1984;4:115–123.
41. Consensus Development Panel. *Diab Care* 1987;10:639–644.
42. Master A, Lasser R. *JAMA* 1960;172:658–662.
43. Larsson B, Svardsudd K, Welin L, Wilhelmsen H, Bjorntorp P, Tibblin G. *Br Med J* 1984;288:1401–1404.
44. Henry RR, Wiest-Kent TA, Scheaffer L, Kolterman OG, Olefsky JM. *Diabetes* 1986;35:155–164.
45. Bauman WA, Schwartz E, Rose HG, Eisenstein HN, Johnson DW. *Am J Med* 1988;85:38–46.
46. Garg A, Bonanome A, Grundy SM. *N Engl J Med* 1988;319:829–834.
47. Coulston AM, Mandelbaum D, Reaven GM. *Am J Clin Nutr (in press)*.
48. Wang JT, Ho LT, Tang KT, Wang LM, Chen YDL, Reaven GM. *J Am Geriatr Soc* 1989;37:203–209.
49. Wood FC, Bierman EL. *N Engl J Med* 1986;315:1224–1227.
50. Jenkins DJA, Woliver TSM, Jenkins AL. *Lancet* 1984;2:388–391.
51. Crapo PA, Reaven G, Olefsky. *Diabetes* 1977;26:1178–1183.
52. Bantle JP, Laine DC, Castle GW, Thomas JW, Hoogwerf BJ, Goetz FC. *N Engl J Med* 1983;309:7–12.
53. Hollenbeck CB, Coulston AM, Reaven GM. *Diab Care* 1989;12:62–66.
54. Crapo PA, Kolterman OG. *Am J Clin Nutr* 1984;39:528–534.
55. Bantle JP, Laine DC, Thomas JW. *JAMA* 1986;256:3241–3246.
56. Bunn HF, Higgens PJ. *Science* 1981;213:222–224.
57. Filer LJ, Stegink LD. *Diab Care* 1989;12:67–74.
58. Anderson JW, Gustafson NJ, Bryant CA, Tietyen-Clark, J. *J Am Dietet Assoc* 87:1189–1197.
59. Munoz JM. *Diab Care* 1984;7:297–300.
60. Caspary WF, Graf S. *Res Exp Med* 1979;175:1–6.
61. Samad AHB, TY Willing TS, Alberti KGMM, Taylor R. *Diab Care* 1988;11:337–344.
62. Glauber H, Wallace P, Griver K, Brechtel G. *Ann Intern Med* 1988;108:663–668.
63. Gammal EB, Carroll KK, Plunkett ER. *Cancer Res* 1967;27:1737–1742.
64. Halpern J, Tso P, Mansbach CM II. *J Clin Invest* 1988;82:74–81.
65. Rosman JB, Terwee PM, Meijer S, Piers-Becht TP, Sluiter WJ, Donker AJ. *Lancet* 1984;2:1291–1296.
66. Nelson RG, Pettitt DJ, Carraher MJ, Baird HR, Knowler WC. *Diabetes* 1988;37:1499–1504.
67. Wylie Rossett J. *Diab Care* 1988;11:143–148.

Geriatric Nutrition, edited by John E. Morley,
Zvi Glick, Laurence Z. Rubenstein.
Raven Press, Ltd., New York © 1990.

20

Nutrition and Cardiovascular Disease

*Roslyn B. Alfin-Slater and †David Kritchevsky

*Department of Nutrition, UCLA School of Public Health,
Los Angeles, California 90024 and †Wistar Institute,
Philadelphia, Pennsylvania 19104

Cardiovascular disease is the most prevalent chronic disease in the United States today. As the leading cause of death, it is responsible for about 53% of all fatalities or approximately 500,000 lives each year (1).

The heart muscle supplies the tissues with oxygen and nutrients and helps dispose of waste products via the blood. However, the heart itself requires a supply of nutrients to function properly; these nutrients are carried to the heart muscle by two blood vessels—the right and left coronary arteries. Normally, the walls of these arteries are smooth and elastic; they can expand or contract to accommodate the flow of blood. However, for a number of reasons, both known and unknown, atheromatous deposits that contain cholesterol, other lipid material, mucopolysaccharides, minerals, and fibrous materials may adhere to and accumulate on the normally smooth arterial wall. This process results in the narrowing of the artery, the subsequent loss of its elasticity, and possibly in complete blockage. If the arteries are severely occluded and the heart muscle is deprived of sufficient oxygen and nutrients, part of the heart may be injured irreversibly. This injury may occur either as a result of the accumulated atheromatous deposits (coronary occlusion) or may be caused by the entrapment of a blood clot (thrombus) in the narrowed, inelastic arteries.

The development of atherosclerosis and its manifestation, coronary heart disease, is multicausal. Actually, the relationship between atherosclerosis and coronary heart disease is not well defined. Whether coronary thrombosis is caused by or whether it is independent of atherosclerosis is still controversial, and the causes of atherosclerosis are still being debated. Many studies have been undertaken and a number of risk factors have been identified as being associated with an increased susceptibility to coronary disease. These risk factors include, among others, genetic inheritance; male gender; certain endocrine and pathologic disease states such as hypertension and hyperglycemia (diabetes); environmental factors (sedentary living and psychosocial tensions); hypercholesterolemia; hypertriglyceridemia; smoking; and obesity.

Most of the investigations into the association of risk factors with cardio-vascular disease have been done on hypercholesterolemic, middle-aged men for several well-documented and understandable reasons: (a) This is the age group that has a high incidence and prevalence of cardiovascular disease, (b) men are at higher risk for coronary heart disease (CHD) than are women; (c) serum cholesterol levels in men are subject to fewer physiologic changes; and (d) large numbers of subjects in this category are available for study. The incidence of coronary disease in women is relatively low, and it occurs later in life (2,3).

Although the elderly segment of the U.S. population is growing rapidly, treatment of cardiovascular disease in the elderly is based on an extrapolation of that which is advised for a younger adult population. It is known that changes in the cardiovascular system accompany aging and that these changes may promote the decline in function and health of other organs in the body. However, because of the relatively small amount of data available on the effect of "normal" aging on organ systems, including the heart, it is difficult to separate the effects of simple aging from pathologic changes. Age-related changes include enlargement of the heart, thickening of the closure of the cardiac valves, calcium deposits, and atheroma in various areas in the coronary arteries being studied (4).

Autopsy data derived from U.S. Army facilities during the Korean War have suggested that the process of atherogenesis is initiated in young adults (5). For reasons not fully elucidated, the atherogenic process continues in most people at differing rates and to different degrees. It therefore is of importance to examine the clues; i.e., the risk factors which have been identified as being associated with increased susceptibility to coronary disease; the effect of various components of the diet on these risk factors; the epidemiological studies and feeding trials which have been undertaken in an attempt to discover the cause(s); and thereafter to recommend changes in diet and life style to minimize or prevent the disease process.

Probably the most important of the risk factors is genetic inheritance (6). The risk of developing heart disease in an individual is enhanced if either of his/her parents has a history of coronary disease.

Smoking in men but not women is associated with a significantly higher rate of coronary heart disease compared with non-smokers (7). Whether smoking is an independent risk-factor or whether it reflects stressful living conditions, and whether stress is an important risk factor, all need further definition. This increased risk seems to decrease with age (8).

Certain disease, e.g., elevated blood pressures, diabetes, and obesity, also seem to be predisposing factors to coronary heart disease (9). The role of obesity is not as clear as are some of the other factors. For example, obesity may be a risk factor because it is associated with the increased incidence of high blood pressure and adult onset diabetes and these, in turn, may be the actual risk factors involved in increased susceptibility to coronary disease.

The association of dietary cholesterol with hypercholesterolemia and atherosclerosis is based on results of experiments with animals and on results of epidemiological surveys. It has been shown that feeding diets high in cholesterol and saturated fats to some animal species can result in elevations in blood cholesterol levels and in experimental atherosclerosis. Some animal species are particularly susceptible, e.g., the rabbit and the chicken; some are particularly resistant, e.g., the dog and the cat. In fact, cholesterol has been found in atheromatous plaques, and epidemiological evidence supports the theory that hypercholesterolemia is associated with a greater risk of coronary disease. However, the cause of hypercholesterolemia in humans is not clear. For example, it is known that serum cholesterol levels increase with age; they are higher in men than in women; they increase in women after the menopause, even though there may be no apparent changes in the diet.

Whether dietary cholesterol is a major cause of hypercholesterolemia in a human population is controversial and investigators are divided in their opinions as to whether the ingestion of cholesterol-containing foods contributes significantly to increases in serum cholesterol levels.

The effects of other dietary factors on serum cholesterol levels has also evoked a series of contradictory reports. In attempts to resolve these controversies, two types of investigations have been pursued, i.e., dietary experiments using both experimental animals and human volunteers, and epidemiological surveys in which diets and general health of various populations have provided clues.

EXPERIMENTAL FEEDING STUDIES

As early as 1913, Anitschkow and Chalatow reported that feeding cholesterol to rabbits resulted in hypercholesterolemia and in deposits on the arterial wall (10). Rabbits fed cholesterol-free diets also developed atherosclerosis. Criticism of the use of rabbits as an animal model for human atherosclerosis (rabbits are herbivores and therefore possibly not able to utilize dietary cholesterol, an animal product, as well as do omnivores) led to cholesterol feeding experiments with rats, chickens, dogs, pigeons, pigs and non-human primates as well as further extensive investigations with rabbits (11). A variety of experimental conditions were used, i.e., feeding cholesterol with and without various types of fat, different levels of dietary fat, different kinds of proteins, with and without certain vitamins, minerals, water, and alcohol. The results of some of these feeding trials implicated hypercholesterolemia and increases in β-lipoproteins (low density lipoproteins (LDL)) with the development of atherosclerosis. However, there were marked species differences, genetic differences and individual differences within species. Rats and dogs were found to be relatively resistant to atherosclerosis, whereas chickens as well as rabbits were highly susceptible. In pigeons, there was a marked species difference. Some animals required drastic manipulations in diet, i.e., reductions in protein and in essential fatty acids before hypercholesterolemia and atherosclerosis could be induced. The situation with primates was also complicated in that certain vitamin deficiencies (e.g., vitamin B_6 deficiency) were required before lesions were obtained. Experiments with animals point out the need for caution before extrapolating these results to humans.

The problem which still remains to be solved is where human beings fit into this scheme. Early experiments done on humans in which hypercholesterolemia was induced, involved few subjects, usually incarcerated, who were fed semisynthetic or formula diets containing abnormally high levels of cholesterol for short periods of time. In one such investigation, six prison volunteers, divided into three groups of 2 each, were fed different levels of egg yolk powder incorporated into a diet sufficient in all required nutrients (12). Egg yolk powder is often used as a dietary source of cholesterol in these experiments, since one large egg contains approximately 250 mg of cholesterol. The design of the experiment was first, the feeding of a cholesterol-free diet, followed by the egg yolk diet; again a cholesterol-free diet; and then a diet containing crystalline cholesterol. Each diet was fed for 3 weeks. The serum lipids responded by decreasing on the cholesterol-free diet and increasing on the cholesterol-containing diets. However, in view of the limited number of subjects, an experimental period too short to allow equilibrium to be established between plasma and tissue cholesterol levels, and the use of a semi-synthetic liquid diet deficient in fiber and in plant sterols, nutrients known to interfere with cholesterol absorption, these experiments could not be considered definitive and are certainly not a true reflection of the normal dietary situation. It is possible that elevations in serum cholesterol levels as a result of feeding crystalline cholesterol may be due to the presence of oxidized cholesterol (13).

Studies on male students and on an older male population given 500 mg or 250 mg of dietary cholesterol (as eggs) per day, respectively, superimposed on an otherwise normal diet over an 8-week period revealed no significant changes in serum cholesterol and triglyceride levels as a result of the additional cholesterol load. It was concluded that, in these selected subjects, physiologic mechanisms enabled them to compensate for the increased dietary cholesterol (14).

Investigations at the University of Missouri confirmed these results in experiments with men aged 32 to 62 years who were fed their normal diet supplemented with either one or two eggs per day for 3 months. No significant differences were observed in their serum cholesterol levels at the end of the experimental period (15,16).

O'Brien and Reiser studied 30 scientists who were fed diets of red meat either alone or with three eggs per day, and of fish and poultry either alone or with three eggs daily for 6 weeks each. The fish-poultry-egg group responded with the highest serum cholesterol, 216 mg/dl, as compared with 199, 194, and 198 mg/dl in the other groups, respectively. Although none of these values could be considered hypercholesterolemic, one subject in this group responded with a serum cholesterol of 273 mg/dl (17).

In another study, physically active men eating varying amounts of eggs were followed over a 7-day period (18). Despite a very large increase in cholesterol intake (from 480 to 3,464 mg), there was hardly any change in total plasma cholesterol levels (from 183 to 191 mg/dl), again showing no correlation between cholesterol intake and plasma cholesterol levels (18).

On the other hand, Mattson and coworkers (19) fed graded doses of egg yolk cholesterol (106, 212, and 317 mg/day) to 56 male prison inmates for 6 weeks and observed proportional increases in serum cholesterol levels, which were estimated to be a 12 mg/100 ml increase for each 100 mg cholesterol in 1,000 kcal of diet. It is possible that these contradictory results may arise from the fact that egg yolk cholesterol and whole eggs differ in their effects on serum cholesterol values or from a comparison of free living and incarcerated subjects.

Sacks et al. (20) fed one extra large egg per day for 3 weeks, and similar but eggless foods for an additional 3 weeks, in a randomized double-blind crossover trial to 17 lacto-ovo vegetarian college students. They found an increase in LDL cholesterol (12%), but no significant change in total plasma cholesterol, ie, from 175 ± 27 to 182 ± 35 mg/dl. The authors cited studies with both confirmatory and opposing results, explaining these contradictory results by the suggestion that the addition of eggs to a diet already high in cholesterol might not affect serum cholesterol levels further.

A review of data from the Framingham study also revealed that, in men whose egg intake was as low as 1.4 or as high as 10.6 per week, there were no differences in serum cholesterol levels or in coronary disease (21).

Grundy (22) has reported that all individuals respond to the ingestion of dietary cholesterol by elevations, albeit widely varied, in serum cholesterol levels. In contrast, a recent study by McNamara et al. (23) of 50 middle-aged men fed either a low-cholesterol (250 mg/day) or a high-cholesterol diet (800 mg/day), with 35% of total calories either from polyunsaturated or saturated fat in a crossover experiment, showed no increases in plasma cholesterol levels in most of the men (two-thirds of the subjects), regardless of the amount of cholesterol ingested. It was concluded that these men were able to compensate for the increased dietary load by changes in their metabolism, ie, decreased cholesterol absorption or decreased biosynthesis. Therefore, generalized recommendations to decrease cholesterol intake will be of value to only a limited number of persons, and further dietary trials to identify these individuals are necessary.

Nutrients other than fat and cholesterol may also affect serum cholesterol levels. Foods that contain soluble fibers, such as pectin, have been reported to decrease serum cholesterol levels, whereas bran and cellulose have no effect (24). In animal experiments fructose and sucrose were shown to be more atherogenic than glucose or lactose. When complex carbohydrates, such as starch, were substituted for simple sugars, there was a decrease in cholesterol levels (25). Animal protein, such as casein, has been found to be more atherogenic than vegetable proteins, eg, soy protein. Vegetarians have lower serum cholesterol levels than the general population. When animal proteins were replaced in the diet by vegetable proteins, serum cholesterol levels were reduced in some individuals (26,27). In areas where the water is soft, there seems to be more atherosclerosis, possibly indicating a role for certain minerals in protecting against atherosclerosis (28,29). A high ratio of zinc/copper in serum has been found to be associated with hypercholesterolemia and may be a risk factor (30). Milk, both skim and whole, and yogurt lower serum cholesterol levels by a mechanism that is not known (31). Beer and wine in moderation raise high-density lipoproteins. With increased alcohol ingestion, there seems to be decreased cardiovascular disease (32). Although fish oils contain cholesterol in amounts varying from 32 mg/100 g for halibut to 90 mg/100 g for yellow perch (33), they have been shown to reduce both hypertriglyceridemia and hypercholesterolemia (34). Cholesterol in foods occurs in association with other lipids and other nutrients, and therefore separating the effects of cholesterol from those of the other nutrients is difficult. It is possible that interactions among the various components of the diet may be involved in the regulation of serum cholesterol levels and atherogenesis.

Furthermore, Kritchevsky (35) described seasonal variations in serum cholesterol levels, with the highest levels occurring in October and December and the lowest in June. Low-density lipoproteins were also highest in October, but were lowest in July. The highest values for high-density lipoproteins were found in January, March, and December and lowest in July (35).

These controversial reports point out the heterogeneity of the populations studied and the need for more standardized conditions before meaningful conclusions can be drawn. Furthermore, more research is needed to fill the gaps in our knowledge of various phases of cholesterol metabolism under these varying experimental conditions.

The absorptive capacity of the human intestine for dietary cholesterol is not definitely known. It has been reported that only 50% of dietary cholesterol is absorbed. Net cholesterol absorption may be limited to 400 mg/day, and therefore, any cholesterol ingested above this amount may not be absorbed. Also, the efficiency of cholesterol absorption depends on many variables, including the amount of cholesterol ingested at any one time, the type of cholesterol-containing food ingested, the type and amount of the fat vehicle, other nutrients in the diet, and the contribution of biosynthesized cholesterol from endogenous sources.

EPIDEMIOLOGIC STUDIES

Many populations have been studied in order to elucidate the possible relationship between diet, primary dietary cholesterol and fat, and serum cholesterol levels. Some of these studies support a role for dietary cholesterol as a cause of the risk factor, hypercholesterolemia, whereas others suggest no role for dietary cholesterol but implicate other dietary factors, primarily saturated fat, as causative agents. However, although epidemiologic studies provide clues, associations, and correlations, they provide no cause-and-effect relationships.

In 1970, a report on the Framingham Study (Massachusetts) found little correlation between diet and serum lipid levels. Subjects who ate more or less than the median cholesterol intake had the same cholesterol levels (36). The 1976 Tecumseh Study (Michigan) concluded that cholesterol and triglyceride levels were unrelated to the quality, quantity, or proportions of fat, carbohydrate, or protein consumed in a 24-hour recall period (37). Similarly, no significant relationship between nutrient intake and serum cholesterol levels was reported in the 1969 Israel Ischemic Heart Disease Study (38).

In the 1985 Honolulu Heart Study the relationship of dietary fat and dietary cholesterol to mortality over a 10-year period in Japanese men in Hawaii was investigated (39). Although there was support for the diet-heart hypothesis, the men ingesting low-fat diets had a higher mortality than the men ingesting the higher-fat diets. The increased mortality was a result of a higher cancer and stroke incidence (39). In another study, Scotsmen with serum cholesterol levels of 249 mg/dl were found to have three times as many coronaries as did Swedish men of the same age whose serum cholesterol levels were 254 mg/dl, indicating that there were obviously causes other than serum cholesterol levels for the increase in coronary heart disease (40).

In our laboratory, we have measured serum lipid levels in a heterogeneous male and female population (600 men, 400 women) at the University of California, Los Angeles. Dietary histories were obtained, and a possible association between diet and serum lipid levels was explored. The results confirmed previous reports that serum cholesterol levels increased with age, regardless of the level of cholesterol intake. In many cases, individuals with similar serum cholesterol levels had markedly different dietary cholesterol intakes, and some individuals ingesting similar amounts of cholesterol had very different serum cholesterol levels. It was concluded that an association between dietery and serum cholesterol levels, if present, was indeed weak (Slater, unpublished data).

Although some studies support a relationship between hypercholesterolemia and atherosclerosis, the cut-off point for hypercholesterolemia is still controversial. The Pooling Project Research Group (41) suggested an upper limit of 220 mg/dl. Other investigators (42) suggest an ideal range of 130 to 190 mg/dl, which would mean that 50 to 60% of adult men in the United States are at high risk for CHD. Still others recommend that other risk factors should be considered before a cut-off value can be given (44). It is suggested that the so-called desirable range for plasma cholesterol may be more appropriate for populations than for individuals (43). Of interest are the findings of the Framingham study that total cholesterol levels may not be the best indication of risk for the development of CHD, but rather it is high-density lipoprotein cholesterol that has shown a marked inverse association with CHD (44).

The increase in plasma cholesterol levels with age has been shown repeatedly. Whether this increase in aging individuals is associated with accelerated atherogenesis or is a normal accompaniment of the aging process needs further research. In a study of blood lipids of young college students of the University of Minnesota followed over a 32-year period, the increase in serum cholesterol that occurred was related to the increase in the degree of overweight during that period (45).

Of course it is of interest to determine whether reducing elevated serum cholesterol levels can modify or prevent coronary heart disease. This has been tested in two large epidemiologic studies sponsored by the National Institutes of Health, the MRFIT (Multiple Risk Factor Intervention Trial) and the CPPT (Coronary Primary Prevention Trial). The latter study used the drug cholestyramine to effect the reduction in elevated serum cholesterol levels in hypercholesterolemic, middle-aged men who had not responded to a cholesterol-lowering diet.

In the MRFIT study (46), 12,000 hypercholesterolemic men were divided into two groups. In one group, there was intervention to reduce hypercholesterolemia with diet (ie, a modified "prudent" diet), drugs to reduce blood pressure, and smoking cessation. In the control group, there was no intervention. Results of the 10-year study showed no difference in mortality between the groups (46).

In the Coronary Primary Prevention Trial (47) 480,000 men were screened to find 3,806 men, aged 35 to 59, with blood cholesterol levels higher than 265 mg/dl, initially free from heart disease, who had not been responsive to a moderate cholesterol-lowering diet (400 mg cholesterol/day). They were divided into two groups of 1,903 each, both receiving the same "prudent" diet. The experimental group received the drug cholestyramine, a resinous compound that has been shown to reduce serum cholesterol levels; the control group received a placebo. After 10 years, the experimental group showed lower serum cholesterol levels, fewer fatal heart attacks (30 versus 38), fewer nonfatal heart attacks (159 versus 187), but a higher incidence of stroke, cancer, accidents, suicides, and homicides so that mortality in both groups was comparable (47). The cholestyramine-treated subjects also reported side effects, including constipation, allergic reactions, and interference with certain drug therapy and with the absorption of fat-soluble vitamins.

The Minnesota Coronary Survey (48) was a 4.5-year open enrollment, double-blind, randomized clinical trial involving 4,393 men and 4,664 women in mental hospitals and a nursing home. The effect of a 39% fat diet containing 18% saturated fat, 5% polyunsaturated fat, 16% monounsaturated fat and 446 mg cholesterol/day was compared with the effects of a diet containing 9% saturated fat, 15% polyunsaturated fat, 14% monounsaturated fat, and 166 mg cholesterol/day. No differences were observed between groups in terms of cardiovascular events, cardiovascular deaths, or total mortality (48).

PRESENT STATUS OF THE PROBLEM

Although the role of dietary cholesterol in the etiology of hypercholesterolemia and atherosclerosis is still controversial, various health agencies are recommending a reduction in dietary fat and cholesterol for the entire U.S. population, including women, children from age 2 onward, and the elderly, on whom testing has not been done. The recommendation to reduce fat to 30% of the diet and cholesterol to 300 mg/day has met with mixed responses from the scientific establishment. Some investigators feel that to change serum cholesterol levels effectively, a further reduction to 20% in fat content may be necessary, a level that may not be entirely safe, especially for the young and the elderly. Very low-fat diets change the composition of cell membranes, making them more rigid, make the plasma more viscous, and reduce the effectiveness of the immune system. In addition, a comprehensive evaluation of the data on which these recommendations are based indicates that the recommended dietary changes have not been tested over sufficiently long periods of time, and therefore, their long-range possible consequences are unknown.

Data available are *not* strong enough to recommend that the entire population, including children and the elderly, eat a low-fat, low-cholesterol diet. Extrapolation of recommendations from the CPPT, a study done on hyper-cholesterolemic middle-aged men, to the whole population seems to be unwarranted at this time and should be done with caution. There is *no* evidence that cholestyramine treatment would be of benefit to hyperlipemic women, to younger men, to older men and women, to children, or to those whose serum cholesterol levels are lower than 265 mg/dl. The recommendation to reduce the cholesterol intake to 300 mg/day will result in a decrease intake of eggs, milk, liver, shellfish, and red meat, and may, if closely followed, lead to nutrient deficiencies, especially in children and in the elderly, rather than the reduction of risk factors for heart disease in these populations.

Many foods, including human milk, that contain cholesterol are good sources of high-quality protein and excellent sources of vitamins and minerals. To reduce fat in the diet to less than 30% of total calories and to increase carbohydrate (CHO) to 50 to 60% will increase the CHO:fat ratio from the present 1.2 to 2.4. High CHO diets have been shown to depress HDL cholesterol levels and to raise very low-density lipoproteins (VLDL) and low-density lipoproteins (LDL) levels.

The Committee on Nutrition of the American Academy of Pediatrics warns that the recommended increase in cereal grains at the expense of animal products might result in a decrease of some protective micronutrients (eg, vitamins and minerals) and thereby pose health risks to children. Human milk, a high-cholesterol-containing product, is still considered the ideal food for infants. Children at age 2 are in an active growth phase, and a change to a low-fat, low-cholesterol diet may neither promote optimum growth nor maintain health.

In a heterogeneous American population there will be a mixed response to any cholesterol-lowering diet, ranging from none to moderate to large; high-risk individuals should not be led to believe that diet is the cure-all for coronary heart disease or its precursors. McNamara (49) has stated, "For the 80% of the population with cholesterol levels below 230 mg/dl, modification of the diet seems both premature and of questionable value since such treatment of the many to benefit the few may not really benefit the high-risk patients and may affect everyone's nutrition pattern in as yet unknown ways."

If reductions in serum cholesterol levels do decrease the incidence and/or prevalence of coronary heart disease, it becomes important to determine to what extent serum cholesterol levels should be reduced. In a study of the MRFIT volunteers, Iso et al. (50) reported a threefold higher death rate from intracranial hemorrhage in men with serum cholesterol levels under 160 mg/dl than in those with higher levels, although these authors did add that there was a positive association of high serum cholesterol levels with death from nonhemorrhagic stroke and total cardiovascular disease.

Epidemiologic data have shown an inverse relationship between serum cholesterol levels and colon cancer and gallbladder disease. Furthermore, recommendations for a cholesterol-lowering diet that restrict dairy products, which are excellent sources of calcium, may contribute to the increased prevalence of osteoporosis in postmenopausal women. For many people, the recommended diet is too restrictive; for low-risk persons, the rationale for changing the diet is difficult to explain, especially in view of Taylor and colleagues' (51) recent estimate of the possible increases in life expectancy as a result of long-term cholesterol reduction. They incorporated two assumptions into a model: (a) that lowering cholesterol levels reduces risk and (b) that cholesterol reduction is safe in that it will not produce an increased risk of dying from other causes. They concluded that, for low-risk persons aged 20 to 60 years, a lifelong program of cholesterol reduction would increase life expectancy from about 3 days to 3 months and for high-risk persons, 18 days to 12 months. They point out that smoking cessation and control of blood pressure have a much greater effect on life expectancy than does reducing serum cholesterol levels.

Other theories of atherosclerosis have been proposed that require further investigation. In particular, in vitamin B_6 deficiency, one particular amino acid, homocystine, which is produced by the amino acid methionine, is not metabolized properly to cystathionine and becomes a toxic substance shown to be associated with atherosclerosis. There is the possibility that vitamin B_6 may be destroyed in food processing and may therefore be limited in the diet (52).

Despite a number of conflicting reports and opinions (53,54,55), Garber et al. (56) have made recommendations based on the hypothesis that total cholesterol and the lipoproteins, HDL and LDL, are risk factors for coronary disease and early mortality in middle-aged men. The evidence is weaker for women and for elderly men, as well as for the role of hypertriglyceridemia. They have concluded that a reduction in serum cholesterol levels reduces the incidence of and death from CHD in asymptomatic middle-aged men who are hypercholesterolemic, particularly in those whose serum cholesterol levels are above 246 mg/dl. This is a rather select population. They do point out, however, that results from the Framingham study indicate a "statistically significant negative association of hypercholesterolemia with overall mortality in men and women 65 years of age and older." The reasons for this lack of association in the elderly is unclear; it may be a result of elevated levels of HDL, or there may be other still unknown reasons why the elderly resist the cardiac effects of hypercholesterolemia.

At present there are suggestions, but no absolute agreement, that dietary cholesterol and/or many dietary fats cause heart disease for most individuals. Although those at high risk need to be identified, advised, and treated, there is little reason to impose very restrictive diets on the entire population, especially the elderly in whom hypercholesterolemia does not appear to be an important risk factor. For most of the population, a varied diet is recommended that includes protein from various sources, complex carbohydrates, fiber, and fat from both vegetable and animal sources in moderation and is sufficient in vitamins and minerals but restricted in total calories to prevent weight increases. Attention to other facets of lifestyle, such as smoking cessation, initiation of an exercise program, and weight management, and treatment of predisposing disease conditions (eg, hypertension and diabetes) are also indicated in helping to prevent CHD.

In the last 25 years, the age-adjusted death rate from CHD has decreased by 30%, whereas the age-adjusted death rate from all causes has decreased by 10% (57). This reduction in mortality from heart disease has occurred at all ages, in all races, and in both men and women for reasons not fully understood. Smoking cessation and the control of hypertension, diabetes, and other hormonally related conditions no doubt play a major role. Treatment of obesity through any number of methods may also make a positive contribution.

Longevity in the United States has been extended so that the adjective "old" is now being redefined. The number of people of 85 years and older is increasing rapidly. A recent survey found that 15% of those aged 65 to 74 years, 5% of those between 74 to 84 years, and 2% of those 85 years of age and older were still at work (58). Extending the life span, however, should include the maintenance of a high-quality lifestyle, free of debilitating disease conditions, both physical and mental. The prevention and treatment of coronary disease should be done on an individualized basis involving the physician and the dietitian/nutritionist (59).

REFERENCES

1. National Heart, Lung and Blood Institute. *Tenth report of the director, Heart and vascular diseases,* vol 2. Bethesda, MD: National Institute of Health, 1984;84–2357.
2. Hazzard WR. *Geriatrics* 1985;40:42–54.
3. Bush TL, Fried LP, Barrett-Connor E. *Clin Chem* 1988;34:B60–69.
4. Waller BF. *Clin Cardiol* 1988;11:513–517.
5. Enos WF, Beyer JC, Holmes RH. *JAMA* 1955;158:912–914.
6. Dahlen G, Ericson C, de Faire U, Iselius L, Lundman J. *Int J Epidemiol* 1983;12:32–35.
7. Fielding JE. *N Engl J Med* 1985;313(8):491–498.
8. Gordon T, Kannel WB, McGEE D, Dawber TK. *Lancet* 1974;2:1345–1348.
9. Kannel, WB. *Nutr Rev* 1988;46:168–178.
10. Antischkow N, Chalatow S. *Zentr allgem Pathol u pathol* 1913;24:1–9.

11. Kritchevsky D. In: Paoletti R, ed. *Lipid pharmacology,* vol. 2. New York: Academic Press, 1963;63–130.
12. Connor WE, Hodges RC, Bleiler RA. *J Clin Invest* 1961;40:894–901.
13. Imai H, Werthessen NT, Taylor CB, Lee KT. *Arch Pathol Lab Med* 1976;100:565–572.
14. Slater G, Mead J, Dhopeshwarkar G, Robinson S, Alfin-Slater RB. *Nutr Rep Int* 1976;14:249–260.
15. Porter MW, Yamanaka W, Carlson SD, Flynn MA. *Am J Clin Nutr* 1977;30:490–495.
16. Flynn MA, Nolph GB, Flynn TC, Kahns R, Krause G. *Am J Clin Nutr* 1979;32:1050–1057.
17. O'Brien BC, Reiser R. *Am J Clin Nutr* 1980;33:2573–2580.
18. Faber WM, Benade ATS. *S Afr J Sci* 1982;78:90–91.
19. Mattson FH, Frickson BH, Kligman AM. *Am J Clin Nutr* 1972;25:589–594.
20. Sacks FM, Miller L, Sutherland M, et al. *Lancet* 1984;1:647–649.
21. Dawber TR, Nickerson RJ, Brand PN, Pool J. *Am J Clin Nutr* 1982;36:617–625.
22. Grundy SM. *JAMA* 1966;256:2849–2858.
23. McNamara DJ, Kolb R, Parker TS, et al. *J Clin Invest* 1987;79:1729–1739.
24. Kritchevsky D, Tepper SA, Story TA. *Nutr Rep Int* 1974;9:301–308.
25. Kritchevsky D, Davidson LM, Kim HK, et al. *Am J Clin Nutr* 1980;33:1869–1887.
26. Carroll KK, Giovanett PM, Huff MW, et al. *Am J Clin Nutr* 1978;31:1312–1321.
27. Kritchevsky D. *J Am Oil Chem Soc* 1979;56:135–146.
28. Crawford MD, Gardner MJ, Morris JN. *Lancet* 1971;2:327–329.
29. Crawford MD, Gardner MJ, Morris JN. *Br Med Bull* 1971;27:21–24.
30. Klevay LM. *Am J Clin Nutr* 1975;28:764–774.
31. Hepner G, Fried R, St. Jeor S, Fasetti L, Morin R. *Am J Clin Nutr* 1979;32:19–24.
32. Castelli WP, Doyle JT, Gordon T, et al. *Lancet* 1977;2:153–155.
33. Hepburn FN, Exler J, Weihrauch JL. *J Am Dietet Assoc* 1986;86:788–793.
34. Nestel PJ. *Am J Clin Nutr* 1986;39:752–757.
35. Kritchevsky D. In: Weininger J, Briggs G, eds. *Nutrition update,* vol 2. New York: John Wiley & Sons, Inc. 1985;91–103.
36. Kannel W, Gordon T. *Diet and regulation of serum cholesterol.* Washington, DC: US Government Printing Office, 1970.
37. Nichols AB, Ravenscroft C, Lanphiear DE. *Am J Clin Nutr* 1976;29:1384–1392.
38. Kahn H, Medalie J, Neufeld H, Riss E, Balogh M, Groen J. *Israel J Med Sci* 1969;5:1117–1127.
39. McGee D, Reed D, Stimmerman G, Rhoads G, Yano K, Feinleib M. *Int J Epidemiol* 1985;14:97–105.
40. Oliver MF, Nimmo IA, Cooke M, Carlson LA, Olsson AG. *Eur J Clin Invest* 1975;5:507–514.
41. Pooling Project Research Group. *J Chron Dis* 1978;31:201–306.
42. Stamler J. *Prev Med* 1979;8:733–759.
43. Heiss G, Tamir I, Davis CE, et al. *Circulation* 1980;61:302–315.
44. Kannel WB, Castelli WP, Gordon J. *Ann Intern Med* 1979;90:85–91.
45. Gillum RF, Taylor HL, Brozek J, Anderson J, Blackburn H. *J Chron Dis* 1982;35:635–641.
46. Multiple Risk Factor Intervention Trial Research Group. *JAMA* 1982;248:1465–1477.
47. Lipid Research Clinics Program. *JAMA* 1984;251:365–374.
48. Frantz ID, Dawson EA, Ashman PL, et al. *Arteriosclerosis* 1989;9:129–135.
49. McNamara D. *Nutr & MD* 1985[1]:1–2.
50. Iso H, Jacobs DR Jr, Wentworth D, Neaton JD, Cohen JD. *N Engl J Med* 1989;320:904–910.
51. Taylor WC, Pass TM, Shepard DS, Komaroff AL. *Ann Intern Med* 1987;106:605–614.
52. Beier RC. *Nature* 1984;310:18.
53. Stehbens WE. *Nutr Rev* 1989;47:1–12.
54. Ahrens EH Jr. *Lancet* 1985;1:1085–1089.
55. Ahrens EH Jr. In: Hallgren B, et al, eds. *Diet and prevention of coronary heart disease and cancer.* New York: Raven Press, 1984:81–94.
56. Garber AM, Sox HC Jr, Littenberg B. *Ann Intern Med* 1989;110:622–639.
57. Kannel WB. *JAMA* 1982;247:877–880.
58. Kovar MG. *Advance data from vital and health statistics.* 1984;115:86–1250.
59. Enloe CF Jr. *Nutr To* 1984;12–13.

Geriatric Nutrition, edited by John E. Morley,
Zvi Glick, Laurence Z. Rubenstein.
Raven Press, Ltd., New York © 1990.

21

Nutritional Interventions as Antihypertensive Therapy in the Elderly

*Dalila B. Corry and †Michael L. Tuck

*†VA Medical Center, Sepulveda, California 91343 and †Department of Medicine,
UCLA School of Medicine, Los Angeles, California 90024*

With advancing age, blood pressure, particularly systolic blood pressure, tends to increase, placing the aging patients at higher risk for developing hypertension (1). In fact, there is a gradual increase in mean arterial pressure in every age group over 35 years old. Approximately two-thirds of all Americans over age 65 have systolic blood pressure levels greater than 140 mm Hg and/or diastolic pressures greater than 90 mm Hg (2,3). The prevalence of hypertension in the elderly is also evident from recent data indicating that close to half of all patients who visit physicians' offices for antihypertensive therapy are at least 60 years old. Hypertension can be as severe in the elderly as in the young and is an important risk factor for morbidity from cardiovascular and cerebrovascular diseases. Three principal types of hypertension afflict the elderly population—isolated systolic hypertension, diastolic hypertension, and renovascular hypertension.

TYPES OF HYPERTENSION IN THE ELDERLY

Systolic Hypertension

Isolated systolic hypertension was found in 6.8% of the patients between 60 and 69 years of age by the Hypertension Detection and Follow-Up Program (4). Two recent consensus groups on hypertension in the elderly—the Working Group on Hypertension in the Elderly (2) in the United States and the Consensus Conference on Hypertension in the Elderly (5) in Canada—have emphasized the difficulty in measuring and defining systolic hypertension in older patients. Thirty percent of geriatric patients have systolic hypertension in part because of a reduced compliance in the aorta and peripheral arteries. This increased rigidity caused by a loss of elastic fibers, when mixed with an increase in collagen and calcium deposition in the media, may result in overdiagnosis of hypertension and inappropriate therapy. These sclerotic changes give rise to the pseudohypertension syndrome in which cuff pressure levels are inappropriately elevated when compared to intra-arterial pressure recordings. Pseudohypertension should be suspected if the vessels are rigid to palpation, if there is no end-organ damage, and if there are inordinate postural symptoms while the patient is taking antihypertensive drugs. The use of the Osler maneuver can help detect the phenomenon. Because some elderly subjects have orthostatic changes in blood pressure, it is recommended that blood pressure be recorded when subjects are both sitting and standing with at least 2 minutes of standing before measurement. It has been shown that measurements made with a sphygmomanometer with the arm dependent by the side were consistently higher than those made with the arm horizontal at heart level and that both systolic and diastolic blood pressure could be changed by 20 mm Hg simply by moving the arm through a 90° angle (6).

Once the diagnosis of hypertension has been firmly established, treatment should be instituted because the data suggests that untreated systolic hypertension puts patients at as great a risk for morbidity and mortality as does diastolic hypertension. Because of the many physiologic changes associated with aging, such as reduced plasma volume, decreased adrenergic responsiveness with normal or high cathecholamine levels, diminished cardiac output, reduced plasma renin activity, markedly increased peripheral resistance, and reduced renal function, it is much more difficult to treat this condition without producing adverse effects from drugs. In contrast to younger adult hypertensives, elderly hypertensive patients are also likely to have other diseases. Given the risks associated with the prescription of powerful medications in patients who also have chronic obstructive pulmonary disease, ischemic heart disease, cerebrovascular disease, diabetes mellitus, or chronic renal failure, a strong argument can be put forth for alternative modes of therapy.

NONPHARMACOLOGIC ANTIHYPERTENSIVE THERAPY

Nonpharmacologic approaches to the management of hypertension—namely, through dietary manipulation—are difficult to assess in term of feasibility or efficacy in the geriatric population. The requirements of the elderly for specific nutrients are relatively ill defined and based almost entirely on extrapolations from data on younger populations (fig. 1). Intake of such nutrients as sodium, potassium, calcium, and magnesium has been found to affect the level of blood pressure, as well as caloric restriction. In older Americans, the National Health and Nutrition Examination Survey (NHANES) (7) found that alcohol consumption and dietary calcium and phosphorus intake were associated with high blood pressure but dietary so-

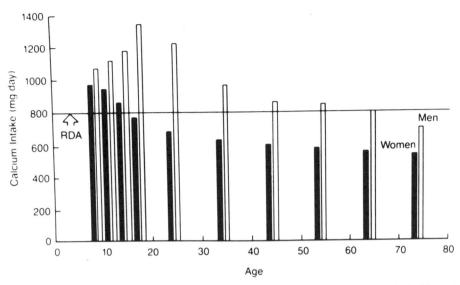

FIG. 1. Decrease in average calcium intake of North Americans from National Health and Nutrition Examination Survey. (Data from ref. 7, with permission.)

dium was not. In this population, body mass had the strongest relationship with blood pressure of all the nutritional variables.

Sodium Restriction

Epidemiologic studies (8) have suggested that the age-associated increase in blood pressure observed in most Westernized societies may be secondary to high sodium intake. This conclusion is based on evidence that hypertension is virtually nonexistent in primitive societies. It was supported mainly by experimental work in some strains of rats in which the introduction of high-sodium diets at a young age influenced the rate of development of hypertension with time (9). Other evidence was provided by a few clinical studies (10) comparing populations in which estimates of salt intake and methods of blood pressure measurement were not uniform. Intersalt (11), a recently completed international study on the association between urinary electrolyte excretion and blood pressure, provides evidence that prescriptive reductions in dietary sodium chloride intake may not have a significant impact upon hypertension in a given society.

Grobbee and Hofman (12) have recently reviewed the results of 13 clinical trials of dietary salt restriction in patients with hypertension. From these results emerged a relationship between age and fall in blood pressure after sodium restriction. In a study by Myers and Morgan (13) the effect of high .

and low sodium intake on blood pressure was examined in relation to age in normotensive and hypertensive subjects. Although the variation in blood pressure response was large, older normotensive and hypertensive subjects had greater blood pressure increments in response to high sodium intake and greater reductions with sodium restriction (fig. 2). The results indicate that blood pressure in the elderly may be more sensitive to dietary sodium intake than in the young adult. This finding might be explained in part by the physiologic changes that age imposes on the kidney. A progressive age-related decline in the glomerular filtration rate (GFR) is known to occur in both sexes (14,15). This decline is a true aging phenomenon and does not result from superimposed renal or extrarenal diseases (16). Follow-up studies in the Baltimore longitudinal study on aging (17) with multiple serial creatinine clearance determinations between 1958 and 1981 revealed a mean decrease in creatinine clearance of 0.75 ml/min/year and an increase in the rate of loss of creatinine clearance with age. This age-related decline in creatinine clearance was found to be much steeper in blacks than whites (18). Under normal circumstances, age has no effect on sodium concentration or on the ability to maintain normal extracellular fluid volume. However, the response to stress is impaired in the aged. Sodium-excreting ability is diminished in the elderly, and excessive sodium retention and volume overload are commonly encountered problems. This lack of natriuretic efficiency is probably secondary to the decrease in GFR. There is also evidence that blood pressure

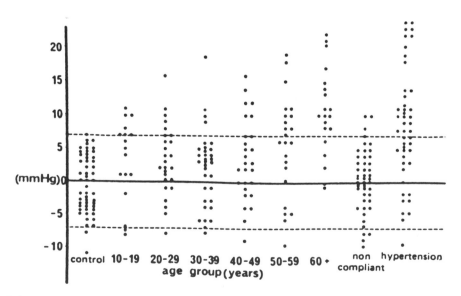

FIG. 2. Changes in the mean arterial pressure when a normotensive person changes from a low to a high sodium intake plotted against age of the patient. (Data from ref. 13, with permission.)

response to sodium restriction correlates inversely with the level of plasma renin activity. As the basal plasma renin activity of most elderly subjects decreases by 30 to 50%, despite a normal level of renin substrate (19), these studies imply a better blood pressure response to sodium restriction in older hypertensive patients. However, the ability of the aged kidney to conserve sodium in response to deprivation is diminished (20). Clearance studies in young and elderly subjects have shown a decrease in sodium reabsorption by the distal tubule, which could be in part explained by the 30 to 50% decrease in plasma aldosterone levels described in the older subjects during recumbency and normal sodium intake (21). This defect is more pronounced during upright posture and sodium restriction (22) and, during severe sodium restriction, can result in dehydration, postural hypotension, and further decline in renal function.

Given the data, the current recommendation in the treatment of geriatric hypertension is to initiate only moderate reductions in sodium intake in the area of 80 mmol/day of sodium or 5 g of table salt.

Potassium Supplementation

An inverse relationship between potassium intake and blood pressure has been suggested by several epidemiologic studies (23–25). The effect of potassium on blood pressure is modest, with an estimated decrease of 0.10 to 0.12 mm Hg in systolic blood pressure and 0.3 to 0.7 mm Hg decrease in diastolic for each 1 mmol increase in potassium intake (26). Earlier data (27) demonstrated that administration of potassium had a more dramatic antihypertensive effect in a small number of individuals with salt-sensitive hypertension. This effect has been confirmed by MacGregor et al. (28) in a double-blind, randomized study. The mechanism of the antihypertensive effect of potassium in humans appears to be related to natriuresis (29).

In a recent study, Krishna et al. (30) investigated the effect of dietary potassium restriction on blood pressure. They found that both mean arterial and diastolic pressure are significantly higher in subjects on a low-potassium diet. They also reported an increase in salt sensitivity in normal healthy volunteers after potassium depletion. Their data also supported a natriuretic effect of potassium supplementation because a significant decrease in urinary sodium was found in the group with a low-potassium diet.

Two studies conducted 30 years ago suggest that total body potassium (31) and total exchangeable potassium (32) decrease with age in both sexes and that the decrease is more pronounced in women than in men. However, the risk of hyperkalemia might be a drawback of potassium supplementation in the elderly, even though studies on the effects of aging on renal and extrarenal adaptation to potassium loads are lacking. The effects of aging on potassium adaptation have been studied in aged rats (33). After a period of dietary high potassium intake, the efficiency of the kaliuretic response to intravenous KCL was impaired in the aged rat, and the rise in plasma potassium was significantly higher. The impairment in potassium adaptation is thought to be caused by a decrease in renal and colon Na^+, K^+ ATPase activity in the older rat. Whether these findings apply to aging humans remains to be determined, but in the face of a relatively low renin state, which is common in this group, most authors promote caution in relation to potassium supplementation (34).

Dietary Calcium and Phosphorus

Recently, there has been considerable interest in the use of dietary calcium to prevent and treat hypertension. MacCarron (35) has provided evidence that low dietary calcium intake and alterations in calcium metabolism predispose to hypertension. However, the potential beneficial impact of increasing dietary calcium intake on blood pressure is still controversial (36).

The first NHANES study (7) has revealed an association between calcium and blood pressure not only in entire population samples but also in specific subgroups that encompassed diverse geographic areas and various ethnic and racial backgrounds. It has been suggested that there is a threshold of approximately 400–600 mg/day of dietary calcium. Below this level the risk of elevated blood pressure increases sharply; above it, the effect of increasing calcium intake is modest.

Numerous calcium intervention trials (37–40) in humans have been reported. A modest antihypertensive response was detected in about two-thirds of these trials, with an average decrease of 4.7 mm Hg systolic and 2.4 mm Hg diastolic blood pressure (41). A blood-pressure-lowering effect of calcium has been reported in some hypertensive subjects independently of age (42,43), race, and basal levels of blood pressure (44), but the response is heterogeneous and no consistent predictors of this response have been described.

In experimental models of hypertension, a variety of metabolic disturbances related to calcium have been identified (45). The abnormalities include the chronic depression of serum ionized calcium associated with elevated levels of parathyroid hormone, low 1,25 $(OH)_2$ D_3 (46), and reduced serum phosphate concentrations.

Similarly, calcium metabolism has been found to be subtly abnormal in a subset of individuals with essential hypertension. Parathyroid hormone levels are modestly increased in hypertensive subjects (47). Serum ionized calcium has been found to be lower (48) or not different in hypertensives compared to normotensive controls while serum phosphates are always reduced (49). Increased urinary calcium excretion has also been reported (50). A number of these biochemical markers of calcium metabolism have been studied in order to determine if any of the variables measured could help predict blood pressure response to calcium supplementation in healthy normotensives, as well as in hypertensives.

Lyle et al. (51) compared subjects whose blood pressure decreased with calcium supplementation with those who had no significant blood pressure changes with calcium supplementation in an effort to determine criteria that could define a "calcium-sensitivity" state analogous to Na-sensitivity. In a well-conducted, 12-week calcium supplementation trial in normotensive males, they observed that the responders were older than nonresponders, had higher mean arterial pressures and serum parathyroid hormone levels, and had lower serum total calcium at baseline. Further analysis of the data revealed that mean arterial pressure and serum total calcium were the most important predictors of blood pressure reduction in this normotensive population.

Grobbee and Hofman (42) reported that mildly hypertensive young adults with greater than median baseline parathyroid hormone experienced a larger fall in diastolic blood pressure on calcium supplementation than the placebo group. They also reported a parallel reduction in plasma parathyroid hormone level in the calcium group, which was absent in the placebo group. Resnick et al. (52) reported a decrease in blood pressure in subjects with essential hypertension who had a profile of low renin, lower ionized calcium, and higher $1,25 (OH)_2 D_3$, but not in subjects with opposite metabolic findings. Strazullo et al. (53) found that individual blood pressure changes were inversely related to basal 24-hour urinary calcium excretion in a group of hypertensive subjects.

In summary, from these studies a number of biochemical parameters have emerged that could be used as potential predictors of a "calcium-sensitive" subpopulation of hypertensives. These parameters are lower serum ionized calcium and/or lower serum total calcium, somewhat higher plasma parathyroid hormone levels, lower renin, and increased 24-hour urinary calcium excretion.

Most nutritional surveys of the elderly in North America have shown a deficiency in dietary calcium intake (54) that is even more pronounced in women. Calcium metabolism is also significantly impaired with aging. In humans the age-related decline in 1,alpha-hydroxylase activity results in decreased levels of $1,25 (OH)_2 D_3$ (55) and reduced intestinal absorption of calcium. Moreover, the intestinal adaptation to the dietary restriction of calcium is impaired, whereas the renal tubular reabsorption is not affected as almost all the bulk of the filtered calcium is reabsorbed (56).

Given these pathophysiologic changes, it would be appealing to emphasize the role of calcium deficiency in geriatric hypertension, and further studies are indicated to examine this relationship. Meanwhile, because the level of calcium intake required to show a reduction in arterial pressure in humans falls within the range of the recommended daily allowance for dietary calcium, it is legitimate to encourage calcium intake at this level. Calcium consumption above a range of 800–1,200 mg per day either for prevention or treatment of hypertension is not currently advised.

There is some epidemiologic evidence suggesting a possible relationship between dietary phosphorus and hypertension. In normotensive humans, serum phosphate is inversely related to blood pressure (49) and in essential hypertension, serum levels of phosphorus have been found to be consistently decreased (48). Bindels and coworkers (57) have reported in the spontaneous hypertensive rat (SHR) that administration of potassium phosphate attenuated hypertension, whereas potassium chloride supplementation did not decrease blood pressure. However, in humans it remains to be determined whether supplemental dietary intake of phosphorus will attenuate hypertension.

The age-related decrease in 1,25 (OH$_2$) D$_3$ production causes a decreased intestinal absorption of phosphorus, as well as impaired intestinal adaptation to dietary phosphorus restriction (58). In aged humans, renal tubular reabsorption of phosphate is also impaired, both during normal and restricted dietary intake of phosphorus; the phosphate leak persists even when the decline in the GFR is calculated (59). These abnormalities in calcium and phosphorus metabolism related to the aging process demonstrate the crucial role of vitamin D and its metabolism. However, no supplementation in this nutrient is presently recommended.

Magnesium is another cation that has been associated with the pathogenesis of hypertension. Some investigators have reported that serum or tissue levels of magnesium are inversely related to blood pressure (60). In normotensive rats, hypertension can be induced by magnesium depletion (61), but inconsistently (62). Massive intake of magnesium has been found to decrease blood pressure in the SHR (63). In human essential hypertension, few trials have been conducted and no consistent results obtained (64–66). As with potassium, the increased urinary excretion of sodium could explain the effect of magnesium supplementation on blood pressure. The exact role of this nutrient in the prevention or the amelioration of hypertension, however, is still to be defined, and no recommendation to increase the daily intake above the RDA of 96 mEq has been formulated for young adults or the elderly.

Dietary Fat and Blood Pressure

Although the dietary intake of protein and carbohydrates appears to have little or no effect on blood pressure, an increased intake of unsaturated fat may be antihypertensive. Available data suggest that increasing the dietary polyunsaturated to saturated fat ratio (P:S) to 1, without salt or caloric restriction, lowers blood pressure (67). This effect on blood pressure is thought to be prostaglandin-mediated. Production of prostaglandins in the kidney and the vessel walls is known to contribute to the regulation of arterial reactivity. Some prostaglandins operate to increase sodium excretion and induce peripheral arteriolar dilatation. Because prostaglandins are synthesized from arachidonic acid, it has been postulated that increasing the dietary intake of its precursor, linoleic acid, would enhance urinary prostaglandin excretion and sodium excretion in rats and humans. By affecting renal sodium excretion and vascular tone, the increased intake of polyunsaturated fats could attenuate hypertension in salt-sensitive subjects.

Norris et al. (68) added an oil derivative of marine fish rich in omega-3 polyunsaturated fatty acids to the diet of eight women and eight men with mild essential hypertension and obtained a significant reduction in systolic blood pressure. In a recent study, Knapp and Fitzgerald (69) report a mean systolic decrease of 6.5 mm Hg and diastolic pressure decrease of 4.4 mm Hg in eight men with mild hypertension at the completion of a 4-week supplementation of high-dose fish oil. No changes in blood pressure were reported in three other groups receiving other types of unsaturated fats or an average American diet.

The true mechanism of the antihypertensive action of fish oil is unclear. Hypotensive effects of fish oil in normotensive subjects have not been found to be related to changes in plasma renin concentration or sodium balance (70). Furthermore, Jorgensen et al. (71) reported that, in Eskimos on a high n-3 polyunsaturated fatty acid intake, plasma renin concentrations were significantly higher than in a group of Caucasian subjects with comparable levels of systolic and diastolic blood pressure. The authors suggest that this renin status of the Eskimos might reflect either a state of decreased sensitivity to angiotensin II not different from that of the pregnant woman or an increased production of vasodilator prostaglandins.

Although promising results have also been reported in the elderly (72), the clinical usefulness and the safety of fish oil in the prevention or treatment of hypertension are not yet conclusively demonstrated in the young adults and the elderly alike.

Weight Reduction

Many cross-sectional population-based studies have shown a positive correlation between body weight and hypertension. The efficacy of weight reduction in decreasing blood pressure in obese hypertensive subjects has been demonstrated (73), including its effect independent of sodium intake (74). Body weight generally increases through the sixth decade of life and thereafter levels off or declines. Body composition also changes with age. Lean body mass can decrease by 2.3% every decade after age 25. The accumulation of excess body weight over the following 30–40 years, which averages 5.1 kg for men and 4.5 kg for women, is due to both absolute and relative increases in the amount of body fat and an absolute decrease in lean body mass.

Even though weight reduction is considered to be the single most effective nonpharmacologic approach to the control of arterial pressure in humans, virtually all of the studies on weight reduction using such strategies as total caloric reduction or isolated reductions in fat, carbohydrate, or protein intake have involved only young to middle-aged subjects. Thus, we still lack guidelines as to the efficacy or safety of this nondrug method of blood pressure control in the elderly, and more specific clinical trials are needed.

Alcohol Consumption

Data from the NHANES I study demonstrated the important effect of alcohol intake on blood pressure among American adults (75). Consumption of more than 2 oz/day of ethanol has been shown to cause significant elevations in blood pressure (78). Potter and Beevers (76) studied the effect of alcohol in hypertensive subjects. A reduction in alcohol consumption resulted in a decrease in both systolic and diastolic pressure. When alcohol was reinstituted, blood pressure increased. In 1984, West et al. (77) reported that the prevalence of hidden alcoholism in the geriatric population is high. On the basis of these studies and considering the fact that drinking can also interfere with pharmacologic therapy, alcohol intake should be carefully evaluated and any excess discouraged in elderly hypertensives (78).

Although 30% incidence of adverse effects of antihypertensive medications in the elderly (74,79) compared to an incidence of 5% in patients between the ages of 25 and 40, speaks strongly for the use of nonpharmacologic methods of therapy, several factors in this population may affect compliance adversely (80). In many elderly patients adherence to low-salt and low-calorie diets may be difficult because of limited access to fresh foods, resulting in a reliance on processed foods. In others, behavioral intervention, such as alcohol restriction, may be more difficult to achieve because the desire to adopt lifestyle changes may be lacking (75). Thus in attempting to manage hypertension with nondrug strategies, elderly patients, as should younger ones, should be offered the range of modalities available and assisted in choosing those best suited for each case. If the nondrug trial is too burdensome or results in only partial success, simple schedules of standard therapy should be considered.

REFERENCES

1. Drizd T, Dannenberg A, Engel A. *Vital Health Stat* 1986;234:1–68.
2. Working Group on Hypertension in the Elderly. *JAMA* 1986;256:70–74.
3. United States Public Health Service Hospitals Cooperative Study. *Circulation* 1979;40 (suppl II):110–124.
4. Freeman DH, Ostfeld AM, Hellenbrand K, et al. *J Chron Dis* 1985;38:157–164.
5. Larochelle P, Bass MJ, Birkett NJ, De Champlain J, Myers MG. *Can Med Assoc J* 1986;135:741–746.
6. Webster J, Newham D, Petrie JC, Lovell HG. *Br Med J* 1984;288:1574–1575.

7. Harlan WR, Hull AL, Schmouder RL, Landis JR, Larkin FA, Thompson FE. *Hypertension* 1984;6:802–809.
8. Freis ED. *Circulation* 1976;53:589–594.
9. Rascher W. In: Ganten D, Ritz E, eds. *Lehrbuch Der Hypertonie.* Stuttgart: Schattaver Verlag, 1985:49.
10. Dahl LK. In: Bock KD, Cottier PT, eds. *Essential hypertension.* Berlin: Springer Verlag, 1960:53.
11. The Intersalt Cooperative Research Group. *Br Med J* 1988;297:319–328.
12. Grobbee DE, Hofman A. *Br Med J* 1986;293:227–229.
13. Myers J, Morgan T. *Clin Exp Hypertens (A)* 1983;5:99.
14. Davies DF, Shock NW. *J Clin Invest* 1950;29:496.
15. Rowe JW, Andres R, Tobin JD, Norris AH, Shock NW. *Ann Intern Med* 1976;84:567.
16. Friedman SA, Raizner AE, Rosen H, Solomon NA, Wilfredo SY. *Ann Intern Med* 1972;76:41.
17. Lindeman RD, Tobin J, Shock NW. *J Am Geriatr Soc* 1985;33:278.
18. Luft FC, Fineberg NS, Miller JZ, Rankin LI, Grim CE, Weinberger MH. *Am J Med Sci* 1980;279:15.
19. Weidmann P, De Myttenaere-Bursztein S, Maxwell NH, De Lima J. *Kidney Int* 1975;8:325.
20. Epstein M, Hollenberg NK. *J Lab Clin Med* 1976;87:411.
21. Maclas Nunez JF, Igleslas G, Bonda Roman A, et al. *Age Aging* 1978;7:178.
22. Hagstad R, Brown RD, Jiang N-S, et al. *Am J Med* 1983;74:442.
23. Tannen RL. *Kidney Int* 1987;32(suppl 22):S242–S248.
24. Walker WG, Whelton PK, Saito H, et al. *Hypertension* 1979;1:287–291.
25. Langford HG. *Ann Intern Med* 1983;98(part 2):770–772.
26. Khaw KT, Barrett-Connor E. *Am J Clin Nutr* 1984;39:963–968.
27. Morgan TO. *Clin Sci* 1982;63:407S–409S.
28. MacGregor GA, Markando ND, Smith SJ, Banks RA, Sangnella GA. *Lancet* 1982;2: 567–570.
29. Overlack A, Stumpe KO, Moch B, et al. *Klin Wochenschr* 1985;63:352–360.
30. Krishna GG, Hiller E, Kapoor S. *N Engl J Med* 1989;320:1177–1182.
31. Allen TH, Anderson EC, Langham WH. *J Gerontol* 1960;15:348.
32. Saglid U. *Scand J Clin Lab Invest* 1956;8:44.
33. Bengele HH, Mathias R, Perkins JH, McNamara ER, Alexander EA. *Kidney Int* 1983;23:684.
34. Suki WN. *Kidney Int* 1988;34;525:5175–5176.
35. McCarron DA. *Kidney Int* 1989;35:717–736.
36. Kaplan NM, Meese RB. *Ann Intern Med* 1986;105:947–955.
37. McCarron DA, Morris CD, Cole C. *Science* 1982;217:267–269.
38. Ackley S, Barrett-Connor E, Suarez L. *Am J Clin Nutr* 1983;38:457–461.
39. Garcia Palmier HR, Coseas R, Cruz Vidal M, et al. *Hypertension* 1984;6:322–328.
40. Belizan JM, Villar J, Pineda O, et al. *JAMA* 1983;249:1161–1165.
41. McCarron DA, Morris CD. *Ann Intern Med* 1985;103:825–831.
42. Grobbee DE, Hofman A. *Lancet* 1986;2:703–706.
43. Tabuchi Y, Ogibara T, Hashizume K, Saito H, Kumabara Y. *J Clin Hypertens* 1986;3:254–262.
44. Lyle RM, Melby CL, Hyner GC, Edmondson JW, Miller JZ, Weinberger MH. *JAMA* 1987;257:1772–1776.
45. Young EW, Bukowski RD, McCarron DA. *Proc Soc Exp Biol Med* 1986;8:45–49.
46. Lau K, Eby B. *Hypertension* 1985;7:657–667.
47. Grobbee DE, Hackeng WHL, Birkenhager JC, Hofman A. *Br Med J* 1988;296:814–816.
48. McCarron DA. *N Engl J Med* 1982;307:226–228.
49. Ljunghall S, Hedstrand H. *Br Med J* 1977;1:553–554.
50. Strazzullo P, Nunziata B, Cirillo M, et al. *Clin Sci* 1983;65:137–141.
51. Lyle RM, Melby CL, Hyner GC. *Am J Clin Nutr* 1988;47:1030–1035.
52. Resnick LM, Nichelson JP, Laragh JH. *Fed Proc* 1986;45:2739–2745.
53. Strazzullo P, Siani A, Guglielmi S, et al. *Hypertension* 1986;8:1084–1088.
54. Bowman BB, Rosenbert IH. *Am J Clin Nutr* 1982;35:1142–1151.
55. Armbrecht H, Forte LR, Halloran BP. *Am J Physiol* 1984;246:E266.

56. Armbrecht HJ, Zenser TV, Bruns MEH, Davis BB. *Am J Physiol* 1979;236:E769.
57. Bindels RJM, Van den Broek LAM, Hillebrand SJW, Wokke JHP. *Hypertension* 1987;9:96–102.
58. Armbrecht HJ, Zenser TV, Gross CJ, Davis BB. *Am J Physiol* 1980;239:E322.
59. Marcus R, Madvig P, Young G. *J Clin Endocrinol Metab* 1984;58:223.
60. Resnick LM, Gupta RK, Laragh JH. *Proc Natl Acad Sci USA* 1984;81:6511–6515.
61. Altura BM, Altura BT, Gebrewold A, et al. *Science* 1984;223:1315–1317.
62. Luthringer C, Rayssiguier Y, Gueux E, Berthelot A. *Br J Nutr* 1988;59:243–250.
63. Altura BT, Altura BM. *Magnesium Bull* 1987;9:6–21.
64. Cappucio FP, Marrandy ND, Beynon GW, et al. *Br Med J* 1985;291:235–238.
65. Heyderson DG, Schierup J, Schodt T. *Br Med J* 1986;293:664–665.
66. Dyckner T, Wester PO. *Br Med J* 1983;286:1847–1849.
67. Comberg HV, Heyden S, Hames CG, et al. *Prostaglandins* 1978;15:193–197.
68. Norris PG, Jones CJG, Weston MJ. *Br Med J* 1986;293:104–105.
69. Knapp HR, Fitzgerald GA. *N Engl J Med* 1989;320:1037–1043.
70. Mortensen JZ, Schmidt EB, Nielsen AH, Dyerberg J. *Thromb Haemost* 1983;50:543–546.
71. Jorgensen KA, Nielsen AH, Dyerbert J. *Acta Med Scand* 1986;219:473–479.
72. Fleischman AI, Bierenbaum ML, Stier A, et al. *J Med Soc NJ* 1979;76:181–183.
73. Havlik RJ, Habert HB, Fabsitz RR, Feinleib M. *Ann Intern Med* 1983;98:855–859.
74. Tuck ML, Sowers JL, Dornfeld L, Maxwell M. *N Engl J Med* 1981;304:930–934.
75. Saunders JB, Beevers DO, Paton A. *Lancet* 1981;2:653–656.
76. Polter JF, Befveis DG. *Lancet* 1984;1:119–122.
77. West IJ, Maxwell DS, Noble EP, Solomon DH. *Ann Intern Med* 1984;100:405–416.
78. Scanlan BC. *Drug Ther* 1988;3:63–67.
79. Curb JD. *JAMA* 1985;253:3263–3268.
80. Tscham JM, Adamsen TE, Coates TJ, Gullion DS. *J Comm Health* 1988;13:19–32.

Geriatric Nutrition, edited by John E. Morley,
Zvi Glick, Laurence Z. Rubenstein.
Raven Press, Ltd., New York © 1990.

22

Obesity

John E. Morley and Zvi Glick

*Geriatric Research, Education and Clinical Center, Sepulveda VA Medical Center,
Sepulveda, California 91343 and Department of Medicine, UCLA School of
Medicine, Los Angeles, California 90024*

Obesity is an important public health problem for younger individuals. The relative importance of mild to moderate overweightedness as a health risk is less clear in older individuals. However, regardless of age, it is clear that those individuals with excessive adipose tissue accumulation (*morbid obesity*) suffer from clear-cut health risks and an impaired quality of life.

Obesity is defined as an excess of adipose tissue for a given weight. Unfortunately, controversy exists over the definition of what constitutes an excess. In addition, the pattern of distribution of body fat may be more important than the total adipose tissue mass when assessing the metabolic effects and health risks associated with obesity (1). In middle-aged individuals (age 54 at measurement), abdominal, rather than lower body, adiposity has been associated with an increased risk of stroke and ischemic heart disease (1). In addition, both cross-sectional and prospective studies have shown an association between an increased weight to hip ratio (android obesity) and Type II diabetes mellitus (2).

It should be remembered that fat plays an important role in the survival of an individual, particularly at times of chronic stress. The major function of fat is to act as a storage organ for excess calories (Fig. 1). This storage function can be particularly important in an older person who develops an acute illness associated with a decreased caloric intake and increased metabolic demands. Fat also plays a role as a protective organ, protecting vital internal organs from injury. Again, in an older person who is at increased risk of falling, this protective function of fat may be critical. Fat softens the contours of the body. Loss of subcutaneous fat with advancing age may lead to an altered body image, with adverse social and psychologic consequences.

This chapter reviews briefly the methods available for assessing body adipose tissue and then examines the available data on the prevalence of obesity and the alterations in body fat content that occur with advancing age.

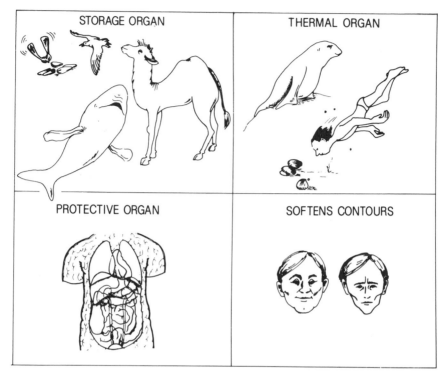

FIG. 1. Functions of fat.

The health hazards associated with obesity are described, with special emphasis on the data available in older individuals. Finally, the management of obesity in older individuals is examined and contrasted to the management strategies utilized in younger individuals.

TECHNIQUES FOR BODY FAT ASSESSMENT

The classical method for calculating body fat is to use hydrodensitometry, in which body density is obtained by dividing body mass by body volume (obtained by weighing first in air and then underwater). The percentage fat is then calculated by utilizing the known densities of fat (0.90) and fat-free mass (1.10). This method has a 3 to 4% error rate. Total body potassium can be calculated by measuring the amount of the naturally occurring radioactive isotope of potassium (^{40}K) in the body. Assuming a constant amount of intracellular potassium in the fat-free mass (63.9 mEq per kg), the fat-free mass can then be calculated and body fat obtained by subtracting the latter from body weight. In older subjects, the use of diuretics that deplete body potassium may confound this measurement. Clearly, both of the above measurements assume a normal state of hydration of the individual; a decreased total body water with advancing age may alter the reliability of these measurements in the elderly.

Total body water can be determined by measuring the concentration of tritium or deuterium in body water 3 to 4 hours after administering an oral dose of labeled water. Water is assumed to constitute a constant fraction of fat-free mass (0.72), thus allowing the calculation of fat-free mass. Steen (3) has demonstrated that 70- to 80-year-old men have less water compared to mature adults. This change is predominantly caused by a decrease in extracellular fluid with advancing age. In addition, measurement of total body water gives an erroneous calculation of fat-free mass in older subjects with heart failure.

A number of other methods for body fat determination that are used experimentally are available. These include ultrasound techniques, computed tomography, and nuclear magnetic resonance, all of which provide pictures from which the amount of fat is calculated. A new method for estimating body composition that has great promise is body impedance measurements in response to a 50-kHz current. This method relies on the principle that electrical conductivity of fat-free tissue mass is much greater than that of fat. This method is portable and relatively inexpensive. Both altered hydration and altered electrolyte balance may alter the results obtained.

In clinical settings, adipose tissue mass is most often obtained by anthropometric measures. The most common measurements are height and weight. A standard for patients of all heights can be obtained by dividing weight, expressed in kg, by the square of height in meters (W/H^2), which is known as the body mass index. Measurement of skinfold thickness is commonly used to determine body fat and its distribution. Correlations between anthropomorphic measures and body fat have been found to be fairly good in the elderly. Studies in 70-year-old individuals have suggested that, on the whole, the correlation between body fat and anthropomorphic measurements was higher in women than in men (4). In older men, the subscapular skinfold appears to be the best available measurement for estimating body fat. In older women, thigh and triceps skinfold were better determinants of body fat.

Body circumference measurements are easy to do and appear to have less interobserver error than skinfold determinations. They are best used to determine body fat distribution. The waist-to-hip ratio has already been mentioned in this regard. When this ratio is above 0.9 in men or 0.8 in women, they are said to have android fat distribution, whereas lower values indicate a gynoid fat distribution.

OBESITY, FAT DISTRIBUTION, AND AGING

The percent of overweight white American men peaks at 30.5% in the years 45 to 54 and then declines slightly to 25.8% by ages 65 to 74 (5). Middle-aged black men have a higher prevalence of overweight, but there are only minimal differences by the time they reach 65 to 74 years of age. In contrast, overweightedness tends to increase in white American women, peaking at 36.5% at ages 65 to 74 years. Sixty percent of black American women are overweight in the 65- to 74-year age group (Fig. 2).

In Austria, there is little difference in the prevalence of obesity before 40 years of age (6). Thereafter, there is a marked increase in obesity in women compared to men. The prevalence of obesity in men peaks at age 55 to 60 and then declines to under 20% in those over 74 years of age. Female obesity peaks at 60 to 65 years of age and declines to under 30% in those over 74 years. Overall, these figures suggest excess adiposity is less common in older than middle-aged individuals.

In a longitudinal study in older men and women from Sweden, body weight declined between 70 and 81 years, with the decrease averaging 7 kg in men and 6 kg in women over the decade (3) (Fig. 3A). The major changes seen were in body cell mass in men, body fat in women, and total body water in both sexes (Fig. 3B). A cross-sectional study in the United States sug-

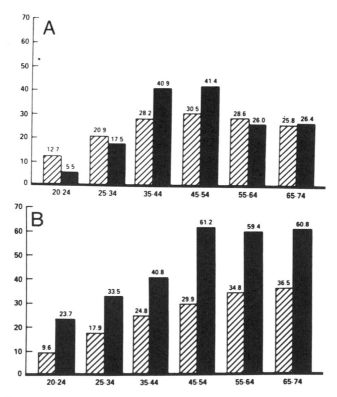

FIG. 2. The percentage of overweight males **(A)** and females **(B)** by age and race. Cross-hatched bars, whites; black bars, blacks. (From Van Italie, ref. 5, with permission.)

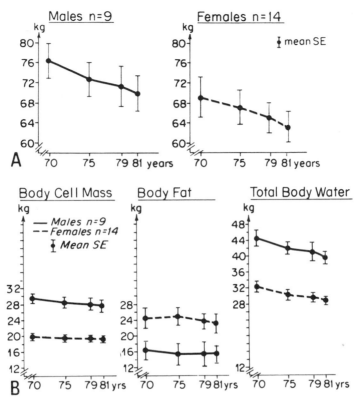

FIG. 3. A: Longitudinal changes in body weight. **B:** Body cell mass, body fat, and total body water content in the same men and women. (From Steen, ref. 30, with permission.)

gested that a similar decrease in body weight is seen in subjects between 65 and 95 years of age (7). Similarly, body mass index declines between 65 and 90 years (8). This decrease is more marked in men than in women. However, body mass index tends to be greater in the 65-year-olds than in the 19- to 24-year-olds.

Frisancho (9) has developed standards for skinfold measurements (triceps and subscapular) for subjects aged 55 to 74 years. In comparison with those aged 25 to 54 years, there is little difference in men, whereas older women tend to have greater triceps skinfold measurements. Another study has suggested that, in subjects over 80 years old, the triceps skinfold falls in women and the subscapular skinfold decreases in both men and women (10).

Fat distribution tends to change with age, with the waist-to-hip ratio increasing in both sexes from ages 20 to 29 to ages 60 to 69 (11). A similar finding has been reported over the ages 17 to 96, with a continued increase in upper and central body fat distribution throughout life (10). In women, there is an acceleration of this trend after menopause. A computed tomography study has suggested that in older men, there is an increase in intra-abdominal fat with a decrease in subcutaneous abdominal fat compared to younger men (12). There is also an increased infiltration of fat into lean tissues with advancing age.

PATHOGENESIS OF OBESITY WITH ADVANCING AGE

Obesity develops when energy intake exceeds energy output. For practical purposes, energy intake is equal to the food eaten, as calorie malabsorption does not appear to occur (nonpathologically) with aging. Data from three studies—the NHANES I, the Lipid Research Clinics, and the U.S. Department of Agriculture—all show that food intake peaks in the twenties and then declines at least to the age of 70 years [reviewed by Bray and Gray (11)]. This decrease in food intake over the lifespan is more marked in men than in women.

Energy output is the sum of the resting metabolic rate, thermogenesis, and physical activity. There is a small decrease in the resting metabolic rate with advancing age (11,13,14). The thermic effect of glucose has also been shown to decrease with advancing age (14). In addition, there is a marked decrease in physical activity in most older individuals. Thus, older individuals are constantly required to adjust their food intake downward to avoid becoming obese. It is easy to see how in this situation minor malfunctions in normal feedback systems involved in the regulation of hunger or satiety could lead to obesity.

An area of energy utilization that is often ignored is the differing resting activity of an individual. "Fidgeting" or purposeless physical activity may expend from 100 to 600 Kcal/day (15). This is dramatically illustrated in parkinsonian patients whose tremors can continuously expend energy. The sight of a fat patient with Parkinson's disease is extremely rare! Similarly, weight gain in an older patient may be related to loss of movement on one side after a cerebrovascular accident or a general paucity of movements when a person becomes chair- or bedbound.

In younger subjects, the available data suggest that genes account for approximately one-quarter of the total body fat and play a similar role as a determinant of fat disposition (16). Genotype appears to account for a greater proportion (approximately 40%) of individual differences in the resting metabolic rate, the thermic effect of a meal, and the thermic effect of exercise.

Although most forms of obesity are caused by an interaction of psychosocial and environmental factors with the genotype, it is important to rule out specific etiologies for obesity. Of these, the most common are the endocrine disorders. Hypothyroidism can occur in up to 5% of individuals over 60 years of age and is commonly associated with weight gain (17). The diagnosis of hypothyroidism is excluded by the measurement of thyrotropin level. Hypogonadism (both primary and secondary) may be present in 30% or more of normal male subjects over 50 years of age (Korenmen and Morley, unpublished data). Hypogonadism is clearly associated with weight gain in younger men. The role of low bioavailable testosterone in the pathogenesis of obesity and perhaps altered fat distribution in older men remains to be determined. Determination of a bioavailable testosterone (non-sex-hormone globulin-bound testosterone) and a luteinizing hormone may help define the etiology of obesity in some older males. Both Cushing's syndrome and hypopituitarism are causes of obesity, but occur rarely in older individuals. Growth hormone deficiency and low insulin-like growth factor I (somatomedin C) levels are common with advancing age, but their role in the obesity of the elderly has not been determined.

Tumors of the ventromedial nucleus of the hypothalamus may lead to obesity. Although depression in older subjects is classically associated with weight loss, a subset of depressed patients will present with weight gain. Treatment of depression with tricyclic antidepressants or monoamine oxidase inhibitors has been known to cause weight gain in older subjects. Glucocorticoid (cortisol) treatment is also associated with obesity. Phenothiazines and butyrophenones can either increase or decrease weight in older subjects.

HEALTH HAZARDS OF OBESITY

The major complications associated with obesity in individuals under 60 years of age are listed in Table 1. The majority of these health hazards of obesity are well recognized, and only those in which differences occur with aging are discussed in this section. In addition, the distribution of body fat may be more important than the actual fat mass in determining the effects of obesity. Based on the 1960 to 1962 Health Examination Survey in a group aged 18 to 79 years, the ratio of upper body to lower body fat increased steadily with age, and increases in this ratio were associated with hypertension, heart disease, and postload serum glucose (18).

A number of studies have examined the relative risk of mortality associated with adiposity (19). When all ages are examined, the curves tend to be U- or J-shaped, with the greatest mortalities occurring at the extremes of under- or overweight. In these studies, extreme overweight tends to confer a greater risk of mortality than does low body weight. Both of the two largest studies that included subjects into their eighties showed U-shaped mortality curves (20,21), whereas two smaller studies including subjects in their seventies failed to show a weight-mortality association (22,23). This raised the question of the importance of weight as a predictor of mortality in older subjects.

In the American Cancer Study (20), there was evidence for an attenuation of death rates with advancing years at higher weights (Fig. 4). Thus, in 30-

TABLE 1. *Complications of obesity in individuals under 60 years of age and the possibility that these complications are also important in older individuals*

Complication	Importance in individuals over 60 years of age[a]
Decreased longevity	± (only with morbid obesity)
Hypertension	+
Hypercholesterolemia	−
Increased triglycerides	+
Diabetes mellitus	+
Coronary artery disease	±
Cancer	
Female	
Endometrial	+
Breast	+ (association seen after 50 years)
Gallbladder	+
Cervix	+
Ovaries	+
Male	
Colon	±
Prostate	+
Pulmonary embolism	+
Sleep apnea	+
Osteoarthritis	+
Gallbladder disease	+
Pickwickian syndrome	± (only with morbid obesity)
Deep vein thrombosis	+
Poor wound healing— bed sores	+ +
Increased surgical risk	+
Diagnostic problems	+ +
Intertrigo	+
Gout	±
Impaired functional status	+ +
Psychosocial problems	±

[a] + +, more prevalent in the elderly; +, probable; ±, possible; −, unlikely.

to 39-year-old males, the mortality rate for those 140% or above of average weight was 1.71 compared to 1.65 in 70- to 79-year-olds and 1.53 in 80- to 89-year-olds. A more marked difference was seen in those 130 to 139% of average weight where the mortality ratio was 1.81 for 40- to 49-year-olds, falling to 1.30 for 70- to 79-year-olds and 0.83 for 80- to 89-year-olds. Similar trends were present in female subjects. Overall, in the older age groups a broad plateau of acceptable weight appeared to be present, ranging from 90 to 130% of average weight.

Recently, the Framingham Heart Study data were examined for the relationship of body mass index to mortality of older nonsmokers (24). In this

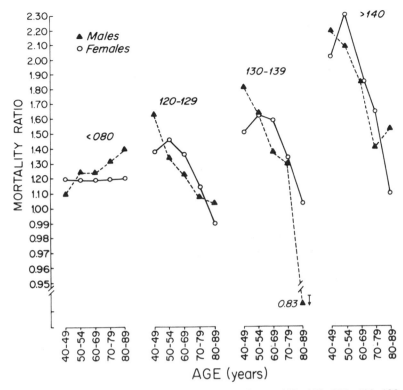

FIG. 4. Mortality ratios from all causes for weight index < 080, 120–129, 130–139, and 140+ . Death rates were compared to those of 90–109% of average weight. Age group 30–39 is not illustrated because of the small number of deaths in this age group. Data adapted from the Framingham Heart Study. (From Lew and Garfinkel, ref. 20, with permission.)

study, the relationship of weight at age 65 to subsequent mortality was examined. In men, the greatest mortality was seen in those who were less than the 10th percentile (body mass index < 28.5 Kg/m²). These data are illustrated in Fig. 5. Those who were over the 70th percentile of body mass index at both ages 55 and 65 years had almost twice the mortality rate of those who were above the 70th percentile only at the age of 65 years. Overall, these data support the notion that morbid obesity (above 130 to 140% of average body weight) is associated with increased risk of death even at extreme ages. However, moderate overweightedness (110 to 130% of average weight) appears to confer minimal increased risk of mortality in the older population.

Fatness is clearly associated with hypertension and elevated systolic blood pressure, and this relationship has been shown to be present in 50- to 75-year-olds (25). Recently, it has been suggested that this increased prevalence of hypertension may be associated with hyperinsulinemia (2). Mortal-

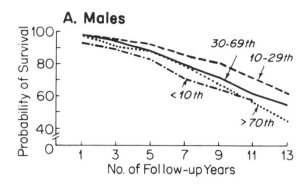

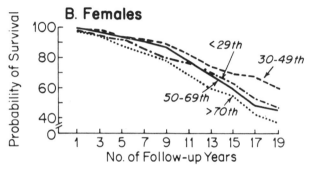

FIG. 5. Probability of surviving based on uneven quartiles of body mass index for nonsmoking men **(A)** and women **(B)** who were 65 years at entry. Data from the Framingham Heart Study. (From Harris et al., ref. 24, with permission.)

ity rates for diabetes mellitus are increased at least up to 79 years even in those with only mild increases (110 to 119%) above average weight; however, these increased mortality rates are less than those seen in 40- to 59-year-old diabetics (20). Increased mortality ratios for a number of cancers are associated with increased weight, and for the most part, these findings appear to be independent of age (26). The relationship of breast cancer to overweightedness appears to be unique to postmenopausal women (2).

Sleep-disordered breathing has been demonstrated to be associated with obesity in older individuals (27). Increases in weight of 10 to 20 pounds may be sufficient to precipitate this syndrome. Sleep-disordered breathing should be suspected in any overweight older patient with daytime somnolence or snoring.

Overweightedness in older subjects may seriously impede functional status. An overweight elderly person with osteoarthritis can have markedly impaired mobility. In addition, in long-term care settings, obesity is related to an increased prevalence of decubiti, presumably related to problems with turning such patients (28). Incontinent overweight patients are less likely to have their linen changed because of the difficulties associated with moving them. Intertrigo can be particularly difficult to treat in overweight patients. Silent or atypical presentations of disease are common in older individuals. These diagnostic dilemmas can be compounded by the problems in examining the obese older patient.

MANAGEMENT ISSUES

The first question is whom to treat? In view of the above review of relative risks, it appears that weight reduction should be mandatory in any subject over 65 years of age who is greater than 130% of average body weight. In addition, subjects with diabetes mellitus who are more than 110% of average body weight should be advised to lose weight. Because the major identifiable etiologic factor in obesity in older individuals is a decrease in physical activity, it seems reasonable to begin with an exercise program as a weight reduction tool in overweight seniors.

In most cases a walking program is the easiest to institute. Walking 1 mile utilizes approximately 100 kcal. A relatively easy program is to require walking 2 to 3 miles a day four times a week and 1 mile a day on the other days of the week. In addition, we encourage our patients to increase their "fidgeting" when at rest. Although such a program is unlikely to result in significant weight loss, it will, if maintained, result in significant improvement in cardiovascular fitness and possibly in carbohydrate tolerance. For such a program to succeed, the subjects often need at the start to walk with a therapist at least three times per week. A minimum induction program appears to be 5 weeks. Maintenance of these programs is problematic, and close lifetime follow-up by a motivated physician and therapist is essential for such programs to succeed. Patients should be made aware that excess weight gain may occur on termination of an exercise program. Alternative exercise programs, such as swimming or Tai Chi, may be particularly appropriate in some groups of elderly.

Diets in older subjects should never provide less than 800 to 1000 kcal/day. At this level of caloric intake, maintenance of adequate micronutrient intake is difficult, and patients should therefore receive a multivitamin and trace element supplementation. Care should be taken to see that an older subject who is dieting and may have the hypodipsia of aging should ingest sufficient fluids. A minimum prescription should be 1 liter/day of fluid drunk separately from meals. Increasing the fiber content of the diet may assist in weight loss. It should, however, be remembered that immobile older patients lose their gastrocolic reflex and that in these patients high-fiber diets may lead to severe constipation.

In many cases, starting a diet in an older individual represents an attempt to change the habits of a lifetime. Such interventions require major behavior modification skills and the intervention of a skilled team, including a dietitian and a psychologist. Behavioral modification techniques should be used in elderly subjects (29). These include self-monitoring and lifestyle changes, such as putting the fork down between bites, avoiding snacking between meals, and eating in only one designated place. Attitude techniques, such as focusing on behavior rather than weight, recognizing high-risk situations, learning to recognize and avoid cravings, and learning to cope positively with lapses, form an important part of any behavior program. Reinforcement techniques and rewards are another facet of the program. In older individuals, praise from the physician may be particularly useful in this regard. In addition, quality-of-life scales allowing the patient to focus on the improvement in general well-being that is associated with weight loss should be used. Awareness of caloric values of food is another part of this program.

In older subjects, dealing with attitudes of the spouse may be particularly important. Many older women feel insulted and/or unloved when their spouse fails to eat their food. Their guilt that they are partially responsible for a spouse's weight problem can lead to denial. In some cases, the spouse finds it difficult to accept the obesity as a problem. It is thus extremely important that the patient's partner be included in the behavior modification process. When it is obvious that the partner is sabotaging the weight reduction program, he or she should be openly confronted with this by the therapist, and the patient should be taught how to deal with pressures to eat. In addition, the partner, whether overweight or not, should be encouraged to exercise with the patient.

Magical diets, such as the "Beverly Hills Diet" and the "grapefruit diets," may have short-term success, but rarely result in long-term weight reduction. Low and very low caloric formula diets have not been adequately tested in the elderly and should be avoided.

In general, drugs should be avoided in the elderly, and there seems little reason to utilize drug therapy for obesity in older subjects. Phenyl propanolamine, which is a common constituent in over-the-counter antiobesity drugs, theoretically may aggravate postural or meal-associated hypotension in older individuals. Drugs that modulate serotonin metabolism, such as fenfluramine and fluoxetine, can cause effective weight loss in some younger individuals. However, cessation of therapy is often associated with rapid regaining of weight. Information on the safety of these drugs in older individuals is generally lacking. However, the use of these serotonergic reuptake blockers may be justified in older obese diabetic patients who either refuse to take insulin or require excess insulin dosage. Opiate antagonists, such as naltrexone, were ineffective in younger subjects and, in view of the fact that the opioid feeding system appears to be absent in older individuals, are unlikely to be useful. Thermogenic drugs, such as thyroid hormone and beta-adrenergic agents, all have some effects on the heart and, as such, should

TABLE 2. *Utility of weight loss techniques in old subjects*

Technique	Utility in elderly
Exercise	Yes
Diet	Yes (if over 130% of average weight or associated with diabetes mellitus)
Behavior modification	Yes
Low and very low calorie diets	Potentially dangerous
Drugs	
Anorectic agents	Rarely indicated
Thermogenic agents	Potentially dangerous
Gastric balloon	Not useful
Surgery	
Gastric restriction	Only when massive obesity is associated with sleep apnea
Jejunoileal bypass	Never used

not be used in older subjects who are at increased risk for arrhythmias. The utility for weight reduction and safety of long-term use of fat substitutes, such as sucrose polyester (Olestra), remain to be determined in both the young and elderly.

Gastric balloons were supposed to decrease feeding by increasing stomach satiety signals after smaller caloric loads. As this technique failed to be effective in younger obese patients, there seems to be no reason to use it in older subjects. Surgical treatments for obesity are not recommended in patients over 60 years of age. An exception to this rule may be in very obese patients with severe sleep apnea.

Massively obese older subjects whose obesity is interfering with their ability to carry out their activities of daily living may benefit from short-term (2 to 4 months) nursing home admission to allow the weight reduction process to be established. In such a therapeutic decision as this one, the effects of the nursing home admission on quality of life need to be carefully weighed against the possible long-term benefits of this approach. The patient and spouse should be made fully aware of the choices and should make an informed decision. Table 2 summarizes the management options in older obese subjects compared to techniques used in younger obese subjects.

CONCLUSION

There are few good studies of obesity in individuals over 70 years of age. Nevertheless, it appears that, even in this age group, morbid obesity (greater than 130% of average body weight) represents an important health risk that should be treated. Treatment involves exercise, diet (with adequate vitamin and mineral supplements), and behavior modification. Drug and surgical treatments should be avoided in the majority of obese elderly. There is a need for a careful evaluation of the success of weight loss programs in older individuals and their long-term outcomes, particularly in regard to quality of life, mortality, and morbidity.

REFERENCES

1. Larsson B, Svardsudd K, Welin L, et al. *Br Med J* 1984;288:1401–1404.
2. Kissebah AH, Freedman DS, Peiris AN. *Med Clin North Am* 1989;73:111–138.
3. Steen B. *Nutr Rev* 1988;46:45–51.
4. Steen B, Bruce A, Isaksson B, et al. *Acta Med Scand* 1977;611(suppl):87–112.
5. Van Italie TB. *Ann Intern Med* 1985;103(part 2):983–988.
6. Kluhte R, Schubert A. *Ann Intern Med* 1985;103(part 2):1037–1042.
7. Master AM, Laner RP, Beckman G. *JAMA* 1960;172:658–662.
8. Chumlea WC, Roche AF, Murherjee D. *J Gerontol* 1986;41:36–39.
9. Frisancho AR. *Am J Clin Nutr* 1984;40:808–819.
10. Shimokata H, Tobin JD, Muller DC, et al. *J Gerontol* 1989;44:M66–73.
11. Bray GA, Gray DS. *West J Med* 1988;149:429–441.
12. Borkan GA, Hults DE, Gerzof SG, et al. *J Gerontol* 1983;38:673–677.
13. Owen OE. *Mayo Clin Proc* 1988;63:503–510.
14. Golay A, Schutz Y, Broquet C, et al. *J Am Geriatr Soc* 1986;31:144–148.
15. Ravussin E, Lillioja S, Anderson TE, et al. *J Clin Invest* 1986;78:1568–1578.
16. Bouchard C. *Med Clin North Am* 1989;73:67–81.
17. Mooradian AD, Morley JE, Korenman SG. *Dis a Month* 1988;7:395–461.
18. Gillum RF. *J Chron Dis* 1987;40:421–428.
19. Manson JE, Stampfer MJ, Hennekens CM, et al. *JAMA* 1987;257:353–358.
20. Lew EA, Garfinkel L. *J Chron Dis* 1979;32:563–576.
21. Waaler HT. *Acta Med Scand* 1984;679(suppl):1–56.
22. Bottiger LE, Carlson LA. *Atherosclerosis* 1980;36:389–408.
23. Borhani NO, Hechter HH, Breslow L. *J Chron Dis* 1963;16:1251–1266.
24. Harris T, Cook EF, Garrison R, Higgins M, et al. *JAMA* 1988;259:1520–1524.
25. Garn SM, Sullivan TV, Hawthorne VM. *J Gerontol* 1988;43:M170–174.
26. Garfinkel L. *Ann Intern Med* 1985;103:1034–1036.
27. Bliwise DL, Feldman DE, Bliwise NG, et al. *J Am Geriatr Soc* 1987;35:132–141.
28. Silver AJ, Morley JE, Strome LS, et al. *J Am Geriatr Soc* 1988;36:487–491.
29. Brownell KD, Kramer FM. *Med Clin North Am* 1989;73:185–201.

Geriatric Nutrition, edited by John E. Morley,
Zvi Glick, Laurence Z. Rubenstein.
Raven Press, Ltd., New York © 1990.

23

Cancer and Malnutrition

David Heber

*Department of Medicine, UCLA School of Medicine,
Los Angeles, California 90024*

Cancer incidence clearly increases with age, and age has been identified as the single most important factor in cancer incidence. In fact, in the United States, overall cancer incidence doubles with every 5-year increase in age (1). This increase is most likely due to an accumulation of premalignant changes occurring over a long period of time so that cancer comes to exist primarily in the elderly (2).

Epidemiologists have identified at least two patterns by which cancer incidence increases with age (3). The most common pattern is an uninterrupted relatively steep increase with age from adulthood into the eighth decade. This pattern is exemplified by the data in Fig. 1 taken from the Third National Cancer Survey for rates of prostate, colon, and stomach cancer in men (4). This pattern is usually found with cancers of epithelial origin. A second pattern is exemplified in Fig. 2 which shows the incidence rates of breast cancer in black and white women, also from the Third National Cancer Survey (4). Although the incidence of breast cancer increases with age, the slope of the incidence curve changes after the age of 45. This change in slope has been attributed to the hormonal changes occurring at the time of menopause, the exact reason for this alteration has not been determined.

Thus, although many other factors clearly affect cancer incidence and not all cancers become more common with advancing age, it is clear that aging is associated with an increased incidence of most common forms of cancer. Cancer has a profound effect on nutritional status, and nutritional status has a profound effect on survival in cancer patients. This chapter outlines the pathophysiology of cancer cachexia, as well as indicates some of the hopeful avenues being investigated to develop effective treatment strategies for this condition.

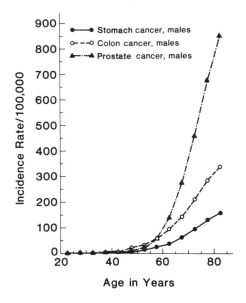

FIG. 1. Incidence of prostate, colon, and stomach cancer among men aged 20 to 80 years from the Third National Cancer Survey rates. (From Devita et al., ref. 4.)

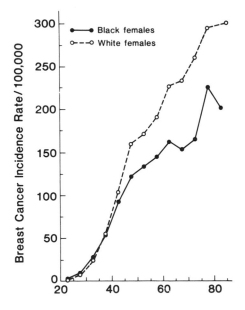

FIG. 2. Incidence of breast cancer among white and black women aged 20 to 80 years from the Third National Cancer Survey rates. (From Devita et al., ref. 4.)

MALNUTRITION AND CANCER

Malnutrition is a frequent and serious problem in patients with cancer. Patients with some types of cancers, such as lung, prostate, head and neck, and gastric cancer, are more frequently malnourished, but the overall incidence of malnutrition ranges between 30 and 87% of different populations studied (5,6). The advanced starvation state resulting from decreased food intake and hormonal/metabolic abnormalities characteristic of the interaction between tumor and host has been called *cancer cachexia* (7). A retrospective analysis of patient body weight at the beginning of cooperative chemotherapy trials determined that the presence of a 6% weight loss from usual body weight was a significant prognostic factor for survival. The apparent effect of weight loss at the time of diagnosis on median survival for certain common cancers was greater than the impact of chemotherapy. Despite the development of advanced technology and costly delivery systems for total parenteral nutrition and continuous enteral nutrition, nutrition therapy alone has had little impact on this problem. Although nutritional rehabilitation can be demonstrated in selected patients who respond to antineoplastic therapy, the routine use of parenteral or enteral nutrition as an adjunct to chemotherapy in cancer patients has not resulted in increased survival or predictable weight gain (8,9). Over the last 15 years, research on the basic pathophysiology of cancer cachexia has identified a number of specific metabolic and hormonal abnormalities that could impair renutrition, but none of the hormonal or metabolic agents tested has resulted in predictable weight gain.

It has been estimated that up to 30% of the 200,000 patients receiving home parenteral nutrition in the United States have cancer. Decreased food intake alone is not likely to account for the phenomenon of progressive weight loss in cancer patients because cancer patients with active disease who ingest adequate calories may still fail to gain weight.

In 1986, Tchekmedyian et al. (10) observed increased appetite and weight gain in 30 of 33 patients with advanced breast cancer treated with a high dose of megestrol acetate, a progestational steroid. Preliminary observations have also demonstrated weight gain in 13 of 14 AIDS patients (11). Patients with cancer have been shown to have decreased activity of lipoprotein lipase (12), the enzyme responsible for hydrolysis of chylomicron and VLDL triglycerides to fatty acids for uptake into adipocytes where they are used for triglyceride synthesis. If these abnormalities of fat metabolism can be reversed by megestrol acetate treatment and fat stores increased predictably in cancer patients, an important advance in combating cancer malnutrition will have been achieved.

PATHOPHYSIOLOGY OF CANCER CACHEXIA

Based on autopsy studies performed in the 1920s (13,14) and animal studies done in the 1950s (15), it was postulated that tumors acted to siphon off needed energy and protein from the host. However, because most tumors in humans seldom exceed 5% of body weight at autopsy, a simple nutrient-trapping mechanism is an unlikely cause of cachexia. In the 1970s and 1980s, specific abnormalities of intermediary metabolism were identified in cancer patients that could account for the common observation that such patients lost weight even in the face of apparently adequate nutrition. The following metabolic abnormalities occur frequently in patients with cancer: (a) increased glucose production in the fasting state, (b) increased whole body protein breakdown, (c) increased lipolysis and decreased fat mass, (d) hypogonadism in male cancer patients, and (e) abnormalities of insulin secretion and action in patients with localized and disseminated cancer. In 1983, we demonstrated that adequate calories and protein administered to six patients with active localized head and neck cancer via forced continuous enteral alimentation under metabolic ward conditions for 29 days failed to lead to significant weight gain (9).

The failure to gain weight, despite adequate caloric intake under metabolic ward conditions, supports the concept that malnourished cancer patients are hypermetabolic. However, it has been difficult to demonstrate consistently increased metabolic rates using either direct or indirect calorimetry (16). Our group and others have consistently demonstrated increased rates of whole body glucose production in the fasting state in cancer patients with non-small-cell lung cancer, head and neck cancer, and colorectal cancer (17,18). It has been estimated that this increase in whole body glucose production could consume enough energy to lead to a weight loss of 0.9 kg/month. In addition, under carefully controlled metabolic ward conditions we have demonstrated increased whole body protein breakdown rates in non-small-cell lung cancer patients (19).

The serendipitous discovery of weight gain as a side effect of megestrol acetate treatment of women with metastatic breast cancer has opened a promising new avenue for the development of an effective agent to treat cancer cachexia (10). In fact, these patients gained weight regardless of whether they responded to the hormonal treatment, and recently AIDS patients have also gained weight during treatment with this hormonal drug.

Lipid Metabolism and Cancer Cachexia

Hypertriglyceridemia, depletion of carcass fat stores, and decreased lipoprotein lipase levels have all been observed in patients with cancer malnutrition (12,20–23). In animals bearing a mammary adenocarcinoma (AC33) for 18 days, decreased adipose tissue lipoprotein lipase activity was observed together with a decrease in fat cell size but not number, and a decrease in serum insulin levels compared to non-tumor-bearing control animals consuming similar amounts of food (24). Increased serum free fatty acids, cholesterol, and triglycerides were observed consistent with the decrease in lipoprotein lipase activity.

Tumor necrosis factor/cachectin (TNF) is a 17,000 m.w. protein secreted by macrophages in response to infection which has been implicated as a mediator of tumor necrosis and cachexia (25). In cell culture studies, TNF has been shown to inhibit the transcription of a number of enzymes promoting lipogenesis in adipocytes, including lipoprotein lipase (26). In fact, the inhibition of LPL activity in cultured 3T3L1 cells has been used as a bioassay for TNF (27). Circulating TNF has been detected in some but not all cancer patients by radioimmunoassay (28), and its presence has not been correlated with weight loss. As a cytokine, it is likely that it is produced locally by macrophages near a tumor or infection and may not always be found in the circulation secondary to its rapid metabolic clearance rate.

In vitro studies of the mechanism of action of megestrol acetate have demonstrated that this agent can induce differentiation of 3T3L1 fibroblasts to adipocytes when combined with insulin, fetal bovine serum, and methylisobutylxanthine as a substitute for dexamethasone (29). These studies monitored the morphologic accumulation of lipid and the activity of glycerol-3-phosphate dehydrogenase, a specific and sensitive indicator of lipogenesis. In other studies, fibroblast transformation to adipocytes has been shown to be accompanied by increases in other enzymes concerned with fat synthesis, including ATP:citrate lyase, fatty acid synthase, and lipoprotein lipase.

Adipose tissue lipoprotein lipase hydrolyzes the core of triglyceride-rich lipoproteins into free fatty acids and monoacylglycerol (30). These fatty acids are the major source of substrate for adipocyte triglyceride synthesis, because adipocytes synthesize very small amounts of fatty acids *de novo* (31).

PHARMACOLOGIC INTERVENTIONS TO TREAT CACHEXIA

Hydrazine sulfate is an inhibitor of phosphoenolpyruvate carboxykinase, the key enzyme in gluconeogenesis. When a group of non-small-cell lung cancer patients were treated with hydrazine sulfate in a placebo-controlled, randomized fashion, both whole body glucose production and whole body protein breakdown decreased together (32). These results suggest that the increased glucose production observed in non-small-cell lung cancer may increase protein breakdown to obtain glucogenic amino acids. Despite this measurable tendency toward normalization of the intermediary metabolism, patients treated with hydrazine sulfate only demonstrated a statistical tendency to maintain weight, but no demonstrable weight gain (33).

In separate studies, male cancer patients were found to be hypogonadal (34). When non-small-cell lung cancer patients were treated with anabolic androgens, only a tendency toward weight maintenance was observed (35).

Abnormalities of insulin action and metabolism have also been observed (36), and in animals insulin administration has been found to reverse cachexia (37). The assessment of insulin action is complex, and in a separate study of patients with head and neck cancer, we are attempting to quantitate the effects of abnormalities of insulin action or metabolism on glucose metabolism in cancer cachexia.

Abnormalities in LPL are present in numerous metabolic disorders other than cancer cachexia. In obesity there is increased adipose tissue LPL when expressed as activity per cell (38,39), suggesting that this enzyme may play a role in the accumulation of excess body fat by stimulating delivery of free fatty acids to adipose tissue for lipid synthesis. Deficiencies in LPL are noted in renal failure (40), diabetes mellitus (41), and hypertriglyceridemia and are similar to that noted with cancer malnutrition.

Administration of recombinant human TNF has resulted in multiple systemic effects, including elevated oxygen consumption, temperature, whole body protein breakdown, increased glucose production, and increased serum triglycerides (42,43). Several groups are studying the potential role of TNF in cancer cachexia. *In vitro* studies have shown that TNF-mediated suppression of lipogenic enzymes in mouse 3T3L1 adipocytes is not reversed by exposure to megestrol acetate (29), but the clinical observation of increased body fat suggests that these observations may not pertain to humans. In fact, in recent studies Kern and coworkers have demonstrated that, in contrast to the suppressive effects of TNF on mouse fibroblast LPL activity, there was no inhibition by human TNF of LPL activity in primary cultures of human adipocytes (44). These more recent findings are supportive of the observations in cancer and AIDS patients to date of weight gain and increased fat mass after treatment with megestrol acetate.

SUMMARY

Malnutrition is a common complication of cancer that affects both morbidity and mortality. Because the occurrence of cancer is much more common in the elderly, some knowledge of the pathophysiology, manifestations, and potential treatments being developed for this serious complication of many common forms of cancer is important for any health care professionals concerned with nutrition in the elderly. It is also possible that some of the lessons learned may be applied to malnutrition occurring in other chronic diseases in the elderly. In both groups of elderly, simple administration of calories alone does not appear to be predictably effective for the treatment of malnutrition. An improved understanding of pathophysiology and the development of effective pharmacologic means to deal with this problem may ultimately lead to practical solutions.

REFERENCES

1. Miller DG. *Cancer* 1980;46:1307–1318.
2. Doll R. *J Roy Stat Soc* 1971;134–155.
3. Kelsey JL. *Epidemiol Rev* 1979;1:74–109.

4. Devita VT, Hellman S, Rosenberg SA, eds. *Cancer principles and practice of oncology.* Philadelphia: JB Lippincott Co, 1986;16.
5. Nixon DW, Heymsfield SB, Cohen AE, et al. *Am J Med* 1980;68:683–690.
6. Shils ME. *Cancer Res* 1977;37:2366–2372.
7. Brennan MR. *Cancer Res* 1977;37:2359–2364.
8. Heber D, Byerley LO, Chi J, Grosvenor M, Bergman RN, Coleman M, Chlebowski RT. *Cancer Res* 1986;58:1867–1873.
9. Nixon D, Rudman D, Heymsfield SB. *Am Assoc Cancer Res Abstr* 1978;698.
10. Tchekmedyian NS, Tait N, Aisner J. *Semin Oncol* 1986;13:20–25.
11. Von Roenn JH, Murphy RL, Weber KM, Williams LM. *Ann Intern Med* 1988;109:840–841.
12. Vlassara H, Spiegel RJ, Doval S, Cerami A. *Hormon Metab Res* 1986;18:698–703.
13. Warren S. *Am J Med Sci* 1932;184:610–615.
14. Terepka AR, Waterhouse C. *Am J Med* 20:225–228.
15. Fenninger LD, Mider GB. *Adv Cancer Res* 1954;2:229–253.
16. Young VR. *Cancer Res* 1977;37:2336–2341.
17. Heber D, Byerley LO, Chlebowski RT. *Cancer* 1985;55:225–229.
18. Chlebowski RT, Heber D. *Surg Clin North Am* 1986;66:957–969.
19. Tayek JA, Heber D, Chlebowski RT. *Lancet* 1987;2:241–244.
20. Mays T. *J Surg Oncol* 1971;3:487–499.
21. Axelrod L, Costa G. *Nutr Cancer* 1980;2:81–83.
22. Costa G. *Cancer Res* 1977;37:2327–2335.
23. Weinhouse S. *Adv Cancer Res* 1955;3:269–325.
24. Lanza-Jacoby S, Lansey SC, Miller EE, Cleary MP. *Cancer Res* 1984;44:5062–5067.
25. Beutler BA, Milsark IW, Cerami A. *J Immunol* 1985;135:3972–3977.
26. Torti F, Dieckmann B, Beutler B, et al. *Science* 1985;229:867–869.
27. Beutler B, Mahoney J, Le Trang N, Pekala P, Cerami A. *J Exp Med* 1985;161:984–995.
28. Aderha D, Fisher S, Levo Y, Holtmann H, Hahn T, Wallach D. *Lancet* 1985;2:1190.
29. Hamburger AW, Parnes H, Gordon GB, Shantz LM, O'Donnell KA, Aisner J. *Semin Oncol* 1988;15:76–78.
30. Robinson DS. In: Florkin M, Stotz EM, eds. *Comprehensive Biochemistry,* vol 18. Amsterdam: Elsevier/North-Holland Biomedical Press, 51.
31. Taskinen MR, Nikkila EA. *Acta Med Scand* 1977;202:399–408.
32. Heber D, Chlebowski RT, Ishibashi DE, Herrold JN, Block JB. *Cancer Res* 1982;42:4815–4819.
33. Chlebowski RT, Heber D, Richardson B, Block JB. *Cancer Res* 1984;44:857–861.
34. Chlebowski RT, Heber D. *Cancer Res* 1982;42:2495–2497.
35. Chlebowski RT, Herrold J, Oktay E, Chlebowski J, Ponce D, Heber D, Block JB. *Cancer* 1986;58:183–186.
36. Byerley LO, Chi J, Grosvenor M, Bergman RN, Chlebowski RT, Heber D. *Fed Proc* 1986;45:1078.
37. Moley JF, Morrison SD, Norton JA. *Cancer Res* 1985;45:4925–4931.
38. Schwartz RA, Brunzell JD. *J Clin Invest* 1981;67:1425.
39. Yost TJ, Eckel RH. *Clin Res* 1987;35:520A.
40. Goldberg A, Sherrard DJ, Brunzell JD. *J Clin Endocrinol Metab* 1978;47:1173.
41. Taskinen MR, Nikkila EA. *Diabetologia* 1979;17:351.
42. Warren RS, Jeevanandam M, Brennan MF. *J Surg Res* 1987;42:43.
43. Starnes HF, Warren RS, Jeevanandam M, Gabrilove JL, Larchian W, Oettgen HF, Brennan MF. *J Clin Invest* 1988;82:1–5.
44. Kern PA. *J Lipid Res* 1988;29:909–914.

Geriatric Nutrition, edited by John E. Morley,
Zvi Glick, Laurence Z. Rubenstein.
Raven Press, Ltd., New York © 1990.

24

Cardiac Cachexia

Martin J. Gorbien

*Section of Geriatric Medicine, The
Cleveland Clinic Foundation, Cleveland, Ohio 44195*

A clear understanding of the entity of cardiac cachexia has eluded medical practitioners and research scientists for some time. One should consider the clinical condition of cardiac cachexia when congestive heart failure exists concomitantly with weight loss, anorexia, cardiomegaly, malabsorption and a protein-losing enteropathy. Despite an awareness of this syndrome that dates to ancient times, a unifying explanation is still missing. Neither sophisticated investigational techniques and nutritional therapies nor a modern pharmacopeia and advanced cardiothoraciac procedures have provided a comprehensive understanding of the subject. Existing prevalence data are based on small series of patients, and comorbidity among elderly populations confounds attempts to clarify current estimates, which are likely outdated. Modern-day physicians continue to rely on anecdotal experiences with such patients.

The number of patients suffering from cardiac cachexia in the United States is probably diminishing, in part, because of a decreasing prevalence of valvular heart disease and ever-improving treatment for chronic congestive heart failure (CHF). Nevertheless, CHF remains a serious and common problem for elderly populations. In reviewing disability and function in elderly patients with heart disease, we are reminded of the heterogeneity of the population; decreased exertional capacity does not necessarily produce severe impairment of functional status (1). Information from the Framingham Disability Study illustrates the predictive significance of certain cardiovascular risk factors, such as hypertension, for disability (2). Hypertensive heart disease is a common cause of CHF. The coexisting burden of age and heart disease can, of course, result in significant functional impairment. In cardiac patients over the age of 95, 85% of men and 50% of women are known to be suffering from disease-related limitations (3). Yet, Pearlman and Uhlman (4) point out that elderly patients with chronic heart disease caused by atherosclerosis or hypertension frequently rate their quality of life as good as average or even better than that of individuals their age. In contrast, the physicians' rating of their patients' quality of life tends to be significantly worse than the perception held by the patient.

Despite the often-stoic nature of patients with chronic cardiac disease, chronic CHF remains a common sequela of ischemic, valvular, and hypertensive heart disease. Over 400,000 new cases of CHF are diagnosed annually with a commensurate rise in hospitalizations due to CHF (5). Additional information from the Framingham study reveals that, within 5 years of the diagnosis of CHF, 62% of men and 42% of women had died (6).

Hippocrates described cardiac cachexia as "dropsy" in the fifth century B.C.; "the flesh is consumed and becomes water, . . . the abdomen fills with water, the feet and legs swell, the shoulders, clavicles, chest, and thighs melt away." In describing patients with CHF and cirrhosis, he wrote, "The whole body is edematous; in the same day at sometime he may appear better while at others he is suffering acutely and may be on the verge of dying" (8).

Recently, Ansari (9) reviewed the syndrome of cardiac cachexia. He describes a typical patient as being a woman in the fifth to ninth decade with a history of rheumatic valvular heart disease. Nevertheless, patients with cardiac cachexia are a diverse group of individuals with heart failure (often severe right-sided failure) accompanied by weight loss. Both body fat and lean body weight are lost. Quinn (10) describes two types of cardiac cachexia. In "classic" cardiac cachexia, malnutrition develops in the face of CHF that has existed for many months. In contrast, the acute or "nosocomial" type may develop in cardiac patients postoperatively because of their inability to ingest sufficient protein and calories. Clearly, there is a marked overlap between the two groups.

When malnutrition and chronic CHF coexist, a work-up targeting the nutritional deficit should be completed while the cardiac issues are being studied. One must keep in mind the social, psychologic, and physical factors that may result in anorexia in elderly people and may be closely interwoven with the pathophysiology of the specific disease state. Body weight may be 15 to 20% below ideal standards. In elderly patients, age-adjusted height-weight tables should be consulted while noting the possibility that peripheral edema and/or ascites may confound interpretation (11). Measurement of triceps skinfold thickness and midarm muscle circumference is helpful in elderly patients and will be less than 60 to 70% of normal in cases of cardiac cachexia (9,12). When these two measurements are low, there is a decreased likelihood that the associated water retention is responsible for the change. Hypoproteinemia, hypoalbuminemia, and low serum transferrin may be seen, depending on the duration or severity of the condition. Patients may be anergic as reflected by skin testing. However, anergy may not be related to malnutrition, but rather to the underlying disease process or to aging *per se*. A chest x-ray may reveal cardiomegaly and, in certain cases, pulmonary venous congestion.

TABLE 1. *Proposed factors in the pathogenesis of cardiac cachexia*

Generalized cellular hypoxia
Decreased caloric intake
  Anorexia due to gastric and hepatic congestion
  Depression
Decreased calorie assimilation
  Malabsorption due to small bowel congestion
  Nephrotic syndrome
  Protein-losing enteropathy
Increased calorie expenditure
  Increased myocardial oxygen consumption
  Increased work of breathing
  Increased metabolic rate
  Low-grade fever
Iatrogenic factors
  Excessive and rigid restriction of salt and water intake
  Aggressive use of diuretics
  Cardiac glycoside excess
  Therapeutic phlebotomy, thoracentesis, and paracentesis

From Ansari, ref. 9.

PATHOGENESIS OF CARDIAC CACHEXIA (TABLE 1)

In their 1964 landmark review of cardiac cachexia, Pittman and Cohen (13) examined the existing thinking on the pathogenesis of the syndrome. Anorexia, malabsorption, hypermetabolism, and iatrogenic factors were considered to be the significant causative factors. In contrast, they felt that cellular hypoxia was of essential importance to the mechanism of cardiac cachexia. The addition of this important but inconclusive concept was based on the biochemical consequences of the "stagnant anoxia" or large oxygen debt that was thought to exist in CHF. Extrapolating information from arterial and mixed venous hypoxia and low oxygen saturation, Pittman and Cohen argued that incomplete and inefficient intermediate metabolism led to elevation of pyruvate and lactate levels. They speculated that a persistent myocardial insult with subsequent hypoxia would trigger the metabolic cascade that would result in changes in various stages of carbohydrate metabolism. These alterations would lead to the proposed changes at the peripheral level. A variety of measurements led them to believe that cellular hypoxia was the cause of the catabolic process.

The work of Krasnow et al. (14) suggested that serum pyruvate and lactate as measures of intracellular events be used with caution because of their possibly remote sensitivity to such metabolic activity. Despite a thorough appreciation of other contributing factors, they felt that the biochemical consequences of cellular hypoxia were primarily responsible for the genesis of cardiac cachexia.

Payne and Peters (15) studied serum proteins in 24 patients with varying degrees of CHF, which they classify as a wasting disease. They found that serum albumin is frequently reduced in patients with CHF and that, although edema can occur with varying levels of serum proteins, it tends to be seen with lower serum albumin. They felt that hypoalbuminemia is directly related to malnutrition in these patients. The authors (15) concluded from their modest study that the "histories leave no doubt that anorexia is the chief cause of malnutrition, with nausea and vomiting frequently acting as contributing factors."

In a study of six patients with cardiac cachexia, Jaenike and Waterhouse (16) studied nitrogen balance, fluid distribution, and clinical course. The patients had varying degrees of CHF, and consistently the excess fluid was extracellular. They found that nitrogen balance was most closely a function of dietary intake. Interestingly, they observed that alterations in nitrogen potassium balance are more likely related to chronic disease, rather than specifically to CHF.

In an attempt to evaluate gastrointestinal (GI) absorption, anorexia, and cellular hypoxia, Buchanan et al. (17) studied 11 young black patients with rheumatic heart (mitral valve) disease and cardiac cachexia. All patients were New York Heart Association (NYHA) Class IV and were treated with digoxin, furosemide, and potassium. D-xylose studies, arterial blood gases, blood lactate and pyruvate, serum albumin, and bilirubin levels were completed. In this undertaking the authors wished to see if they could isolate a factor for malnutrition in a small but homogeneous study population. They found essentially no evidence of malabsorption or cellular hypoxia as measured in this very indirect way. In all patients the preoperative nutritional status was poor and was thought to be a reflection of anorexia. They concurred with the 1932 conclusion of Payne and Peters, once again citing anorexia as the chief cause of malnutrition.

In another study, 11 subjects, 5 of whom were hypoproteinemic, were evaluated for jejunal absorption of an amino acid mixture (18). Two of the 5 hypoproteinemic patients had cardiac failure, and 10 of 11 patients had generalized edema. Using a closed jejunal loop system it was revealed that the hypoproteinemic subjects absorbed 27.9% of the nitrogen available versus 36.8% in the normal subjects (18).

Davidson (19) examined four patients with chronic CHF and hypoproteinemia. Radioactive-labeled isotope studies revealed a protein-losing gastroenteropathy in all four patients. From the design of this study one cannot infer a mechanism for the development of the deficit. A common theory is that increased venous pressure in patients with CHF results in the excessive filtration of fluid from the capillaries and local edema of the intestinal wall, causing a flux of proteins.

In a study of 20 patients with CHF, fat absorption was evaluated by measuring fecal I-131-labeled triolein after an oral dose of the isotope in arachis oil (20). Five of the 20 patients had evidence of fat malabsorption with the suspicion of false-normal triolein tests when compared to conventional fecal fat measurements. Mayer and Schomerus (21) investigated synthesis rates of albumin and fibrinogen in patients with cardiac and pulmonary cachexia. Based on their study of five patients, they concluded that the liver is able to maintain normal or increased rates of protein synthesis in the face of significant protein loss.

We studied a number of nutritional parameters in young and old cardiac patients. Looking at lymphocyte counts, serum albumin, percent ideal body weight, skinfold measurements, and midarm muscle circumference we were able to compare nutritional status in different age groups. Not only did we find that the prevalence of malnutrition is very low, but we also saw little difference among the young and old subjects (Gorbien & Morley, unpublished data).

Drugs and Anorexia

The complicated issue of appetite loss in aging patients is frequently encountered by those involved in the care of the elderly. Anorexia in the elderly is in many ways a paradigm for geriatric medicine in that its etiology may be quite simple or esoteric, yet its impact is always of great clinical importance. Morley and Silver (7) present an extensive list of reasons for anorexia in the elderly, which includes the issues of functional status that are related not only to various disease states and mood but also to the various neurochemical pathways involved.

Dietary restrictions for patients with CHF often result in meals that are unappetizing. In addition, patients may develop electrolyte imbalances while on diuretic therapy and severe salt and water restriction. In fact, when such individuals are on maximal therapy and begin to retain fluid they experience the "sodium dilution syndrome." In a 1964 study, five patients with intractable heart failure were put on a 5- to 7-day fast. Three of the five patients showed marked improvement in their symptoms of congestive heart failure (22).

Over the last 40 years, digoxin has been incriminated in the pathogenesias of cardiac cachexia. Even though new and effective agents for preload and afterload reduction may have resulted in less utilization and smaller doses of digoxin and diuretics, modern agents still carry the risk of appetite loss for elderly patients. The frequency of this response may be low or idiosyncratic, but suspicion levels should nevertheless remain high.

Digoxin is well known for its GI side effects. It is important to remember that patients with CHF receiving digoxin will likely have other possible causes of anorexia, such as metabolic disturbances and polypharmacy. Anorexia due to digoxin has been reported to be dramatic and insidious (23). Even if appetite loss is not a complaint of the patient, the desire for food may dramatically reappear soon after withdrawal of the agent. This effect may be caused by removal of the anorexigenic effect of the cardiac glycoside or the proposed myocardial depression that may result in catabolism and malabsorption (24).

In Pittman and Cohen's (13) review, they discuss the effect of cardiac glycosides on myocardial membrane transport, which they feel to be of fundamental importance. They attribute the GI effects of digitalis to its inhibitory action on amino acid and sugar transport, which may subsequently affect intestinal absorption. The cardiac glycosides also have vasoconstrictive properties at cellular and subcellular levels. They note that ouabain results in decreased amino acid transport in rodent diaphragms. However, myocardial amino acid transport and kinetics were studied in great detail by Lesch et al. (25) in 1970 who concluded that ouabain inhibits alpha-aminoisobutyric acid at high concentrations, such as 10^{-5}M. This level is extremely high and exceeds the concentration that would be seen in clinical use.

When digitalis was still commonly used, nausea and anorexia were sometimes reported in 80% of patients receiving therapy (26). Despite newer preparations, digitalis toxicity remains quite common, with estimates ranging from 5 to 15% of hospitalized individuals receiving the drug. It is now understood that the nausea, vomiting, and loss of appetite caused by digoxin are usually mediated by chemoreceptors in the medulla. Too, many drugs interact with digoxin, and such agents as quinidine, verapamil, and amiodarone can raise the serum digoxin level (27).

We studied approximately 100 patients with NYHA Class II and III disease. As part of a larger study we examined the relationship between the use of digoxin and anorexia, early satiety, nausea, and vomiting. Of the 33% of patients receiving digoxin, very few had any of the four complaints listed above (Gorbien & Morley, unpublished data). Not only were symptoms of digoxin toxicity quite rare, alterations in appetite were similarly uncommon in patients with long-standing congestive heart failure.

As mentioned previously, newer agents have offered more flexibility in the treatment of heart failure (28,29). The newer and more sophisticated modalities with which we can study cardiac contractility will help us define the patient population that can truly benefit from digoxin therapy and will make it easier to withdraw therapy in patients who had been receiving digoxin for vague indications (30). Although morbidity and mortality rates (26) vary dramatically, we continue to consider digoxin an important agent in carefully selected patients.

Diuretics may cause anorexia by inducing zinc loss in the urine. The effect of calcium channel antagonists on appetite has been poorly studied. However, animal studies do suggest that calcium is necessary for feeding to occur. Similarly, angiotensin-converting enzyme inhibitors also alter the degradation of a number of endogenous neuropeptides, including the endorphins, which have been implicated in appetite regulation. There is a need for careful evaluation of the effects of some of the newer cardiac drugs on appetite. This is particularly true in *the elderly,* who are more prone to exhibit drug-induced side effects.

In addition to drugs, patients with cardiac cachexia may have anorexia secondary to generalized fatigue and malaise; feelings of abdominal bloating related to hepatosplenomegaly, ascites, and/or edema of the stomach wall; and dyspnea during eating. Patients with atherosclerotic heart disease may have abdominal angina that can present as early satiety.

MANAGEMENT OF CARDIAC CACHEXIA

Because of the insidious onset of cardiac cachexia and malnutrition in general, often patients are unfortunately recognized at a point where the syndrome is far advanced. Table 2 lists a number of diagnostic criteria to be considered.

The controversy regarding the treatment of cardiac cachexia centers around the nature of nutritional therapies, rather than the therapeutic modalities related to the treatment of the underlying cardiac disease. Clearly, the choices of interventions are growing and include pharmacologic, surgical, and invasive procedures, eg, valvuloplasty, angioplasty.

Much of the available information regarding the nutritional support of malnourished individuals with cardiac disease comes from the surgical literature. Refeeding starving patients is known to be associated with highly significant morbidity and mortality. An interesting study by Abel et al. (31) is one of several reports to recognize that, even though nourished and malnourished patients have dissimilar postoperative courses, postoperative hyperalimentation did not have a significant effect on morbidity and mortality in the malnourished group. Furthermore, the authors speculate that 1 in 15 patients in a surgical intensive care unit has "nosocomial" cardiac cachexia.

TABLE 2. *Diagnostic criteria of cardiac cachexia*

Chronic congestive heart failure—often biventricular (with a history of valvular heart
    disease)
Deficient nutritional status
  Serum albumin
  Serum total protein
  Total lymphocyte count
  Anergic to skin testing
  Decrease in midarm circumference
  Decrease in triceps or subscapular skinfold thickness
Supporting information regarding cardiac status that is often derived from
  Electrocardiogram
  Chest x-ray
  Nuclear scan
  Cardiac catheterization

Adapted with modification from Ansari, ref. 9.

In a study of 350 hospitalized patients, it was found that 50 patients with cardiac disease had severe protein-calorie malnutrition. Of this group 28% were in NYHA Class III and IV. The study points out that undernourished patients can be identified with ease, but nevertheless the results of hyper-alimentation were ambiguous and not very promising (32). The mortality rates in Abel's (31) study were 0% in well-nourished patients and 16% in malnourished patients undergoing cardiac surgery. However, there are little data to suggest that delaying cardiac surgery for the purpose of repletion is helpful (33). The amounts of fluid necessary for total parenteral nutrition are great and particularly hazardous for this population of patients.

Clearly, the goal of treatment in cardiac cachexia is to achieve positive nitrogen balance through the route of refeeding that is determined to be saf-est for the particular patient. Refeeding, of course, must be carried out in concert with the treatment of the condition that is responsible for the chronic CHF.

CONCLUSION

We must assiduously search for cases of anorexia and malnutrition in older individuals, particularly as nutritional disorders can present atypically or be masked by coexisting medical illness, such as CHF. The multiple etiol-ogies for cardiac cachexia must be kept in mind as they have been elusive over the years. Of course, prudent evaluation of drug doses, dosing sched-ules, and drug combinations is of particular importance in these patients.

The example of developing nations provides, at least qualitatively, infor-mation regarding the burden of malnutrition and heart disease. The conse-quence of these entities observed in young black South Africans is likely not very different from that seen in older patients in industrialized countries. Cardiac cachexia is a rare syndrome that does not appear to be any more common in old than young subjects. The incidence of cardiac cachexia may be decreasing because of better detection and treatment of heart failure dis-ease. However, we should continue to vigilantly watch for that syndrome that Hippocrates described so well so many centuries ago.

REFERENCES

1. Neill WA, Branch LG, DeJong G, et al. *Arch Intern Med* 1985;145:1642–1647.
2. Pinsky JL, Branch LG, Jette AM, et al. *Am J Epidemiol* 1988;122:644–656.
3. Feinleib M, Gillum RF. In: Wegner NK, Farberg CD, Pitt E, eds. *Coronary heart dis-ease in the elderly.* New York: Elsevier, 1986;25–29.
4. Pearlman RA, Uhlman RF. *Qual Life Cardiovasc Care* 1986;2:142–158.
5. Furberg CD, Yusuf S. *Am J Cardiol* 1985;55:1110–1113.
6. McKee PA, Castelli WP, McNamara PM, et al. *N Engl J Med* 1971;285:1441–1446.
7. Morley JE, Silver AJ. *Neurobiol Aging* 1988;9:9–16.

8. Katz AM, Katz PB. *Br Heart J* 1962;24:256–264.
9. Ansari A. *Progr Cardiovascular Dis* 1987;30:45–60.
10. Quinn T, Ashkanaz J. *Crit Care Clin* 1987;3:167–184.
11. Master AM, Lasser RP, Beckman G. *JAMA* 1960;172:658–662.
12. Morley JE, Silver AJ, Fiatarone M, Mooradian AD. *J Am Geriatr Soc* 1986;34:823–832.
13. Pittman JG, Cohen P. *N Engl J Med* 1964;271:403–409.
14. Krasnow N, Neill WA, Messer JV, Gorlin R. *J Clin Invest* 1962;41:2075–2085.
15. Payne SA, Peters JP. *J Clin Invest* 1932;11:103–112.
16. Jaenike JR, Waterhouse C. *J Lab Clin Med* 1958;52:384–393.
17. Buchanan N, Cane RD, Kinsley R, Eyberg CD. *Intens Care Med* 1977;3:89–91.
18. Hardy J, Schultz J. *J Applied Physiol* 1952;4:789–792.
19. Davidson JD, Waldman TA, Goodman DS, Gordon RS. *Lancet* 1961;1:899–902.
20. Jones RV. *Br Med J* 1961;1:1276–1278.
21. Mayer G, Schomerus H. *Acta Hepatogastroenterol* 1976;24:82–85.
22. Merrill AJ. *Am Heart J* 1964;433–436.
23. Anorexia [editorial]. *Br Med J* 1974;5932:639–640.
24. Banks T, Ali N. *N Engl J Med* 1974;291:746.
25. Lesch M, Borlin R, Sonnenblick H. *Circ Res* 1970;28:445–458.
26. Lely AH, van Enter CHJ. *Am Heart J* 1972;83:149–152.
27. Smith TW. *N Engl J Med* 1988;318:358–365.
28. The Captopril-Digoxin Multicenter Research Group. *JAMA* 1986;259:539–544.
29. Guyatt GH, Sullivan MJ, Fallen EL. *Am J Cardiol* 1988;61:371–375.
30. Sueta CA, Carey TS, Burnett CK. *Arch Intern Med* 1989;149:609–612.
31. Abel RM, Fischer JE, Buckley MJ, et al. *Arch Surg* 1976;111:45–50.
32. Blackburn GL, Gibbon GW, Bathe A, et al. *J Thoracic Cardiovasc Surg* 1977;73:489–496.
33. Gibbons GW, Blackburn GL, Harken DE, et al. *J Surg Res* 1976;20:439–444.

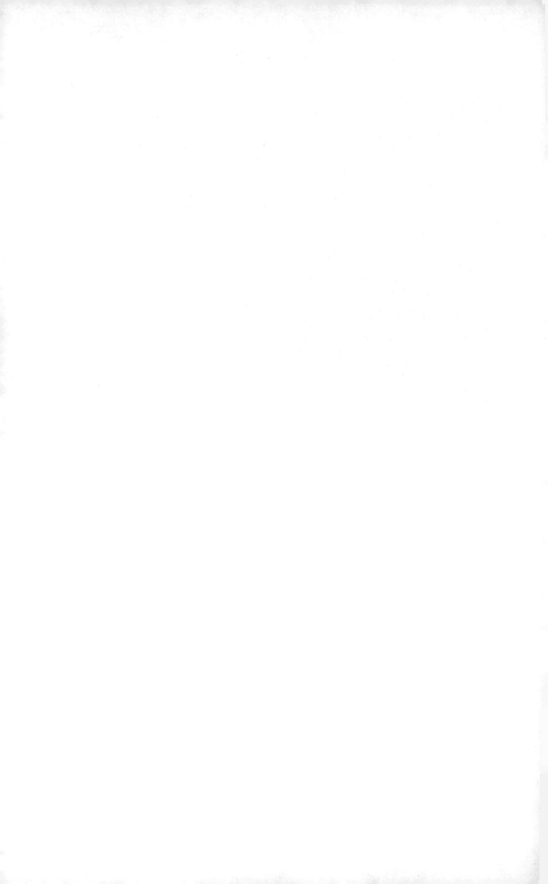

Geriatric Nutrition, edited by John E. Morley,
Zvi Glick, Laurence Z. Rubenstein.
Raven Press, Ltd., New York © 1990.

25

Epidemiology of Malnutrition in Nursing Homes

Daniel Rudman, Vasu D. Arora, Axel G. Feller,
Hoskote S. Nagraj, Parde Y. Lalitha, and Norma P. Caindec

*Medical Service, VA Medical Center, Milwaukee, Wisconsin 53295,
Department of Medicine, The Medical College of Wisconsin,
Milwaukee, Wisconsin 53295, and The Medical and Dietetic Services
VA Medical Center, North Chicago, Illinois 60064*

There are approximately 20,000 nursing homes in the United States, representing 50% more bed capacity than the acute hospitals in this nation. Within the nursing homes reside about 1.5 million Americans over 65 years old, who represent 5% of the elderly population. It is projected that 20% of Americans who reach the age of 65 will experience nursing home life before their demise.

In the 20th century, socioeconomic improvements have largely eliminated nutritional deficiencies in the general American population. It comes as a surprise, therefore, that the nursing home population is now recognized as a major reservoir of undernutrition.

The objectives of this chapter are to describe the prevalence of protein-calorie undernutrition in the nursing home population, its causes and consequences, and to suggest measures to alleviate this nutritional deficiency state.

DEMOGRAPHY

With declining birth rates, a favorable economic climate, and improved treatment of the medical problems of late adulthood, the elderly population of the United States is expanding at the most rapid rate of any age group. By the year 2000, 1 in every 8 Americans will be over 65 years old. By contrast, in 1900 only 1 in 25 Americans was over 65. Current usage defines elderly persons as 65 and older (65+). Categories of the elderly are the "young old" who are 65 to 74, the "old old" who are 75 to 84 years of age, and the "oldest old" who are 85 and over (1).

The elderly population is more heterogeneous than the younger age seg-

TABLE 1. *Elderly population in the United States, 1987*

Category	Location	Approximate number (million)
Total		25
Fully independent	Community	14
Impaired independent	Community	6
Dependent ("homebound")	Community[a]	3–4
Dependent	Nursing homes	1.4

[a]Includes sheltered residences.

ment of the population. This heterogeneity is reflected not only in the 3.5 decade age span but also in numerous other attributes affecting their health: marital status, social support system, finances, place of residence, number of continuing drugs, number of chronic illnesses, and ability to perform independently activities of daily living (2,3). Three main dimensions of heterogeneity—residence, function, and state of health—are depicted in Tables 1 and 2.

In the two decades after World War II, comments appeared frequently in the literature concerning nutritional problems of the elderly population. The resulting concern led to a series of systematic surveys of the nutritional status of older Americans. Two strategies were used. Some investigators focused on the nutritional intakes of the study groups as measured by diet recall or diet diary. Other observers measured the anthropometric and biochemical indicators of nutritional status.

Surveys of the Healthy Elderly Population

When the study group was a random sample of the entire elderly population, with its wide range of clinical conditions, the resulting data understand-

TABLE 2. *Classification of the elderly according to residence, functional status, and medical condition*

Category	Place of residence	Subcategory	Degree of dependence	Physical impairment	One or more chronic diseases
	Community	a	None	0	0
	Community	b	None	0	+
A	Community	c	None	+	+
	Community	d	Partial	+	+
	Community	e	Total	+	+
B	Sheltered residence	f	None	0	+
	Sheltered residence	g	Partial	+	+
	Long-term care	h	None	0	+
C	Long-term care	i	None	+	+
	Long-term care	j	Partial	+	+
	Long-term care	k	Total	+	+

ably portrayed great variability in nutritional status. A more coherent picture, however, was provided by surveys on more sharply defined elderly subgroups.

Table 3 summarizes surveys of the independent community elderly (4–11). In about one-third of the subjects, energy intake was below the recommended daily allowance (RDA). Body weight, adipose mass, and muscle mass, however, were rarely depleted, and protein intake was generally adequate. The consumptions of minerals and vitamins were below the RDA in up to 50% of subjects, and the blood levels were subnormal in 10 to 30%. The interpretation of these findings is as follows. The diminishing energy expenditure of the elderly leads to a lower energy requirement and therefore a reduced food intake. Unless the nutrient density of the diet is simultaneously increased, subclinical mineral and vitamin deficiencies will tend to occur. Because the American diet tends to be high in protein, however, the intake of protein usually remains adequate even at the lower level of calorie consumption.

Surveys of the Nursing Home Population

The nutritional picture in this subgroup of the American elderly people is less favorable (Table 4) (12–23). Intakes are frequently low for both calories and protein. Thirty to 50% of the residents are substandard in body weight, midarm muscle circumference, and serum albumin level, indicating wide-

TABLE 3. *Nutritional status of the healthy elderly*

	Low intakes (%)	Subnormal nutritional indicators (%)
Calories	29–33	3
Protein	2–15	3
Calcium	37	
Iron		4
Zinc	76	
Vitamin A	11	
Vitamin D	72	15
Ascorbic acid	5	4–24
Thiamine	8	2–5
Riboflavin	4	2–3
Vitamin B_6	85	18
Folate	77	8–9
Niacin	0	13
Vitamin B_{12}	31	3–31
Zinc	76	
Phosphorus	3	
Vitamin E	44	4
Biotin		1
Panthotenic acid		4

From refs. 4–11.

TABLE 4. *Nutritional status of the institutionalized elderly*

	Low intakes (%)	Subnormal nutritional indicators (%)
Calories	5–18	30–66
Protein	0–33	15–60
Calcium	0–54	2
Iron	5–35	10–31
Vitamin A	5–13	0–18
Vitamin D	63–77	48
Ascorbic acid	0–40	0–83
Thiamine	7–30	4–23
Riboflavin	0–34	2
Vitamin B_6	57–100	28–49
Folate	37	7–57
Vitamin B_{12}		0–20
Niacin	0	33
Vitamin E		3–40
Biotin		0
Pantothenic acid		3
Zinc	21	

From refs. 12-23.

spread protein-calorie undernutrition (PCU). Blood levels are frequently low for both water-soluble and fat-soluble vitamins.

We conclude that, despite the federal, state and Veterans Administration regulations designed to ensure adequate nutrition within nursing homes, nutritional deficiencies are common. The prevalence rates vary between institutions, depending on their case mix, especially the proportion of total care cases.

RELATION OF PCU TO MORTALITY RATE IN THE NURSING HOME

The adverse effect of PCU on clinical outcome in the acutely ill general hospital population of all ages has been recognized since the 1970s (24–27). Only recently, however, has the linkage between PCU and death rate in the nursing home been documented. In 1986, Phillips (28) reported a reciprocal correlation of midarm muscle circumference and albumin level to the mortality rate in the nursing home. Dwyer et al. (29) in 1987 reported that the recent loss of weight was a sensitive predictor of death in nursing home residents.

The present authors have conducted an epidemiologic survey during the year 1985 in the 200-bed nursing home of the North Chicago Veterans Administration Medical Center (30–33). At the beginning of the year of surveillance, a 67-item clinical data base was compiled that included diagnoses, drugs, and measures of nutritional, metabolic, hematologic, hepatic, and renal function. Deaths were recorded during the year of observation. We then sought correlations between the items of the annual data base and the mortality rate.

Fifty-five deaths occurred during the year, for which infection was usually the immediate cause (50 cases) and chronic organic brain syndrome was usually the underlying cause (42 cases). Of the 67 attributes in the data base, only 7 were significant predictors of death in the univariate analysis: age, functional level, and five nutrition-related variables: triceps skinfold, mid-arm muscle circumference, albumin, cholesterol, and hematocrit. The decedents were older, more dependent, depleted in adipose and muscle, hypoalbuminemic, and hypocholesterolemic.

For each mortality-related nutritional indicator, there was a threshold at which the risk of death increased (30–33). For albumin, cholesterol, or hematocrit, the threshold occurred within the conventional "normal range." Thus, death rate rose significantly when the albumin concentration declined below 4.0 g/dl, when the cholesterol level declined below 160 mg/dl, or when the hematocrit declined below 41%. Evidently, the "desirable ranges" for nutritional indicators (and perhaps for other clinical tests) in the nursing home elderly are not the same as the normal ranges, which are usually defined as the 95% confidence limits in the general population of overtly healthy adults.

When multivariate analysis was applied to the seven mortality-related variables, the statistical model selected cholesterol first and hematocrit second (34). These analyses demonstrated the dire prognostic significance of a serum cholesterol level below 160 mg/dl in the nursing home.

CAUSES OF PCU IN THE NURSING HOME

Because the prevalence of PCU in our nursing homes (Table 4) is similar to that in many poverty-stricken underdeveloped nations, it behooves us to recall the causes of PCU in the Third World. There, inadequate food intake caused by poverty is compounded by the catabolic effects of repeated infections caused by poor hygiene.

Analogous mechanisms of poor intake and frequent infections operate in the nursing home. In these institutions, food intake is frequently inadequate, although unlike the underdeveloped Third World, proper diets are provided. The causes of nursing home hypophagia are complex (35–48). The psychosocial environment is often below par. Taste, smell, and appetite are often blunted. Many patients are affected by mental confusion, emotional depression, loss of agility in the hands, loss of teeth, and impaired swallowing. For a time, assistance by staff can compensate for these handicaps of the "eating-dependent" individuals, but eventually the dysphagia, anorexia, or both prevent further oral nutrition. Survival then will require force-feeding via a nasogastric tube, gastrostomy tube, or jejunostomy tube. In the authors' nursing home, the proportion of force-fed residents averages 10%.

The struggle of nursing home patients to maintain their dietary intake is compounded by the catabolic effect of repeated infections. The prevalence and incidence of infections in the nursing home population are high (34,35,39,42–44,49–51). The common sites are the respiratory tract, urinary tract, skin, and eye. Point-in-time surveys show a 15 to 30% prevalence of active infection. New episodes of fever and infection occur on the average every 3 months in nursing home residents. Each febrile episode causes hypermetabolism and negative nitrogen balance, lowering the patient to the next level of PCU. The difficulties in eating tend to prevent the convalescent "catch-up hyperphagia," which enables younger unimpaired subjects to replete their body composition after acute wasting illnesses.

INTERVENTION MEASURES

Although it is unlikely that PCU can be eliminated from the nursing home, a series of measures can be proposed to limit the prevalence and severity of the problem.

1. Maintain a surveillance of the nutritional status of each resident. Involuntary weight loss is the most sensitive early warning signal. Body weight <95% of ideal or substandard values for albumin, cholesterol, or hematocrit require intervention. Further work is needed on the threshold values of the latter three variables, which should activate nutritional support intervention measures. The authors' experience suggests that albumin <4.0 g/dl, cholesterol <160 mg/dl, or hematocrit <39% in male nursing home residents warrants attention.
2. Review promptly such cases for correctible dental, medical, or emotional problems or interfering drugs, which could tend to impair nutrition. Modification of the diet, including diet supplements, and provision of adequate eating assistance by dedicated capable staff should be considered.
3. Strive to optimize the physical and psychosocial aspects of the dining areas.
4. Maintain a vigorous anti-infection program. The components are (a) education of staff regarding protection of patients from sources of infection (either staff or patients), including handwashing, environmental sanitation, handling of fomites, sick leave when ill, and health screening of staff; (b) early detection and treatment of acute infections; and (c) vaccination against the pneumococcus and the influenza virus.

ACKNOWLEDGMENTS

This work was supported in part by a grant from the Veterans Administration.

REFERENCES

1. Kane RL, Ouslander JG, Abrass IB. *Essentials of Clinical Geriatrics.* New York: McGraw-Hill, 1984;17–33.
2. Allan CA, Brotman H, comp. *Chartbook on aging in America.* Washington, DC: The 1981 White House Conference on Aging, 1981.
3. Federal Council on the Aging: *The need for long-term care: A Chartbook of the Federal Council on the Aging.* Washington, DC: US Government Printing Office, 1981 (OHDS Publ. No. 81-20704).
4. Baker H, Frank O, Thind IS, Jaslow SP, Louria DB. *J Am Geriatr Soc* 1979;27:444–450.
5. Garry PJ, Goodwin JS, Hunt WC, Gilbert BA. *Am J Clin Nutr* 1982;36:332–339.
6. Garry PJ, Goodwin JS, Hunt WC, Hooper EM, Leonard AG. *Am J Clin Nutr* 1982;36:319–331.
7. Garry PJ, Goodwin JS, Hunt WC. *J Am Geriatr Soc* 1984;32:719–726.
8. Garry PJ, Goodwin JS, Hunt WC. *Am J Clin Nutr* 1982;36:902–909.
9. Morgan DB, Newton HMV, Schorah CJ, Jewitt MA, Hancock MR, Hullin RP. *Age Aging* 1986;15:65–76.
10. Munro HN, McGandy RB, Hartz SC, Russell RM, Jacob RA, Otradovec CL. *Am J Clin Nutr* 1987;46:586–592.
11. Omdahl JL, Garry PJ, Hunsaker LA, Hunt WC, Goodwin JS. *Am J Clin Nutr* 1982;36:1225–1233.
12. Asplund K, Normark M, Pettersson V. *Age Aging* 1981;10:87–94.
13. Chen LH, Fan-Chiang WL. *Int J Vitam Nutr Res* 1981;51:232–238.
14. Hontela S, Vobecky J, Shapcott N, Vobecky JS. *Nutr Rep Int* 1983;27:1101–1111.
15. Justice CL, Howe JM, Clark HE. *J Am Dietet Assoc* 1974;65:639–646.
16. Munice HL, Carbonetto C. *J Fam Pract* 1982;14:1061–1064.
17. Pinchcofsky-Devin GD, Kaminski MV. *J Am Geriatr Soc* 1986;34:435–440.
18. Sandman PO, Adolfsson R, Nygren C, Hallmans G, Winblad B. *J Am Geriatr Soc* 1987;35:31–38.
19. Shaver HJ, Loper JA, Lutes RA. *JPEN* 1980;4:367–370.
20. Smith JL, Wickiser AA, Korth LL, Grandjean AC, Schaefer AE. *J Am Coll Nutr* 1984;3:13–25.
21. Stiedemann M, Jansen C, Harrill I. *J Am Dietet Assoc* 1987;73:132–139.
22. Vincent M, Gibson RS. *Gerontology* 1982;28:245–251.
23. Vir SC, Love AHG. *Am J Clin Nutr* 1979;32:1934–1947.
24. Bistrian BR, et al. *JAMA* 1976;235:1567.
25. Butterworth CE. *Nutr Tod* 1974;9:4.
26. Buzby GP, Mullen JL, Mathews DC, Hobbs CL, Rosato EF. *Am J Surg* 1980;139:160–167.
27. Weinsier RL, Hunker EM, Krumdieck CL, Butterworth CE. *Am J Clin Nutr* 1979;32:418–426.
28. Phillips P. *Age Aging* 1986;15:53–56.
29. Dwyer JT, Coleman KA, Krall E, et al. *J Gerontol* 1987;42:246–251.
30. Rudman D, Feller AG, Nagraj HS, Jackson DL, Rudman IW, Mattson DE. *JPEN* 1987;11:360–363.
31. Rudman D, Mattson DE, Feller AG, Nagraj HS. *JPEN* (in press).
32. Rudman D, Mattson DE, Nagraj HS, Caindec N, Rudman IW, Jackson DL. *J Am Geriatr Soc* 1987;35:496–502.
33. Rudman D, Mattson DE, Nagraj HS, et al. *JPEN* (in press).
34. Nicolle LE, McIntyre M, Zacharias H, MacDonell JA. *J Am Geriatr Soc* 1984;32:513–519.
35. Davies AD, Snaith PA. *Age Aging* 1980;9:100–105.
36. Donner M, Silbiger M. *Am J Med Sci* 1966;251:600–616.
37. Feldman RS, Kapur KK, Alman JE, Chauncey HH. *J Am Geriatr Soc* 1980;28:97–103.
38. Garfinkel PE, Garner DM, Kaplan AS, Rodin G, Kennedy S. *Can Med Assoc J* 1983;129:939–945.
39. Henrikson B, Cate HD. *J Am Dietet Assoc* 1971;59:126–129.

40. Lieberman AN, Horowitz L, Redman P, Pachter L, Lieberman I. *Am J Gastroenterol* 1980;74:157.
41. Linden P, Siebens AA. *Arch Phys Med Rehabil* 1983;64:281–284.
42. MacLennan WJ, Martin P, Mason BJ. *Age Aging* 1975;4:175–180.
43. Miller MB. *Gerontologist* 1971;11:329–336.
44. Nguyen NH, Flint DM, Prinsley DM, Wahlqvist ML. *Hum Nutr Applied Nutr* 1985;39:333–338.
45. Schiffman SS, Covey E. In: Ordy JM, ed. *Nutrition in gerontology*. New York: Raven Press, 1984;43–64.
46. Siebens H, Trupe E, Siebens A, et al. *J Am Geriatr Soc* 1986;34:192–198.
47. Veis SL, Logemann JA. *Arch Phys Med Rehabil* 1985;66:372–375.
48. Wayler AH, Kapur KK, Feldman RS, Chauncey HH. *J Gerontol* 1982;37:294–299.
49. Farber BF, Brennen C, Puntereri AJ, Brody JP. *J Am Geriatr Soc* 1984;32:499–502.
50. Franson TR, Duthie EH, Cooper JV, VanOudenhoven G, Hoffmann RG. *J Am Geriatr Soc* 1986;34:95–100.
51. Garibaldi RA, Brodine S, Matsumiya S. *N Engl J Med* 1981;305:731–735.

Geriatric Nutrition, edited by John E. Morley,
Zvi Glick, Laurence Z. Rubenstein.
Raven Press, Ltd., New York © 1990.

26

Nutrition Management in Nursing Homes

Ann M. Coulston

*General Clinical Research Center, Stanford University Hospital,
Stanford, California 94305*

"We have added years to life; now we must add life to those years"

Author unknown

With the steady increase of persons over 65 years of age and the realization that approximately 5% of that population, 1.5 million persons today, reside in a long-term care or nursing home facility, the public and health care community are concerned about the quality of nutrition services and the nutritional status of nursing home residents (1). The average nursing home resident is more than 80 years old and will be in the institution from 2 to 3 years until transfer to an acute care facility, recovery, or death (2). Older adults move to the nursing home when independent living is no longer possible because of chronic physical or mental illness, loss of home, or impairment of activities of daily living. For example, the recent National Nursing Home Survey indicates that 63% of residents are disoriented or have impaired memory, and 91% require help with bathing (2,3). In reality, most of the elderly residents will live the remainder of their life in this setting.

Most residents have at least one of several chronic conditions that can affect nutritional status (Table 1). However, nursing home residents are a generally clinically stable population, despite considerable chronic disease and drug therapy. A recent review indicated that each patient receives an average of five drugs per day (4). The most frequently prescribed drugs are antihypertensives (especially diuretics), cathartics, and vitamin and mineral supplements.

Elderly persons of the same chronologic age may differ appreciably in functional capacities and health status. Because older adults are a very heterogeneous population, nutritional management of each resident must be individualized and evaluated periodically.

This chapter reviews and discusses three aspects of nutritional care for nursing home residents: food service, nutritional status, and therapeutic dietary needs. A review of the food service system provides information about the meal service and nutritive quality of the food provided. Nutritional sta-

TABLE 1. *Chronic conditions of nursing home residents that can affect nutritional status*

Physical conditions
   Nutrition-related chronic diseases
   Constipation or incontinence
   Poor eyesight or hearing
   Poor dentition, ill-fitting or missing dentures
   Inability to feed self
Psychosociologic conditions
   Psychologic conditions (Alzheimer's disease, depression)
   Confusion due to change in environment
   Anorexia or loss of interest in eating
   Lack of socialization at mealtimes
   Change in long-established food habits and preferences
Medical conditions
   Atherosclerotic heart disease
   Hypertension
   Dementia
   Cerebrovascular accident
   Diabetes mellitus
   Chronic obstructive pulmonary disease
   Neurologic disorders

tus is determined by periodic nutritional assessment and provides an outcome measure of overall nutrition care. Nutritional status reflects not only the food or nutrient intake but also the person's ability to utilize nutrients, which varies with chronic or acute medical and mental disease. Finally, the clinical utility of restrictive therapeutic diets is discussed.

FOOD SERVICE MANAGEMENT

Food service standards for skilled nursing facilities were first published in 1966 by the Federal Conditions of Participation for Skilled Nursing Facilities for participation by Medicare. These standards are currently under review by the Health Care Finance Administration; the final rule was published early in 1989 and is expected to be accepted later in the year (5). Interpretive guidelines and regulations are specified in each state, which must meet the federal rule. Because approximately 90% of nursing homes are Medicare or Medicaid certified, these federal guidelines regulate the majority of food service programs in long-term care facilities.

Meals must provide food of the quality and quantity to meet the Recommended Dietary Allowances (RDA) and individual physician diet orders (6). Not less than three meals must be served, with no more than 14 hours between the evening meal and breakfast. Bedtime nourishments must be offered to all residents unless contraindicated by physician order. Patient food preferences must be adhered to as much as possible and substitutes from the same food group offered for foods refused. For example, in California the daily menu pattern established to meet these guidelines includes two cups of milk; at least 6 oz of lean meat; at least four servings of fruits and vegetables, including a daily choice from a vitamin C rich food and a vitamin A rich food three to four times per week; at least four servings of bread, cereals, or starch foods; and other foods to satisfy caloric requirements (7).

Fiscal constraints have a direct impact on the quality of food and nutrition services. Governmental financial reimbursement for care is determined by a formula, which is adjusted periodically to reflect increased costs. However, the allocation of funds to various services, such as nursing, housekeeping, supplies, and dietary, is left to the discretion of the facility. Because most long-term care facilities are operated for profit, any increase in costs that exceeds the increase in reimbursement usually must be offset by reductions in other expenses, such as food budgets. Inadequate food budgets may result in patient food of lesser quality and potentially marginal nutritional adequacy.

As mentioned earlier, the nutrient standard for the food service is the National Research Council's RDA (6). The most recent edition has one nutrient standard for ages 51 years and older. This is felt by many to be inadequate, and revisions in nutrient standards more in concert with nutrient requirements of older adults have been recommended. The current 9th edition notes that, with the decrease in energy expenditure that accompanies aging and with the consequent reduced caloric requirement, food choices must be made carefully to ensure that amounts of essential nutrients consumed do not fall below desired levels. The smaller quantity of food consumed must be selected carefully to provide the needed amounts of essential nutrients.

Menus of 14 nursing homes in Wisconsin were analyzed for calories, protein, calcium, iron, magnesium, zinc, vitamins A, C, B_6, B_{12}, thiamine, riboflavin, niacin, folic acid, and pantothenic acid (8). None of the nursing homes had a menu plan that met the RDA for both sexes for all nutrients. The most common deficiencies were for magnesium, zinc, vitamin B_6, and folic acid. Given the nutrient density of the menus, a resident would have had to consume more than the recommended caloric requirement to meet the RDA for all nutrients. Changes identified to improve the nutrient density included reducing the amounts of high-calorie, low-nutrient foods and increasing the quantities of such foods as legumes, nuts, bananas, dry cereal, and green leafy vegetables. As a result of this survey, Allington and associates developed a Model Food Plan that would provide 100% of the RDA without exceeding 110% of the RDA for calories (9). The Model Food Plan can be used as a food service management tool to identify quantities and types of foods to be used in menu planning to increase the nutrient level of food served to the residents.

Ideally, food service evaluation should be based upon the nutritional status of residents and go beyond nutrient requirements and the health and safety standards of state and federal regulations.

NUTRITIONAL STATUS OF NURSING HOME RESIDENTS

Despite seemingly appropriate food service standards and regulations for dietary supervision, patients in nursing homes remain at risk for developing malnutrition. For example, only approximately 20% of nursing home residents consume diets below recommended caloric levels, yet up to 50% demonstrate decreased adipose reserves (1). Historically, malnutrition in the elderly has been a complex and poorly understood phenomenon. Nursing home residents generally have a less favorable nutrition profile than age-matched, healthy, independent elderly. For example, an unexplained 34% of healthy nursing home residents were found to be anergic to skin testing as compared to only 17% of healthy, independent-living elderly and 0% of a healthy, younger population (10).

A combination of physiologic and psychosocial factors is involved in determining nutritional status. Standard nutritional assessment parameters include body weight and height, skinfold thickness, arm circumference, serum albumin, serum lymphocyte count, hemoglobin and hematocrit, and skin testing for cell-mediated immunity. These techniques for the assessment of individual nutritional status have been applied to various populations over the past several years (11).

When individual nutritional assessment techniques have been applied to nursing home residents, the incidence of malnutrition varies between 40 and 85%. An earlier study by Shaver et al. (12) found that 85% of residents demonstrated some indication of decreased nutritional status. Forty percent were below weight for height standards, 32% had serum albumin levels below 3.5 mg/dl, and 20% did not react to skin testing. Later, Silver et al. (4) reported that 46% of long-term care residents had body weights that were at least 10% below average body weight. Eighteen percent had albumin levels below 3.5 mg/dl, and 44% were anergic. Pinchcofsky-Devin and Kaminiski found a 52% rate of malnutrition (13). Serum albumin was low in 41%, and 28% were anergic. They also reported a 76% prevalence of anemia and marked decreases in adipose reserves. Sandman and associates reported a 50% prevalence of malnutrition in institutionalized individuals with Alzheimer's disease or multi-infarct dementia (14). In a survey of a rural nursing home, Stephens and associates (15) found that 72% of the residents fulfilled the criteria for the diagnosis of at least mild malnutrition, and 30% had serum albumin levels less than 3.5 mg/dl. Rudman and associates (16) examined nutritional assessment parameters to identify those predictive of mortality. The mortality-related nutritional indicators were age, functional level, adipose reserves, skeletal muscle reserves, serum albumin, low plasma cholesterol concentration, hemoglobin, and hematocrit (see Chapter 15).

The lack of concordant results among investigators may be due to several methodologic factors, including different criteria for the definition of malnutrition. Accepted standards for evaluation of nutritional assessment measurements vary from study to study and have yet to be agreed upon for the elderly. According to the extensive review of nutrition-related laboratory values and the correlation with morbidity in nursing home residents, "desirable ranges" for these parameters cannot be equated with the normal ranges described for healthy, younger adults (1). Only by standardization of a nutritional assessment protocol can results be compared from facility to facility and a true picture of the problem of malnutrition in long-term care facilities be obtained. Nevertheless, it is clear from these and other studies that malnutrition does exist in the nursing home setting, and attention must be paid to correction of this problem.

Despite the seemingly alarming reported incidence of malnutrition, studies that have documented dietary intakes in this population report less startling results. For example, although constipation is a commonly reported problem for nursing home residents, they are reported to be consuming as much dietary fiber as their independent-living peers (18). Sandman et al. (14) reported mean intakes for calories that were significantly higher than calculated energy needs. Most patients had nutrient intakes well above recommended dietary intakes. A dietary intake survey of healthy, institutionalized elderly free of clinically apparent terminal or wasting illness in the Boston area demonstrated that, with the exception of total calories, vitamin B_6, folate, and zinc, mean dietary intakes were above the RDA for both men and women (17).

How can this information be applied to the individual nutritional management of nursing home residents? A major recommendation is the development and implementation of a standardized nutritional risk protocol to identify high-risk patients in all nursing homes. Documentation of the nutritional assessment upon admission to the skilled nursing facility is essential. The author's recommendations are: measurement of height and body weight, triceps skinfold and mid upper arm circumference, serum albumin, total lymphocyte count, hemoglobin and hematocrit, plasma glucose and cholesterol, and skin testing for immunocompetence. Standards for each of these assessment parameters have been outlined in Chapter 6, "Nutritional Assessment of the Elderly."

In the nursing home setting, anthropometric data, specifically height and body weight, are the most accessible and most descriptive parameters of nutritional assessment. These data can be used to evaluate nutrition care, to anticipate nutrition problems, and identify residents at risk to develop nutritional problems. Nursing home regulations in most states require monthly body weights. Height can be more difficult to obtain because many nursing home residents cannot stand erect due to curvature of the spine or do not have the strength to stand for a measurement. Recently, a technique has been validated by which knee height can be used to estimate stature with good accuracy (19).

The more costly laboratory tests can be performed every 6 months or annually. Of course if a patient's diagnostic condition changes, laboratory assessment may be obtained more frequently. Dietary intake evaluation should be recorded in a qualitative manner daily by the nursing staff. A more careful evaluation could be completed in conjunction with the monthly anthropometric evaluation.

There are two main causes of malnutrition: factors that result in inadequate food or nutrient intake and, conditions that cause an increase in nutrient requirements, such as fever, infection, or catabolic illness. A recent examination of nutritional assessment parameters and their correlation with nutritional status revealed that poor appetite and food acceptability, inability to feed self, early weight loss, low total lymphocyte count, increased numbers of infection, age on admission, and admission body weight were most often associated with a decreased nutritional status (20).

One factor that has been related to a decrease in food acceptability is the dentition status of residents. Taste and texture acceptability correlates highly with ease of chewing (21). Not surprisingly, persons with compromised dentition (less than 20 to 26 teeth) avoid hard-to-chew foods. Also, 30 to 80% of residents may be edentulous (22). The recent National Nursing Home Survey reported that 40% of residents require assistance with eating (1). Eating dependency does not correlate with age or weight loss, but with impaired mobility, impaired cognition, and increased mortality (23). To feed an eating-dependent patient properly can take 30 to 45 minutes of personnel time three times per day. So, although the numbers of residents requiring eating assistance are lower than for such activities as bathing, when one considers that eating occurs at least three times per day, the personnel costs are high. Interestingly, those who require assistance at mealtime consume a diet that more closely meets the RDA than do independent residents (24).

Dwyer and associates (25) reviewed the weight records of nursing home residents at admission and at 1 and 2 years later. They calculated a 4-year survival rate based on weight change seen in the first 2 years of residency. Those who gained 4.5 kg or more had the highest survival rate, whereas those who lost 4.5 kg or more the lowest. It is not always possible to prevent weight loss in the case of severe catabolic illness, such as aggressive neoplastic disease, however, weight loss due to circumstances mentioned earlier, which can result in decreased food intake, can be prevented.

Harris et al. (26) studied the relationship of body weight, the using body mass index (kg/m2), at age 65 years and subsequent mortality. Body mass index between 23 and 25 kg/m2 for men and 24 and 26 kg/m2 for women was associated with the lowest relative risk for mortality. In healthy adults, these levels would be considered above the desirable weight range.

DIET THERAPY FOR NUTRITION-RELATED CHRONIC DISEASES

When patients with nutrition-related chronic diseases, such as diabetes, hypertension, or atherosclerotic heart disease, are admitted to long-term care facilities, they are frequently prescribed a "special" or "therapeutic" diet following the acute hospital model. For example, patients with diabetes might be prescribed a calorie-controlled diet or a "no concentrated sweets" diet, those with hypertension or heart disease might be prescribed a specific sodium level (ie, 2-g sodium diet) or "no added salt" diet, and those with hyperlipidemia a low-cholesterol, modified-fat diet.

The specifics of the foods provided for these diets vary as a function of the institution, but at least two characteristics of the prescribed diets are constant. First, it is unlikely that the dietary approach instituted will have been shown under experimental conditions to be clinically useful in the nursing home setting. Second, the initiation of a special diet will restrict the variety of foods available to the patient.

Special or therapeutic diets for nursing home residents with nutrition-related chronic diseases are viewed as being beneficial. However, the therapeutic benefit of a restrictive diet at this stage of life needs to be evaluated. Entry into a nursing home is rarely viewed as desirable, and the majority of individuals greatly regret the loss of independence. In this context, therapeutic intervention should be instituted only when the alternative would risk the health of the patient.

Sodium-Restricted Diets

Restriction of sodium intake has been the primary intervention in treating expanded cellular volume conditions, regardless of the clinical setting. For patients with severe heart failure, sodium restriction is critical. Yet, the benefit of sodium-restricted diets for mild disease in a group of patients for whom transfer to acute hospitals is frequently due to dehydration and for whom the thirst threshold is impaired, especially in addition to diuretic or antihypertensive therapy, must be questioned (27).

A 6-month trial of a less restrictive sodium diet has been described by Hadler (28). All patients from a 220-bed nursing home who were prescribed a 2-g sodium diet were identified. These 39 patients were observed for 6 months on a 4-g sodium diet with no change in medication. At the sixth month there was no significant change in body weight, blood pressure, electrolyte level, serum creatinine, blood urea nitrogen, or general clinical status.

This is not to imply that restricted sodium diets are not beneficial in the acute care or outpatient setting. However, institutionalized populations are more compliant with dietary restriction and drug therapy by the nature of the nursing home routine. If there is no clinical benefit to be gained from restrictive sodium diets, then these patients can be spared less palatable meals and the elimination of preferred foods.

Diabetic Diets

Diet therapy is an important component of the medical management of patients with diabetes. The dietary prescription for patient management is based on a total calorie level, with specific percentages allocated to carbohydrate, protein, and fat. In addition, regular spacing of meals and similarity of meal patterns are recommended dietary guidelines for patients with diabetes (29).

Several groups have documented that the severity of symptoms among patients with diabetes mellitus in nursing homes is considerably less than observed in an older ambulatory population with diabetes (30–32). As mentioned earlier, compliance with dietary and medication regimens is improved in the nursing home setting. In addition, meals for all residents are planned in a pattern so that similar types and amounts of foods are served at each meal, and the availability of foods is limited to meals and planned snacks. This is in marked contrast to the food availability of the independent-living older patient with diabetes.

We tested the clinical utility of calorie-controlled diabetic diets as compared to the regular diet in nursing home patients with diabetes (32). When patients with diabetes had access to regular diets, they consumed more calories because of increased intake of carbohydrate- and fat-containing foods, mainly simple desserts and a greater variety of breakfast foods. Fasting plasma glucose was significantly increased during the 2 months that patients consumed the regular diet, although the absolute increase in glucose concentration was from 121 mg/dl (6.7 mmol/liter) to 131 mg/dl (7.3 mmol/liter) on the regular diet. Glycosylated hemoglobin remained unchanged—7.8% on the diabetic diet and 8.1% on the regular diet. This indicates that day-long plasma glucose concentrations were within acceptable limits. Body weight did not change over the course of the study.

Data from our study and others demonstrate that the majority of patients with diabetes in nursing homes are in relatively good glycemic control and the therapeutic advantage of a diabetic diet in such a population must be questioned (30–32). Based upon the expected life span of nursing home patients, it is necessary to wonder if substitution of a regular for a diabetic diet would lead to differences in either acute or chronic complications of hyperglycemia.

Fat-Modified Diets

No data exist on the treatment efficacy of patients with hyperlipidemia who are more than 70 years of age (33). The rationale for treating hyperlipidemia is based on the association between blood lipid levels and risk for coronary heart disease. The association between serum cholesterol and heart disease weakens with age. Total cholesterol level does not consistently predict heart disease risk in the elderly and may have a negative relation to overall mortality in the nursing home population (34). Until there is stronger evidence that cholesterol-lowering interventions are likely to benefit elderly persons, fat-modified diets may not be clinically useful in the nursing home setting.

If the liberalization of diet has little metabolic impact, there seems to be a great deal of positive gain that will accrue to the patient and institution. It is less complex and more economical for the nursing home to prepare meals if they can minimize the variety of special foods required for each meal. In addition, there is the positive benefit of permitting patients the luxury of eating a regular diet and participating fully in social activities.

In order to meet the dietary needs of the majority of residents, the regular diet for a facility should be based on the RDA for nutrient requirements without containing excessive amounts of high-caloric, low-nutrient foods. The food should be seasoned to be palatable, but not be "salty." Fat-foods should be selected to favor poly- and monounsaturated fatty acids. Modifications of the regular diet for consistency, from soft to ground to puree, would further meet the needs of residents unable to chew or swallow normally. Periodic nutritional assessment of residents would verify the nutritional outcome of such a regimen.

REFERENCES

1. Rudman D, Feller AG. *J Am Geriatr Soc* 1989;37:173–183.
2. National Center for Health Statistics. *Advance Data from Vital and Health Statistics* 1987; May 14, no. 135.
3. National Center for Health Statistics. *Advance Data from Vital and Health Statistics* 1987; March 27, no. 131.
4. Silver AJ, Morley JE, Strome LS, Jones D, Vickers L. *J Am Geriatr Soc* 1988;36:487–491.
5. *Medicare and Medicaid requirements for long term care facilities. Fed Reg* 1989;54:5316.
6. Committee on Dietary Allowances, Food and Nutrition Board. *Recommended dietary allowances,* 10th rev. ed. Washington, DC: National Academy of Sciences, 1989.
7. *Regulations, guidelines, survey procedures for skilled nursing facilities.* California Administrative Code, 1982, Title 22, Div. 5, Ch. 3.
8. Sempos CT, Johnson NE, Elmer PJ, Allington JK, Matthews ME. *J Am Dietet Assoc* 1982;81:35–40.
9. Allington JK, Matthews ME, Johnson NE. *J Am Dietet Assoc* 1983;82:377–384.
10. Rodysill KJ, Hansen L, O'Leary JJ. *J Am Geriatr Soc* 1989;37:435–443.
11. Blackburn GL, Bristrian BR, Maini BS, et al. *JPEN* 1977;1:11–22.
12. Shaver HJ, Loper JA, Lutes RA. *JPEN* 1980;4:367–370.
13. Pinchcofsky-Devin GD, Kaminski MV. *J Am Coll Nutr* 1987;6:109–112.
14. Sandman PO, Adolfsson R, Nygren C, Hallmans G, Winblad B. *J Am Geriatr Soc* 1987;35:31–38.
15. Stephens ND, Messner RL, Neitch SM. *Nutr Supp Serv* 1988;8:5–11.
16. Rudman D, Mattson DE, Nagraj HS, Caindec N, Rudman IW, Jackson DL. *J Am Geriatr Soc* 1987;35:496–502.
17. Sahyoun NR, Otradovec CL, Hartz SC, et al. *Am J Clin Nutr* 1988;47:524–533.
18. Johnson EJ, Roth CA, Reinhardt JT, Marlett JA. *Am J Clin Nutr* 1988;48:159–164.
19. Chumela WC, Roche AF, Steinbaugh ML, *J Am Geriatr Soc* 1985;33:116–120.

20. Cooper JW, Cobb HH. *Nutr Supp Serv* 1988;8:5–7.
21. Wayler AH, Kapur KK, Feldman RS, Chauncey HH. *J Gerontol* 1982;37:294–299.
22. Feldman RS, Kapur KK, Alman JE, Chauncey HH. *J Am Geriatr Soc* 1980;28:97–103.
23. Siebens H, Trupe E, Siebens A, et al. *J Am Geriatr Soc* 1986;34:192–198.
24. Nguyen NH, Flint DM, Prinsley DM, Wahlqvist ML. *Human Nutr: Applied Nutr* 1985;39(A):333–338.
25. Dwyer JT, Coleman KA, Krall E, et al. *J Gerontol* 1987;42:246–251.
26. Harris T, Cook F, Garrison R, Higgins M, Kannel W, Goldman L. *JAMA* 1988;259: 1520–1524.
27. Phillips PA, Rolls BJ, Ledinghan JGG, et al. *N Engl J Med* 1984;311:753–759.
28. Hadler MH. *J Am Geriatr Soc* 1984;32:235–236.
29. American Diabetes Association. *Diab Care* 1987;10:126–132.
30. Zimmer JG, Williams TF. *J Am Geriatr Soc* 1978;26:443–452.
31. Mooradian AD, Osterweil D, Petrasek D, Morley JE. *J Am Geriatr Soc* 1988;36: 391–396.
32. Coulston AM, Mandelbaum D, Reaven GM. *Am J Clin Nutr* 1990;51:67–71.
33. Garber AM, Sox HC, Littenberg B. *Ann Intern Med* 1989;110:622–639.
34. Rudman D, Mattson DE, Nagarj HS, et al. *JPEN* 1988;12:155–158.

Geriatric Nutrition, edited by John E. Morley,
Zvi Glick, Laurence Z. Rubenstein.
Raven Press, Ltd., New York © 1990.

27

Nutritional Support for Elderly Patients

Dennis H. Sullivan

*Department of Geriatrics, University of Arkansas School of Medicine,
Little Rock, Arkansas 72206*

Over the last 20 years tremendous advances have been made in the field of nutritional support therapy–the provision of nutrients to person unable to ingest adequate food by mouth. A wide array of new nutritional support products have become available, including the relatively recent introduction of new sources of energy (such as intravenous fat emulsions and medium chain triglycerides), protein (for example, dipeptide and amino acids, as well as essential amino acids and their keto-analogs) and micronutrients (such as trace minerals and specific vitamin preparations). Improved methods of administering these products have also been developed, such as the technique of percutaneous endoscopic gastrostomy. Through these advances, it is now possible to tailor nutritional intervention strategies more effectively to meet the specific needs of the elderly patient. The purpose of this chapter is to present a general overview of this complex array of both enteral and parenteral nutritional support products and to provide some general guidelines for utilizing these products effectively to treat elderly patients in need of nutritional support.

Most of the information presented in this chapter is based on studies of general medicine and surgical patient populations. Unfortunately, there are only limited data available that are related specifically to the use of nutritional support therapy for elderly patients. Further research dealing with the many complex issues of providing nutritional support to the elderly is clearly needed.

ENTERAL NUTRITIONAL SUPPORT

Indications and Contraindications

In general, if the gastrointestinal (GI) tract is functioning and can be used effectively without undue morbidity, enteral nutritional support is preferred over parenteral therapy. Specific contraindications would include uncon-

TABLE 1. Commonly available enteral feeding products

Formula	Calories[a] (per ml)	Protein[b] (g/liter)	Nonprotein (kcal/g N)	Carbohydrate[b] (g/liter)	Fat[b] (g/liter)	Na[b] (mEq/liter)	K[b] (mEq/liter)
0.5–1.4 kcal/ml lactose free							
Attain (Sherwood Medical)	1.0	40	131:1	120	40	30	29
Ensure (Ross)	1.1	37	153:1	145	37	37	40
Entra-Life (Corpak)	1.1	35	153:1	137	35	37	40
Entrition (Biosearch)	1.0	35	154:1	136	35	31	31
Entrition HN (Biosearch)	1.0	44	117:1	114	41	37	41
Isocal (Mead Johnson)	1.1	34	167:1	133	44	23	34
Isocal HN (Mead Johnson)	1.1	45	127:1	125	42	35	27
Isolife (Navaco)	1.0	42	124:1	138	34	35	38
Isotein HN (Sandoz Nutrition)	1.2	68	86:1	156	34	27	27
Nutren 1.0 (Clintec Nutrition)	1.0	40	131:1	127	38	22	32
Osmolite (Ross)	1.1	37	153:1	145	39	28	26
Osmolite HN (Ross)	1.1	44	124:1	141	37	41	40
Pre-Attain (Sherwood Medical)	0.5	20	131:1	60	20	15	15
Replete (Clintec Nutrition)	1.0	62	75:1	113	33	22	40
Resource (Sandoz)	1.1	37	153:1	145	37	37	40
Sustacal liquid (Mead Johnson)	1.0	61	79:1	145	23	41	53
Sustacal HC (Mead Johnson)	1.5	61	134:1	190	58	36	38
Travasorb MCT Powder (Travenol)	1.0	49	102:1	123	33	15	26
0.5–1.4 kcal/ml lactose free, fiber-containing[c]							
Enrich (FC: 14) (Ross)	1.1	40	148:1	158	37	37	40
Jevity (FC: 14) (Ross)	1.1	45	125:1	152	37	40	40
Profiber (FC: 12) (Sherwood Medical)	1.0	40	131:1	132	40	32	32
Sustacal with fiber (FC: 6) (Mead Johnson)	1.1	46	120:1	141	35	31	36

344

	kcal/ml[a]		ratio	Osm	[b]	[b]	[c]
0.5–1.4 kcal/ml with lactose							
Compleat (Sandoz)	1.1	43	131:1	128	43	57	36
Vitaneed (Sherwood Medical)	1.0	40	131:1	128	40	30	32
Meritene liquid (Sandoz)	1.0	69	67:1	119	34	48	72
Sustacal Powder (Mead Johnson)	1.3	77	80:1	180	34	54	87
1.5–2.0 kcal/ml lactose free							
Comply (Sherwood Medical)	1.5	60	131:1	180	60	44	44
Ensure Plus (Ross)	1.5	55	146:1	200	53	50	54
Ensure Plus HN (Ross)	1.5	63	125:1	200	50	52	47
Isocal HCN (Mead Johnson)	2.0	75	145:1	200	102	35	43
Magnacal (Sherwood Medical)	2.0	70	154:1	250	80	44	32
Nutren 1.5 (Clintec Nutrition)	1.5	60	131:1	168	65	33	48
Nutren 2.0 (Clintec Nutrition)	2.0	80	131:1	196	106	43	64
Resource Plus (Sandoz)	1.5	55	146:1	200	53	39	45
Sustacal HC (Mead Johnson)	1.5	61	134:1	190	58	36	38
Travasorb MCT Liquid (Travenol)	1.5	74	102:1	185	50	23	36
Two Cal HN (Ross)	2.0	84	125:1	217	91	46	59
1.5–2.0 kcal/ml with lactose							
Sustagen (Mead Johnson)	1.7	112	77:1	312	17	55	87

From Blackburn GL et al., ref. 6. *Nutritional medicine: A case management approach*. Philadelphia: WB Saunders, 1989.

[a]Figures rounded to the nearest 0.1 kcal/ml.
[b]Figures rounded to nearest whole number.
[c]FC, Fiber content in g/liter.

trolled GI hemorrhage, obstruction or fistulas distal to the feeding site, peritonitis, ileus, intractable vomiting, or insufficient functional small bowel to absorb the delivered nutrients. Intractable diarrhea and high risk of aspiration are relative contraindications.

Several studies have concluded that enteral and parenteral therapy are equally efficacious in meeting the nutritional needs of patients (1–3). However, if its use is not contraindicated, enteral support has several advantages. The most significant advantages relate to cost, safety and the apparent trophic effect of enteral therapy on the gut. Because of less stringent requirements for preparation and delivery and the need for less sophisticated equipment, the cost of enteral therapy is often one-third to one-fourth that of parenteral support. In certain groups of patients, the risks of septic, metabolic, and pleural-pulmonary complications are also reduced. When patients are starved, or all nutrients are delivered parenterally, atrophic changes develop rapidly in the gut and the pancreas. Enteral feedings are needed to maintain or replete normal mucosal cellular mass and gut enzyme activity. This trophic effect is mediated by both hormonal and neurovascular mechanisms and through the direct stimulatory effect of the nutrients in contact with the mucosal surface (4,5). Whether enteral feeding has advantages in terms of endocrine, immune, or cardiovascular function remains controversial.

Amount and Type of Solution

A number of important factors must be considered in selecting a nutritional formula. Of special importance are the patient's nutrient requirements and metabolic limitations, the functional capacity of the patient's GI tract, the presence of any food allergy or intolerance, and the cost, availability, convenience, osmolarity, viscosity, and anticipated route of delivery of the solution. One or a combination of several products can be used to meet the patient's needs (6) (Table 1).

Patient's Nutrient Requirements

Among other factors, an important consideration in choosing an enteral feeding product is the formula's ratio of protein to total nonprotein calories. Seriously ill patients requiring repletion of both protein and energy stores usually benefit the most from a solution with a calorie-to-nitrogen ratio of approximately 150:1. However, this is only an estimate. The actual requirements, which can be determined from the nutritional assessment, may range from 100:1 to 200:1 (7,8). Patients in need of protein repletion and weight reduction may do well with a solution containing a high protein-to-total energy concentration. To meet this need, products are available with a calorie-to-nitrogen ratio of less than 100:1. Alternatively, modular protein powder can be added to a standard formula to increase the total protein content. Formulas are also available with very high calorie-to-nitrogen ratios for patients unable to tolerate significant protein loads. For seriously ill patients, it is often advisable to reassess protein requirements after initiating therapy. Nitrogen balance studies may be useful in this regard.

In addition to protein and calorie requirements, it is important to meet the patient's requirements for vitamins, essential fatty acids, and minerals. Products that are classified as nutritionally complete usually meet or exceed the recommended daily allowances (RDA) for the essential fatty acids, most vitamins, and many minerals. Some products contain vitamin K, which may be a concern for patients on warfarin-type anticoagulants. Additional needs can be met by vitamin and mineral supplements.

The requirements for trace minerals are not well defined. Nine trace minerals are regarded as essential for humans: iodine, copper, zinc, manganese, selenium, chromium, iron, cobalt, and molybdenum. Many authorities recommend that all enterally fed patients routinely receive the RDA of zinc, copper, iodine, manganese, and chromium and that all patients requiring long-term nutritional support be provided with safe and adequate amounts of selenium (Table 2). The routine use of cobalt and molybdenum is controversial. The need for iron should be determined on an individual basis.

Although often not considered a nutrient, water is an essential component of the enteral feeding formula. As a general rule, patients require 1.5 liters/ m^2/day. Adjustments to this formula should be made based on the clinical circumstances.

Patient's Metabolic Limitations

For patients with metabolic dysfunctions, such as those caused by hepatic, renal, or cardiac failure, consideration can be given to the use of either modular or disease-specific enteral feeding formulas. Several nutritionally complete, ready-to-use, disease-specific formulas are available commercially. Although their efficacy has never been proven, these products are designed to meet the exceptional metabolic needs of patients with particular

TABLE 2. *Recommended daily doses of trace elements*

	Oral	Intravenous
Chromium	50–290 μg	10–20 μg
Copper	1.5–3.0 mg	0.5–1.5 mg
Iodine	100–200 μg	1–2 μg/kg
Manganese	1–5 mg	1–3 mg
Selenium	50–200 μg	40–120 μg
Zinc	10–15 mg	2.5–4.0 mg

disease states. Several of the products designed for patients with hepatic or renal disease have high carbohydrate-to-nitrogen ratios and substitute branched chain essential amino acids or their ketoanalog for the protein component of the formula. To avoid the restrictions of fixed composition preparations, modular components can be used either as supplements or by mixing several type of modules together to create a formula to meet exact specifications. Various types of fat, carbohydrate, and protein modules are available commercially (Tables 3–5), as are vitamin, mineral, and trace mineral preparations.

Functional Capacity of the Patient's Gastrointestinal Tract

Fats, whole proteins, and complex carbohydrates require effective digestive and absorptive processes for utilization. Patients with severe exocrine pancreatic insufficiency, biliary obstruction, short bowel syndrome, severe mucosal abnormalities, or other disease of the digestive tract are often unable to assimilate some or all of these complex nutrients. To meet the nutritional needs of these compromised patients, a number of products are available that contain modified or predigested components. These products can be obtained in either modular form or as nutritionally complete fixed composition formulas. If proteins cannot be digested, amino acids or dipeptides are equally effective substitutes ("elemental" or "peptide" diets) because both can be absorbed directly even through a limited mucosal surface (9). Likewise, medium chain triglycerides (MCT), which are also absorbed di-

TABLE 3. *Examples of modular enteral feeding products—fat modules*

Formula	/100 ml Calories	g/100 ml formula			mEq/100 ml	
		Protein	Carbohydrate	Fat	Na	K
		Fat Modules				
Lipomul (Upjohn)	600	0	0	66.6		
MCT Oil (Mead Johnson)	767	0	0	93.4		
Microlipid (Sherwood Medical)	450	0	0	50.0		
Nutrisource LCT (Sandoz)	216	0	0	24.0	0	0
Nutrisource MCT (Sandoz)	201	0	0	24.0	0	0

From Blackburn et al., ref. 6.

TABLE 4. *Examples of modular enteral feeding products—protein modules*

Formula	/100 g	g/100 gm formula			mEq/100 g	
	Calories	Protein	Carbohydrate[a]	Fat[a]	Na	K
Casec (Mead Johnson)	370	88	0	2	6.5	0.3
Nutrisource Amino Acids (Sandoz)	390	97	0	0	0.0	0.0
Nutrisource High BCAA (Sandoz)	390	97	0	0	0.0	0.0
Nutrisource Protein (Sandoz)	402	76	9	7	11.7	14.6
Pro-mix (Navaco)	360	75	5	4	10.0	21.0
Promod (Ross)	420	75	10	9	0.6	1.7
Propac (Sherwood Medical)	395	75	0	8	9.8	12.8

From Blackburn et al., ref. 6.
[a]Figures rounded to nearest whole number.

rectly into the portal circulation, can be supplied to patients unable to digest whole fats. MCTs do not provide essential fatty acids and, because they are ketogenic, must be used cautiously in acidotic patients (10). For patients with lactase deficiency, formulas low in lactose are often useful. Lactase deficiency is an extremely common condition among persons of African or Asian descent, and is often found in association with bowel disease, starvation, protein deficiency, and advanced age.

TABLE 5. *Examples of modular enteral feeding products—carbohydrate modules*

Formula	/100 ml	g/100 ml formula			mEq/100 ml	
	Calories	Protein	Carbohydrate[a]	Fat	Na	K
		Liquids				
Hycal (Beecham)	246	0	60	0	0.4	0.02
Liquid Carbohydrate (Navaco)	250	0	63	0	2.5	0.5
Nutrisource Carbohydrate (Sandoz)	320	0	80	0	0.1	0
Polycose Liquid (Ross)	200	0	50	0	3.0	0.15
		Powders				
Moducal Powder (Mead Johnson)	380	0	95	0	0	0
Polycose Powder (Ross)	380	0	94	0	0	0
Pure Carbohydrate (Navaco)	400	0	97	0	0	0
Sumacal (Sherwood Medical)	380	0	95	0	0	0

From Blackburn et al., ref. 6.
[a]Figures rounded to nearest whole number.

Other Considerations

Although in an institutional environment product selection may be limited to what is on the formulary, cost, availability, and convenience are important considerations in choosing an enteral feeding formula. The difference in price between products can be substantial. In some situations the convenience of a ready-to-use product may offset the labor costs involved in mixing solutions. However, patients with limited income requiring long-term enteral support may find the inconvenience of preparing blenderized feedings worth the savings.

Solution osmolarity is an important concern, especially for patients receiving enteral feedings directly into the small bowel. With increasing osmolarity there is a greater potential to develop diarrhea and other GI symptoms. In response to this problem, most commercial products available today use starches, dextrins, and glucose oligosaccharides as the carbohydrate source in place of the more osmotically active simple sugars. Elemental or predigested products tend to be more osmotically active.

Methods of Enteral Nutritional Support

A strategy for providing enteral nutritional support should be formulated based on the specific needs of the elderly patient. The anatomic site to which nutrients are to be delivered; the route, mode, and schedule of nutrient delivery; and the nutrient formula to be used should be chosen only after careful consideration is given to the elderly patient's physiologic needs, physical comfort, safety, psychologic welfare, and desires. The provision of enteral nutrition support to the elderly person is as much an art as it is a science.

Site of Nutrient Delivery

Nutrients can be delivered either to the stomach, duodenum, or jejunum. The advantages and limitations of each of these alternatives must be weighed carefully. Because the stomach physiologically controls the rate of nutrient delivery to the small bowel, there are a number of advantages to intragastric feedings. Formula osmolarity and, with large gastrostomy tubes, viscosity are of less concern, thereby making bolus feedings possible. These advantages are offset by the greater danger of aspiration, particularly for the patient who maintains high gastric residuals, has a depressed sensorium, or has an absent gag reflex. Intraduodenal feedings reduce the risk of aspiration and obviate the need to check gastric residuals constantly. As with all feedings distal to the stomach, the rate of nutrient delivery and the choice of formula may be restricted by the development of diarrhea or manifestations of the dumping syndrome. The initial placement of the distal end of the feeding tube into the duodenum and its maintenance in this location can be exceedingly difficult in some patients. Intrajejunal feedings almost completely eliminate the risk of pulmonary aspiration. In addition, this location for nutrient delivery may be suited for patients with postoperative ileus, which primarily affects the stomach and colon, and obstruction or inflammation of the stomach and duodenum (11).

Route of Nutrient Delivery

Intubation of the upper GI tract can be accomplished either transnasally, percutaneously, or surgically. The transnasal approach is well suited for select patients, especially those who require enteral nutritional support for a relatively brief period of time. A variety of enteral feeding tubes are commercially available that are specifically designed for this purpose. The soft, small-bore tubes are least irritating to the patient and can be obtained in the desired length for gastric, duodenal, or jejunal feeding. Some of the tubes have a radiopaque weighted tip that facilitates tube insertion and allows x-ray verification of placement. However, insertion of these tubes and proper tip placement, even for the skilled clinician, are sometimes difficult if not impossible, especially in the agitated patient. Packing the tube in ice before insertion or using a tube with a stiff removable inner stylet may facilitate its introduction. If all else fails, a small diameter feeding tube can be passed attached to a larger diameter nasogastric tube. Two variations of this technique are popular. The two tubes can be held together during insertion by a gelatin capsule that subsequently dissolves, allowing independent removal of the larger tube. Alternately, a portion of the small-bore tube, proximal to its weighted tip, can be placed inside a larger tube that has been spliced open lengthwise. As the larger tube approaches body temperature it becomes more pliable, allowing it to be removed independently. Extreme caution must be exercised when using these techniques to avoid complications.

Percutaneous endoscopic gastrostomy (PEG) is an intubation technique that is ideally suited for many elderly patients who do not tolerate a nasoenteral tube or who require long-term enteral nutritional support. This technique is performed under local anesthesia that is occasionally supplemented with mild intravenous sedation. Patients who are unable to undergo endoscopy or who have a coagulopathy are not candidates for this procedure. Upper GI bleeding, ascites, massive obesity, and varices are relative contraindications. When performed by a skilled endoscopist, the procedure has an acceptably low complication rate in properly selected patients (12,13). One version of this technique is described in Fig. 1. A technique of percutaneous gastrostomy is also performed by invasive radiologists (14,15).

Intubation of the upper GI tract can be accomplished by a variety of surgical techniques. Patients who are not candidates for percutaneous or transnasal intubation techniques and those undergoing general anesthesia for

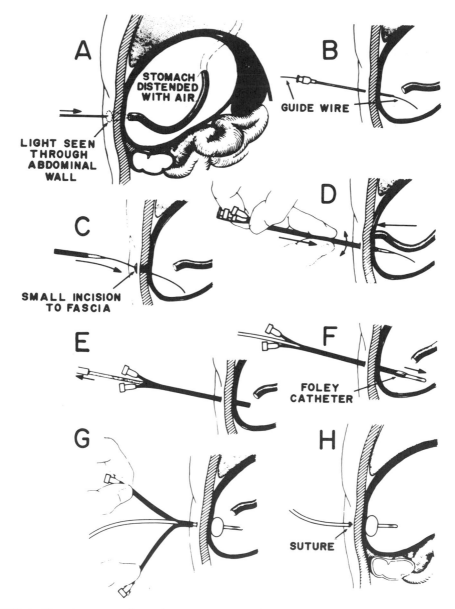

FIG. 1. Percutaneous endoscopic gastrostomy, method of Russell and associates. **A:** Gastric distention with needle directed at light source. **B:** Guidewire passed through the needle into the stomach followed by needle removal. **C:** Small incision is made along the guidewire to the peritoneum. **D:** Dilator and sheath over the guidewire are advanced as a unit into stomach (gastric distention, rotary motion, and counterpressure aid this maneuver). **E:** Wire and dilator removed with sheath observed remaining in stomach. **F:** Lubricated Foley catheter advanced through the sheath. **G:** Foley balloon inflated (leakproof) and sheath peeled away. **H:** Catheter is sutured to the skin under slight tension to appose the stomach and anterior abdominal wall. (From Russell TR, et al. *Am J Surg* 1984;148:132–137, with permission.)

other reasons are often candidates for one of these approaches. Esophagostomies, gastrostomies, and jejunostomies can be constructed depending on the needs and the desires of the patient.

Mode of Nutrient Delivery

Enteral feedings can be given as a bolus or by slow continuous drip. There does not appear to be a physiologic advantage of one method over the other (16,17). Bolus feeding into the stomach may be the ideal method of feeding for patients who are active, as this approach allows for more freedom of movement. When there is a high risk of aspiration, uncontrolled diarrhea, or persistence of dumping symptoms or when nutrients are delivered directly into the small bowel, feedings must be given by slow infusion. Infusion pumps offer many advantages over a simple gravity drip; however, high cost and limited availability often preclude their use.

Regardless of the method of nutrient delivery employed, complications can best be avoided by initiating enteral nutritional support with small volumes of a isotonic solution. If this approach is successful, solution strength and rate of delivery should then be increased slowly. Many institutions have standardized protocols that can be used as guidelines when starting enteral feedings. However, each time a change in therapy is made, the patient's response should be assessed and modifications to the protocol made as necessary.

Schedule of Nutrient Delivery

Feedings can be given intermittently or as a constant infusion 24 hours per day. As mentioned above, a bolus feeding regimen may be optimal for select patients, especially when there is a desire to maximize the patient's independence and to encourage a resumption of volitional food consumption. The frequency of the bolus feedings can be from every 2 to every 6 hours, depending on the needs and tolerance of the patient. An alternate approach is to provide a constant infusion of enteral tube feedings only for part of the day. An example of this approach is to infuse nutrients over a 12-hour period each night and then provide regular meals during the day. When not in use, the tube can either be disconnected or, as some patients prefer, removed each morning and reinserted at night.

Complications of Enteral Feeding and Their Prevention

A variety of complications can occur as a consequence of tube placement or infusion of the nutrient formula. These complications can be classified as feeding tube intolerance, mechanical, septic-metabolic, pleural-pulmonary, and gastrointestinal.

Patient Intolerance to Enteral Feeding Tubes

In our experience, intolerance to enteral feeding tubes is a common problem, especially for elderly patients who are confused or agitated. This view is confirmed by a study recently conducted by the author at a major teaching center (18). The study reveals that many elderly patients assessed to be at high risk for nutrition-related complications never receive an optimal level of nutritional support. Intolerance to the enteral feeding tubes, particularly nasoenteral tubes, is the most common contributing factor for this suboptimal level of care. In addition, an increased rate of enteral-support-related complications can be linked to intolerance of enteral feeding tubes. Patients are often restrained or sedated to enable passage of the enteral tube or in an effort to prevent the tube from being pulled out. The restrained patient, who is more likely to remain confused, agitated, and immobile, is at an increased risk of complications.

A skilled clinician who is well versed in the proper technique of tube placement and subsequent management can minimize the problem of patient intolerance to enteral feeding tubes. However, for many patients it is best to avoid nasoenteral tubes, as these tubes are often the least well tolerated and the most difficult to keep in place. On occasion, it is advisable to utilize parenteral nutritional support if intravenous catheters are better tolerated until the patient stabilizes and can resume adequate oral intake or becomes a candidate for a percutaneous endoscopic gastrostomy.

Mechanical Complications

The most commonly encountered mechanical complications include tube obstruction, displacement, or rupture. All small-bore enteral feeding tubes are susceptible to becoming clogged, particularly when the tubes are used as conduits for the delivery of pulverized medications. The best way to prevent this problem is to limit their use to liquids. Occasionally the tube knots itself in the stomach, a problem that can be avoided by confirming proper placement before initiation of infusion. In addition to being pulled out deliberately or accidentally, occasionally a tube is dislodged from the small bowel when the patient vomits. It is always important to recheck tube placement after a patient has an episode of vomiting or retching. Rupture of the tube can occur when an attempt is made to clear an obstruction forcefully using a small-gauge syringe or by reinserting a stylet. Both of these approaches are potentially dangerous and should be strongly discouraged.

Septic-Metabolic Complications

While receiving enteral nutritional support, elderly patients need to be monitored closely for the development of metabolic complications, including congestive heart failure secondary to excessive salt and water retention, hyperkalemia, hyper- and hyponatremia, and severe hyperglycemia. Although they can arise at any time during the course of therapy, these complications are most likely to develop soon after initiation of enteral feedings, especially in patients who are critically ill or chronically starved. The risk also rises any time that a patient's clinical status deteriorates; for example, with the development of a complicating acute medical problem.

Potentially serious complications can arise as a result of microbial contamination of an enteral nutrient formula. Such a situation is likely to occur if a preservative-free product is left at room temperature for prolonged periods after the sterile container is opened. The delivery system can also be colonized with bacterial pathogens during prolonged use, but the significance of this problem to the development of contaminated formula is less clearly defined. Administering a contaminated enteral feeding formula can cause severe diarrhea and other symptoms of gastroenteritis (19,20). It may also lead to the development of generalized sepsis in immunocompromised patients (20).

Pleural-Pulmonary Complications

A variety of pleural-pulmonary complications can develop as a result of enteral feeding tube placement or nutrient delivery. The frequency with which these problems arise is related both to the skills and vigilance of the attending health care team and the severity of the patient's illness. When using the transnasal approach there is always a danger of inadvertent placement of the feeding tube into the lungs, pleural space, or, rarely, mediastinum. The risk is greatest when the patient is agitated, confused, or obtunded; there is an inflammatory or obstructing lesion of the esophagus; or an attempt is made to pass a relatively rigid tube forcefully. Using a cuffed endotracheal tube does not provide adequate assurance that tracheal intubation will not occur. Although it is probably not necessary to confirm tube placement radiographically in every case, such a precaution is mandatory should there be any doubt of the tube's location or when difficulties are encountered during tube placement because of the presence of any of the above risk factors. Aspiration of gastric contents or auscultating for the tube's location while insufflating with air is not a fail-proof safeguard. An enteral feeding tube should always be removed completely before any attempt is made to reinsert a stylet.

All enterally fed patients are at risk for aspiration of nutrient formula into the lungs. Patients at greatest risk are those who are obtunded or who have a diminished cough and gag reflex. As outlined previously, the risk can be minimized by elevating the head of the patient's bed, using a constant infusion pump, and delivering the nutrients into the duodenum or jejunum.

Gastrointestinal Complications

Although rare, the most serious GI complications of enteral feeding are bowel perforation and rupture. These complications usually develop during the process of intubating the GI tract and are often the result of inappropriate technique. Nausea, vomiting, and diarrhea occur more commonly and on occasion limit the use of enteral feedings.

Diarrhea is often a relatively minor problem that can be resolved by making simple changes to the feeding regimen. However, in some cases, particularly in patients who are seriously ill, the etiology of the disorder is multifactorial, and the problem is difficult to control. In these cases, a planned approach to therapeutic intervention should be formulated based on a careful assessment of the patient.

As a first step in the evaluation process, conditions that could potentially contribute to the development of clinically significant enteral-feeding-associated diarrhea should be identified. Chronic starvation or prolonged periods of alimentation exclusively by the parenteral route, concomitant drug administration, severe hypoproteinemia, inflammatory bowel disease, and the use of hyperosmolar formula or bolus feedings are all risk factors. It is also important to consider lactose intolerance and microbial contamination of the enteral feeding formula as a potential source of diarrhea.

Chronic starvation and prolonged parenteral alimentation produce atrophy of the intestinal epithelium, resulting in a diminution of the digestive capacity of the gut. With rapid reinstitution of enteral feedings, malabsorption occurs and severe diarrhea develops. To attenuate the risk of producing diarrhea in these patients, enteral feedings should be introduced slowly. A reasonable approach would be to initiate therapy with one-quarter strength formula delivered at a rate of 25 cc/hr. If this regimen is tolerated, the formula osmolarity and rate of delivery can be advanced every 24 to 48 hours. Nutrients in contact with the intestinal mucosa stimulate epithelial regeneration by both direct and systemic mechanisms and eventually result in improved bowel function. Until full therapeutic requirements are reached, concomitant parenteral nutritional support can be utilized to supplement the enteral feedings. If the diarrhea cannot be controlled using this regimen, the rate of nutrient delivery can be reduced, or an elemental diet formula can be tried. In some cases, it is necessary to postpone the use of enteral feedings until the patient's condition improves.

The concomitant use of various medications is often overlooked as a cause of diarrhea in enterally fed patients. Many liquid pharmaceutical preparations are hyperosmolar and cause diarrhea when administered through an enteral feeding tube. Magnesium-containing antacids are another easily overlooked potential source of diarrhea. Consideration should always be given to the possibility that diarrhea in an enterally fed patient receiving antibiotics is caused by pseudomembranous colitis.

Patients with severe hypoproteinemia often have problems with diarrhea while receiving enteral feedings (21). The mechanism by which diarrhea develops in these patients is not defined.

PARENTERAL NUTRITIONAL SUPPORT

It is beyond the scope of this chapter to provide a complete discussion of parenteral nutritional support therapy. Instead, the goal is to emphasize how parenteral therapy can be used to complement enteral support. Recent advances in the use of peripheral alimentation have particular relevance in this regard. Using a combination of techniques, it is possible to provide optimal nutritional support therapy to a wide spectrum of elderly patients in a variety of clinical settings.

Indications

The enteral route is the preferred method for alimentation for most elderly patients who have a functioning GI tract. Patients who have contraindications to or cannot be managed safely and effectively with enteral feedings are potential candidates for parenteral alimentation. As discussed previously, parenteral alimentation can also be used in combination with enteral therapy. Combination therapy is particularly effective for patients who require optimal nutritional support or who are candidates for enteral therapy yet have severe diarrhea or other problems that limit temporarily the quantity of nutrients that can be delivered by that route.

General Principles

Parenteral alimentation must be formulated to provide the correct ratio of water, electrolytes, protein, calories, essential fatty acids, vitamins, and trace elements to meet the specific nutritional requirements of the elderly patient. This goal can be accomplished most economically by using commercially available modular parenteral nutrition products. After a complete nutritional assessment of the patient is performed and the requirement for each nutrient calculated, the desired parenteral nutrition formula is prepared by mixing the appropriate modular units in the correct proportions.

The protein component of parenteral alimentation is usually provided in the form of crystalline amino acids. Standard, commercially available amino acid solutions contain all the necessary essential and nonessential amino acids in a ratio that is optimal for most hospitalized patients. Although of unproven efficacy, special formulas designed specifically for use in patients with advanced hepatic or renal disease are also available.

The required nonprotein calories can be provided by a combination of carbohydrates and lipids. Of the various forms of carbohydrate available, glucose is used most frequently. All patients should receive at least the equivalent of 150 g/day of glucose in order to ensure maximal protein sparing, to supply a ready source of energy for the nervous system and other glucose-dependent tissues, and to prevent certain complications, such as ketosis, that develop when 100% of the nonprotein calories are furnished as fat. Patients should also be provided with an appropriate amount of lipid to meet their daily requirement for essential fatty acids. Beyond these minimal requirements, any combination of glucose and lipid can be utilized to provide the required nonprotein calories. For most patients, there does not appear to be any significant advantage of one caloric source over the other (22–24).

Glucose is the traditional source of nonprotein calories in parenteral nutrition formulas. It is relatively inexpensive and can be given in large amounts and in high concentration (greater than 20% solution), and its administration is associated with few complications when appropriate measures are taken to avoid hyperglycemia. A disadvantage of using glucose is that it is a relatively small, osmotically active molecule. To meet the caloric needs of most patients, it is necessary either to infuse large volumes of a 5 or 10% glucose solution or to use a more concentrated formula that must be administered through a central vein.

The most commonly used sources of intravenous lipids are emulsions consisting of long chain triglycerides (LCT) held in suspension by egg phospholipids. The emulsions also contain glycerol, which is added to make the solution isosmotic. The LCT are derived from soybean and safflower oils and contain high concentrations of the essential fat, linoleic acid. Both 10 and 20% lipid emulsions are available commercially supplying 1.1 kcal/ml and 2.0 kcal/ml, respectively. An amino acid, electrolyte, and glucose solution can be mixed with the lipid emulsion during administration or in the pharmacy before administering it.

For some elderly patients, there are advantages of using lipids as the primary source of nonprotein calories. A nutritionally complete parenteral alimentation formula that can be administered safely and efficaciously by peripheral vein can be derived using a 10% fat emulsion in combination with a solution of amino acids, electrolytes, and glucose (25). Using this approach, the nutritional requirements of most elderly patients can be reached with the administration of less than 4 liters/day of formula. Intravenous lipids are not recommended as the primary caloric source for patients who have uncontrolled hyperlipidemia, are recovering from a recent myocardial infarction, or require fluid restriction.

Route of Administration

The nonprotein calorie source used and the desired final solution volume are the major determinants of whether the resulting formula must be administered through a central as opposed to a peripheral vein. With the introduction of high caloric density lipid emulsions, peripheral alimentation is a viable choice for many elderly patients. This route is a particularly attractive option for patients who require temporary parenteral nutritional supplementation during the introduction of enteral feedings.

Patient Care and Monitoring

Parenteral nutritional support is being offered to patients in a wide range of clinical settings. Formerly limited to acute care hospitals, patients receiving parenteral alimentation are now being managed successfully in intermediate and long-term care facilities and in their own homes. The decision to use this form of therapy in either an institutional or outpatient setting requires careful consideration of the patient's needs, associated risks, and capabilities of both the caregiver and the provider. A reliable system must be in place to monitor the patient closely, obtain solutions rapidly, store solutions appropriately until used, handle all intravenous tubing safely, and change dressings as required. Monitoring capabilities need to include the accurate determination of weights, inputs and outputs, patient's hydration status, blood chemistries, and vital signs. The complexity of the patient's care is another consideration in determining the appropriateness of parenteral alimentation in a particular clinical setting. Relatively stable patients on well-formulated regimens of parenteral nutrition with either surgically implanted central lines or reliable peripheral access can be managed safely and effectively in a wider range of clinical settings.

Limitations to the Use of Parenteral Nutritional Support

A number of factors limit the effectiveness of parenteral nutritional support therapy for elderly patients. The costs of therapy, patient intolerance, lack of adequately skilled supporting personnel, and the development of supervening complications are just a few.

Elderly patients are particularly susceptible to the development of parenteral-nutrition-related complications. Such complications can arise as a consequence of the procedures used to establish venous access, the indwelling venous catheters, or the administration of the nutrient formula. The most common complications related to nutrient formula administration include fluid and electrolyte imbalance, hyperglycemia, and, with abrupt discontinuation of the feedings, potentially life-threatening hypoglycemia. Sepsis can develop if either the nutrient solution or the intravenous tubing becomes contaminated.

A number of potentially serious complications can develop as a result of use of the indwelling venous catheters. Localized thrombophlebitis is the most common complication of peripheral venous catheters. Venous thrombosis, air embolization, infection at the insertion site, and generalized sepsis are more likely to complicate the use of central venous catheters. The incidence of central venous catheter-related sepsis is related to both the type of catheter and the manner in which it is utilized. Multilumen catheters, which often serve several functions, are associated with a much greater risk of sepsis than are single-lumen catheters (26,27). Catheters that are tunneled under the skin before entering the vein do not appear to reduce the risk of sepsis compared to percutaneously placed catheters that are properly cared for and dedicated solely to parenteral nutrition (28). However, when optimal sterile technique cannot be maintained, as in the outpatient setting, or when the central line is used for more than parenteral alimentation, a catheter that is tunneled subcutaneously may be the best method of maintaining central venous access. Compared to percutaneous central lines, subcutaneously placed catheters are easier to maintain and, in less than optimal clinical conditions, are associated with a lower risk of catheter-associated complications. Even when receiving proper care, elderly patients with centrally placed catheters remain at significant risk of developing septic complications.

SUMMARY

For the elderly patient who requires nutritional support therapy, a strategy of intervention should be carefully formulated based on the results of the clinical assessment. Thoughtful consideration should be given to choosing the most optimal site and route of alimentation, composition of the nutrient formula, rate and schedule of formula delivery, and duration of therapy. While receiving nutritional support, the patient should be monitored carefully for complications and changing metabolic requirements. As necessary, modifications to the original regimen should be made to meet the patient's changing needs.

REFERENCES

1. Bennegard K, Lindmark L, Wickstrom I, et al. *Am J Clin Nutr* 1984;40:752–757.
2. Fletcher JP, Little JM. *Surgery* 1986;100:21–24.
3. McArdle AH, Palmason C, Morency I, Brown RA. *Surgery* 1981;90:616–623.

4. Levine GM, Deren JJ, Steiger E, Zinno R. *Gastroenterology* 1974;67:975–982.
5. Tilson MD. *Surg Clin North Am* 1980;60:1273–1284.
6. Blackburn GL, Bell SJ, Mullen JL, et al. *Nutritional medicine: A case management approach*. Philadelphia: WB Saunders, 1989.
7. Long CL. *Contemp Surg* 1980;16:29–42.
8. Wilmore DW. *The metabolic management of the critically ill*. New York: Plenum Medical Book Co, 1977.
9. Sleisenger MH, Kim YS. *N Engl J Med* 1979;300:659–663.
10. Sucher KP. *Nutr Clin Prac* 1986;1:146–150.
11. Dunn EL, Moore EE, Bohus RW. *JPEN* 1980;4:393–395.
12. Miller RE, Kummer BA, Tiszenkel HI, Kotler DP. *Ann Surg* 1986;204:543–545.
13. Ponsky JL, Gauderer MWL, Stellato TA, Aszodi A. *Am J Surg* 1985;149:102–105.
14. Alzate GD, Coons HG, Elliott J, Carey PH. *AJR* 1986;147:822–825.
15. Ho C-S, Gray RR, Goldfinger M, et al. *Radiology* 1985;156:349–351.
16. Fitzpatrick GF, Meguid MM, O'Connell RC, et al. *Surgery* 1975;78:105–113.
17. Pinchofsky-Devin GD, Kaminski MV. *JPEN* 1985;9:474–476.
18. Sullivan DH, Moriarty MS, Chernoff R, Lipschitz DA. *JPEN* 1989;13:249–254.
19. Anderson KR, Norris DJ, Godfrey LB, et al. *JPEN* 1984;8:673–678.
20. De Leeuw IH, Vandewoude MF. *Gut* 1986;27(suppl 1):56–57.
21. Zagoren AJ, Waters DW, Beck S, Rose N. *J Am Coll Nutr* 1984;3:260.
22. Gazzaniga AB, Bartlett RH, Shobe JB. *Ann Surg* 1975;182:163–168.
23. Jeejeebhoy KN, Anderson GH, Nakhooda AF, et al. *J Clin Invest* 1976;57:125–136.
24. Wolfe BM, Culebras JM, Sim AJW, et al. *Ann Surg* 1977;186:518–540.
25. Brown R, Quercia RA, Sigman R. *JPEN* 1986;10:650–658.
26. McCarthy MC, Shives JK, Robison RJ, Broadie TA. *JPEN* 1987;11:259–262.
27. Pemberton LB, Lyman B, Lander V, Covinsky J. *Arch Surg* 1986;121:591–594.
28. Von Meyenfeldt MM, Stapert J, de Jong PC, et al. *JPEN* 1980;4:514–517.

Geriatric Nutrition, edited by John E. Morley,
Zvi Glick, Laurence Z. Rubenstein.
Raven Press, Ltd., New York © 1990.

28

Pressure Sores and Nutrition

Bruce A. Ferrell and Dan Osterweil

*Division of Geriatric Medicine, UCLA School of Medicine,
Los Angeles, California 90024 and Jewish Homes for the Aging
of Greater Los Angeles, Reseda, California 91335*

Pressure sores are a common and serious problem associated with malnutrition (1). Moreover, they are associated with significant morbidity, mortality, and resource expenditure. The prevalence of pressure sores is 3 to 11% in patients in acute care hospitals and nursing homes (2–4). Ninety percent of pressures sores occur below the waist, and 50% occur in patients over the age of 70 (5). Among geriatric nursing home residents, pressure sores are associated with a fourfold increased risk of death (6). The inhospital mortality rate for patients with pressure sores has been reported to be between 23 to 37% (1,7).

NUTRITION AS A RISK FACTOR FOR PRESSURE SORES

A variety of variables have been associated with the occurrence of pressure sores, and multiple reviews have summarized the available literature on the pathogenesis and management of pressure sores (8–11). Clinical experience suggests that most pressure sores are multifactorial in etiology. Table 1 summarizes the factors commonly associated with the development and healing of pressure sores. Conceptually, pressure and shear forces are considered the primary factors because of their implications for direct causality (8,12,13). Other factors, such as nutritional status, immobility, anemia, sensory impairment, vascular insufficiency, and concurrent infection are considered secondary or permissive factors because of their role in indirect causality (14,15). Although it has been accepted that these factors are associated with the development and healing of pressure sores, little prospective data exist on the predictive vaule of these individual factors. Clinical risk assessment based on identifying these factors has, in fact, been disappointing. The Norton Pressure Sore Risk Assessment Scale, which has been used most extensively to identify patients at risk, has been reported to have only 50% predictive value in some settings (16).

TABLE 1. *Factors associated with pressure sore development and healing*

Primary factors	Secondary factors
Pressure over bony prominence	Malnutrition
Shear forces	Immobility
	Moisture
	Anemia
	Vascular insufficiency
	Sensory impairment

Nutritional factors have been associated with the healing of pressure sores in a variety of studies. Bergstrom and Braden have shown that baseline nutritional status is one of the best predictors of pressure sore healing (14). Allman et al. have demonstrated that increased protein intake alone is associated with a 1.4-fold increased odds ratio for healing pressure sores (7). Other studies have focused on vitamin and mineral supplementation. In a randomized, placebo-controlled trial, vitamin C (ascorbic acid, 500 mg bid) produced a significant reduction in pressure sore surface area, even in the absence of a true deficiency state (17). Although an effect of zinc supplementation has also been reported (18), its use in the absence of true deficiency remains controversial (9).

The effect of nutritional factors on pressure sore healing at the cellular and biochemical level have not been specifically studied. Most of our knowledge on how nutritional factors may play a role in pressure healing has been extrapolated from studies of surgical wound healing and of chronic wounds other than pressure sores. In order to understand better the role of nutrition in pressure sore healing, a review of the basic biology of wound healing is in order.

BIOLOGY OF WOUND HEALING

The major biologic processes that are important in tissue repair and wound healing are shown in Fig. 1. They include inflammation, collagen metabolism, wound contraction, and epithelialization (19). A clear understanding of these processes is vital for a rational approach to management of pressure sores. Nutritional factors play an important role in each of these processes.

The *inflammatory* response to injury is a vital process in wound healing. All tissue injury is followed immediately by a cascade of molecular and cellular events that are clinically observed as inflammation. With tissue injury, altered vascularity results in coagulation, and platelet mediators are released. Small blood vessels dilate, capillary permeability increases, and leukocytes migrate into the wound. Monocytes and macrophages ingest necrotic material, as well as bacteria. It is now known that macrophages also play a role in collagen synthesis. Indeed, it has been shown that depletion of wound macrophages decreases significantly the deposition of wound collagen (20).

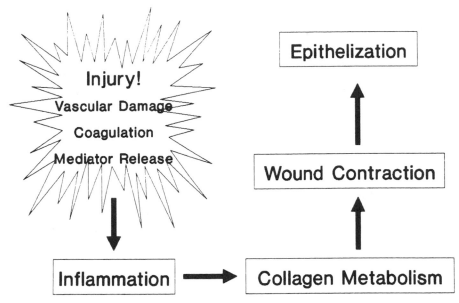

FIG. 1. Schematic representation of the major events in tissue repair and wound healing.

Collagen metabolism provides strength and integrity to healing wounds. Collagen is secreted from cells in a triple-helical structure. The formation of this procollagen requires the specific enzymes, lysyl and prolyl hydroxylase. The activity of these enzymes requires oxygen, vitamin C, and iron as co-factors. After collagen has been secreted from the cell, glycosolation occurs through the action of the enzyme, O-lysyl glactosyltransferase. This enzyme is known to depend on manganese as a cofactor (21). However, it is not collagen synthesis but collagen cross-linking that is critical for the strength and integrity of healing wounds. For the final cross-linking of collagen, the enzyme, lysyl oxidase, requires copper as a critical factor (21). Theoretically, nutritional deficiency of any of these cofactors may therefore result in diminished collagen formation.

Wound contraction may be the most important process in the spontaneous closure of large wounds. Unless contraction occurs, bringing the dermal structures together, the granulating surface is covered by a layer of epithelial cells that is ineffective in providing adequate strength and integrity. It is thought that the myofibroblast is the cell responsible for contraction while collagen holds the newly contracted tissue in place (22). The relationship between this process and the development of contractures remains unclear.

Epithelialization results from epithelial cell propagation and migration in a partial-thickness wound, the final result of which is the restoration of a barrier function similar to normal skin. It has been shown that a moist environment and oxygen are essential for epithelialization to take place (10).

Thus, dressings that are both gas permeable and hydrophobic are most useful at this stage of healing (10).

Studies of specific age-related changes associated with wound healing have been quite limited. In animals and humans there appears to be an age-associated decrease in wound healing (23). Epithelialization and cellular proliferation proceed more slowly (24,25) with advancing age, and collagen strength and overall wound strength often do not reach the same level as in younger subjects (23,26). These age-associated findings appear to be more qualitative than quantitative. Events begin later, proceed more slowly, and often do not reach the same level.

SPECIFIC NUTRITIONAL REQUIREMENTS

Table 2 summarizes the function of the various nutritional elements in tissue repair and wound healing.

Protein

Protein deficiency prolongs the inflammatory phase and impairs cellular proliferation. Studies have shown reduced fibroblastic proliferation, collagen synthesis, neoangiogenesis, and wound remodeling in the presence of

TABLE 2. *Function of various nutritional elements in wound healing*

Element	Function	Deficiency effect
Protein	Cell proliferation, collagen metabolism	Delayed healing
Carbohydrate	Energy source	Altered WBC function
Fats	Membrane function	Not known
Vitamin C	Enzyme cofactor in collagen metabolism	Altered collagen formation, delayed healing, scurvy
Vitamin A	Antagonizing effect of steroids	Not well known
Thiamine	Energy metabolism	Decreased cell proliferation and collagen metabolism
Vitamin E	Stabilization of membranes	None known
Vitamin K	Coagulation cofactor	Excessive bleeding, hematoma, wound disruption
Water and salts: Na^+, K^+, Cl^-	Membrane function, hydration	Volume depletion, decreased tissue profusion
Phosphorus	ATP metabolism	Altered cell replication and protein metabolism
Ca^{++}, Mg^{++}, Mn	Enzyme cofactors in collagen metabolism	Altered collagen formation, delayed healing
Zinc	RNA metabolism	Altered cell replication, delayed healing
Iron, copper	Enzyme cofactors in collagen metabolism	Delayed healing, anemia

hypoproteinemia (27). It has been possible to single out at least one amino acid that is a critical factor in these processes. Methionine, which is converted to cysteine, may act as a cofactor for a number of enzymes in collagen synthesis. Moreover, cysteine is critical in the collagen molecule, providing disulfide bridges to align the triple-helical structure of collagen (27). Other important functions have been postulated for histidine (28) and arginine (29); however, their exact roles in wound healing have not been well characterized.

Carbohydrate and Fat

Glucose is needed as an energy source for most tissues. Moreover, glucose is essential for white blood cell function. Fats are constituents necessary for membrane synthesis in proliferating cells. No significant wound impairment has been associated with essential fatty acid deficiency (27).

Vitamins

Vitamin C has been shown to have a dominant role in wound healing. Vitamin C deficiency results in abnormal collagen synthesis as described above. Abnormal amino acid sequences are produced, procollagen is not secreted from cells, appropriate cross-linking cannot occur, and the clinical picture of scurvy occurs. New wounds do not heal appropriately, and old wounds may break down. Administration of vitamin C rapidly corrects these problems. Recently, it has been suggested that administration of vitamin C may enhance wound healing, even in the absence of a deficiency state (17).

Vitamin A may also play an important role in wound healing. Vitamin A can counteract some of the effects of steroids, presumably by reversing the stabilizing effect that steroids have on lysosomal membranes (30). Although poor wound healing as a result of vitamin A deficiency has not been well isolated and described clinically, animals on steroids have shown improved healing when concurrently treated with vitamin A (30).

Thiamine (vitamin B_1) deficiency has been shown to have a dramatic effect on collagen synthesis in animals. It is postulated that thiamine's role is played at a cellular level related to energy metabolism in rapidly proliferating cells that secrete collagen (31).

The effect of vitamin E on wound healing similar to that of steroids, is to interfere with collagen metabolism and wound healing (32). Studies to date have failed to show any beneficial effect of either systemic or topical administration of this vitamin.

Other vitamins, including pyridoxine and riboflavin, may contribute to wound healing through either their effects as cofactors in collagen metabolism or in more basic cellular energy and protein metabolism (21). Vitamin K plays an indirect role by preventing disorders of coagulation that may result in excessive bleeding or subsequent wound disruption.

Minerals

Macrominerals, such as sodium, potassium, chloride, calcium, and phosphorus, are all required for efficient cellular processes that are vital to healing tissues. Salt and water balance is critical for maintaining adequate intravascular volume and local tissue perfusion. Phosphorus provides necessary substrates for ATP energy metabolism. Finally, calcium is a necessary cofactor for many cellular enzyme systems, including various collagenases, and for contractile mechanisms.

Zinc deficiency results in a variety of adverse effects on the healing process. There is a reduction in the rate of epithelialization, the rate of gain in wound strength, and collagen strength. Zinc acts as a cofactor in RNA polymerase and reverse transcriptase, which are vitally important in cell proliferation. Zinc deficiency probably impairs the proliferation of inflammatory cells, epithelial cells, and fibroblasts essential for synthesis of sufficient amounts of collagen. Whether zinc administration in the absence of true deficiency results in enhanced healing remains controversial (18).

In theory, iron deficiency can impair hydroxylation of the collagen molecule as described above. In practice, however, iron deficiency and anemia have never been shown to alter this process. Anemia, however, can result in hypovolemia and decreased oxygen delivery to healing tissues. Anemia, hypovolemia, and tissue hypoxia appear to have far more potent delayed healing effects than iron deficiency *per se* (33).

Other trace elements, including copper, manganese, and magnesium, are important in the synthesis of the collagen peptide chain. Although deficiency states of these minerals are extremely rare, production of trace element deficiencies have been observed during prolonged total parenteral nutrition (34). Wound healing abnormalities might be important in such cases.

MANAGEMENT OF NUTRITIONAL FACTORS ASSOCIATED WITH PRESSURE SORES

In addition to mobilizing patients and controlling pressure, management of nutritional factors is essential for prevention and rapid healing of pressure sores. Nutritional assessment should be an integral part of the evaluation of all patients at risk for pressure sore development, as well as of those with existing pressure sores. Nutritional assessment may be derived from a variety of sources, including the history, physical exam, and laboratory evaluations as described in Chapter 6.

Once the patient's nutritional status has been assessed, appropriate intervention must occur. Protein and calories should be supplied based on the expectation of increased requirements for the correction of existing deficits and for increased catabolic states, such as fever, infection, and healing wounds. The use of enteral and/or parenteral hyperalimentation may be required in patients whose appetite or disability impairs adequate intake. Vitamin, mineral, and trace element deficiencies must be anticipated and corrected in this population. A multivitamin and mineral supplement providing the Recommended Daily Allowances is probably reasonable. Although administration of vitamin C and zinc in the absence of a deficiency state remains controversial, there may be a benefit observed, and toxicity of these nutrients is reasonably low (17,18). Finally, nutritional reassessment should continue throughout the treatment course to ensure replenishment of deficits and prevent complications of hyperalimentation, including hyperglycemia and fluid volume disturbances. These issues are covered in more detail in other chapters.

CONCLUSION

Pressure sore problems can be expected to increase with the growing number of frail elderly. The maintenance of good nutrition is critical for patients at risk or with existing pressure sores. Appropriate management of nutritional factors plays a dramatic role in the overall comfort, quality of care, and cost of the management of pressure sores in the elderly.

REFERENCES

1. Pinchofsky-Devin GD, Kaminski MV. *J Am Geriatr Soc* 1986; 43:435–440.
2. Allman RM, Laparade CA, Noel LB, et al. *Ann Intern Med* 1986; 105:337–342.
3. *National nursing home survey, United States, May-Dec. 1977,* Vital and Health Statistics, series 13:51. Washington, DC: Government Printing Office, 1981 (DHHS Pub. No. (PHS):81-1712).
4. Schakle WE, Peterson PJ. *Arch Intern Med* 1986; 146:1981–1984.
5. Peterson NC, Bittman S. *Scand J Plast Reconstr Surg* 1971; 5:26–66.
6. Michocki RJ, Lamy PP. *J Am Geriatr Soc* 1976; 24:323–328.
7. Allman RM, Wallace JM, Hart MK, Laprake CA, Noel LB, Smity CR. *Ann Intern Med* 1987; 107:641–648.
8. Reuler JC, Cooney TG. *Ann Intern Med* 1981; 94:661–666.
9. Allman RM. *N Engl J Med* 1989; 320:850–853.
10. Seiler WO, Stahelin HB. *Geriatrics* 1985; 40:30.
11. Ferrell BA, Azain G, Osterweil D. *Geriatr Med Tod* 1989; 8:81–88.
12. Kosiak M. *Arch Phys Med Rehabil* 1959; 40:62–69.
13. Bennet L, Kavner D, Lee BK, Trainor FA. *Arch Phys Med* 1969; 60:309–314.

14. Bergstrom N, Braden BJ, Laguzza A, Holman V. *Nurs Res* 1987; 36:205–210.
15. Krouskop TA. *Medi Hypoth* 1983; 11:255–267.
16. Lincoln R, Roberts R, Maddox A, Levine S, Patterson C. *J Enterost Ther* 1986; 13:132–138.
17. Taylor TV, Rimmer S, Day B, Butcher J, Dymock IW. *Lancet* 1974; 2:544–546.
18. Pories WJ, Henzel JH, Rob CG, Strain WH. *Lancet* 1967; 1:121–124.
19. Carrico TJ, Mehrhof AI, Cohen IK. *Surg Clin North Am* 1984; 64:721–733.
20. Dieglemann RF, Cohen IK, Kaplan AM. *Plast Reconstr Surg* 1981; 68:107–113.
21. Ruberg RL. *Surg Clin North Am* 1984;64:705–714.
22. Majno G, Gappiani G, Hirshcel BJ, et al. *Science* 1971; 173:548.
23. Eaglstein WH. *Clin Geriatr Med* 1989; 5:183–188.
24. Olerud JH, Gown AM, et al. *J Invest Dermatol* 1988; 90:845–850.
25. Staatz WD, Van Horn DL. *Invest Opthalmol Vis Sci* 1980; 19:983–986.
26. Holm-Pederson P, Zenderfildt B. *Scand J Plast Reconstr Surg* 1971; 5:13–16.
27. Pollack SV. *J Dermatol Surg Oncol* 1979; 5:615.
28. Fitzpatrick DW, Fisher H. *Ann Surg* 1982; 91:56–60.
29. Barbul A, Rettiture G, Levenson SM, et al. *Surg Forum* 1977; 28:108.
30. Ehrlich HP, Hunt DK. *Ann Surg* 1968; 167:324.
31. Alvarez OM, Gilbreath RL. *J Surg Res* 1982; 32:24–31.
32. Erlich HP, Tarver H, Hunt TK. *Ann Surg* 1972; 175:235.
33. Heughan C, Grislis G, Hunt TK. *Ann Surg* 1974; 179:163.
34. Ruberg RL, Mirtallo J. *Ohio State Med J* 1981; 77:725.

Geriatric Nutrition, edited by John E. Morley,
Zvi Glick, Laurence Z. Rubenstein.
Raven Press, Ltd., New York © 1990.

29

Drug-Food/Food-Drug Interactions

Christine Hamilton Smith

*Division of Food Science, Nutrition and Dietetics, Home Economics Department
California State University, Northridge, Northridge, California 91330*

Aging is not a homogeneous process nor a disease with a course of action that can be reversed or cured by medications or nutrients. In each person, an inevitable decline in physiologic function will occur, which will ultimately affect the well-being of the individual. The prevalence of chronic disease conditions is likely to increase in this growing segment of the American population, as demographic projections into the 21st century indicate that longevity will continue to rise over the next three decades.

At present, persons 65 years of age and over represent about 12% of the total population, yet they use close to 30% of all prescribed and over-the-counter (OTC) medications; undoubtedly, their drug usage is related to the frequency of chronic illnesses and disabilities. The therapeutic armamentarium used to treat these conditions is made up of numerous prescription medications and nonprescription drugs. The average older person with multiple concurrent problems may be using from three to seven (or more) different medications at any given time (1). Some patients in long-term care institutions are prescribed up to 23 drugs (2). In addition to cardiovascular, psychotropic, antimicrobial, gastric, and other agents, commonly used OTC preparations by the elderly include analgesics, vitamins, and laxatives (3). In fact, laxatives are regularly used by the elderly and were found to be the single largest class of drugs prescribed for the largest number of nursing home patients (2).

Drugs often influence nutrient disposition through their effects on nutrient absorption, metabolism, and excretion. In addition to these effects, food itself or specific constituents in food or beverages, as well as vitamin, mineral, and other food supplements, can influence drug behavior (4).

Nutrient (food) and drug interactions are likely to occur in elderly patients not only because of drug- or food-induced alterations in nutrient and drug disposition, respectively, but also because of nonuniform organ deterioration, underlying chronic diseases, dietary regimens, an already compromised nutritional state, and other factors related to aging. Multiple drug use too can affect the health of patients and potentially reduce the quality of their life. A variety of commonly prescribed medications and nonprescription drugs deserve special consideration because of their influence on nutritional status or the effect of diet on drug response. Without proper nutritional management of the elderly patient, use of gastric medications, cardiovascular agents or blood modifiers, anti-inflammatory agents, analgesics, respiratory tract agents, central nervous system (CNS) medications, and food supplements can ultimately result in either nutrient depletion or food-induced, altered drug efficacy.

CARDIOVASCULAR DRUGS AND BLOOD MODIFIERS

Digitalis Glycosides

Digoxin is a frequently prescribed drug in the United States. Because of its narrow therapeutic index, this drug is known to produce a number of adverse effects in older adults.

Loss of appetite, gastrointestinal (GI) disturbances, or diet- or diuretic-induced changes in plasma electrolytes can influence the likelihood of digitalis toxicity, which occurs frequently and can be life threatening. Although anorexia and GI effects may be early signs of drug intoxication, diminished food intake resulting from these effects is considered a significant risk factor in the frail elderly for whom digoxin is prescribed (5).

In addition, nausea (a symptom of either the disease itself or drug intoxication), vomiting or diarrhea, and other disturbances can further compromise food intake and result in nutrient depletion. Because of a multitude of factors in the aged population that can alter their dietary habits and appetite or even affect food procurement, knowledge of the patient's dietary habits is not only helpful but also essential in order to avoid possible situations that may compromise the health of the aging adult.

Of equal importance, hypokalemia and hypomagnesemia (possible effects of faulty nutrition), concomitant diuretic therapy, or both increase the patient's sensitivity to digitalis, thus enhancing its toxicity. Also, concurrent use of calcium or vitamin D supplements (6) needs to be evaluated carefully in digitalized, elderly patients as such combined therapies may lead to hypercalcemia and cause severe toxic reactions. Nutritional implications and dietary suggestions pertaining to the use of digoxin are described in Table 1.

Diuretics

Other nutrient-drug interactions worthy of special notice include the effects of diuretics on mineral excretion. These drugs are prescribed to treat a number of cardiovascular disorders, including hypertension, edema associated with congestive heart failure, and other conditions. Nutritional implications associated with them center around electrolyte disturbances and the use of prescribed diet therapies to treat hypertension.

Potassium-depleting diuretics—furosemide, thiazide—enhance the renal excretion of potassium, as well as magnesium. With either of those drugs, sodium-restricted diets and foods rich in potassium are usually prescribed. However, caution needs to be exercised in prescribing a high potassium intake for patients with renal impairment. Patients should also be encouraged to incorporate magnesium-rich foods into their diet. Similar dietary suggestions are important for patients who are being concomitantly treated with digitalis; decreased plasma concentrations of potassium or magnesium may predispose the patient to digitalis toxicity.

Yet, not all patients treated with diuretics need to consider the increased intake of potassium-rich foods in their diet; some diuretics, such as spironolactone, spare potassium. Because of the common association of diuretic therapy with the depletion of potassium, patients treated with other diuretics (potassium-sparing) or diuretic combinations may not be aware that dietary mineral recommendations vary, depending on the action of the drug. Patients must be counseled about the importance of their personal diet prescription and cautioned about following the dietary advice of well-meaning friends and acquaintances.

Numerous nutritional implications and dietary suggestions associated with the use of diuretics in the treatment of disease are listed in Table 1. Elderly patients should be advised to take single-dose preparations in the morning to minimize the inconvenience of nocturnal diuresis, which may increase the risk of falling and injury.

Beta-Adrenergic Blocking Agents

Several dietary concerns pertaining to the use of propranolol, the beta-adrenergic blocking agent, are listed in Table 1. As a nonselective beta blocker, this drug is used to treat hypertension, cardiac arrhythmias, and other conditions. Because food enhances its bioavailability and the intake of propranolol with food may also improve compliance, it is recommended that this drug be taken with meals (7). The concurrent ingestion with food may temporarily reduce firstpass hepatic metabolism of the medication, an effect believed to be caused by the inhibition of presystemic primary conjugation in the liver.

Vasodilators and Antiarrhythmic Agents

The predominant effect of hydralazine, a nondiuretic antihypertensive agent, is direct anteriolar dilatation. Its use in the elderly may be limited because of intolerable side effects, such as increased sensitivity to the hy-

TABLE 1. *Cardiovascular drugs and nutritional concerns*

| Drug (usage) | Nutritional implications | | Dietary suggestions |
	Gastrointestinal side/ adverse effects	Other effects	
Cholestyramine (antihyperlipemic agent, bile acid sequestrant)	Constipation Flatulence Indigestion Nausea/vomiting Steatorrhea Stomach pain	Malabsorption of lipids, carotene, calcium, iron, vitamins A, D, K, B_{12}, & folacin Hypoprothrombinemia Possible weight changes Gritty texture Unpalatable taste Anorexia	**Drug:** 1. Hydrate thoroughly drug with at least 120- to 180-ml water, milk, fruit juice, or noncarbonated or other beverages before ingestion. 2. Disguise gritty texture and unpalatable taste by mixing with highly flavored liquids, thin soups, milk in cereals, or pureed foods. **Diet Rx:** 1. If permissible, include a high-bulk diet with increased fluid intake to counter constipation. 2. Monitor and control or reduce weight. 3. Take food supplements at least 1 hr before or 4 to 6 hrs after drug. **Other:** Before drug therapy, attempt to control serum cholesterol by diet therapy. During drug therapy, advise patient of the importance of following a prescribed diet, as effects of diet and drug are additive.
Digoxin (cardiotonic)	Nausea/vomiting Stomach pain Diarrhea (signs of toxicity)	Anorexia Weakness (signs of toxicity)	**Drug:** 1. Drug absorption can be delayed by the presence of food in gastrointestinal tract (GI) or by delayed gastric emptying 2. Take with water 1/2 hr before or 2 hrs after high-fiber foods (fiber may delay absorption). **Diet Rx:** 1. Monitor for adequate food intake. 2. Maintain diet high in potassium, low in sodium, and adequate in magnesium. 3. Caution patient about calcium and vitamin D supplements; may lead to hypercalcemia.

374

Drug	Effects	Instructions
		4. Caution patient about herbal teas; may be made from plants with digitalis-like activity.
		5. Limit natural licorice.
		6. Provide medical attention to any patient presenting anorexia, unusual tiredness or weakness, or GI disturbances.
Furosemide (potassium-depleting diuretic)	Enhanced excretion of potassium, calcium, magnesium, sodium, chloride, and water Fluid and electrolyte disturbances Dry mouth Thirst Anorexia Dizziness Peculiar sweet taste Diarrhea Nausea/vomiting Stomach cramps/pain	**Drug:** 1. Take on empty stomach with water. Food decreases drug absorption. 2. To minimize effect of nocturnal diuresis, take single daily dose in morning. **Diet Rx:** 1. If appropriate, emphasize the importance of a decreased kcal/low-sodium diet for the treatment of hypertension. 2. Maintain diet high in potassium and magnesium. 3. Monitor and control or reduce weight. 4. Limit alcohol. 5. Limit natural licorice. 6. Monitor diabetics as drug impairs glucose tolerance. 7. Advise patient that dry mouth, increased thirst, or severe nausea, vomiting, or diarrhea may indicate or contribute to fluid and electrolyte imbalance. **Other:** Avoid OTC preparations containing sympathomimetics (cold/cough medications and some forms used for weight control).
Hydralazine (nondiuretic antihypertensive)	Vitamin B_6 antagonism (may result in peripheral neuropathy) Anorexia Dizziness Diarrhea Nausea/vomiting Constipation (rare)	**Diet:** 1. Take consistently with food (may enhance drug bioavailability). **Diet Rx:** 1. If appropriate, emphasize the importance of a decreased kcal/low-sodium diet for the treatment of hypertension. 2. Monitor and control or reduce weight. 3. Limit alcohol.

continued

375

TABLE 1. Continued

Drug (usage)	Nutritional implications		Dietary suggestions
	Gastrointestinal side/ adverse effects	Other effects	
			4. Limit natural licorice.
			5. May prescribe vitamin B$_6$ supplementation if signs of peripheral neuropathy develop.
			Other: See furosemide.
Propranolol (antiarrhythmic, nondiuretic antihypertensive, beta-adrenergic blocking agent)	Constipation or diarrhea Nausea/vomiting Gastric discomfort	Dry mouth Impaired glycogenolysis	**Drug:** 1. Take consistently with food (enhances drug bioavailability). **Diet Rx:** 1. If appropriate, emphasize the importance of a decreased kcal/low-sodium diet for the treatment of hypertension. 2. Limit alcohol. 3. Monitor and control or reduce weight. 4. Limit natural licorice. **Other:** See furosemide.
Quinidine (antiarrhythmic)	Diarrhea Nausea/vomiting Stomach cramps/pain	Anorexia Bitter taste Dizziness Suppression of vitamin-K-dependent clotting factors	**Drug:** 1. Take with 250 ml water on an empty stomach, preferably 1 hr before or 2 hrs after meals to enhance absorption. 2. To reduce gastric irritation, take with food or milk. 3. Swallow tablet whole; do not chew, crush, or break tablet. **Diet Rx:** 1. Avoid excessive intake of large amounts of citrus juices; may alkalinize urine, enhance renal drug reabsorption, and increase serum quinidine levels. 2. Maintain adequate intake of vitamin K as need may be increased.

376

Drug	Side effects	Recommendations
Spironolactone (potassium-sparing diuretic)	Abdominal cramps Diarrhea Nausea/vomiting Fluid and electrolyte changes (enhanced excretion of sodium chloride, magnesium, calcium, and water) Dry mouth Thirst Anorexia Altered taste	**Drug:** 1. Take with meals or milk to minimize gastric irritation. May also enhance bioavailability. 2. Take at least 6 hrs before bedtime to minimize inconvenience of nocturnal diuresis. **Diet Rx:** 1. If appropriate, emphasize the importance of a decreased kcal/low-sodium diet for the treatment of hypertension. 2. Monitor and control or reduce weight. 3. Caution against potassium-containing salt substitutes, low-sodium foods with high potassium content, and potassium supplements. 4. Limit potassium-rich foods. 5. Limit natural licorice. 6. Advise cautious use by diabetics; as it may increase blood glucose. 7. Advise patient that dry mouth, increased thirst, or severe nausea, vomiting, or diarrhea may indicate or contribute to fluid and electrolyte imbalance. **Other:** See furosemide.
Thiazide diuretics (potassium-depleting)	Diarrhea Nausea/vomiting Upset stomach or cramping Enhanced excretion of potassium, magnesium, sodium, zinc, and water Fluid and electrolyte disturbances Decreased urinary calcium excretion Dry mouth Thirst Anorexia	**Drug:** 1. Take with meals or milk to minimize gastric irritation. 2. To minimize the effect of nocturnal diuresis, take single dose early in morning. **Diet Rx:** 1. If appropriate, emphasize the importance of a decreased kcal/low-sodium diet for the treatment of hypertension. 2. Monitor and control or reduce weight. 3. Maintain diet high in potassium and magnesium.

continued

TABLE 1. *Continued*

| Drug (usage) | Nutritional implications | | Dietary suggestions |
	Gastrointestinal side/ adverse effects	Other effects	
		Dizziness	4. Caution against the use of large doses of calcium and vitamin D supplements. 5. Limit alcohol. 6. Limit natural licorice. 7. Advise patient that dry mouth, increased thirst, or severe nausea, vomiting, or diarrhea may indicate or contribute to fluid and electrolyte imbalance. **Other:** See furosemide.
Warfarin (anticoagulant)	Diarrhea Nausea/vomiting Stomach cramps/pain	Inhibition of vitamin-K-dependent coagulation factors Hypoprothrombinemia	**Diet Rx:** 1. Maintain an adequate, balanced diet; prolonged dietary insufficiency enhances anticoagulant response. 2. Limit foods high in vitamin K and green tea; may decrease anticoagulant response. 3. Limit fried or boiled onions; may enhance anticoagulant response. 4. Limit alcohol. 5. Caution against the use of large doses of ascorbic acid and vitamins A, E, and K. 6. Caution against the use of some herbal teas; may contain naturally occurring coumarin derivatives.

378

potensive effects of the drug, the development of peripheral neuropathy, and other effects. Consistent intake with meals is suggested, which may enhance drug bioavailability by decreasing first-pass hepatic metabolism. In addition, this drug is believed to have an antipyridoxine effect that may cause peripheral neuropathy in patients for whom the drug is prescribed. Pyridoxine requirements may be increased, and often supplemental pyridoxine is taken to counter this side effect. Other dietary suggestions and nutritional implications associated with the use of hydralazine are shown in Table 1.

Drug-food interactions should be of particular concern in the elderly for whom quinidine is prescribed. A large intake of citrus fruit juices (>1 liter/day) has been found to increase urinary pH, an effect believed to be responsible for increasing the proportion of un-ionized quinidine. Because quinidine is a weak base, renal clearance may be decreased in a slightly alkaline urine, thus increasing the serum concentration of the drug. The concurrent intake of large amounts of citrus fruit juices may increase the potential for toxic effects, thus predisposing the elderly patient to an increased risk of cardiac arrhythmias, depressed myocardial contractility, hypotension, cinchonism (a cluster of adverse effects, such as nausea, vomiting, diarrhea, tinnitus, dizziness, and blurred vision), and other adverse effects. Dietary and other concerns pertaining to its use are included in Table 1.

Anticoagulants

Warfarin, a coumarin derivative, prevents the formation of vitamin-K-dependent blood clotting factors by inhibiting procoagulation factors II, VII, IX, and X in the liver. Anticoagulants are used for prophylaxis against the development of thromboembolic events in elderly, high-risk patients. After such an episode, anticoagulation therapy may also be indicated in the treatment of immobilized patients or other high-risk patients with underlying or coexisting disorders.

Dietary suggestions (Table 1) for the use of oral anticoagulants focus on dietary habits and the use of some vitamin supplements. Resistance to the hypoprothrombinemic effects of the anticoagulant warfarin may be a reflection of several factors, including the availability of vitamin K in foods. Patients who are undergoing anticoagulation therapy are usually stabilized while on hospital diets; therefore, they should be questioned about their usual dietary habits at home and cautioned about the overuse of certain foods, especially those that are high in vitamin K content, as well as their use of food supplements.

Cholesterol-Lowering Agents

Although intensive dietary treatment is the primary therapy for treating patients with elevated cholesterol, drug therapy may be added after strict adherence to dietary changes has proven to be inadequate (8). Cholestyramine, a bile acid sequestrant, has been shown in clinical trials to be effective, when combined with fat-modified diets, in reducing elevated cholesterol levels. This drug, as well as colestipol, also a bile acid sequestrant, however, must be cautiously used in elderly patients because it is likely to cause GI disturbances and nutrient malabsorption. Specific nutrients can bind to the cholestyramine in the intestinal lumen, or potentially, the drug may inhibit the absorption of fat-soluble nutrients because of decreased availability of bile acids. Because of its side effects, especially constipation or a delayed or reduced absorption of nutrients, nutrition counseling is deemed necessary to advise patients about the concurrent intake of food, food supplements, and the drug. Patients need to know how to take the drug in order to disguise its undesirable taste and texture. Too, patients should be encouraged to incorporate dietary fiber into their diet in order to counter the constipating effects of the drug (Table 1).

The National Cholesterol Education Program-Adult Treatment Panel recommends that cholesterol-lowering agents, such as bile-acid resins, lovastatin, and nicotinic acid, be added to, but not considered as a substitute for dietary therapy. Patients must be informed that the combined effects of diet and drug therapy have been shown to be necessary and effective in lowering blood cholesterol.

GASTROINTESTINAL MEDICATIONS

Laxatives

Laxative use is common in the elderly, mainly as an agent to correct constipation or what may be perceived to be constipation. A variety of factors, such as aging itself, sedentary habits, diet, constipating medications, and confinement to bed, may all contribute to the development of this disorder. The overuse of laxatives too may contribute to constipation because of altered colonic motility. Of concern is the loss of nutrients resulting from drug-induced hyperperistalsis (bisacodyl, phenolphthalein) or the trapping of fat-soluble nutrients in the laxative itself (mineral oil). In addition to these effects, bulk-forming preparations (psyllium) or even dietary fiber may reduce appetite and result in decreased food intake because of a feeling of fullness.

Table 2 shows the various effects of laxatives on nutrient absorption and the dietary suggestions associated with the use of these drugs. If a laxative is deemed necessary in the older adult, the patient needs to be educated about its proper use. For most types of orally administered laxatives, the patient must drink at least 1.5 to 2.0 liters/day of water or other liquids. Not only does this help prevent the formation of hard, dry stools but it also aids in stool softening. Furthermore, patients should not be using such drugs more often than recommended by the manufacturer and should not be using these medications unnecessarily, eg, to clean out "toxins" in the GI tract or to aid in a bowel movement if one is missed for 1 or 2 days. In order to avoid the laxative habit and to re-establish normal bowel habits (and to reduce the cost of medications), older adults need to be encouraged to institute, if possible, some changes in the types of foods consumed, their meal patterns, and their activity levels. Some simple measures that may help restore normal colonic activity are outlined in *Food Medication Interactions* by Powers and Moore (9).

Cimetidine

Cimetidine is a histamine H_2-receptor antagonist indicated in the treatment of peptic ulcers and to decrease gastic secretions. Dietary concerns (Table 2) associated with the use of this agent center around its ability to inhibit hepatic microsomal drug metabolism, thus decreasing the metabolism of methylxanthines, eg, caffeine. In addition, it is important that the drug be taken with or just after meals to prolong its effect during the postprandial period. The diet prescription should also incorporate the dietary principles associated with the treatment of ulcer disease.

MUSCULOSKELETAL AGENTS

Common joint diseases seen in older patients include osteoarthritis, gout and pseudogout, and rheumatoid arthritis. Although these disorders are frequently seen in the elderly, some joint disorders (gout, rheumatoid arthritis) can occur at any age. However, as patients age, these conditions become increasingly disabling. Aspirin, as well as nonsalicylate, nonsteroidal anti-inflammatory agents (NSAIA), are commonly taken by the elderly and are effective drugs for the relief of such diverse ailments as headaches, aches, pains, and musculoskeletal stiffness. However, because their potential to produce adverse reactions is not well known by older adults, they need to be educated about the responsible use of these medications.

Contrary to popular belief, special diets or food supplements play no role in the progression or treatment of arthritis, other than a possible kilocalorie-restricted diet for weight reduction. Nutritional implications and dietary suggestions for the use of aspirin in the treatment of this disorder center around potential nutrient deficiencies and dietary means to reduce or prevent gastric disturbances and altered nutrient status. Low serum folacin levels, reflecting perhaps vitamin redistribution, have been found in rheumatoid arthritic patients for whom aspirin has been prescribed (10). Reduced platelet and plasma ascorbic acid levels have also been reported in rheumatoid arthritic patients receiving aspirin (11). Until additional information is available

TABLE 2. *Gastrointestinal medications and nutritional concerns*

| Drug (usage) | Nutritional implications | | Dietary suggestions |
	Gastrointestinal side/adverse effects	Other effects	
Bisacodyl (stimulant laxative)	Belching Cramping Diarrhea Nausea	Electrolyte imbalance (hypokalemia with chronic use)	**Drug:** 1. Take with 250 ml water on an empty stomach. 2. Administer at least 1 hr apart from milk; concurrent use may dissolve enteric coating. 3. Swallow tablet whole; do not chew, crush, or break. **Diet Rx:** 1. Drink at least 1.5 to 2.0 liters/day of fluid. 2. Inform patient of dietary principles associated with the treatment of constipation. **Other:** 1. Avoid chronic misuse; may cause electrolyte loss or exacerbate incoordination, orthostatic hypertension, and weakness. 2. Avoid chronic misuse; may cause dependence on drug for bowel function.
Cimetidine (histamine H_2- receptor antagonist; antiulcer)	Diarrhea Decreased gastric acid and intrinsic factor secretion Nausea/vomiting	Inhibition of hepatic cytochrome (P450 and P448) mixed-function oxidase system Dizziness	**Drug:** Take with food or meals. **Diet Rx:** 1. Limit caffeine. 2. Inform patient of dietary principles associated with the treatment of ulcer disease; avoid foods and beverages known to cause GI irritation.

382

Drug			
Mineral oil (lubricant laxative)	Flatulence Indigestion	Malabsorption of carotene; vitamins A, D, E, and K; calcium; and phosphorus Disagreeable consistency Anorexia, weight loss, and hypokalemia with chronic use	**Drug:** Take 2 hrs apart from food. **Diet Rx:** See bisacodyl. **Other:** Avoid chronic misuse; may cause dependence on drug for bowel function.
Phenolphthalein (stimulant laxative)	See bisacodyl	See bisacodyl	**Drug:** 1. Take with 250 ml water on an empty stomach. 2. Chew chewable tablets or wafer well before swallowing; follow with 250 ml water. **Diet Rx:** See bisacodyl. **Other:** See bisacodyl.
Psyllium hydrophilic mucilloid (bulk-forming laxative)	Diarrhea Flatulence Nausea/vomiting	Decreased appetite (abdominal fullness) Electrolyte imbalance (hypokalemia with chronic use)	**Drug:** Dissolve or mix dry form in 250 ml water or other fluids before swallowing. **Diet Rx:** 1. See bisacodyl. 2. Advise cautious use by diabetics; some preparations contain sugar. **Other:** See mineral oil.

to clarify the mechanisms by which aspirin affects vitamin status, well-balanced diets containing optimum amounts of these vitamins should be encouraged, rather than the use of supplements unless, of course, reduced blood levels indicate a need for supplementation. Of concern too is simple iron-deficiency anemia caused by occult blood loss from aspirin-induced GI bleeding. Other concerns associated with the use of aspirin and of ibuprofen are listed in Table 3.

PSYCHOTHERAPEUTIC AND OTHER CNS MEDICATIONS

Psychotherapeutic agents—tricyclic antidepressants, antipsychotics, and anxiolytic sedatives—are a commonly prescribed category of medications for elderly persons. These drugs are frequently given to nursing home residents or taken by older persons in the community to treat a variety of organic (dementia) and affective (depression) disorders, as well as anxiety and neurotic behaviors. Depression may be caused by multiple changes within the psychologic and social environment and, if untreated, may result in anorexia and significant weight loss. It is also important to look for medical or pharmacologic causes of the illness and the overuse or abuse of alcohol.

Tricylic Antidepressants

Table 3 lists nutritional implications and dietary suggestions associated with the use of the tricyclic antidepressant amitriptyline. Elderly patients should be warned of the potential anticholinergic effects of amitriptyline, as well as of other tricyclic antidepressants. Because of this effect, older adults who are already troubled with constipation may notice a worsening of the condition, which may subside after several weeks of therapy. However, aged patients who are particularly affected by the anticholinergic effects of some of these drugs should be advised that dry mouth or constipation is usually related to drug effects and not the diet. The inclusion of fiber in the diet, if tolerated, may diminish the significance of bowel disturbances. On the other hand, dry mouth and a diminished flow of saliva may contribute to the development of dental caries, periodontal disease, and other problems. The elderly patient should be encouraged to use sugarless gum or candy or ice, rather than increasing the intake of fluids high in kilocalories, which may contribute to weight gain.

Weight changes may also be indirectly related to an improved mental state or enhanced perception of taste, the effect of which then may lead to an overall increase in food consumption. An increased craving for specific foods, such as sweets, has also been found to be a causative factor in weight gain in patients for whom tricyclic antidepressants have been prescribed (12).

Lithium

A significant number of elderly patients receive lithium for the treatment of manic-depressive illness. Their intake of sodium and fluid may need to be adjusted as restriction of either one decreases renal clearance of the drug and predisposes the patient to lithium toxicity. Constancy of daily sodium intake and ample fluid intake (2.5 to 3 liters/day) are essential means to maintain stable lithium levels (13). Patients also need to be aware of the sodium content of common foods, especially highly processed foods. Other risk factors that may cause toxic drug reactions include low-salt diets, profuse sweating, and dehydration. Not only should elderly patients be advised about their diets but their initial body weight should also be determined at the time of drug stabilization and then monitored periodically. Bothersome side effects of lithium treatment include drug-induced increased appetite, polyuria, dry mouth, and excessive thirst. Patients may increase their intake of foods or fluids in an attempt to overcome these problems, which may contribute to an increase in body weight. Other concerns pertaining to the use of lithium are outlined in Table 3.

Antiparkinson Agents

Parkinsonism occurs most frequently in late middle age; the peak incidence is during the seventh decade of life. This disease is incurable, caused by a disruption of dopaminergic neurotransmission, and is a progressive degenerative condition affecting the central nervous system. Clinical features include tremor, rigidity, slowness of voluntary motion (bradykinesia), and a disturbance of posture. In addition, the patient also suffers from difficulties with mastication, swallowing, and other problems.

Levodopa may be prescribed alone or in combination with the dopa decarboxylase inhibitor (carbidopa). Dietary concerns associated with use of levodopa are listed in Table 3 and focus on the concurrent use of the drug with high-protein foods or with pyridoxine supplements. In the parkinsonian patient for whom this drug is prescribed, concomitant intake of pyridoxine with levodopa is not recommended as peripheral metabolism of the drug is thereby enhanced, thus reversing its therapeutic effect. Relatively modest amounts (5 mg) of supplemental pyridoxine, only slightly in excess of the Recommended Dietary Allowances (RDA) of 2 mg, are contraindicated for these patients, and they should be advised that many multivitamin preparations contain pyridoxine in excess of 5 mg (14).

Of concern too is inclusion of high-protein foods in the diet. Products resulting from protein digestion, especially the aromatic amino acids, compete for absorption sites in the small intestine and interfere with the bioavailability of levodopa (15). The suggested protein intake of 0.5 g/kg body weight for these patients (16) is below the RDA for protein (0.8 g/kg); however, if

TABLE 3. *Central nervous system medications and nutritional concerns*

| Drug (usage) | Nutritional implications | | Dietary suggestions |
	Gastrointestinal side/ adverse effects	Other effects	
Acetylsalicylic acid (aspirin) (analgesic, antipyretic, antiinflammatory)	Gastric pain Heartburn Nausea/vomiting Ulcerogenic potential	Increased excretion of ascorbic acid Altered folacin blood levels Potassium depletion (large doses) Iron-deficiency anemia (prolonged use/overuse)	**Drug:** 1. Take with food and 250 ml water to reduce GI irritation. 2. Swallow enteric-coated tablets whole; do not chew, crush, or break tablet. 3. Use buffered effervescent preparations cautiously for patients on low-sodium diets. **Diet Rx:** 1. Maintain a diet adequate in ascorbic acid and folacin. 2. Limit alcohol. 3. Maintain adequate fluid intake, especially if high dosages have been prescribed. 4. Advise cautious use for patients prone to vitamin K deficiency. 5. Advise patient that drug may contribute to or aggravate iron-deficiency anemia.
Amitriptyline (tricyclic antidepressant)	Constipation (or diarrhea) Nausea/vomiting	Increased appetite for carbohydrates Weight changes Dry mouth Peculiar taste Anorexia Dizziness	**Drug:** Take with or immediately after food to minimize GI irritation. **Diet Rx:** 1. Avoid alcohol. 2. Inform patient about possible appetite changes, especially for sweets. 3. Monitor and control or reduce weight. 4. Encourage the intake of high-fiber foods to counter constipation. 5. Limit caffeine. 6. Suggest the use of sugarless gum or candy, ice, or cold nonkilocaloric fluids as measures to relieve dry mouth.

386

Drug	Side effects	Instructions
Ibuprofen (analgesic, antipyretic, antiinflammatory)	Nausea/vomiting GI irritation Constipation (or diarrhea) Abdominal cramps (or pain) Bloating Flatulence Ulcerogenic potential	Decreased appetite Dry mouth Dizziness	**Drug:** Take with food and 250 ml water to reduce GI irritation. **Diet Rx:** Avoid alcohol; concurrent use may increase ulcerogenic potential.
Levodopa (antiparkinson agent)	Constipation (or diarrhea) Epigastric distress Nausea/vomiting	Anorexia Dry mouth Bitter taste Dizziness	**Drug:** Take food shortly after drug to minimize gastric distress (concurrent intake may alter drug effect); do not take with high-protein foods. **Diet Rx:** 1. Limit dietary protein intake to 0.5 g high biologic value protein/kg body weight/day or delay intake of protein foods until evening. 2. Avoid use of food supplements containing pyridoxine; 5-mg dose may abolish drug effect. 3. Avoid the use of amino acid or protein supplements. 4. Avoid caffeine. 5. Monitor diabetics; drug may alter blood glucose. 6. Suggest the use of sugarless gum or candy, ice, or cold nonkilocaloric fluids as measures to relieve dry mouth. **Other:** High gastric acidity or delayed stomach emptying may delay drug absorption.
Lithium (antimanic)	Bloated feeling Mild nausea Diarrhea, nausea/vomiting (signs of toxicity)	Increased thirst Dry mouth Metallic taste Weight gain Edema Hypothyroidism Dizziness	**Drug:** 1. Take with food. 2. Swallow extended- or slow-release dosage form whole; do not chew, crush, or break. **Diet Rx:** 1. Avoid dietary extremes. Maintain constant intake of sodium; avoid foods high in sodium.

continued

TABLE 3. *Continued*

| Drug (usage) | Nutritional implications | | Dietary suggestions |
	Gastrointestinal side/ adverse effects	Other effects	
		Altered glucose tolerance Hypercalcemia Hypophosphatemia Anorexia (toxic effect)	2. Advise cautious use for patients on low-sodium diets. 3. Caution against self-prescribed reducing diets. 4. Maintain adequate water or fluid intake (2.5 to 3.0 liters/day). 5. Monitor intake of kilocaloric-containing fluids. 6. Limit caffeine. 7. Monitor weight; obtain baseline weight before drug therapy. 8. Suggest the use of sugarless gum or candy, ice, or cold nonkilocaloric fluids as measures to relieve dry mouth. **Other:** 1. Educate patient about treatment and dietary guidelines, benefits, side effects, risk situations, and precautions. 2. Avoid situations that may result in severe dehydration or profuse perspiration.
Phenelzine (antidepressant, monoamine oxidase inhibitor [MAOI])	Constipation GI distress	Appetite changes Weight changes Dry mouth Dizziness	**Diet Rx:** 1. Avoid foods and beverages high in tyramine and other pressor amines, eg, cheese, Chianti and vermouth wines, beer and ale, smoke or pickled fish, and other foods and beverages. 2. Avoid alcohol. 3. Limit caffeine. 4. Use tryptophan supplements cautiously. **Other:** Avoid OTC preparations containing sympathomimetics (cold/cough medications and some forms used for weight control).

the diet includes protein foods of high biologic value, this amount of protein should be adequate, especially in those patients for whom the levodopa-carbidopa combination is prescribed. Another suggestion is to delay eating protein foods until evening so that the drug can produce the desired effect at least for most of the day (17).

Concurrent administration of levodopa with carbidopa (dopa decarboxylase inhibitor) diminishes peripheral tissue decarboxylation of levodopa, thus increasing availability of the drug for uptake by the brain. Other advantages associated with coadministration of these drugs include decreased nausea and vomiting and elimination of the antagonism of the therapeutic efficacy of the drug by pyridoxine.

Monoamine Oxidase Inhibitors (MAOI)

Experience with the use of MAOI in the elderly is limited (18). The overall effect of these drugs is to increase the concentration of selected neurotransmitters, which is thought to be the basis for their antidepressant activity. However, they have potentially serious side effects resulting from interactions with foods or other drugs. Concurrent intake of tyramine- or other high pressor amine-containing foods or beverages with these drugs can precipitate sudden severe hypertensive episodes that can be fatal. A critical review of the literature on amine composition in food and relevant case reports provides rational guidelines for diet planning and counseling of patients on MAOI (19). Nutritional implications and dietary suggestions pertaining to the use of MAOI, such as phenelzine, are listed in Table 3.

RESPIRATORY TRACT AGENTS

Bronchodilators

Theophylline (xanthine-derivative bronchodilator) and albuterol (beta-adrenergic agonist) are examples of drugs indicated for the treatment of a variety of respiratory diseases, such as bronchial asthma, bronchitis, emphysema, and other chronic pulmonary obstructive diseases, that are common in the elderly.

The ingestion of high-protein, low-carbohydrate diets may enhance the metabolism of theophylline, thus increasing its clearance and decreasing its maximal effect. On the other hand, low-protein, high-carbohydrate diets may produce an opposite effect. Thus, dosage adjustments may be necessary to avoid drug side effects (20). Furthermore, concurrent use of caffeine-containing beverages during drug therapy may result in additive CNS stimulation and may predispose the elderly patient to undesirable side effects, such as insomnia, irritability, nervousness, and possible cardiac disturbances.

ALCOHOL

Elderly patients may tend to overuse or abuse alcohol as a coping mechanism during stressful periods of boredom, bereavement, depression, or loneliness or during other sudden lifestyle changes (21, 22). Although the therapeutic use of alcohol may be beneficial in some instances, the elderly are more sensitive to the effects of alcohol than younger adults, and its use or overuse by the elderly may cause a variety of adverse and life-threatening effects: altered drug metabolism; malnutrition or vitamin deficiencies; altered physiologic states, such as fluid and electrolyte imbalances, peripheral neuropathy, hypoglycemia, hypothermia, or cerebral degeneration; or aggravation of pre-existing diseases or their conversion to overt diseases. Even casual use can be dangerous, particularly if the older adult is being treated with drugs than interact with alcohol.

The elderly need to be cautioned about mixing alcohol with medications. With concurrent alcohol use, impaired judgment, lack of coordination, and risk of trauma from resulting falls may be increased in individuals for whom antidepressants, diuretics, anticonvulsants, sedatives, or other drugs have been prescribed. In the chronic drinker, alcohol induces hepatic drug metabolism, an effect that results in an enhanced rate of drug clearance during a period of abstinence. In contrast, acute ingestion of alcohol in a medicated person may result in reduced drug clearance due to competition for the same hepatic microsomal enzyme system, thus potentiating drug action and prolonging its half-life.

Other unusual effects of the concomitant intake of alcohol and certain drugs include unpredictable fluctuations of plasma glucose concentrations and a disulfiram-like reaction in those patients for whom oral hypoglycemic agents are prescribed. Alcohol abuse in the elderly, especially in late-onset alcoholics, may be managed by the use of medications or by emotional support systems, socialization programs, or education. Appropriate therapeutic aids in the treatment of alcoholism may also be considered. Disulfiram, as an adjunct in the treatment of chronic alcoholism, has few side effects when administered alone. However, during concomitant intake with alcohol, this drug effectively alters the intermediary metabolism of alcohol, thus causing an accumulation of acetaldehyde. The signs and symptoms of this interaction—flushing, pulsating headache, respiratory difficulties, nausea, vomiting, hypotension, and other effects—are collectively known as a disulfiram-alcohol reaction (acetaldehyde syndrome). Depending on the mental status and motivation of the elderly patient, disulfiram may be a useful deterrent in the treatment of alcohol abuse. However, education of patients is of utmost importance. They must be warned to avoid not only obvious forms of alcohol but also hidden forms—uncooked fermented foods and sauces, OTC medications containing alcohol, or certain extracts or flavoring agents added to food after cooking—and must be informed that concurrent intake may endanger their lives.

FOOD SUPPLEMENTS AND DRUG INTERACTIONS

When food supplements are used indiscriminately, a variety of undesirable effects on drug disposition can occur (Table 4). Even though vitamin, mineral, and other supplements are widely used by the geriatric population, primarily as a form of "nutrition insurance," these agents are generally thought to be safe, and little consideration is given to possible adverse effects resulting from their interactions with drugs (4). Because of these perceptions, a careful history of supplement usage is needed in order to advise the patient about their proper use and potential interactions with concurrently prescribed medications. Contrary to popular belief, the efficacy of large vitamin doses to prevent cancer, combat chronic degenerative illnesses, rejuvenate age-related physiologic changes, or extend life has not been demonstrated. (See Chapter 30.) Other concerns pertaining to their use have been recently reviewed by the Council of Scientific Affairs, American Medical Association (23).

Interactions between warfarin anticoagulants and vitamin supplements have been reported. Decreased prothrombin times have been shown in patients taking warfarin and large amounts of ascorbic acid (24, 25). However, Feetam et al. (26) suggest that the altered hypoprothrombinemic response occurs only when extremely large doses of ascorbic acid (>10 g/day) are ingested with the drug. Indiscriminate use of vitamin E (800 to 1,200 IU/day) has been found to enhance the hypoprothrombinemic response to warfarin (27–29). Also, to prevent a possible hypoprothrombinec response (30), large doses of vitamin A should be avoided in patients for whom oral anticoagulants are prescribed. Thus, patients who choose to ingest large amounts of vitamin supplements while they are being treated with oral anticoagulants need to be alerted about possible serious complications (Table 4).

Vitamin supplementation, however, may be in the best interest of elderly patients who develop or are susceptible to drug-induced peripheral neuropathy. This neurologic side effect has been reported with the use of hydralazine, isoniazid, and penicillamine, but can be corrected by pyridoxine supplementation (31–33).

Thiazide diuretics are known to lower urinary calcium excretion, an effect that may elevate serum calcium to hypercalcemic levels. Concurrent use of thiazide diuretics with large doses of calcium supplements, combined with vitamin D, could potentially result in hypercalcemia, particularly in elderly patients with compromised renal function (Table 4).

The use of amino acid supplements as "natural remedies" to treat mental

TABLE 4. *Food supplements and drug interactions*

Supplement	Drug	Effect
Vitamins		
Vitamin A	Aluminum hydroxide	Drug-induced precipitated bile acids may decrease vitamin absorption.
	Cholestyramine	Concurrent use may impair vitamin absorption.
	Mineral oil	Concurrent use may interfere with vitamin absorption.
	Warfarin	Large doses may enhance anticoagulant activity.
Vitamin D	Digoxin	Vitamin-D-induced hypercalcemia may sensitize the patient to toxic effects of the drug.
	Mineral oil, aluminum hydroxide, cholestyramine	Concurrent use may decrease vitamin absorption.
Vitamin E	Warfarin	Megadoses may enhance anticoagulant activity.
	Mineral oil, aluminum hydroxide, cholestyramine	Concurrent use may decrease vitamin absorption.
Vitamin K	Warfarin	Concurrent use inhibits hypoprothrombic effect of drug.
	Mineral oil, aluminum hydroxide, cholestyramine	Concurrent use may decrease vitamin absorption.
Ascorbic acid	Haloperidol	Concurrent use may enhance antipsychotic effect of drug.
	Warfarin	Megadoses may decrease prothrombin time.
Folacin	Phenytoin	Vitamin replacement in folate-deficient patients may increase drug metabolism.
Pyridoxine	Levodopa	Concurrent use reverses antiparkinsonian effect.
	Phenytoin	Large doses may reduce anticonvulsant activity.
	Hydralazine, isoniazid, penicillamine	Concurrent use may reverse drug-induced peripheral neuropathy.
Minerals		
Calcium	Digitalis	Concurrent use with vitamin D may result in hypercalcemia and may enhance toxic effects of drug.
	Hydrochlorothiazide	Concurrent use with vitamin D may result in hypercalcemia.
	Phenytoin	Concurrent use may decrease both drug and calcium bioavailability.
	Verapamil	Concurrent use with vitamin D may counter the antidysrhythmic effect of drug.
Iron	Penicillamine	Concurrent use may decrease drug effectiveness.
	Calcium carbonate	Concurrent use may impair iron absorption.

TABLE 4. *Continued*

Supplement	Drug	Effect
Other Supplements		
Protein or amino acids	Levodopa, methyldopa	Concurrent use may potentially inhibit drug absorption.
	Theophylline	Concurrent use may potentially decrease plasma half-life of drug.
Tryptophan	Fluoxetine	Concurrent use may intensify agitation, restlessness, and GI problems.
	Monoamine oxidase inhibitors (MAOI)	Concurrent use may result in confusion, a deterioration in mental status, headaches, agitation, and other adverse effects.
	Tricyclic antidepressants	Variable results are observed when used to augment antidepressant effects.

illness or other disorders may not be in the best interest of medicated patients. Despite the appeal of tryptophan to treat depression or sleep disturbances, which are common in the elderly, not all patients respond to it similarly. Such interactions may cause hyperexcitability, headache, severe hypertension, and hallucinations (34). Deterioration in mental status has also been described when tryptophan is given alone or in combination with MAOI (35). Other interactive effects among drugs and tryptophan are listed in Table 4.

In addition, treatment failure might occur in patients who use amino acid supplements concurrently with the antiparkinsonian agent, levodopa, or the nondiuretic antihypertensive agent, methyldopa, because dietary amino acids are known to competitively inhibit the absorption of these drugs. The use of protein supplements by patients receiving theophylline might also result in altered drug efficacy. In this case, studies have indicated that a high-protein diet in children and adults decreases the plasma half-life of theophylline, an effect believed to be due to an increase in drug metabolism (36). Although treatment failure from such interactions has yet to be reported in the elderly, medicated patients should be cautioned about the use of amino acid or protein supplements during drug therapy until further information is available.

GUIDELINES FOR COUNSELING—DIET AND DRUGS

Although modified diets are a valid part of medical care for several diseases, these diets are of no value unless they are followed by the patient. In order to ensure some degree of patient compliance, the medicated elderly must receive and continue to receive effective nutritional counseling. Modified diets are usually nutritionally adequate when they have been individually designed by a competent health professional. However, exacerbation of underlying problems can occur when the older adult (a) is not advised properly how to take drugs in relation to the diet or specific foods, (b) is not medically supervised during dietary and drug treatment, (c) modifies either the drug or dietary regimens, or (d) is influenced by well-meaning friends who are prescribed similar drugs but have different diet prescriptions (37). Helping the elderly establish and maintain good eating habits is a complex problem that is influenced by their total life experiences. Cultural, religious, ethnic, physical, economic, social, and other factors must be taken into consideration in counseling patients as any one of these can affect dietary intake directly or indirectly.

The causes of poor compliance with drug and diet regimens are multiple and complex. Balancing diet and drug regimens, especially in patients taking a number of drugs and attempting to adhere to diet instructions, may be complicated and a burden and next to impossible. Unpleasant effects that are associated with medications, unpalatable special diets, or bland food can discourage a patient from following a medication schedule or a diet prescription. Multiple chronic disease processes, including decreased mobility and failing vision, may limit the ability of a person to prepare food or to read instructions about how to take the medications. Economic and social factors may inhibit the procurement of food or medications. Diverse conditions within the elderly patient's living environment must also be considered.

In the development of diet and drug regimens, a failure to provide knowledge about the reasons for and the uses of the individualized diet and the drug may contribute to misconceptions about the treatment that may result in nonadherence. Adequate communication between the health care practitioner and the elderly patient is essential and needs to include both verbal and written instructions that are easy to understand. These schedules must be individualized, kept as simple as possible, and designed in such a way that they will not overwhelm the patient. It is also important to keep in mind that simply handing a patient printed instructions and/or providing only short-term counseling are poor education techniques. Because compliance is known to decrease with a lack of follow-up (38), patients need to be counseled early in the treatment of the disorder, and regular follow-up is essential to reinforce the importance of nutritional support during drug therapy.

CONCLUDING REMARKS

The frequency of adverse effects arising from nutrient (food) and medication incompatibilities in the elderly has not been well documented. In the many situations discussed here, various dietary suggestions must be interpreted in relationship to the patient's dietary habits, need for therapeutic diets, underlying illness, physiologic state, or other variables that affect nutrient utilization and drug efficacy. These suggestions are also intended to reinforce rather than replace any information in the diet prescription or provided by the physician.

It is generally not justified to assume that nutrient supplementation is needed on the basis of drug therapy alone. Laboratory data are needed to verify possible changes in nutritional status. A nutritious diet, however, will make an important contribution to the health of the elderly for whom drugs are prescribed and will reduce the risk of nutritional disorders or food-induced, altered drug efficacy. Furthermore, such a diet will provide a sense of well-being because eating is such a significant aspect of life. Even though the frequency of adverse effects arising from food-induced drug changes or altered nutritional status is in need of further clarification and consideration, an understanding of reported and potential interactions is a step forward in preventing undesirable and often serious drug effects in this population group.

REFERENCES

1. Tideiksaar R. *Hosp Physician* 1984; 20:92–101.
2. Department of Health, Education and Welfare. *Long-term care facility improvement campaign. Monograph No 2. Physicians' drug prescribing patterns in skilled nursing facilities.* Washington, DC: US Government Printing Office, 1976 (Office of Long Term Care, Publ. No. (OS) 76-50050).
3. Lamy PP. *Prescribing for the elderly.* Littleton, MA: PSG Publishing, 1980.
4. Smith CH, Bidlack WR. *J Am Dietet Assoc* 1984; 84:901–914.
5. United States Pharmacopeial Dispensing Information. In: *Drug information for the health care provider,* vol IA, 9th ed. Rockville, MD: The United States Pharmacopeial Convention, Inc, 1989; 1026–1032.
6. Haynes RC Jr, Murad F. In: Gilman AG, Goodman LS, Rall TW, Murad R, eds. *Goodman and Gilman's: The pharmacological basis of therapeutics,* 7th ed. New York: Macmillan Publishing, 1985; 1517–1543.
7. Liedholm H, Melander A. *Clin Pharmacol Ther* 1986; 40:29–36.
8. National Cholesterol Education Program. *Arch Intern Med* 1988; 148:36–69.
9. Powers DE, Moore AO. *Food medication interactions,* 6th ed. Phoenix: FMI Publishing, 1988.
10. Alter HJ, Zvaifler NJ, Rath CE. *Blood* 1971; 38:405–416.
11. Sahud MA, Cohen RJ. *Lancet* 1971; 1:937–938.
12. Paykel ES, Mueller PS, De La Vergne PM. *Br J Psychiatry* 1979; 123:501–507.
13. United States Pharmacopeial Dispensing Information. In: *Drug information for the health care provider,* vol IB, 9th ed. Rockville, MD: The United States Pharmacopeial Convention, Inc, 1989; 1528–1533.
14. Yahr MD, Duvoisin RC. *JAMA* 1972; 220:861.
15. Bianchine JR. In: Gilman AG, Goodman LS, Rall TW, Murad R, eds. *Goodman and Gilman's: The pharmacological basis of therapeutics,* 7th ed. New York: Macmillan Publishing, 1985; 473–490.
16. Giilespie NG, Mena I, Cotzias GC, Bell MA. *J Am Dietet Assoc* 1973; 62:525–528.
17. Pincus JH, Barry K. *Arch Neurol* 1987; 44:270–272
18. Ashford JW, Ford CV. *Am J Psychiatry* 1979; 136:1466–1467.
19. McCabe BJ. *J Am Dietet Assoc* 1986; 86:1059–1064.

20. United States Pharmacopeial Dispensing Information. In: *Drug information for the health care provider,* vol IB, 9th ed. Rockville, MD: The Unites States Pharmacopeial Convention, Inc, 1989; 623–637.
21. Pattee JJ. *Geriatrics* 1982; 37:145–146.
22. Blum L, Rosner F. *J Natl Med Assoc* 1983; 75:489–495.
23. Council on Scientific Affairs. *JAMA* 1987; 257:1929–1936.
24. Rosenthal G. *JAMA* 1971; 215:1671.
25. Smith EC, Skalski RJ, Johnson GC, Rossi GV. *JAMA* 1972; 221:1166.
26. Feetam CL, Leach RH, Meynell MJ. *Toxicol Appl Pharmacol* 1975; 31:544–547.
27. Vitamin K, vitamin E and the coumarin drugs. *Nutr Rev* 1982; 40:180–182.
28. Corrigan JJ, Marcus FI. *JAMA* 1974; 230:1300–1301.
29. Schrogie JJ. *JAMA* 1975; 232:19.
30. Olson RE. *Ann Rev Nutr* 1984; 4:281–337.
31. Bhagavan HN, Brine M. In: Winick J, ed. *Nutrition and drugs.* New York: John Wiley & Sons, 1983:1–12.
32. Raskin NH, Fishman RA. *N Engl J Med* 1965; 273:1182–1185.
33. Snider DE Jr. *Tubercle* 1980; 61:191–196.
34. Brotman AW, Rosenbaum JF. *Biol Ther Psychiatry* 1984; 7:47.
35. Blackwell B. *Drug* 1981; 21:273–282.
36. Anderson KE, Conney AH, Kappas A. *Nutr Rev* 1982; 40:161–171.
37. Bidlack WR, Smith CH. *CRC Critical Rev Food Sci Nutr* 1989; 27:189–218.
38. Eckerling L, Kohrs MB. *J Am Dietet Assoc* 1984; 84:805–809.

Geriatric Nutrition, edited by John E. Morley,
Zvi Glick, Laurence Z. Rubenstein.
Raven Press, Ltd., New York © 1990.

30

Nutrition Misinformation:
Health Fraud and the Elderly Population—
Creation of Food Fads for Profit

Wayne R. Bidlack

*Department of Pharmacology and Nutrition, University of Southern California
School of Medicine, Los Angeles, California 90033*

To Claude Pepper (1901–1989)
Champion of the poor and the elderly

The elderly population spends billions of dollars each year on health products and services that may not only be useless but may also cause harm or result in death. These senior citizens are victims of health fraud.

HEALTH FRAUD COSTS

In 1984, the House Subcommittee on Health and Long-Term Health Care published a report entitled, "Quackery: A $10 Billion Scandal," which presented the findings of a 4-year investigation examining the national problem of health fraud (1). The $10 billion figure was felt to be a conservative underestimate of wasted monies because most quackery goes undetected and unreported. At the hearings, Victor Herbert estimated that the total cost of health fraud in the United States was at least $25 billion per year and noted that the elderly were victims of $10 billion alone. In either case, nutrition and health quackery has become a serious health care problem for the elderly population.

The subcommittee identified several major target areas to which quacks focus their phony cures: fake cancer cures costing $4 to 5 billion per year, antiaging remedies costing $2 billion per year, and questionable arthritis cures costing $2 billion annually. A host of other areas comprise the remainder of the total cost of health fraud.

Pepper (2) estimated that the elderly account for 40% of all health fraud victims. Thus, about 30 million elderly people account for $4 billion of the total amount spent on fraudulent and unproven health products, services, and treatments. This relationship would suggest that the average expenditure was about $130 per person. However, depending on the actual percentage of the elderly population being deceived, this amount would be significantly increased. If only one-tenth to one-fifth of the elderly are directly involved, the amount becomes $650 to $1300 per person, which would have a major financial impact on individuals living on fixed income.

QUACKERY

By definition, a quack is a person who practices medicine fraudulently, pretending to have knowledge or skill that he does not have in a particular field. The term "fraud" is used in many definitions of quackery; fraud is deceit, trickery, or cheating. In the legal sense, an individual operating fraudulently must employ deception to cause a person to give up property or some legal right. However, some well-meaning people, including many health professionals, have themselves been deceived and believe in the products they sell.

The New York State Assembly on Health Fraud (3) used the following definition of quackery: "the promotion, for financial gain, of fraudulent devices, treatments, services, plans, or products (including but not limited to food, diet, and nutritional supplements) which alter or claim to alter the human condition." The definition is too restrictive because many people promoting quackery have themselves been deceived and may well believe the product is efficacious and are sincerely trying to help others independent of financial gain. Unfortunately, such action is still quackery and poses a health risk to the unsuspecting elderly population.

The hawking of fraudulent cures has become much more sophisticated since the days of the "medicine wagon" (3). Today's quacks push their cures and wares through modern methods, including treatment and testing centers, clinics, slick advertisement of products, diagnoses by unqualified doctors and, unfortunately in some cases, the promotion of unproven or fraudulent remedies by licensed physicians. Quacks and companies promoting quack products use testimonials of satisfied (or paid) users, including movie stars and athletes, and tricky labeling tactics in their advertising.

VULNERABILITY OF THE ELDERLY POPULATION

The vulnerability of the elderly to nutrition and health quackery is enhanced relative to the rest of society for a variety of reasons:

1. The process of aging has become a focal point of health fraud. Growing old is generally perceived to be an undesirable physiologic process, to be socially unacceptable, and to result in reduced economic status. From middle age life on, it has become desirable to alter the visible changes associated with aging, such as graying hair, baldness, and wrinkles.

2. The lack of nutrition education makes the elderly population susceptible targets for authentic-sounding but fraudulent health information. Quacks create and use medical terms that have no meaning, but unfortunately, the jargon communicates a sense of knowledge to the patient. In addition, many quacks use medical terms that the patients have heard before, and when these terms are integrated with meaningless jargon, the patients become convinced that they are receiving competent care.

3. A large number of elderly people have chronic medical problems for which there are no cures, such as arthritis, Alzheimer's disease, cancer, and the like. The possibility that an unknown product may be able to provide either relief or a "miracle" cure for the condition is readily attractive. Unfortunately, many patients only need to be told that through testimonials that someone else has been helped, and, even without substantiation provided by scientific testing, they conclude that they may also be the one to be helped.

4. The poor elderly subpopulation appears to be more susceptible to exploitation by individuals better off than they are. They develop a strong identification with successful people, including television and movie stars and especially those of their own age group. They tend to be trusting of other people's advice. Unfortunately, unscrupulous individuals promote a variety of unethical products and business practices, eg, distorted funeral arrangements, phony medical insurance, unnecessary dental work, and promotion of nonefficacious cures for nontreatable problems.

5. People, especially of advanced age, are frequently more lonely as a consequence of the loss of their spouse, friends, and possibly their children as they move away. They need someone with whom they can talk and trust. As such, they are susceptible to individuals with strong personalities who provide them personal attention.

Nutrition and health misinformation should be considered a health hazard because improper diagnosis and treatment delay the identification of a disease at its earliest stages when it would be most responsive to therapy. Too, expenditure of funds on worthless nutritional supplements, nostrums, and treatments reduces the monies that elderly people, especially those on limited incomes, have available to purchase quality foods and health care.

TYPES OF NUTRITIONAL MISINFORMATION AND HEALTH FRAUD

Fear of the Existing Food Supply

Health Foods

The elderly consumer is constantly besieged by material that infers or states that the food supply is unsafe or unhealthy. This is fraud! The U.S. food supply is the most abundant and safest in the world. Yet, persistent repetition of these claims has convinced many elderly people that they must purchase alternative food products and nutritional supplements to ensure good health.

Safety and Chemophobia

The term "natural" has been used to infer safety from harmful chemicals. It should be noted that thousands of toxic compounds, such as aflatoxin, alkaloids, and carcinogens, occur naturally in foods. This does not mean they are unsafe, but rather that most foods contain substances, which if tested at high concentrations, might prove to be toxic or carcinogenic. Thus, as long as these compounds are consumed at very low doses there is *no* health hazard and probably a nonmeasurable health risk.

Chemophobia

Despite the lack of scientific evidence to support these claims, the public has become convinced that many diseases, including cancer and birth defects, and even the life span are affected by the chemicals used to grow and preserve our food supply. Statements about industrial chemicals, pollution, and cancer are constantly issued by self-serving scientists, government agencies, and consumer groups. The relationships between toxic chemicals and health are extrapolated indiscriminately to low-dose exposures that pose no health threat. The media promote these stories and amplify the impact of the claims being made. Unfortunately, these scare stories are not serving the public good (4).

Nutritional Quality

The nutritional quality of the food supply is also frequently challenged. Indeed, processing does cause the loss of nutrients, but the end result is that more foods are available throughout the year to more people than would be possible without existing processing techniques (5). Thus, all people benefit from the availability of these products. As long as persons select a variety of foods from all food groups and watch their total calorie consumption, they can easily meet their nutrient needs and have a balanced, safe diet.

The health food industry takes exception to this statement. However, the health food industry is a multibillion dollar industry (6). It has created and maintained a market based on misinformation. Although their products are promoted as more nutritious and healthier, vitamin and mineral supplements still account for more than one-third of their total sales (7). It is ironic that the use of health foods to improve nutrient intake has not eliminated the need for the industry to sell nutritional supplements.

Promoters (corporate advertising agencies) of nutritional supplements infer that consumption of a greater amount of a nutrient must be proportionately more beneficial to one's health. This philosophy is the primary basis for the selling of nutritional supplements, such as protein, amino acids, vitamins, and minerals. These sales campaigns never explain that the human body can only utilize a given amount of each nutrient and will in fact either discard or store the excess. They do not inform the consumer of the pharmacologic principle, "The dose makes the poison," which was stated by Paracelsus, the father of pharmacology and toxicology, in the 16th century.

Protein and amino acid supplements are claimed to enhance the quality of dietary protein, improve athletic and work performance, and enhance neurofunction. Although 10 to 15% of elderly people do have dietary protein intakes of less than two-thirds of the Recommended Daily Allowances (RDA) (8,9), the dietary intake of protein by the average American is more than 50% above the RDA (10). Excess protein and amino acids are simply deaminated and metabolized for energy. Thus, little need exists for amino acid or protein supplements.

From the National Health and Nutritional Examination Surveys I and II (8,9), certain groups in the United States have been identified as consuming diets containing less than the RDA in vitamins, but these findings are based on 24-hour recall and therefore underestimate actual intake. The specific identification of biochemically defined vitamin deficiencies has been very rare. At best, a simple multivitamin supplement containing the RDA would be more than sufficient to meet the needs of elderly people when taken in addition to their normal dietary intake (11).

Of the nutritional supplements, vitamins are the biggest money maker (12). The deceptions in promoting vitamins are numerous. Claims are made that the American diet is lacking in vitamins, that work and emotional stress increases the need for vitamins, and that vitamins should be taken as insurance to prevent disease (13).

The advertising campaigns and written material begin by describing the deficiency diseases related to each vitamin. If the individual reading these descriptions has any of the symptoms mentioned, he may assume that he is deficient in that vitamin. Many of these books, such as *The Vitamin Bible* by Earl Mindell (14) and *The Right Dose: How to Take Vitamins and Minerals Safely* by Patricia Hausman (15), are sold alongside the vitamins.

The most blatant case of distortion has been the promotion of megadoses (gram amounts) of vitamin C to prevent colds or cancer (16,17). An increased intake of vitamin C results in elevated plasma levels (18). As the level exceeds 125 mg/dl, the vitamin is spilled into the urine just as sugar is spilled by a diabetic. Only 10 to 12 mg/day of vitamin C are required to prevent the onset of vitamin C deficiency, whereas the average intake of vitamin C exceeds the RDA of 60 mg/day. Vitamin C is distributed throughout the body's water space, resulting in a storage pool of 1,200 to 1,500 mg that would last for several months without additional intake. With an intake between 250 and 500 mg/day, the body tissue stores become saturated, and intestinal absorption should become limited (19). Excessive intakes of vitamin C supplements beyond the RDA provide the individual with no health or medical benefit.

Another sleight of hand involves the interpretation of the mean serum vitamin C levels in smokers and nonsmokers. At the same intake, the mean serum vitamin C levels for smokers are consistently 0.2 mg/dl lower than that of the nonsmokers (9). Other researchers have also reported a 30% lower vitamin C level in smokers (20,21). Apparently, because of decreased absorption and increased clearance, smokers require an additional 60 mg/day of vitamin C to meet their vitamin C needs. However, recommendations to take vitamin C supplements ignore the most important factors related to health: to enhance the quality of the diet and to reduce or stop smoking.

Ingesting gram doses of niacin also results in inefficient utilization. High doses cause vasodilatation, which can be harmful if the patient is already hypotensive. However, because of the noticeable physiologic effect, a strong placebo effect results. Although gram doses (1.5–3.0 g/day to 3.0–9.0 g/day) have been used for more than 30 years as therapy for elevated cholesterol levels, not everyone responds positively to this treatment. In clinical trials, there has been some success when niacin is used in combination with other hyperlipidemic drugs, especially the bile acid sequestrants (22). Apparently, niacin lowers low-density lipoprotein (LDL) cholesterol levels by decreasing very low-density lipoprotein (VLDL) synthesis in the liver. However, the mechanism remains unclear, and niacinamide does not produce the same effect. Niacin is not a panacea for high cholesterol nor should it be assumed to be safe. The most common side effects associated with nicotinic acid use include intense cutaneous flushing and pruritis, dry skin, nausea, vomiting, and diarrhea. In most individuals, these effects are transitory. However, even at 1-g doses, liver damage occurs, but reverses in most cases after an adaption response or upon cessation of supplement use.

Fat-soluble vitamins accumulate in the body and can prove to be toxic. Vitamin A is the most toxic vitamin and accounts for many poisonings each year (23,24). The symptoms include spleen enlargement, liver damage, increased cranial pressure, and joint pain (25,26). Yet, the literature sold or given away in the health food stores identifies these symptoms as indicative of the need for greater vitamin A intake!

Many elderly and other consumers believe that nutritional supplements are completely safe. However, nutrients used in excessive amounts become drugs and in some cases toxicants. Interestingly, the vitamin industry through their lobby group, the Council for Responsible Nutrition, is responding by claiming a low incidence of toxicity, rather than arguing or defending the amount needed for efficacy (27).

Claims of Health and Longevity

Media and Popular Publications

Newspapers carry lengthy articles exposing aspects of health fraud and they write editorials to the same effect, yet in the same issue they continue to carry ads promoting the exact nonsense being debunked. It is easier to argue ethical stances than to give up the dollars produced by those same ads.

The quality of nutrition and health articles published in popular magazines varies greatly. Most major magazines are making greater efforts to enhance the quality and accuracy of the health material being published. Still, many magazines carry advertisements that are written and set to look similar to commissioned articles. Although a statement identifying the material as an advertisement is present, the advertisement may cover several pages, which enhances its credibility.

Television and radio stations not only carry ads promoting misinformation and fraud but many program hosts and stars actually lend their name to the material, enhancing its credibility. More recently, on television, full half-hour and hour-long advertisements using an interview format have been aired. The style of the presentation tends to trick the viewer into believing that the questions and responses are spontaneous, rather than designed to promote the product, the name of which is mentioned frequently.

Package labels have also become promotional sales gimmicks. The most recent example is the inclusion on the back of cereal boxes of the claim that fiber *may* prevent cancer. Unfortunately, the public is led to believe that these statements are scientifically established. Credibility has also been enhanced by including an address and telephone number for the National Cancer Institute (NCI). Such an arrangement leads the consumer to believe that the product is endorsed by the NCI. The FDA tried to block this health-label claim, but was overridden by the NCI.

Numerous brochures, booklets, and books have promoted a variety of methods to decrease aging and its associated disease processes. Two books are used to illustrate the widely varying quality of both the scientific material included and the interpretation of their recommendations. The first is *Life Extension* by Durk Pearson and Sandy Shaw (28), and the second is *Maximum Lifespan* by Roy L. Walford, M.D. (29).

The formulas presented in *Life Extension* include a variety of nutrients and other chemicals: zinc; selenium; large doses of vitamins; nonnutrients that occur naturally in foods, such as RNA, choline, and bioflavonoids; and the commercial antioxidant BHT. The authors developed a complete product line of these nutrients to be sold through health food stores, including "Power Maker" and "Personal Radical Shield."

One of the theories of aging presented in *Life Extension* involves free radical mechanisms. However, antioxidant materials in excess of body needs have little benefit. Claims that these agents, such as BHT or vitamin E, protect the cellular nucleic acids, RNA and DNA, have not been well substantiated. The generous comment would be that Shaw and Pearson accumulated but did not interpret the results of the scientific studies they read. However, it might be more accurate to state that they misinterpreted the results and cited only those experiments in support of their premise. Little evidence has surfaced that any nutrient or other chemical can truly interfere with, slow, or stop aging. Once you've picked your grandparents, good nutrition can only optimize your genetic potential.

In contrast, *Maximum Lifespan* (29) is a more professional presentation of a current hypothesis that low-calorie diets can extend the life span in animals. However, similar to the Shaw and Pearson volume, extrapolation of animal data to the human situation is not presented critically.

In animal studies, calorie restriction (60% of *ad libitum* fed controls) decreased degenerative disease and extended both mean life span and, for a few animals, the apparent length of life (30–33). It should be noted that, in the animal studies, sick animals (of an infectious nature, such as colds, wheezing, etc.) are removed from the colony. Would the life span increase if all sick people were isolated from the rest of the population? The animals also have delayed sexual maturation and altered hormonal balance, which may affect the rate of aging, but may not be desirable overall. Finally, the control animals in these studies are sedentary and overweight. Thus, the interpretation of the data could be reversed; obesity and inactivity are detrimental to longevity.

Extrapolation of these results to the human situation could prove harmful. A semistarvation diet involving a 30 to 40% decrease in calorie intake can result in a loss of adipose and provide an increase in lean body mass. However, an individual who becomes too thin lacks sufficient caloric reserves to survive a severe illness. In addition, overrestriction of caloric intake makes it more difficult for the elderly to meet their other nutrient needs.

Nutritional Enhancement of Longevity

One of the earliest claims for decreasing the rate of aging involved the use of free radical scavengers or antioxidants (34,35). In the early animal experiments the dietary antioxidants were greatly decreased in one group compared to another, and then the groups were evaluated for longevity. Increased life span was credited to the beneficial effects of vitamins or antioxidants. However, deficiency of those compounds could have shortened life span for other reasons; for example, the onset of vitamin deficiency. In addition, similar dietary experiments examined these animals after exposure to radiation. Some protection provided by the antioxidants was observed. However, misinterpretation of these results and their extrapolation to the human situation are very common in the promotion of antiaging products.

Vitamin E is an antioxidant that protects cellular membranes from oxidative damage. However, excess intake of vitamin E has not been proven to be of benefit. In addition, although it is an ingredient of face cream and is rubbed directly on the face to decrease wrinkles, there is no scientific evidence to support the claim that vitamin E can reverse wrinkles.

Butylated hyroxytoluene (BHT) is a synthetic antioxidant used in the food industry to decrease oxidative rancidity and the off-flavor of oils and foods deep fried in oil. The health food industry has claimed from its inception that food additives are harmful. Yet, after publication of Pearson's *Life Extension,* this same industry promoted the sales of BHT tablets (250 mg), promising that they would slow or prevent aging. It is very puzzling that BHT as a food additive is harmful, but consumption of 250-mg tablets of BHT is healthful; the most obvious conclusion is that the first claim was fraudulent and the second claim was profitable.

Several types of antioxidant enzyme supplements are currently enjoying widespread use. For example, "Cell Guard" is composed of superoxide dismutase (SOD), catalase, and glutathione peroxidase. Another product contains 2000 IU of SOD, 75,000 IU of catalase, and 2,000 IU of glutathione peroxidase at a cost of $0.85/tablet. The label of this product claims that 10 years of clinical research has proven its absorption. This claim is physiologically impossible. If taken orally, the enzymes are digested just like any food protein, and no enzymes are absorbed in their active state. Therefore, the label is fraudulent!

Zidenberg-Cherr et al. (36) completed an animal experiment that proved that SOD was not absorbed. In addition, analysis of 12 brands of SOD tablets purchased from health food stores indicated that 10 of the samples had less than 20% of the claimed activity, and one had zero enzyme activity (37). Just another example of a product sold for profit and not for efficacy.

Amino acid supplements are promoted for a variety of reasons. L-Arginine, L-ornithine, and L-tryptophan are sold as a combined tablet—at a cost of $0.25/tablet—that is claimed to stimulate the release of growth hormone (GH). However, there are no scientific data to support the claim that these amino acids can elevate GH levels; nor is there evidence that GH alters the aging processes.

Nucleic acids, such as RNA (ribonucleic acid) or DNA (deoxyribonucleic acid), are sold as components of many antiaging products. The ads suggest that RNA/DNA can rejuvenate old cells and wrinkled skin, improve memory, and slow aging. However, there is no dietary requirement for nucleic acids.

Dosages of RNA claimed to be effective in reversing aging processes range between 30 and 300 mg daily; of course, therapeutic vitamin and mineral tablets are needed as well. The brochures promise many benefits, including an increase in energy and well-being, an increase in the smoothness and color of the skin, and a decrease in fine wrinkles—all within 1 to 2 months. Physiologically, this claim is not valid.

The RNA in a cell is synthesized within that cell. Nucleic acids are not transported into the cell from outside. During digestion, nucleic acids are broken down to their requisite purine and pyrimidine bases, which can be absorbed. However, supplemental bases do not differ from the bases provided from nucleic acids within all other foods. For elderly people susceptible to gout, nucleic acid supplements are actually contraindicated.

p-Aminobenzoic acid (PABA) is not a vitamin, but is a growth promoter for bacteria. PABA is included in a variety of antiaging products, ranging from vitamin supplements to hair shampoo. The major claim is that PABA can reverse the graying of hair, but high doses are required to have an effect. Side effects include nausea and vomiting, which usually are sufficient to prevent continuation of the high-dose regimens.

Colon Detoxification

The concept that the intestine is the major source of toxins and disease was first promoted before 1900. The health food industry and the books written by the members of the industry have yet to realize that science and medicine have progressed since that time. In fact, no accumulation of toxins occurs in the intestinal tract.

Enemas have been used to relieve severe problems of constipation for hundreds of years. However, today colonics and enemas are promoted as a means of detoxifying the body. Special devices are sold to be attached to home toilets, including special reclining boards, reservoirs to hold the fluids used in the colonic, and colanders to catch the materials flushed from the colon, which allow personal examination for toxic material.

Self-Medication

Numerous pharmacologic agents are claimed to alter the effects of aging on the human condition. Gerovital (GH-3) has been sold in Europe and the United States since the 1950s to improve brain synaptic function. It can be obtained by mail order and through some health food stores and has been legalized in Nevada.

GH-3 is procaine hydrochoride, which is commonly known as Novocain. In the United States, Novocain is sold as a prescription drug (2% procaine hydrochloride) under a variety of names (38). GH-3 is readily absorbed from muscle and other tissues after parenteral administration and is readily hydrolyzed in the plasma to p-aminobenzoic acid and diethylaminoethanol.

Systemic procaine has been used for treatment of various chronic diseases associated with aging. GH-3 has been claimed to relieve various disorders, including arthritis, arteriosclerosis, angina pectoris, deafness, neuritis, Parkinson's disease, depression, and impotence. It has also been reported to stimulate hair growth, repigment gray hair, and tighten and smooth the skin (39). Although GH-3 has not been shown to be effective in improving the physical or mental status of the elderly (40,41), it is estimated that more than 100,000 people have used the product during the last 30 years.

Many worthless products are sold to cure baldness, such as "New Generation" (California Pacific Research) and the "Helsinki Formula" (Pantron), that have not been approved by the FDA nor demonstrated to be effective (42). Some of these products have been advertised in airline flight magazines and extensively on television. Both media provide access to a large audience of sensitive, aging males.

The interest in natural products has also enhanced the interest in self-therapy using herbs and other natural remedies. Herbal remedies can be produced from any part of a plant, including the leaves, flowers, stems, bark, roots, and seeds. Individual herbs or mixtures of them can contain a variety of pharmacologically active (or toxic) chemicals. The irony of their use is the avoidance of medicinal products evaluated for safety and efficacy and substitution by those which are not well controlled.

Many herbs have been used throughout history to treat a variety of diseases. However, very few records are available concerning the efficacy of their use (37,43,44). If most books on herbal medicine are examined closely, claims are made that a given herb has been used to treat a large variety of disease conditions. In no case do these claims identify the efficacy or lack thereof of the popular herbs.

An example of the problems faced by the FDA in regulating herbal products is provided by a product called Matol, Km, a Canadian product from Matol Botannical International (42). Matol, Km is described as a rich exotic blend of herbs that have been "synergistically combined" to obtain the optimum from each individual plant. It contains chamomile root, celery seed, sarsparilla root, angelica root, horehound root, licorice root, senega root, passion flower, gentian root, and cascara sagrada. Advertising claims made for the product state that it can purify the blood, improve digestion, aid hair growth, and help people sleep better. These claims are typical of the "hype" used for herbal products.

In 1986, the FDA ruled that Matol, Km was a new drug without an approved new drug application (42). However, Km has since been reintroduced into the United States without any health claims. Currently, Km is being promoted by multi-level sales as a nutrient supplement. The FDA has less regulatory control over food items than over pharmaceutical agents. All other claims and promises are communicated orally. No documentation is provided by Matol Botanical International to indicate any level of efficacy! Why then do customers buy the product?

An example of a popular herb that has been believed for thousands of years to provide health benefits is garlic. Garlic (*Alium sativum*) has been claimed to prevent the aging process and a variety of diseases, lower blood pressure, decrease serum cholesterol, and prevent colds. Indeed, some scientific support is provided for a weak antithrombitic effect for a cholesterol lowering effect, and for a weak antibiotic effect (45).

The form of garlic recommended by the health food industry is a capsule or "perle" that contains the garlic oil and can be swallowed without affecting breath odor. Natural tablets with parsley are also sold; the chlorophyll is suggested to offset breath odor as well. There are active components in garlic, but the effective dose of those chemicals has not been determined. It is anticipated that the dose would be greater than available in the commercially available garlic extracts.

Fraudulent Diagnostic Practices

Numerous tests and assays are carried out by pseudo-practitioners in the hopes of deceiving the public into believing that they are valid methods of clinical evaluation. Examples of these distortions are cytotoxic testing, dried blood analysis, live-cell analysis, uncontrolled hair analysis, and iridology.

Remedies for Specific Diseases of Aging

Elderly victims of this type of health fraud are usually suffering from pain and/or the fear of dying. Susceptible people include not only the individual but also their family and friends. Although all diseases are vulnerable to quackery, arthritis and cancer are most often exploited. More recently, AIDS patients have become prime targets of the quacks and their therapies.

To gain the confidence of the ill, the huckster implies that the medical professional has the cure but will not share it for financial reasons. This concept is based on the incorrect assumption that the entire medical profession would be able to hide these secrets. However, too many researchers are working on treatments for both diseases to make it possible for anyone to conceal a cure. Too, the financial rewards and prestige accruing to a major discovery of this magnitude would encourage publicity of any cure. There are lists of unproven "cures" for both arthritis and cancer, which are supported by personal testimonials (46). People are very susceptible to these claims when they are desperately looking for a cure, relief of pain and suffering, and forestalling or prevention of death. Unfortunately, the result is usually the loss of monies with no health benefit and a delay in starting proper medical therapy.

Arthritis

The term "arthritis" refers to more than 100 diseases related to joint inflammation. Thirty-six million people in the United States suffer from some form of arthritic disease (47,48). It has been estimated that, for every $1 spent on arthritis research, $25 is spent on quackery, including unapproved devices, nutritional supplements, useless nostrums, and diet books. Several examples of promoted but noneffective arthritis therapies include copper bracelets, DMSO, irradiation in uranium mines, phony diets and cookbooks, and herbal remedies, some of which are actually toxic (47,49). No nutritional deficiencies are related to arthritis.

"Arth rite," a product imported from Australia but patented in the United States, contains calcium carbonate, cyanocobalamin B_{12}, and potassium iodide. (Obviously, the manufacturer did not know that vitamin B_{12} and cobalamin are two names for the same compound and mistakenly combined the names.) Descriptive literature accompanying the product exaggerates greatly the function of these nutrient supplements. Another product, "Oxycal," is a calcium chelate of vitamin C. Apparently, one of the misunderstood concepts on which these products are formulated is that arthritic pain is related to osteoporosis and therefore indicates a need for calcium. Health food stores have also sold other products having no efficacy, such as "Seatone," an extract of green-lipped mussel from New Zealand, and "Honegar," a mixture of honey and vinegar. None of these products has any therapeutic benefit for arthritis.

A prime example of fraudulent arthritis therapy is "Metabolic Arthritis Therapy," which is promoted by H.W. Manner. His treatment includes detoxification of intestinal toxins using coffee enemas to stimulate bile and restore the "alkaline condition of the small intestine." His diet regimen reduces the consumption of animal protein, red meat, beef, pork, veal, lamb, and high-fat processed foods. He claims that metabolites of digestion are antagonistic to inflamed joints. The patients also supplement their diets with digestive enzymes to aid digestion and increase nutrient availability for absorption. He provides vitamins A in an emulsified form to stimulate the immune system and vitamin C to increase resistance to degenerative disease. He also uses DMSO, topically or intravenously, on his patients. Dr. Manner requires a $200 deposit to review a patient's record and consult on the case. Treatment costs range from $1,000 to $1,500 or more, without providing a chance for benefit.

Quack remedies appear to succeed in arthritis therapy for several reasons, including the placebo effect, the offering of hope provided by a new therapy, and the cyclic nature of the pain. The placebo effect results essentially from the power of the mind over the body. The patient responds because of a faith in the physician, in the treatment, or in himself (50,51). Between 30 and 50% of patients respond to placebo therapy and find relief of pain.

Cancer

Cancer quackery provides no chance for cure, although a variety of claims have been made by unethical groups promoting alternative therapies for the treatment of cancer (52,53). Usually these groups make statements that discredit existing medical science and conventional cancer therapy. Elderly people often become confused by these claims because they do not have the facts to counter the misinformation.

In addition, many healthy patients are misdiagnosed by quacks. They are told they have cancer and then are treated. When the patients "recover" from the disease that they never had in the first place, they frequently become evangelists for the alternative "healers." A recent survey of 660 cancer patients revealed that 8% had never received conventional therapy, whereas 54% of them had taken some unorthodox treatment while undergoing conventional therapy (54). Even worse, 40% of the patients had abandoned conventional care after trying unorthodox therapy.

A brief summary of recent unproven cancer therapies is presented in Table 1. Many of the cancer clinics located in Tijuana, Mexico use these therapies and others. There is no chance for efficacy, but there is an increased chance of harm.

An example of how the treatment of cancer patients by quacks results in distortion and harm is provided by the sad case of Steve McQueen. McQueen was diagnosed as having mesothelioma, a severe form of lung cancer, and it was determined to be so advanced that there was no possibility of successful treatment; it was noncurable. Rather than spending time with his family and loved ones, he went to Mexico for "alternative therapy." He was given Metabolic Therapy by William Kelly, DDS. The treatment regimen consisted of laetrile, pancreatic enzyme tablets, aloe vera, gerovital, mistletoe, megavitamins, DMSO, rectal enzymes, and coffee enemas every hour. However, he was convinced by the charlatans in Mexico that his disease was improving, and he said as much to the press and television reporters. *Newsweek* even interviewed McQueen's wife, who told the reporters that Steve was feeling much better. The doctors reported that his tumor was shrinking. Thus, the message provided to all patients suffering from cancer was that Mexico was ahead of the United States in using new, effective therapies in curing cancer. A few weeks later McQueen was rushed to surgery at which time he died. He was *not* cured.

TABLE 1. *Summary of unorthodox, alternative therapies lacking known efficacy in cancer treatment*

Metabolic therapy: This form of therapy assumes that waste materials in the patient's body interfere with metabolism and healing and that the body's cells lack proper nutrients essential to health. Treatment includes detoxification, colonic cleansing, enemas, special diets, vitamins, minerals, enzymes, and occasionally laetrile or other "special" or secret drugs. In the United States, many of the patients receiving metabolic therapy are being treated by misinformed physicians or chiropractors.

Diet therapies: This form of treatment, which may be part of a "metabolic" regimen, is based on the premise that cancer results from nutrient imbalances or deficiencies. Thus, eating specified foods prepared and consumed in specific ways is supposed to enable the body to ward off the cancer cells.

    The macrobiotic diet, an extreme form of this therapy, consists almost exclusively of whole grains and soybeans, which are purported to have anticancer properties.

    The Kushi macrobiotic diet, the type currently popular, is not as restrictive as the original Ohsawa regimen. It is supposedly based on the Far Eastern concept of Yin and Yang. However, it is so inadequate in nutrient balance that the patient's nutritional status worsens, as does the progression of the cancer.

    The Gerson Diet, which is a strict vegetarian diet, was developed initially to treat migraine headaches, tuberculosis, and cancer. Max Gerson, M.D., developed the therapies that have since been promulgated by his daughter, Charollette Gerson-Strauss, who operates the Vista Medical Center, a clinic in Playas de Tijuana, Mexico.

Megavitamins: This therapy prescribes ingestion of one or more vitamins in large (gram) doses in the belief that the body's defenses against cancer cells will be improved and the cancer cell will be destroyed.

    Vitamin A is being used in doses of 1 million IU/day, which is an extremely toxic level. Although certain analogs of vitamin A, such as 13-cis retinoic acid, have proven to be potent therapeutic agents in treating certain epithelial cancers, consumption of megadoses of vitamin A supplements does not provide the same efficacy.

    Vitamin B_{13} is a fictional vitamin, which is actually composed of calcium orotate. It has no known essential biologic function at all, let alone activity as a therapeutic agent for cancer.

    Vitamin B_{15}, pangamic acid, is also a nonexistent nutrient that was initially promoted for athletic performance. It has no efficacy in treating cancer. Recently, its "active" form has been renamed dimethylglycine (DMG-15). This component is no more active than the original compound, B_{15}.

    Vitamin B_{17}, laetrile or amygdalin, is not a vitamin, but is a cyanoglycoside. Ernest Krebs Sr., a physician, initially promoted the chemical on the hypothesis that a specific enzyme within the cancer cell would hydrolyze the cyanoglycoside, releasing the cyanide within the cancer cell to kill it. Unfortunately, the magic bullet does not work. The cyanide is released, but it is nonselective as it poisons the patient. Although no efficacy can be documented, laetrile is promoted as a natural and safe therapeutic agent.

    Vitamin C was granted anticancer properties by Linus Pauling, Ph.D., even though the results of his initial report have not been confirmed by three additional studies, including two from the Mayo Clinic. Many of the alternative therapy clinics include gram doses of vitamin C as part of their regimens. However, in animal studies carried out in Dr. Pauling's laboratory, test animals fed quantities equivalent to those recommended contracted skin cancer almost twice as frequently as the control group.

    Vitamin F is a nonvitamin supplement, which actually contains the essential fatty acids.

Mental imagery: In this method, the patient is coached to visualize the destruction of his cancer cells. Once he becomes convinced that he is capable of controlling the disease by mental thought, he theoretically is controlling his cancer.

Faith healing: The patient again must have a strong belief in the individual healer. The process combines the spiritual belief of prayer with the added effect of the laying on of hands. No conventional medicines are used.

continued

TABLE 1. *Continued*

Immune therapy: This method is based on the premise that cancer is a result of a defective immune mechanism that allows the tumor to develop. The therapy uses injections of animal fetal tissues and autogenous vaccines made from the patient's own body fluids, eg urine. The therapy is supposed to strengthen the immune system, which in turn kills the cancer cells.

Antineoplastons: Although there are similarities to the immune therapy method, this alternative therapy, promoted by Stanislou Burzynski of Houston, Texas, depends on peptides isolated from the patient's own urine. These peptides are claimed to revert oncogenes back to normal. Theoretically, a deficiency of these compounds in the body predisposes the body to cancer. Over 100 different peptides have been isolated, including those resulting from bacterial degradation, but no specificity toward cancer has been determined. Burzysnki did claim to kill cultured cells with these peptides, but no scientifically controlled experiments have supported his hypothesis.

Rodaquin: This agent was initially promoted by Koch to rejuvenate nerves and the vascular system. Harold Manner, Ph.D., a promoter who heads the "Metabolic Research Foundation" located in San Ysidro, California, has expanded Koch's formulations, primarily using tetrahydroxyquinone to treat stroke, metastatic cancer, and liver cirrhosis.

Tumorex: This agent has been promoted by James Keller and others, who claim that it reduces the size of cancer cells. There are four types composed of various amino acids, peptides, and herbs.

Live-cell therapy: This method has been practiced for several thousand years with the same lack of success. Cells are taken from 3- to 5-month-old calf fetuses. Specific tissues are dissected and matched to the patient's specific tumor site—liver cells for liver tumors, brain cells for brain tumors, etc. The fetal cells are then injected into the patient intramuscularly, apparently in the hope that they will reach the tumor site and replace the tumor cells.

From Bidlack and Lowell, ref. 52.

The National Health Federation, a strong supporter of alternative therapies, reported that Steve McQueen actually died of a heart attack. In reality, this may have occurred because of the electrolyte imbalance produced by the coffee enemas, that was then aggravated by caffeine toxicity. However, whatever the medical record shows, the final cause of death was cancer. When he died, the media never exposed the treatments for the frauds that they were. Instead, thousands of additional cancer patients have now undergone the same or similar treatments. How many have died because of a lack of media concern for the truth?

Dentition

The American Dental Association has confronted quackery in the dental profession, identifying numerous fraudulent practices, including alternative therapies for temporomandibular joint dysfunction (TMJ), toxicity from dental fillings, "cranial osteopathy" (manipulation of skull bones), antifluoridation, "applied kinesiology," reflexology, and nutrition and "holistic dentistry." Several of these diagnostic methods have been reviewed by Lowell et al. (55).

A current problem, as reported by the *Consumer's Union* (56), is the safety of mercury-containing dental amalgam fillings. Phony devices—the Dermatron or the Amalgamater—are used to convince patients that they should replace these fillings. These instruments supposedly measure mercury vapors. Actually, such devices are used in the industrial setting to protect workers from unacceptable occupational exposures. However, blood and urine samples have not supported the claim by these dentists that the fillings are leaking mercury into the patient's circulation.

In several cases, a fine has been levied on dentists using those phony devices. One of the most prominent cases is described here to indicate how quackery can produce harm. The Dermatron device was used by a dentist to convince a 55-year-old patient that six of her amalgam fillings needed to be replaced because they were a liability to her large intestine. Five fillings were then replaced. She subsequently suffered pulpal irritation and had to have two root canals and the extraction of two teeth, all of which had been asymptomatic at the beginning of her treatment. The settlement was $100,000 (53).

Gonzalez et al. (57) reported that there was no relationship between hair mercury levels (an acceptable measurement of body mercury levels when carefully controlled) and dental fillings. The claimed mercury release was overestimated by at least 16-fold. The volumes of air reported previously were larger than the capacity of the mouth. The mercury vapor concentration in the mouth was multiplied by 8,000, theoretically corresponding to the amount of air inhaled in 1 hour. However, chewing only lasts for a few minutes, and very little inhalation occurs through the mouth while eating; thus, the numbers produced are totally incorrect.

Chiropractice

In a book distributed in my community, a series of advertisements appeared from different chiropractors. Many contained information about spinal manipulation. However, there also appeared a major number of ads promoting the following services:

• precision nutritional handling
• vitamins and supplements
• body chemistry analysis
• glandular extracts
• digestive enzymes
• cleansing and detoxification—colonics
• weight loss—lifelong correction

When chiropractors are criticized for promoting the use of nonscientific methods, they protest strongly. If they wish to become credible, then chi-

---

TABLE 2. *Resource agencies and health organizations*

Federal Agencies: Regulation of Fraudulent Sales and Advertising
Food and Drug Administration (FDA)
5600 Fishers Lane
Rockville, MD 20857
Press Office: 301-443-3285
   The FDA has jurisdiction over the content and labeling of foods, drugs, medical devices, and cosmetics. The agency can take enforcement action to seize and prohibit the sale of products that are falsely labeled or pose a threat to health.

Federal Trade Commission (FTC)
Washington, D.C. 20580
Office of Public Affairs:
202-523-3830
   The FTC has jurisdiction over the advertising and marketing of foods, nonprescription drugs, cosmetics, medical devices, and health care services. The FTC Act prohibits unfair or deceptive acts or practices, and the FTC has the authority to prohibit those acts or practices. The agency can seek federal court injunctions to halt fraudulent claims and to seek reimbursement for injured consumers.

U.S. Postal Service (USPS)
Washington, D.C. 20260
Post Inspection Service:
202-268-2000
   The USPS has jurisdiction over fraudulent health care products that are advertised or sold through the mail. Considerable attention is paid to fraudulent mail order scams, especially those involving health products.

Health Associations
American Dietetic Association (ADA)
430 North Michigan Avenue
Chicago, Ill. 60611
Public Relations Office: 312-899-0040
   The ADA is concerned with nutritional topics in general, diet therapies, fad diets, and supplements.

American Cancer Society (ACS)
4 W, 35th Street
New York, N.Y. 10001
212-763-3030
   The ACS is concerned with established cancer therapies, drugs, herbs and nutritional supplements, and fraudulent or unproven cancer therapies.

American Heart Association (AHA)
7320 Greenville Avenue
Dallas, TX 75231
214-373-6300
   The AHA provides information on fraudulent or unproven drugs, supplements, and therapies used to treat heart disease.

American Diabetes Association
National Service Center
1660 Duke Street
Alexandria, VA 22314
703-549-1500

Arthritis Foundation
1314 Spring Street, NW
Atlanta, GA 30309
404-872-7100

TABLE 2. *Continued*

Asthma and Allergy Foundation of America
Washington, D.C. 10036
202-265-0265

American Association of Retired Persons
1909 K Street
Washington, D.C. 20049
202-872-4700

Medical Trade Associations
American Medical Association
535 North Dearborn
Chicago, IL 60610
312-645-5000

American Academy of Dermatology
PO Box 3116
Evanston, IL 60204
312-869-3954

American Academy of Allergy and Immunology
611 East Wells Street
Milwaukee, WI 53202
414-272-6071

Other Resources
Major medical schools or universities, departments of health and nutrition: Contact public relations office
    State Attorney General's Office

    Better Business Bureau

National Council Against Health Fraud
PO Box 1276
Loma Linda, CA 92354
714-824-4690

The American Council on Science and Health
1995 Broadway
18th Floor
New York, NY 10023

---

ropractors should regulate themselves and not tolerate individuals in their midst who commit fraud and do harm.

Physicians tend to regulate themselves to a higher degree than chiropractors. However, there remains room for improvement. In 1985 the Special Committee on Aging of the U.S. Senate reported that Medicare pays about $1 billion a year for unnecessary surgeries on older Americans. Thus, quackery, deceit, and fraud can be practiced by licensed professionals and unlicensed charlatans alike.

CONCLUSIONS

The FDA funds are very limited and only about 0.001% of its budget is used to fight quackery. Most of these funds are spent on public education, leaving very little for investigation and prosecution of fraudulent cases (58). Answers to questions concerning nutritional or health fraud can be obtained from the appropriate government agency or health organization (Table 2).

ACKNOWLEDGMENTS

Support was provided in part by a grant from CALRECO, Inc. The author appreciates interaction with and sharing of information by Jim Lowell and William Jarvis of the National Council Against Health Fraud.

REFERENCES

1. House Subcommittee on Aging. *Quackery: A $10 billion scandal.* Washington, DC: US Government Printing Office, 1984.
2. Pepper C. *Skeptical Inquirer* 1987;12:70–74.
3. New York State Assembly. *Health fraud and the elderly.* New York: Assembly Republican Task Force on Health Fraud and the Elderly, 1987.
4. Jukes TH. *21st Cent* 1988;Sept–Oct:46–48.
5. Tannenbaum SR. *Nutritional and safety aspects of food processing.* New York: Marcel Dekker, 1979.
6. *Health Food Business.* 1984;30:68–78.
7. PR Week, April 18–24, 1988.
8. Abraham S, Carroll MD, Dresser CM, Johnson CL. *Dietary intake source data, United States, 1971–1974.* Washington, DC: National Center for Health Statistics, 1979.
9. Carroll MD, Abraham S, Dresser CM. *Dietary intake source data, United States, 1976–1980.* PHS 83-1681. Washington, DC: US Government Printing Office, 1983 (USDHHS Publ. No. (PHS) 83-1681).
10. *Recommended dietary allowances.* 9th rev Ed. Washington, DC: National Academy of Sciences, 1980.
11. Kirsch A, Bidlack WR. *Nutrition* 1987;3:305–314.
12. Herbert V, Barrett S. *Vitamins and "health" foods: The great American hustle.* Philadelphia: George F Stickley, 1981.
13. Consumer's Union. *Consumer Reports* 1986; March, 150–152.
14. Mindell E. *Vitamin bible.* New York: Warner Books, 1980.
15. Hausman P. *The right dose: How to take vitamins and minerals safely.* Emmaus, PA: Rodale Press, 1987.
16. Cameron E, Pauling L. *Cancer and vitamin C.* Palo Alto, CA: Linus Pauling Institute of Science and Medicine, 1979.
17. Pauling L. *Vitamin C and the common cold.* San Francisco: WH Freeman and Co, 1970.
18. Bidlack WR, Meskin MS. *Cal Pharmacist* 1989;36:34–43.
19. Basu TK, Schorah CJ. *Vitamin C in health and disease.* Westport, CT: AVI Publishing Company Inc, 1982.
20. McClean HE, Dodds PM, Abernathy MH, Stewart AW, Beaven DW. *NZ Med* 1976;83:226–229.
21. Smith JL, Hodges RE. *Ann NY Acad Sci* 1986;498:144–151.
22. Goldstein JL, Brown MS. In: Gilman AG, Goodman LS, Rall TW, Murad F, eds. *Goodman and Gilman's: The pharmacological basis of therapeutics,* 6th ed. New York: Macmillan, 1985;827–845.

23. Herbert V. *Am J Clin Nutr* 1982;36:185–186.
24. Miller DR, Hayes KC. In: Hathcock JN, ed. *Nutritional toxicology,* vol 1, New York: Academic Press, 1982;81–133.
25. Minuk GY, Kelly JK, Hwang W-S. *Hepatology* 1988;8:272–275.
26. Muenter MD, Perry HO, Ludwig J. *Am J Med* 1971;50:129–136.
27. Bidlack WR. *SCIFTS Newsl* 1987;40:5.
28. Pearson D, Shaw S. *Life extension.* New York: Warner Books, 1983.
29. Walford RL. *Maximum lifespan.* New York: Avon Books, 1983.
30. McCay CM, Crowell MF, Maynard LA. *J Nutr* 1935;10:63–79.
31. Ross MH. *J Nutr* 1961;75:197–210.
32. Ross MH. *Am J Clin Nutr* 1972;25:834–838.
33. Ross MH, Bras G. *JNCI* 1971;47:1095–1113.
34. Harman D. *J Gerontol* 1957;12:257–267.
35. Harman D. In: Pryor WA, ed. *Free Radicals in biology* vol V. New York: Academic Press, 1982;255–275.
36. Zidenberg-Cherr S, Keen CL, Lonnerdal B, Hurley LS. *Am J Clin Nutr* 1983;37:5–7.
37. Der Marderosian A, Liberti L. *Natural product medicine.* Philadelphia: George F Stickley, 1988.
38. Kent S. *Geriatrics* 1976;31:95–102.
39. Ostfeld A, Smith CM, Stotsky BA. *J Am Geriatr Soc* 1977;25:1–19.
40. Medical Letter. *Med Lett Drug Ther* 1979;21:4.
41. Olsen EJ, Bank L, Jarvik LF. *J Gerontol* 1978;33:514–520.
42. Jarvis W. *NCAHF Newsl* 1989;12:3.
43. Duke JA. *CRC handbook of medicinal herbs.* Boca Raton, FL: CRC Press, 1985.
44. Lewis WH, Elvin-Lewis MPF. *Medical botany.* New York: John Wiley & Sons, 1977.
45. Lawrence Review of Natural Products. *Garlic. A monograph.* Levittown, PA: Pharmaceutical Information Associates, 1988:1–4.
46. Barrett S, Knight G. *The health robbers: How to protect your money and your life.* Philadelphia: George F Stickley, 1976.
47. Hecht A. *Hocus pocus as applied to arthritis.* Washington, DC: US Government Printing Office, 1981 (DHHS Publ. No. (FDA) 81-1080).
48. Panush R. *Bull Rheuma Dis* 1984;34:5.
49. Consumer's Union. *Health quackery.* Mt. Vernon, NY: Consumer's Union, 1980.
50. Benson H, Epstein MD. *JAMA* 1975;232:1225–1227.
51. Evans FJ. *Adv Inst Adv Health* 1984;1:11–21.
52. Bidlack WR, Lowell J. *SCIFTS Newsl* 1988;41:3–4.
53. Jarvis W. *CA—A Cancer Journal for Clinicians,* 36:293.
54. Cassileth BR, Lusk EJ, Strouse TB, Bodenheimer BJ. *Ann Intern Med* 1984;101:105–112.
55. Lowell JA, Kenney JJ, Rasmussen AL. *Combatting nutritional health fraud. Nutritional assessment: Separating fact, fiction and fraud.* Tucson, AZ: Nutrition Information Center, 1987.
56. Consumer's Union. *Consumer Reports* 1986; March: 170–172.
57. Gonzales MJ, Rico MC, Hernandez LM, Baluga G. *Arch Env Health* 1985;40:225–228.
58. Grossman J. *Hippocrates* 1988;Nov/Dec:50–56.

Geriatric Nutrition, edited by John E. Morley,
Zvi Glick, Laurence Z. Rubenstein.
Raven Press, Ltd., New York © 1990.

31

Nutrition and Behavior

Allen S. Levine

*Neuroendocrine Research Laboratory, VA Medical Center,
Minneapolis, Minnesota 55417 and the
Departments of Medicine, Surgery, Psychiatry, and
Food Science & Nutrition, University of Minnesota,
Minneapolis/St. Paul, Minnesota 55455*

Maimonides, the great Jewish philosopher of the Middle Ages, felt that most disease, including diseases of the mind, should be treated with diet. Cosman (1) wrote in 1983 that "even the most nutritionally enlightened modern practitioners will not find among colleagues nor patients an understanding of the unity between food and health commonplace in medieval hospitals and banquet halls." In our high-tech society few medical practitioners use nutrition as a therapeutic means of treating behavioral problems. In fact, those health professionals who use vitamin therapy and other nutritional therapies as a treatment for disease are often assumed to be shamans. Yet in May of 1986 an entire issue of a respected journal, *Nutrition Reviews,* was devoted to diet and behavior. In this journal, diet was linked to such issues as criminal behavior, hyperactivity in children, and sleep disorders. Thus, it is apparent that seven centuries after people labeled a variety of foods as aphrodisiacs, the public as well as scientists still feel there is a relationship between diet and behavior.

MALNUTRITION AND BEHAVIOR

One of the most convincing sources of information linking nutritional status to behavior is from the literature on starvation. During World War II, it became clear that prisoners who underwent severe starvation were apathetic and had decreased interest in most normal activities. Ancel Keys et al. (2) fed a group of conscientious objectors during World War II a low-calorie diet and found these individuals to be apathetic and less interested in many activities, including sex. Malnutrition that occurs during growth and development can result in poor social and intellectual skills in children. From the animal literature we know that malnutrition in young animals can result in permanent behavioral problems. Rats subjected to severe malnutrition during the first 3 weeks of life have smaller and fewer neurons, resulting in permanent brain damage (3). Poor nutrition later in development does not result in a permanent decrease in brain DNA, which reflects cell number. Some studies in humans have suggested that malnutrition *in utero* or during very early development might lead to permanent brain damage (4). It has also been shown that mild malnutrition is associated with cognitive disturbances in older individuals (5). Unfortunately, in human studies it is difficult to separate malnutrition and undernutrition from other conditions such as increased infectious disease, war, poverty, and the like.

It is well known that vitamin and mineral deficiencies result in various neurologic changes. For example, a deficiency in niacin results in pellagra, which is associated with mental depression, anxiety, memory deficits, and apathy (6). With extreme niacin deficiency one observes mania, delirium, and dementia. The reason for such changes in neural management are not clear, although it is known that certain vitamins and minerals are involved in the synthesis of chemicals that act as neurotransmitters (7) (Fig. 1).

Vitamin B_6 or pyridoxine is involved in amino acid decarboxylations, such as those that occur in the synthesis of gamma amino butyric acid (GABA), 5-hydroxytryptamine (serotonin), and dopamine. In humans, administration of tryptophan to individuals with a pyridoxine deficiency results in increased excretion of tryptophan metabolites, probably because of decreased activity of 5-HT decarboxylase. This is in contrast to pyridoxine-replete humans in whom neither vitamin B_6 nor its metabolites are found in the urine after a loading dose of tryptophan. Vitamin B_6 deficiency can also result in a decrease in GABA concentrations due to the decreased activity of glutamic acid decarboxylase resulting in hypoplasia of myelin and seizures. Although some studies suggest that vitamin B_6 might be involved in depression, the data are inconclusive (7). For example in 23 depressed patients about 17% were pyridoxine deficient, hardly a convincing finding (8). Other vitamins are also involved in the synthesis of neurotransmitters or other substances important to normal neuronal functioning. Thiamine deficiency in animals and humans result in Wernicke-Korsakoff syndrome and beriberi, defects of the central and peripheral nervous systems, respectively.

Minerals are also involved in neural functioning. Zinc deficiency results in lethargy, apathy, and decreased sexual drive, a set of behaviors resembling those that occur with starvation. Kimura and Kumura (9) found that brains of schizophrenic patients, when examined at autopsy, contained less than half the zinc of brains from normal individuals. Penicillamine, which increases zinc concentrations in tissues by binding copper, thereby altering the competition for uptake enzymes in favor of zinc, was said to improve the clinical condition of five schizophrenic patients. Unfortunately, little further work has been conducted in this research arena. Along with ascorbic acid, copper is involved in hydroxylation reactions necessary for catechol-

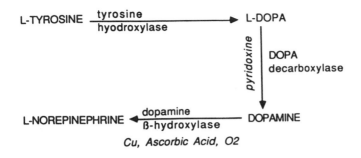

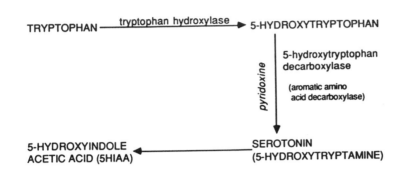

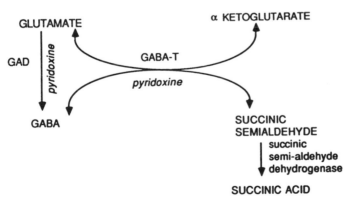

FIG. 1. Synthetic pathways of catecholamines, serotonin, and gamma amino butyric acid. L-DOPA, 3,4-dihydroxy-L-phenylalanine; 5HIAA, 5-hydroxyindoleacetic acid; GAD, glutamic acid decarboxylase; GABA, gamma amino butyric acid; GABA-T, gamma amino butyric acid alpha-oxoglutarate transaminase.

amine synthesis. Thus, both mineral and vitamin deficiencies can alter neurotransmitter synthesis and other chemical reactions involved in normal neural functioning.

NUTRIENTS AS PRECURSORS OF NEUROTRANSMITTERS

Knowing that nutritional deficiencies can lead to altered nervous system functioning, one then wonders if changes in dietary patterns can alter the nervous system as well. Richard Wurtman and his colleagues (10) have championed the notion that diet may alter the synthesis of neurotransmitters, in particular serotonin. Because tryptophan is the precursor of serotonin (Fig. 1), one might assume that feeding tryptophan itself or feeding a diet high in tryptophan would result in an increase in brain concentrations of serotonin. Also, it should be noted that the limiting factor in serotonin synthesis is not the synthetic enzyme activity, but rather the availability of the substrate. A variety of animal studies have demonstrated this to be the case; that is, increasing the ingestion of tryptophan increases serotonin concentration in the brain and the blood. However, feeding a diet high in protein does not result in an increase in serotonin concentration, whereas a diet high in carbohydrate is more effective at achieving this end. This conundrum is due to the manner in which tryptophan is absorbed and transported across the blood-brain barrier (11). Transport of tryptophan across the blood-brain barrier is dependent on the amount of other large neutral amino acids circulating in the blood. When the concentration of other circulating large neutral amino acids is lower, there is less competition for the transport of tryptophan into the brain. After a carbohydrate meal, insulin is released, which results in the uptake of large neutral amino acids, such as valine, isoleucine, and leucine, by various tissues. Ingestion of a high-protein meal increases the concentration of other large neutral amino acids more than tryptophan. This action is partially due to the fact that tryptophan is relatively scarce in high-protein foods compared with other large neutral amino acids. Thus, ingestion of a high-protein meal results in large neutral amino acids competing with tryptophan for enzymatic uptake into the brain.

In 1985, Trulson (12) questioned the idea that diet would alter serotonin-mediated events. He evaluated the effect of the alteration of dietary tryptophan levels on the functional activity of serotonin-containing neurons in the central nervous system. He found changes in the levels of brain serotonin and 5-hydroxyindoleacetic acid in cats after ingestion of tryptophan. However, he also measured the electrophysiologic activity of single serotonergic neurons in the raphe nucleus of awake, behaving cats after the ingestion of diets high in tryptophan and observed no change in the activity of serotonin-containing raphe cells. Trulson then injected labeled tryptophan into the cats and found no change in the amount of tritiated serotonin released into the lateral ventricles; however, there was an increase in tritiated 5-hydroxyin-doleacetic acid. This suggests that the labeled serotonin was intraneuronally catabolized, but never became functionally active.

To complicate matters further, the time of the day when diets are consumed may also alter the levels of serotonin. Ashley et al. (13) found that diets high in carbohydrate or low in protein do not alter the ratio of tryptophan to large neutral amino acids when ingested in the evening unless tryptophan is added directly. In contrast, a high-carbohydrate diet can alter the tryptophan to neutral amino acid ratio when ingested in the morning (14). Inclusion of tryptophan in the high-carbohydrate drink increased this ratio more than twofold.

In spite of the above results, some studies have shown a direct effect on tryptophan feeding on behaviors associated with serotonin, such as sleep, feeding, mood, and pain perception. A large number of studies have been conducted on the effect of tryptophan on sleep (15). L-tryptophan administered in doses of 1 g about 30 minutes before bedtime reduces the latency to sleep and in some individuals with sleep disorders increases total sleep time. Lesions of the raphe in the cat result in insomnia (16). Also inhibition of serotonin synthesis results in insomnia, and serotonergic treatments restore sleep. Tryptophan-free diets given to rats decrease rapid eye movement sleep (17). However, feeding diets that are chronically deficient in tryptophan does not alter sleep (18). Infants fed tryptophan had a shorter sleep latency than those given a diet low in valine and carbohydrate (19). A double-blind study by Lieberman and colleagues (20) demonstrated that a single oral dose of 50 mg/kg of tryptophan increased fatigue and decreased alertness and vigor self-ratings. Hypnotics often impair cognitive test performance, whereas tryptophan does not. Tryptophan may therefore be a useful, safe medication to induce sleep in the elderly, although whether it is more efficacious than a placebo remains controversial.

Another function of serotonin seems to be regulation of appetite. Administration of fenfluramine, which releases serotonin, deceases food consumption in rats and in humans (21). Also, fenfluramine and tryptophan administration has been shown to decrease carbohydrate intake selectively in overweight patients. Such obese people have been labeled as carbohydrate cravers. However, in most studies, foods that have been considered to be high in carbohydrate (potato chips, ice cream, candy) are also very high in fat. Fewer people seem to crave foods very high in carbohydrate, such as pasta, bread, jams, hard candies, soda pop, and licorice.

In a pilot study, Shaw et al. (cited in 22) demonstrated that patients with senile dementia have significantly lower levels of tryptophan present in their plasma than elderly controls. These data suggest that tryptophan or serotonin may in some way alter memory or other behaviors associated with senile dementia. Thomas et al. (22) compared the nutritional status of 23 severely demented patients with that of age-matched controls. They used a 3-day weighed intake of food as their standard. The patient group ingested less energy, protein, ascorbic acid, and nicotinic acid than the control group and had lower plasma levels of ascorbic acid and red cell folate. The demented subjects had reduced fasting plasma concentrations of tryptophan for both total and protein-bound fractions. The relationship between plasma concentration of tryptophan and other metabolic measurements could not explain why tryptophan levels were low. Thus, the low levels of tryptophan found in senile patients may simply be due to their poor diet.

Nutrients, such as choline, tyrosine, and histidine, serve as precursors for such neurotransmitters as acetylcholine, catecholamines, and histamine, respectively. There are fewer studies of the effect of these precursors on behavior than on tryptophan and serotonin. Anyone who reads the newspaper has seen articles suggesting that acetylcholine may be involved in senile dementia associated with Alzheimer's disease. Patients with this type of dementia seem to have a major decrease in the synthesis of acetylcholine in their brains, particularly in areas of the brain involved in memory processing, such as the temporal cortex and the hippocampus. Because increasing dietary choline intake is thought to increase brain levels of acetylcholine, one might predict that scientists would conduct studies administering dietary choline to patients with Alzheimer's disease. Dietary choline does elevate serum choline levels in healthy humans, and one study indicated an improvement in learning in normal volunteers. Sanchez et al. (23) conducted a study evaluating the effect of dietary choline on cognitive function in healthy elderly individuals and also reviewed the literature relevant to the demented patient. Subjects with Alzheimer's disease have decreased choline acetyltransferase activity (as low as one-tenth of normal values) in various brain regions compared with normal controls who were matched for age. Blockade of cholinergic function with scopolamine or atropine seems to impair memory function. When acetylcholinesterase activity is blocked, scopolamine no longer affects memory function. In 1978, Sitarem et al. (cited in 23) showed that a cholinergic agonist could improve learning in young people. Thus, one would like to increase choline brain levels in demented individuals on the hypothesis that doing so might alter memory function.

Many researchers have attempted to increase brain acetylcholine levels by feeding choline supplements. Sanchez et al. (23) found no relationship between choline intake and choline blood levels in 258 healthy volunteers (mean age, 72 years). Also, there was no relationship among choline intake, blood levels, and performance in a variety of cognitive tests. Other trials in the literature have also failed to find a relationship between dietary ingestion of choline and memory retention. Subjects with tardive dyskinesia also have reduced cholinergic transmission, and it has been suggested that choline chloride administration may be somewhat beneficial in treating tardive dyskinesia (24). It does appear to be premature to recommend ingestion of choline supplements or foods high in choline (eggs, fish, meat) for either dementia or tardive dyskinesia. Recent studies examining taurine in combination with lecithin have suggested that this drug-nutrient combination may improve cognition in some patients with Alzheimer's disease. The role of the nutrient in these possible responses remains to be determined.

NUTRITION AND LEARNING

The ability to learn appears to be affected by diet. Iron deficiency is known to alter the ability of children to learn new tasks (25). Unfortunately, these data are obfuscated by other factors, including the socioeconomic status of the individuals and other nutritional deficiencies that accompany iron deficiency. Also, it is unknown whether the iron-deficient state or the presence of any type of anemia results in learning deficits. Children with hemoglobin levels below 10 g/dl display decreased attention span with no change in intelligence quotient. Other studies indicate that children with anemia have low IQ scores (26). It should be noted, however, that these children were educationally and economically disadvantaged. In one study students from similar economic backgrounds who were iron-deficient had lower scores on the Iowa Test of Basic Skills (27). Infants who were iron deficient (between 6 to 18 months) appeared to have problems with neurologic signs, such as repetitive hand to food movements and balancing on one foot, when they reached 6 to 7 years of age. Some data suggests that improving iron status in children may improve cognitive function.

A series of studies conducted at the University of Iowa in the 1950s indicated that breakfast consumption could influence school performance (28). Although no neurologic changes were noted in 25 boys who did not eat breakfast, teachers found that these boys had a lower scholastic record and a poorer attitude about school than boys who ate breakfast. Breakfast intakes of greater than 400 kcal appeared to improve work performance compared with very low-calorie breakfasts (29). Snacks, such as fruit juice, seem to reduce fatigue and irritability, but this simply could be due to a break in routine. In 9- to 11-year-old children, skipping breakfast decreased their problem-solving ability later in the morning. Interestingly, a lack of breakfast enhanced short-term recall. Breakfast cereals together with milk and bread might result in sleepiness because of the high carbohydrate intake.

A recent study by Flood, Smith, and Morley (30) indicates the interrelationships among nutrition, neuroactive agents, and memory. These authors remind the reader of the importance of memory to the success of finding food in a natural environment. To test the relationship between feeding and memory, they studied whether feeding mice after an aversive training session would improve memory retention. Flood et al. (30) exposed three groups of mice to four training trials in which they learned to avoid footshock. One group of mice ate *ad libitum* before the trial, whereas the other two groups were deprived of food. Immediately after the training trial, food was presented to the *ad libitum* fed group and one group of deprived animals, whereas the other deprived mice received food 3 hours later. As expected, the food-deprived rats consumed food when it was presented, whereas the *ad libitum* fed group ate virtually no food. Retention testing was conducted after 1 week of *ad libitum* feeding. The mice that received the food immediately after the training session performed significantly better than either the *ad libitum* fed group or the mice that received the food 3 hours after the training session. These data suggest that eating reinforces memory retention, but only when feeding occurs after the event.

Because eating releases a series of neuroactive agents, it seems likely that such agents may also alter memory retention. To test this hypothesis Flood and colleagues studied the effect of the gut peptide cholecystokinin (CCK) on memory retention. This peptide is known to be released after meals and is thought to be involved in regulating food intake, as well as a number of gastrointestinal (GI) events that follow eating. CCK-8S (the active form of the peptide) was administered intraperitoneally after four training trials. This peptide improved memory retention when evaluated 1 week later. However, when the vagus nerve was cut, the CCK-8S no longer was effective. Thus, this study indicates that eating and at least one neuropeptide may be involved in memory retention. In subsequent studies they have shown that a number of other hormones, such as bombesin, gastrin-releasing peptide, and pancreastation, also enhance memory retention. They have also shown that a CCK antagonist blocks the memory enhancement produced by feeding. Johnson and Morley have preliminary data demonstrating that feeding after learning a task also enhances memory in humans.

NUTRITION AND CRIMINAL BEHAVIOR

Some penal institutions have begun feeding prisoners specialized diets that are thought to decrease violent behavior. It is thought that such aggressive behavior is caused by reactive hypoglycemia, sugar consumption, food-additive ingestion, and vitamin and mineral deficiencies (31,32). Violent criminals are thought to have a more prolonged and marked decrease in blood glucose after ingestion of glucose. Unfortunately, such evidence comes from self-diagnosis and questionnaires answered by the criminals. Also, as most endocrinologists know, hypoglycemic symptoms are variable and not precise. Thus, self-reporting by prisoners is not to be trusted. For example, in one study of 135 patients who were convinced that they were hypoglycemic, only 4 actually had hypoglycemia (33). There has been no substantiation of reports indicating that sugar results in violent behavior. These studies were not double-blind experiments, and furthermore the investigators were ignorant about sugar chemistry (34).

ATTENTION DEFICIT DISORDER AND FOOD

In the 1970s Dr. Benjamin Feingold, a physician employed by a health maintenance organization in California, observed that certain foods seemed to precipitate "hyperactivity" in children. He believed that specific low-molecular weight chemicals present in certain foods resulted in hyperactivity. In his book, *Why Your Child is Hyperactive* (35), he suggested a diet that eliminated all foods containing artificial food colorings or flavorings and salicylates. He knew that aspirin-sensitive individuals also were sensitive to yellow dye #5, also referred to as tartrazine; in fact, labeling for foods containing tartrazine is required for those individuals sensitive to this food dye. Dr. Feingold eliminated such foods as oranges, peaches, tomatos, cucumbers, almonds, apples, and apricots that he thought contained salicylates based on chemical analyses from the 1940s. As is obvious, eliminating such important foods as citrus fruits could result in nutrient deficiencies. The "Feingold diet" no longer limits these foods as it was found that the chemical analyses were incorrect and that these foods do not contain large quantities of salicylates. Feingold and his supporters claimed that the behavior of 50% of hyperactive children improved when they adhered strictly to such a diet. The claims of this one physician, based on anecdotes and simple observation, resulted in a series of very costly studies funded by government agencies.

First, it should be noted that it is very difficult to measure activity levels in children accurately. In one methodology, investigators measure the activity level of the child by placing toys in a room that is divided into segments with tape. The amount of area that the child moves about in is compared with the area covered by a normal, age-matched control group. Another approach is to give teachers and parents questionnaires evaluating the child's ability to focus on one activity. The latter approach is more commonly used, but is somewhat inaccurate because "hyperactivity" is not well defined and teachers and parents differ in their opinions about what is normal. Two types of studies were used to evaluate activity levels of children after the ingestion of specific foods. In one study, referred to as the challenge-type study, the subjects are selected and given a food-additive-free period in which baseline measurements are made. The challenge food or placebo food is then presented and behavior is re-evaluated. In the other type of study the subjects are selected and baseline behavioral measurements are made. Then, the subjects are given either a control or experimental diet for a given period of time, and their behavior is evaluated during this time frame. Harley et al. (36) conducted a study of the latter type in which all foods were removed from the household of the child. Foods eaten by this child, including those eaten at a friend's party, were provided by the study personnel. He evaluated 36 school-aged children and 10 preschool children. Neither the teachers nor the researchers noted any change in the children's behavior during the period of the study; however, some parents claimed to observe a difference. In a study of this type conducted by Conners and colleagues (37), behavioral improvement was seen by the teachers when the control diet was given first, but not when the experimental diet was presented first. In more than 12 studies evaluating 200 children using the challenge design, no differences were noted by the teachers or researchers. In some cases parents seemed to observe increased activity levels when a challenge food was presented. These data convinced most individuals that diet does not alter the ability of children to focus on individual activities.

In spite of these data, large number of "Feingold diet" support groups continue to function, and studies continue to be conducted. In 1985, a study by Egger and colleagues (38) did suggest that diet might influence behavior in children. They gave 76 hyperactive children a diet containing only two meats, two starches, one vegetable, and two fruits for weeks (a micro-nutrient supplement was also supplied). Those children who responded well to the elimination diet were then presented with single challenge foods. During this open trial over 80% of the children showed some type of improvement, and about 30% appeared to resemble normal children. A double-blind study was then conducted on a subset of children. During the control diet, fewer behavioral abnormalities were observed as measured by the Conners scale, and a neurologist found that the behavior improved in 20 of 28 children. Behavior deteriorated during the presentation of certain challenge foods, including tartrazine, the preservative, sodium benzoate, milk, chocolate, eggs, wheat, corn, oats, and fish. However, placing children on an elimination diet and then identifying the specific problematic foods is an extremely difficult task and takes great patience on the part of the parents, as well as the children.

A large part of the population believes that table sugar causes hyperactivity in children. Boys given a high-sucrose diet were found to score lower on a behavioral test measuring attention span (39). Also, there appeared to be a correlation of sucrose intake over 7 days with aggressive, restless and destructive behavior in children with attention deficit disorder. This study was not conducted in a blinded fashion and should be taken as anecdotal. In a double-blind study, it has been shown that sucrose actually calmed children and to support this finding further, saccharin and aspartame had no effect (40).

One study by O'Banion and colleagues (41) suggested that foods could increase disruptive behavior in one 8-year-old autistic child. The child first fasted for a 6-day period and then was given a normal diet. This child would bite, scratch, scream, and laugh inappropriately and increase activity levels after eating wheat. Other foods, including corn, mushrooms, tomatos, and milk, caused less extreme behavior changes, but nevertheless exacerbated the situation. The child did not alter his behavior after ingestion of rice, apples, beef, or eggs. Of course, this study is a case report on one child and should not be extrapolated to all autistic children.

BEHAVIOR AND DIET

From the above discussion, it seems probable that diet can change behavior. We also know that an individual's mental status can alter the ingestion of food. For example, anorexia is often associated with depression, dementia, and other psychiatric illness. Sometimes, anorexia is associated with a medical problem that occurs in tandem with the psychiatric illness. However, it does appear that a "clear mind" is needed to make proper decisions about diet. We also know from the animal and human literature that various stresses can increase or decrease total food intake. Pinching the tail of a rat, a model of stress, results in eating at a time of the day when rats normally do not eat (42). Obese students eat more when under the pressure of school examinations, whereas lean individuals decrease food intake during such stressful situations (43). Corticotropin-releasing hormone, a peptide released from the hypothalamus during stress, causes grooming behavior in rats with a concomitant decrease in eating (44). Psychologic stress can also alter the utilization of nutrients, such as calcium and fat. Stress can even change the bacterial flora of feces. Anger, but not other mood states, has been shown to cause a sudden peak in the presence of *Bacteroides sp.* in fecal specimens of humans (45).

The drugs that are used to treat psychiatric disorders often alter appetite. This is not particularly surprising because these drugs alter the concentration of various neurotransmitters, which as a group are thought to influence food intake. In human studies, it is difficult to differentiate if the change in appetite is due to the drug or to an improvement in the psychiatric state of the patient. Also, most of these studies have only examined food records and other means of self-reporting by subjects, rather than actual measurements of intake. Few studies have evaluated the effects of these drugs on normals because of the difficulty of administering such drugs to individuals not facing psychiatric problems. The literature does suggest that antidepressants, such as amitriptyline, result in weight gain and sweets craving (46). Benzodiazepines and lithium administered for anxiety and manic-depressive illness, respectively, result in weight gain (47). Such antipsychotic drugs as haloperidol, fluphenazine, and thioridazine generally cause weight gain (48). Recently, molindone has been used to treat psychosis and does not appear to result in weight gain.

HEADACHES AND DIET

The pain from headaches can be debilitating and often troublesome to the individual because the etiology of the headache is not always clear. For these reasons, individuals are willing to try any suggested treatment, which at times results in inappropriate use of nutrient therapy. When questioned, 25% of 500 patients believed that their headaches were related to the intake

TABLE 1. *Foods implicated in migraine headaches*

Food	Offending substance
Cheese	Tyramine
Chocolate	Phenylethylamine
Cured meats	Nitrites
Processed foods	Monosodium glutamate
Liquor	Ethanol
Coffee	Caffeine
Ice cream	Cold

of specific foods (see 49). Physicians also believe that diet is an important factor in the etiology of migraine headaches. Hanington (49) and Diamond et al. (50) have reviewed this subject in some detail. Vasoactive substances are present in foods and may precipitate migraine headaches (Table 1). These substances include amines, monosodium glutamate, nitrites, and ethanol. The 500 migraine sufferers interviewed by Hanington listed cheese and chocolate as the major problem foods. Because cheese contains tyramine, Hanington gave tyramine or placebo capsules to patients with migraine headaches. Those subjects receiving the tyramine (40/49 trials) complained of migraine headaches, whereas those receiving placebo generally did not. Hanington also found in a double-blind study that bitter chocolate (2 oz) precipitated migraine attacks. Chocolate contains phenylethylamine, which itself can precipitate migraine attacks in certain individuals. This amine is also present in fermented foods, including Cheddar, Cheshire, and double Gloucester cheese. Amyl nitrite has been said to cause headaches in some people. Cured meats contain nitrites, which also seem to cause headaches in sensitive individuals. Monosodium glutamate (MSG), a flavor enhancer, is well known as a cause of "Chinese restaurant syndrome," symptoms of which include headaches. Sensitive individuals respond within the first hour after ingestion of the MSG.

Other vasoactive substances can cause headaches. These include caffeine, monoamine oxidase inhibitors, and nicotine. Because caffeine is present in many foods ranging from soda pop to candy, sensitive individuals need to read labels carefully. Individuals with reactive hypoglycemia often have headaches associated with their hypoglycemic episode. Even ingestion of cold foods, such as ice cream, can result in headaches.

NONNUTRITIVE SUBSTANCES PRESENT IN FOODS

Morley in 1982 (51) originated the concept of food hormones (formones); that is, hormones present in foods that may alter our physiology. As an example, alfalfa contains a peptide that resembles thyrotropin-releasing hormone, oats contain a peptide related in structure to luteinizing-releasing hormone, and wheat and milk protein contain opioid-like substances. Such peptides could work within the lumen of the GI tract to alter motility and absorption, they might act at peripheral sites if absorbed intact, or they may cross the blood-brain barrier. Our group has shown that opioid-like peptides found in wheat protein alter GI transit time and the concentration of somatostatin circulating in blood (52). In one study, gluten was associated with a worsening of behavior in schizophrenic patients (53). Catecholamines are present in bananas and perhaps may have some physiologic effects either in the gut lumen or after absorption. Thus, foods may not only contain precursors of neurotransmitters, but may also contain neuroactive substances that may alter behavior. Continued research in this area may demonstrate a true "mood-food" connection.

CONCLUSION

The idea that you are what you eat is an ancient concept. Based on the synthetic pathways of neurotransmitters and other neuroactive substances, one would hypothesize that diet should alter behavior. No one questions that a nutritional deficiency can alter behavior, and in fact many individuals were institutionalized for psychiatric disorders associated with vitamin deficiencies before this century. In the present century, these behavioral alterations associated with nutritional deficiencies are most often seen in older subjects with concomitant disease. However, the role that food plays in behavior is not as clear in the well-nourished population. The analysis of behavior is tedious and often inaccurate. The behavior of an organism is influenced by many external and internal factors in addition to nutritional ones. For these reasons, at the present time it is difficult to recommend specific foods for specific behavioral problems, and we must tell our friends and patients that the information is not yet complete. Standardization of methodology for measuring behavior, improved study designs with adequate controls, use of double-blind procedures, and cautious analysis of the data must be done before we can advance our knowledge about this complex research arena. There is a particular need to examine the role of the diet in modulating age-related cognitive changes. The role of the diet in modulating behavioral disturbances observed in long-term care settings is also deserving of study.

REFERENCES

1. Cosman MP. *Annu Rev Nutr* 1983;3:1–33.
2. Keys A, Brozek J, Henschel A, Mickelson O, Taylor HL. *The biology of human starvation, vol II*. Minneapolis: University of Minnesota Press, 1950.
3. Winick M. *Malnutrition and brain development*. New York: Oxford University Press, 1976.
4. Cravioto J, DeLicardie ER, Birch HG. *Pediatrics* 1966;38:319–372.
5. Goodwin JS, Goodwin JM, Gary PJ. *JAMA* 1983;249:2917–2921.

6. Dakshinamurti K. In: Wurtman RJ, Wurtman JJ, eds. *Nutrition and the brain, vol 1: Determinants of the availability of nutrients to the brain.* New York: Raven Press, 1977;249–318.
7. Dreyfus PM, Geel SE. In: Siegel GJ, Albers RW, Agranoff BW, Katzman R, eds. *Basic neurochemistry,* 3rd ed. Boston: Little, Brown and Co, 1981;661–679.
8. Nobbs BT. *Lancet* 1974;1:405–406.
9. Kimura K, Kumura J. *Proc Japn Acad* 1965;41:943–947.
10. Wurtman JJ, Wurtman RJ, Growdon JH, Henry P, Lipscomb A, Zeisel SH. *Int J Eating Dis* 1981;1:2–15.
11. Fernstrom JD, Wurtman RJ. *Science* 1972;178:414–416.
12. Trulson ME. *Life Sci* 1985;37:1067–1072.
13. Ashley DV, Barclay DV, Chauffard FA, Moennoz D, Leathwood PD. *Am J Clin Nutr* 1982;36:143–153.
14. Ashley DV, Liardon R, Leathwood PD. *J Neural Transm* 1985;63:271–283.
15. Hartmann E. *Waking Sleeping* 1977;1:155–161.
16. Jouvet M. In: Iverson LL, Iverson SD, Snyder SH, eds. *Handbook of psychopharmacology, vol. 8: Drugs, neurotransmitters, and behavior.* New York: Plenum, 1977;233–293.
17. Moja EA, Mendelson WB, Stoff DM, Gillin JC, Wyatt RJ. *Life Sci* 1979;24:1467–1450.
18. Clancy JJ, Caldwell DF, Oberleas D, Sangiah S, Velleneuve MJ. *Brain Res Bull* 1978;3:83–87.
19. Yogman MW, Zeisel SH. *Am J Clin Nutr* 1985;42:352–360.
20. Lieberman HR, Corkin S, Spring BJ, Wurtman RJ, Growdon JH. *Am J Clin Nutr* 1985;42:366–370.
21. Blundell JE, Latham CJ, Moniz E, MacArthur RA, Rogers PJ. *Curr Med Res Opin* 1979;6(suppl. 1):34–54.
22. Thomas DE, Chung-A-On, KO, Dickerson WT, Tidmarsh SF, Shaw DM. *Psychol Med* 1986;16:297–305.
23. Sanchez CJ, Hooper E, Garry PJ, Goodwin JM, Goodwin JS. *J Am Geriatr Soc* 1984;32:208–212.
24. Davis KL, Hollister LE, Berger PA, Vento AL. *Psychopharmacol Bull* 1978;14:56–58.
25. Cantwell RJ. *Pediatr Res* 1974;8:342.
26. Howell D. *Summary proceedings, Workshop of the Food and Nutrition Board.* Washington, DC: National Academy of Sciences, 1971.
27. Webb TE, Oski FA. *Pediatr Res* 1973;7:294.
28. Tuttle WW, Daum K, Larsen R, Salzano J, Roloff L. *J Am Dietet Assoc* 1954;30:674–677.
29. Arvedson I, Sterky G, Tjernstrom K. *J Am Dietet Assoc* 1969;55:257–261.
30. Flood JF, Smith GE, Morley JE. *Science* 1987;236:832–834.
31. Hippchen LJ. *Int J Biosoc Res* 1981;2:37–42.
32. Schoenthaler SJ. *Int J Biosoc Res* 1983;4:25–39.
33. Anderson RW, Lev-Ran A. *Psychosomatics* 1985;26:38–47.
34. Gray GE, Gray LR. *Nutr Tod* 1983;18:14–17.
35. Feingold BF. *Why your child is hyperactive.* New York: Random House, 1975.
36. Harley JP, Ray RS, Tomasi L, Eichman PL, Matthews CG, Chun R, Cleeland S, Traisman E. *Pediatrics* 1978;61:818–828.
37. Conners CK, Goyette CH, Southwick DA, Lees JM, Andrulonis PA. *Pediatrics* 1976;58:154–166.
38. Egger J, Carter CM, Graham PJ, Gumley D, Soothill JF. *Lancet* 1985;1:540–545.
39. Prinz RJ, Roberts WA, Hantman E. *J Consult Clin Psychol* 1980;48:760–769.
40. Behar D, Rapoport JL, Adams AJ, Berg CJ, Cornblath M. *Nutr Behav* 1984;1:277–288.
41. O'Banion D, Armstrong B, Cummings RA, Stange J. *J Autism Child Schizophr* 1978;8:325–337.
42. Morley JE, Levine AS, Rowland NE. *Life Sci* 1983;32:2169–2182.
43. Beller AS. *Fat and thin: A natural history of obesity.* New York: Farrar, Straus, 1977.
44. Morley JE, Levine AS. *Life Sci* 1982;31:1459–1464.
45. Holdeman LV, Good IJ, Moore WEC. *Appl Environ Microbiol* 1976;31:359–375.
46. Paykel ES, Mueller PS, de la Vergne PM. *Br J Psychiatry* 1973;123:501–507.
47. Duguay R, Flach FF. *Acta Psychiatr Scand* 1964;40:1–9.

48. Doss FW. *J Clin Psychiatry* 1979;49:528–530.
49. Hanington E. In: Lessof MH, ed. *Clinical reactions to food*. New York: Wiley, 1983;155–180.
50. Diamond S, Praser J, Freitas FG. *Postgrad Med* 1986;79:279–286.
51. Morley JE. *JAMA* 1982;247:2379–2380.
52. Morley JE, Levine AS, Yamada T, Gebhard RL, Prigge WF, Shafer RB, Goetz FC, Silvis SE. *Gastroenterology* 1983;84:1517–1523.
53. Singh MM, Kay SR. *Science* 1976;191:401–402.

Geriatric Nutrition, edited by John E. Morley,
Zvi Glick, Laurence Z. Rubenstein.
Raven Press, Ltd., New York © 1990.

32

Memory Enhancement in Mice with Chronic Menhaden Oil Administration

James F. Flood, Ernesto N. Hernandez, and John E. Morley

Geriatric Research, Education and Clinical Center VA Medical Center, Sepulveda, California 91343 and Departments of Medicine and Psychiatry and Biobehavioral Sciences, UCLA School of Medicine, Los Angeles, California 90024

Fish are a rich source of omega-3 polyunsaturated fatty acids, such as eicosopentaenoic acid (20:5 W3) and docosahexaenoic acid (22:6 W3). Eicosopentaenoic acid and docosahexaenoic acid influence the metabolism of eicosanoids (ie, prostaglandins, thromboxanes, prostacyclins, and leukotrienes) and lipoproteins in a manner that should be protective against coronary heart disease (1). Docosahexaenoic acid constitutes approximately one-third of the fatty acid content of ethanolamine and serine phosphoglycerides (2,3) and is found in particularly high concentrations in synaptosomes (4). Rats specifically depleted of w-3 fatty acid failed to learn a two-choice discrimination problem (5). In view of these findings, we studied whether administration of fish (menhaden) oil would improve retention in mice trained on a simple footshock avoidance task, with retention measured 1 week after training.

METHODS

Subjects

After 1 week in the laboratory, CD-1 male mice obtained at 6 weeks of age from Charles River Breeding Laboratories, Wilmington, MA, were individually caged 24 to 48 hours before training and remained singly housed until retention was tested 1 week later. The median body weight was 35 g, with a range of 33 to 38 g. Animal rooms were maintained on a 12-hour light-dark cycle with light on at 0600. The mice were trained between 0700 and 1500. They were assigned randomly to groups of 15 unless otherwise indicated.

Apparatus and Training Procedure

The T-maze and training procedure have been described previously (6). The maze was made up of a black plastic start alley with a start box at one end and two goal boxes at the other; a stainless steel rod floor ran throughout the maze. The start box was separated from the start alley by a plastic guillotine door that prevented the mouse from moving down the alley until the training started. The intertrial interval was 30 seconds, with a 55-db doorbell-type buzzer as the conditioned stimulus and a nominal footshock of 0.30 ma (Coulbourn Instruments scrambled grid floor shocker model E13-08) unless otherwise indicated. A training trial started when a mouse was placed into the start box. The guillotine door was raised and the buzzer sounded simultaneously; then, 0.5 seconds later, a footshock was applied. At the end of each trial, the mouse was removed from the goal box and returned to its home cage. A new trial began by placing the mouse in the start box, sounding the buzzer, and raising the guillotine door, with footshock beginning 5 seconds later if the mouse did not move into its correct goal box.

The mice received four training trials. On the first training trial only, the mouse continued to receive footshock until it entered the goal box on the opposite side; this was the "correct" goal box for this mouse for the remaining training and retention test trials. As training proceeded, a mouse made one of two types of responses. A response latency longer than 5 seconds was classed as an escape from the footshock. A response latency less than or equal to 5 seconds was considered an avoidance because the mouse avoided receiving a footshock. On the first training trials, mice with escape latencies greater than 20 seconds were discarded.

Retention Test

One week after training and drug administration, the T-maze training was resumed until the mice made five avoidances in six trials. The overall significance of the drug treatment effect was determined by a Student's t-test or two-way analysis of variance (7,8). Dunnett's t-test was used to make multiple comparisons between each drug group and its control group (9). A nonparametric measure of retention was derived to better visualize the effects of drug treatments on retention test performance and to correspond with usual reporting practice. For this measure, the number of trials to the first avoidance response was dichotomized to yield a percent recall score. Those mice making their first avoidance in three trials or less were classed as remembering the original training. This criterion was adopted because it has provided optimal separation between the retention test performance of naive mice (with no T-maze training) and well-trained mice (10).

Drugs

Deodorized menhaden oil and corn oil vehicle were supplied by Zapata-Haynie, Reedsville, VA. Antioxidants (mixed tocopherols) from Eastman-Kodak, Rochester, NY, were added to both preparations. The menhaden oil or vehicle (corn oil) was injected intraperitoneally at a volume of 1 ml per mouse. Menhaden oil contains 13% eicosopentaenoic (20:5) and 6.94% docosahexanoic (22:6) acid, whereas corn oil is predominantly linoleic (18:3, 57.7%) acid.

RESULTS

Experiment 1: The Effect of Menhaden Oil Administered 1, 2, 4, or 7 Days on Retention for T-Maze Footshock Avoidance Training

Pilot studies indicated that acute posttraining administration of menhaden oil had only a slight improving effect on retention. The menhaden oil may not be absorbed rapidly enough into the system to affect memory processing when it is administered immediately after training. The purpose of the first experiment was to determine if chronic administration of menhaden oil facilitates retention test performance for footshock avoidance training in the T-maze. Mice were randomly assigned to groups that received corn oil or 25%, 50%, or 100% of 1 ml menhaden oil. These four dose groups were further divided into groups that received menhaden oil for 1, 2, 4, or 7 days before t-maze training. Retention was tested 1 week after training.

A two-way ANOVA (days by dose) indicated that menhaden oil administration had a significant effect on retention tested 1 week after training. The main effect for both days [$F(3,224) = 6.46$, $p<0.001$] and dose [$F(3,224) = 8.72$, $p<0.001$] was significant. A partitioning of the sum of squares indicated that only 4- and 7-day treatment periods contributed significantly to the effect of menhaden oil on retention test performance. A comparison of treatment means for each dose relative to its control for 4- and 7-day treatment periods indicated that 100% menhaden oil differed from the 4-day treatment control at $p<0.05$ and from the 7-day treatment control at $p<0.01$; 50% menhaden oil only differed significantly at $p<0.05$ from its control in the 7-day treatment group (Table 1).

Experiment 2: Effect of a Single Injection of Menhaden Oil 7 Days Before Training on Retention

The first experiment did not necessarily demonstrate that menhaden oil must be administered chronically to be effective. It is possible that the oil

TABLE 1. *Effect of dose and duration of fish oil treatment on memory retention*

Number of treatment days	Fish oil concentration			
	0	25	50	100
1 mean trials to criterion	9.60	9.53	8.27	9.07
(±SEM)	0.29	0.41	0.44	0.33
Recall score (%)	13	20	33	13
2 mean trials to criterion	9.07	9.07	8.87	8.80
(±SEM)	0.49	0.32	0.39	0.43
Recall score (%)	20	13	27	27
4 mean trials to criterion	9.27	8.33	7.80	7.47[a],*
(±SEM)	0.41	0.43	0.48	0.48
Recall score (%)	20	33	53	67
7 mean trials to criterion	9.60	8.33	7.80[a],*	7.40[a],**
(±SEM)	0.25	0.48	0.31	0.40
Recall score (%)	13	33	60	73

[a]The means differed from their respective control groups (0% menhaden oil) at $p < 0.05$ indicated by * and at $p < 0.01$ indicated by ** using Dunnett's t-test.

was absorbed slowly and that giving a single injection 7 days before training could have been as effective as 7 daily injections. To determine this, 1 ml of 100% menhaden oil or corn oil was administered on day 1. Seven days later, the mice were trained as in the first experiment. Retention was tested 1 week after training.

A single administration of menhaden oil 7 days before training did not significantly affect retention compared to the corn oil control group. The recall scores were 13% for both groups. The mean trials to criterion (±SEM) were $9.27 ± 0.42$ for the menhaden oil injected group and $8.80 ± 0.39$ for the control group ($t < 1$).

Experiment 3: A Test of the Need for Chronic Administration Immediately Before Training for Menhaden Oil Improvement of Retention

In the first experiment (Table 1), four successive injections of 1 ml of 100% menhaden oil before training facilitated retention nearly as much as 7 days of chronic administration. As a further test of the necessity of chronic administration, we administered menhaden oil for 4 days and then waited 3 days to train the mice on the T-maze footshock avoidance task. The training and retention testing were done as in Experiment 1.

Even though 4 successive days of 1 ml of 100% menhaden oil or vehicle immediately before training facilitated retention at 1 week, 4 successive days of treatment followed by 3 days of no treatment failed to improve retention. The recall score for both groups was 13%. The mean trials to criterion (±SEM) were $9.27 ± 0.36$ for the menhaden oil injected group and $9.07 ± 0.28$ for the control group ($t < 1$).

Experiment 4: Effects of Chronic Menhaden Oil Administration on T-Maze Footshock Avoidance Acquisition

Better retention in the mice receiving 1 ml of 100% menhaden oil chronically for 7 days before training may have resulted from an enhanced ability to acquire the footshock avoidance habit, rather than enhanced memory processing. To test this hypothesis, mice were administered 1 ml of 100% menhaden oil or corn oil 7 consecutive days before training and then trained as in the first experiment, except training continued until each mouse made five avoidances in six consecutive trials.

Chronic menhaden oil treatment did not facilitate acquisition compared to the vehicle control. A two-way ANOVA (drug by days) with repeated measures on days indicated no significant effect (F<1). The mean left-right discrimination errors ($\pm$ SEM) were 1.47 ± 0.24 for the menhaden oil group and 1.40 ± 0.14 for the control group. The mean trials to first avoidance ($\pm$ SEM) were 6.20 ± 0.38 for the menhaden oil group and 6.27 ± 0.42 for the control. The mean trials to criterion ($\pm$ SEM) were 10.33 ± 0.34 for the menhaden oil group and 10.40 ± 0.40 for the control. None of these measures of acquisition indicate that facilitation of acquisition resulted from chronic menhaden oil administration.

DISCUSSION

These experiments demonstrate that chronic menhaden oil administration improved retention test performance (Exp. 1) without affecting acquisition of the T-maze footshock avoidance task (Exp. 4). The failure of menhaden oil treatment to alter acquisition argues against the enhanced retention test performance being caused by nonspecific effects in performance, such as altered perception, footshock sensitivity, or motor activity. The study showed that improved retention only occurred when high concentrations of menhaden oil were administered for several days immediately before training. Further, the beneficial effect of menhaden oil administration on retention dissipated rather quickly, considering that 4 consecutive days of 100% menhaden oil administration before training facilitated retention (Exp. 1) but 4 consecutive days of administration of menhaden oil followed by training 3 days later had no significant effect on retention (Exp. 3). It does not seem likely that menhaden oil improved retention by blocking impaired memory processing caused by corn oil administration because the average of the mean trials to the avoidance criterion in the four control groups in Exp. 1 of 9.39 ± 0.36 is similar to the average of the means for six saline-injected controls of 8.97 ± 0.39 described in three of our recent publications (11–13).

Although it is difficult to extrapolate from a mouse model to humans, the results of the study suggest that memory enhancement in humans is likely to be impractical because a very large quantity of fish oil would have to be ingested daily. However, this study does not rule out the possibility of a low-dose effect with more refined polyunsaturated fatty acids. Some evidence suggests that menhaden oil alters membrane fluidity within the central nervous system (14). It remains a question for further study whether menhaden oil enhanced retention by altering membrane fluidity or by altering the metabolism of eicosanoids.

ACKNOWLEDGMENTS

Support of this research was in part supplied by Research Service, Veterans Administration Medical Center.

REFERENCES

1. Sanders TAB. *Br Heart J* 1987;57:214.
2. O'Brien JS, Sampson EL. *J Lipid Res* 1965;6:545.
3. Svennerholm L. *J Lipid Res* 1968;9:570.
4. Cotman C, Blank ML, Moehl A, Snyder F. *Biochemistry* 1969;8:4604.
5. Lamptey MS, Walker BL. *J Nutr* 1976;106:86.
6. Flood JF, Cherkin A. *Behav Neurol Biol* 1986;45:169.
7. Keppel G. *Design and analysis: A researcher's handbook.* Englewood Cliffs, NJ: Prentice-Hall, 1973;402.
8. Winer BJ. *Statistical principles in experimental design,* 2nd ed. New York, McGraw-Hill, 1971;196.
9. Bruning JL, Kintz BL. *Computational handbook of statistics,* 3rd ed. Glenview, IL: Scott, Foresman and Co, 1978;130.
10. Flood JF, Bennett EL, Orme A, Rosenzweig MR. *Physiol Behav* 1975;14:177.
11. Flood JF, Cherkin A. *Psychopharmacology* 1987;93:36.
12. Flood JF, Cherkin A, Morley JE. *Brain Res* 1987;422:18.
13. Flood JF, Smith GE, Roberts E. *Brain Res* 1988;447:269.
14. Kessler AR, Kessler B, Yehuda B. *Life Sci* 1986;38:1185.

Geriatric Nutrition, edited by John E. Morley,
Zvi Glick, Laurence Z. Rubenstein.
Raven Press, Ltd., New York © 1990.

33

Zinc Status and Impotence

*Charles J. Billington, *Rex B. Shafer, *Phillip A. Krezowski,
*Allen S. Levine, and †John E. Morley

*Departments of Medicine and of Food Science & Nutrition,
Minneapolis VA Medical Center and the University of Minnesota,
Minneapolis/St. Paul, Minnesota 55455 and §Geriatric Research, Education, and
Clinical Center, VA Medical Center, Sepulveda, California 91343*

The possibility that an individual's zinc status could affect sexual function was first suggested by the delay in the sexual maturation of boys raised in a zinc-deficient environment (1,2). This possibility was supported by observations (3,4), in dispute (5) that individuals on chronic hemodialysis, who had become zinc deficient as a result of that treatment, also experienced sexual impotence that could sometimes be reversed by administration of zinc. Further, zinc has been reported to partially reverse oligospermia (6). Because a number of other conditions resulting in negative zinc balance have now been described (7–9), we sought to evaluate the zinc nutriture status of patients presenting to a referral clinic with the complaint of sexual impotence, as well as the effect of zinc replacement in a subset of these patients.

METHODS

The patients evaluated were 137 consecutive patients referred to the Impotence Study Clinic at the Minneapolis VA Medical Center. This referral clinic receives the majority of its patients from the medical department. The patients are generally representative of the VA medical clinic population, are of middle to older age (mean age 60 years), and are often afflicted with at least one other medical problem (Table 1).

We have previously analyzed patients from this population and found that the majority of them are suffering from impotence of an organic cause (10). Sexual function at presentation ranges from complete erectile failure to inability to achieve an erection of sufficient turgidity for intercourse. The evaluation of these patients includes a history of sexual function; general medical history; medication list; physical examination and determinations of

TABLE 1. *Principal diagnoses in referred impotent patients*[a]

Hypertension	60
Atherosclerotic cardiovascular disease	51
Diabetes mellitus	30
Chronic lung disease	11
Alcoholism/substance abuse	10
Cancer	7
Low back pain	7
Psychiatric disorders	5
Peptic ulcer disease	5
Prostatism	4
Peripheral venous disease	4
Gout	4
Hyperthyroidism, systemic lupus erythematosus, rheumatoid arthritis, chronic renal failure, tuberculosis, migraine, muscular dystrophy, hepatic failure, primary cardiac rhythm disturbance	Less than 4

[a]Many patients have more than one diagnosis.

testosterone, LH, FSH, prolactin, and thyroid function, and tests for the presence of diabetes.

Samples of serum for determination of zinc levels were collected in zinc-free plastic tubes and held frozen until determinations could be made. Analysis was carried out in duplicate using an atomic absorption spectrophotometer as described by Prasad and colleagues (11). Normal values have previously been established at our institution and range from 70 to 110 μg/dl (8,9). This range for serum zinc concentration is similar to that reported by many others (12–19). A majority of the patients were also able to provide a 24-hour urine collection in zinc-free plastic containers, which was also held frozen until analysis. The upper limit of the normal range established for this determination is a zinc excretion of less than 700 μg/24 hr (8,9). Again, this range is in accord with other published values (16,17,18,20).

RESULTS

Serum zinc determinations in 137 consecutive patients identified 41 patients (30%) with serum zinc values below the lower limit of normal for our laboratory (70 μg/dl). No statistically significant associations could be found between this abnormality and testosterone levels or usage of diuretics, although 34% of these patients with low serum zinc levels did have clinically low testosterone values and 56% of them were taking diuretics. There was no association of serum zinc level and measures of LH, FSH, or prolactin.

Urinary zinc excretion was measured on 82 of the above patients who were able to bring a 24-hour urine collection, and 44 (54%) of these patients were found to have abnormally high urinary zinc levels. Elevated urinary zinc excretion was associated with clinically low serum testosterone levels in 15 of the 44 cases (34%) compared to 6 instances (16%) of low serum

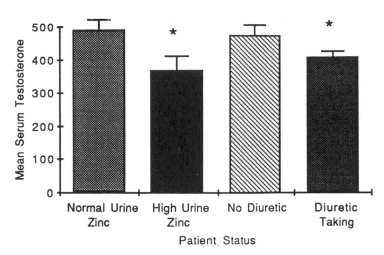

FIG. 1. Relationship of urinary zinc status and diuretic use to mean serum testosterone. *, a significant difference ($p < 0.05$ by t-test) from respective control group.

testosterone among those 38 cases with normal urinary zinc excretion. Although there was a tendency for more frequent hypogonadism in the group with abnormal urinary zinc status, this did not quite reach statistical significance ($p < 0.1$ by chi-square). This association may have been weakened because we did not eliminate other causes of hypogonadism. Patients with exaggerated urinary zinc excretion also had a significantly lower serum testosterone (Fig. 1) than those with normal urinary zinc excretion: 373.8 ± 25.3 vs. 463.8 ± 30.8 ng/dl ($p < 0.05$ by Student's t-test).

In addition there was a significant association, indicated in Fig. 2, between

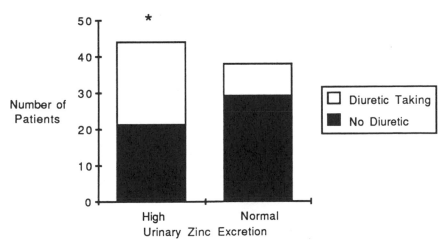

FIG. 2. Association between diuretic use and frequency of elevated zinc excretion. *, a significant difference ($p < 0.05$ by chi-square).

the use of diuretics and elevated urinary zinc excretion ($p < 0.01$ by chi-square). Mean urinary zinc excretion was significantly higher in those taking diuretics: 1077 ± 98 vs. 766 ± 73 µg/24h ($p < 0.01$ by Student's t-test). Further, the mean serum testosterone values (Fig. 1) of those taking diuretics was significantly lower than the mean serum testosterone values of those not so treated: 406.4 ± 27.2 versus 477.0 ± 26.5 ng/dl ($p < 0.05$ by Student's t-test). Measures of LH, FSH, and prolactin were associated with urinary zinc status.

DISCUSSION

It is apparent from these studies that the relationship between zinc status and sexual potency deserves further consideration. The frequency of abnormally high urinary zinc excretion in these patients is striking. The physiologic significance of this observation is underlined by the statistically lower testosterone values seen in the same group. The case for zinc abnormalities as a potential pathogenic factor in impotence could be made stronger by the performance of zinc balance studies. Nonetheless, there are previous investigations that indicate that the general observation is qualitatively accurate.

The link between the zinc status of individuals and the ability to manufacture testosterone has been known for some time. Much of this evidence is inferential, based on studies of natural and induced zinc deficiency states. Nutritional zinc deficiency in the Middle East resulted in a delay in the sexual maturation of young men (1,2). This same observation has been made in experimental animals in which zinc-deficient diets created abnormally low testosterone values (21,22). A strong correlation has been found between serum zinc levels and serum testosterone values in a previous large human study (23). However, two difficulties remain with these studies: First, zinc-deficient diets may also be deficient in other key nutritional elements (notably in the case of the population studies, there may be an element of protein-calorie malnutrition); and second, the exact biochemical site at which zinc is required for testosterone synthesis has not been established. Another type of evidence has been provided by clinical observations of dialysis patients (3,4) and sickle-cell anemia patients (7). Both conditions have a demonstrated propensity to zinc deficiency, and impotence in these cases seems to be partially causable by zinc deficiency and correctable by administration of zinc, although there is some evidence that does not support this conclusion (5). There is also evidence of partial correction of oligospermia by zinc administration (6). Further, there is a recent report that zinc is involved in the binding of the androgen receptor to nuclear acceptance sites (24), thus raising the possibility that zinc is required for the expression of androgen effects. With this background, the recognition of frequent abnormalities of zinc status in impotence clinic patients becomes more expected.

The association of elevated zinc excretion and lower serum testosterone values has not, to our knowledge, been previously reported, but the observation of elevated zinc excretion with diuretics has been previously made in humans (25) and there is experimental literature from animal studies that would indicate that it was likely to be so (26,27). Thiazide-type diuretics, in particular, appear to alter the renal tubular handling of zinc, resulting in net distal tubular secretion of zinc, rather than the normal zinc-conserving reabsorption (27). Thus, although the kidney is not a normal route of significant zinc excretion, when thiazide diuretics are being used it may become so. Even in the absence of balance studies, it is not difficult to hypothesize that if this rate of excretion is large enough or if the dietary provision of zinc is inadequate, either through diet selection or malabsorption, then a negative zinc balance and tissue zinc inadequacy will result. This interpretation is supported by the low testosterone values seen in our impotent patients who had been treated with diuretics.

We are unable to say that these patients are zinc deficient in the same sense that patients experiencing a zinc-deficient diet might be, and we make this caveat in part because the assessment of actual tissue zinc status is difficult. Measurement of serum and urine zinc levels is an imperfect reflection of tissue levels (28). At present, no one test measuring tissue zinc levels exists that could be applied to a population study such as this one. There is some hope that current development work on such studies as neutrophil zinc levels (29,30) may offer the prospect of such a test. For the present it appears that the measurement of urinary zinc excretion may have adequate medical and physiologic correlates for this type of study.

We conclude that there is now evidence supporting the notion that zinc status abnormalities are seen with frequency in patients afflicted with sexual impotence and that there is reason to believe that a fair porportion of such abnormalities may be associated with the use of diuretics, particularly thiazide-type diuretics. The next step in investigating this potential link between zinc status in humans and sexual potency should be a prospective, placebo-controlled study of zinc administration to determine if such an intervention has any important clinical benefits to the population of men experiencing sexual impotence. Further, the use of thiazide diuretics, particularly in the management of such conditions as hypertension, should be evaluated with respect to the potential impact on zinc status, testosterone, and sexual potency. If a link can be better established, there is prospect for a change in medical policy that may benefit a large number of Americans who are facing the prospect of treatment for hypertension and other conditions.

ACKNOWLEDGMENTS

We greatly appreciate the technical assistance of Martha Grace, and thank JoAnn Tallman for preparing the manuscript. This study was supported by grants from the Veterans Administration.

REFERENCES

1. Prasad AS, Miale A, Farid Z, Sandstead HH, Schulert AR. *J Lab Clin Med* 1963;61: 537–549.
2. Sandstead HH, Prasad AS, Schulert AR, et al. *Am J Clin Nutr* 1967;20:422–442.
3. Antoniou LD, Sudhakar T, Shaloub RJ, Smith JC. *Lancet* 1977;2:895–898.
4. Mahajan SK, Abbasi AA, Prasad AS, Rabbani P, Briggs WA, McDonald FD. *Ann Intern Med* 1982;97:357–361.
5. Brook AC, Ward MK, Cook DB, Johnston DG, Watson MJ, Kerr DNS. *Lancet* 1980;2:618–620.
6. Hartoma R, Nahoul K, Netter A. *Lancet* 1977;2:1125–1126.
7. Prasad AS, Abbasi AA, Rabbani P, Dumouchelle E. *Am J Hematol* 1981;10:119–127.
8. Kinlaw WB, Levine AS, Morley JE, Silvis SE, McClain CJ. *Am J Med* 1983;75: 273–277.
9. Allen JI, Bell E, Boosalis MG, et al. *Am J Med* 1985;79:209–215.
10. Slag MF, Morley JE, Elson MK, et al. *JAMA* 1983;249:1736–1740.
11. Prasad AS, Rabbani P, Abbasi A, Bowersox E, Spivey Fox MR. *Ann Intern Med* 1978:89:483–490.
12. Walravens PA. *West J Med* 1979;130:133–142.
13. Davies IJT, Musa M, Dormandy TL. *J Clin Pathol* 1968;21:359–365.
14. Halsted JA, Smith JC. *Lancet* 1970;1:322–324.
15. Kosman DJ, Henkin RI. *Lancet* 1979;1:1410.
16. Voyatzoglou V, Mountokalakis T, Tsata-Voyatzoglou V, Koutselinis A, Skalkeas G. *Am J Surg* 1982;144:355–357.
17. Dawson JB, Walker BE. *Clin Chim Acta* 1969;26:465–475.
18. Johnson HL, Sauberlich HE. In: *Clinical, biochemical, and nutritional aspects of trace elements.* New York: Alan R Liss, 1982;405–426.
19. Shapcott D. In: *Clinical applications of recent advances in zinc metabolism.* New York: Alan R Liss, 1982;121–139.
20. Spencer H, Kramer L, Osis D. In: *Clinical, biochemical, and nutritional aspects of trace elements.* New York: Alan R Liss, 1982;103–115.
21. Root AW, Duckett G, Sweetland M, Reiter EO. *J Nutr* 1979;109:958–964.
22. Lei KY, Abbasi A, Prasad AS. *Am J Physiol* 1976;230:1730–1732.
23. Hartoma R. *Acta Physiol Scand* 1977;10:336–341.
24. Colvard DS, Wison EM. *Biochemistry* 1984;23:3471–3478.
25. Webster PO. *Acta Med Scand* 1973;194:505–512.
26. Pak CY, Ruskin B, Diller E. *Clin Chem Acta* 1979;39:511–517.
27. Victery W, Smith JM, Vander AJ. *Am J Physiol* 1981;241:F532–F539.
28. Prasad AS. *Ann Rev Nutr* 1985;5:341–363.
29. Whitehouse RC, Prasad AS, Rabbani PI, Cossack ZT. *Clin Chem* 1982;28:475–480.
30. Prasad AS, Cossack ZT. *Ann Intern Med* 1984;100:367–371.

Geriatric Nutrition, edited by John E. Morley,
Zvi Glick, Laurence Z. Rubenstein.
Raven Press, Ltd., New York © 1990.

34

Exercise and Muscle Strength

*R. A. Wiswell, †S. Victoria Jaque, and †M. Hamilton-Wessler

*Departments of *Medicine and †Exercise Sciences, University of Southern
California, Los Angeles, California 90089*

In a recent editorial in the *Lancet*, it was suggested that many older adults live perilously close to functional thresholds that, with just minor stress, render them dependent (1). If one accepts the premise that, for many older adults, a large percentage of the reduction in function is not attributable to pathology, it could be concluded that many significant losses are a result of normal aging processes. How much is "true aging" and how much is related to a sedentary lifestyle, at this point in time, cannot be readily discerned. Regardless of the reason, there can be no question that inactivity can accelerate the functional losses associated with aging and that exercise intervention can reduce the rate of loss effectively.

The reluctance of many older people to participate in regular exercise may relate, in part, to the tremendous recognition that jogging and aerobics have received over the past decade. Many people who are not interested in this type of exercise fail to recognize the benefit of other types of physical activity and, as a result, do not exercise at all. The President's Council on Physical Fitness and Sports has identified several important reasons to engage in regular exercise. In addition to an improvement in cardiovascular endurance, exercise can improve and/or maintain strength, flexibility, and body composition. Furthermore, a psychosocial benefit of regular exercise, particularly in older subjects, has been well documented.

Muscle loss and the exercise's potential for strength improvement are the focus of this chapter. We are now recognizing the possible benefit of strength conditioning on aging muscle and bone and, in time, hope to provide more scientific evidence for the possible benefit of strength and/or resistance training on the ability of the older person to maintain functional independence. The issue of the quality of life of older persons is a concern to health practitioners as they look toward the expanding aging population of the future. As more and more people are living longer, it will become more and more important for us as professionals and/or practitioners to stimulate older individuals to maintain optimal function throughout the life span.

A recent study reported that nearly two-thirds of women and one-quarter of men over the age of 70 were unable to lift a 4.5-kg weight (2). When one considers the findings by Aniansson (3) that simply standing up from a stool or low armed chair may require a maximum quadriceps contraction, one realizes that some steps must be taken to reduce the losses of sedentary living and reverse the trend of functional loss in these older individuals. In order to find a solution to the problem of functional decline, one must first identify the specific age-related losses and then evaluate the intervention strategies associated with their improvement.

COMPONENTS OF MUSCULAR STRENGTH

There is evidence of histochemical changes in the muscle fibers that may be responsible for the reduction of strength with increasing age (4). The distribution (size and number) of Type II fibers may decline at a greater rate during aging and disuse than the aerobic, Type I fibers (5,6). The end result of aging appears to be a reduction in both the size and functional number of these fiber types and therefore a diminution in neuromuscular strength potential (7,8). Certain components of muscle control and integration diminish with aging and could account for the decrease in muscle strength (Table 1)(9).

PHYSIOLOGIC CHANGES IN MUSCLE WITH AGING

Various physiologic changes in the muscle have been noted with aging that help explain why function becomes impaired, even though the mechanisms by which this occurs can only be hypothesized. Because of discrepancies among findings in the literature, the picture of muscular adaptations to aging

TABLE 1. *Components of tension production and the effect of aging and strength training*

Component	Effect of aging	Effect of training (hypothetical)
Central integration (nervous system's ability to activate muscle)		
Number of motor units recruited	Increased	Decreased
Frequency of motor unit firing	Decreased	Increased
Synchronization of motor unit firing	?	Improved
Local muscle control		
Muscle mass (cross-sectional area)	Decreased	No change ?
Fiber characteristics		
Percentage of FT/ST fibers	No change	Increased ?
FT/ST fiber area	Decrease	Increased ?

From Wiswell et al., ref. 38. FT, fast twitch; ST, slow twitch.

is unclear at best. However, an examination of the available research can elucidate some aspects of muscular aging and their role in functional loss.

Gross Muscle Size

Muscle size, as determined by thigh circumference, has been reported to remain stable with aging (6). However, this external measure does not account for changes in the amounts of actual muscle tissue, connective tissue, and fat found subcutaneously. More recent research reports suggest that, although the muscle may appear not to diminish in size externally, there is an internal decrease in muscle tissue (10).

Fiber-Specific Changes

Individual fibers of muscles are also reduced in size. Mean fiber length has been seen to diminish with age because of a decrease in the number of sarcomeres in series, not a loss in sarcomere length (11). Fiber number also appears to be affected by the aging process. A 20% decrease in fiber number in the aged human vastus lateralis when compared to a young control muscle has been reported, but caution must be used in interpreting cross-sectional data (10).

Although some reports have found no changes in mean fiber area, (10,11), the majority of research in this area suggests a decrease in fiber size with aging (5,12–14). Of this decrease in mean fiber area, the primary muscle fiber type affected appears to be the fast-twitch fiber type (5,12–14).

This finding suggests two important points. First, individual muscle fibers atrophy, or decrease in cell size, with aging (6,11,14). Second, the selective atrophy of Type II fibers is accompanied by a decrease in the fast twitch/slow twitch fiber area ratio (5,13). Although some have suggested that the number and/or proportion of Type II fibers decreases with age (6,10), the majority of research supports the assumption that the fiber type composition of old muscle remains stable with aging (5,12–14). Thus, the important change with respect to fiber type is the selective atrophy of Type II fibers, not a change in fiber type composition.

There do not appear to be specific changes in the contractile proteins in muscle with aging. Myosin light chains from 9- and 30-month-old rats appear to be similar (15,16). A new type of fiber in the soleus of old rats, intermediate between the fast oxidative glycolytic and the slow oxidative fibers found in the young rat, has been reported; however, some question has arisen as to the significance of this reported fiber type transition (17). Were it truly a case of fiber type transition, aspects of the fiber, such as its myosin light and heavy chains, would be involved, as well as cellular calcium transport mechanisms and metabolic processes. This does not appear to be the case.

Motor Nerves

Motor units, which are composed of a motor nerve and the fibers that it innervates, have been found to undergo functional change with aging. First, there is a decrease in the number of functioning motor units with aging (17,18). Second, there is often an enlargement of the surviving motor units, which is accompanied by a slowing of their twitch response. A decrease in maximum impulse velocity has also been demonstrated (18). Together, these factors suggest changes in the functional abilities of motor units with aging that, in turn, may affect muscle contraction characteristics.

These changes in the motor units with aging may help explain the morphologic alterations that were described earlier. In an experiment on aged rat gastrocnemius muscles, Kanda et al (19) reported a preferential degeneration of the faster motor neurons, causing a reorganization of the motor unit. There is also a greater decrease in conduction velocity in the faster type motor unit than in the slower type. These motor unit changes may account for the selective atrophy of fast-twitch fibers and the subsequent decreases in the fast twitch/slow twitch fiber area ratio.

Electromyographic (EMG) Changes

Human EMG values have been found to decrease in amplitude with aging (20). This reduction can probably be explained by the decreases in both fiber number and size that accompany aging. An increase in polyphasic activity has also been reported in the EMG values of the elderly, which suggests a delay in end-plate transmission of the electrical signal (20). These changes may help explain the decrease in maximal EMG voltage and the reduced efficiency of electrical activity reported by Moritani and deVries (21).

Changes in nerve terminal morphology may also help explain the alterations found in neuromuscular activity. Muscle activity has been demonstrated to reduce the detrimental changes at the nerve terminal associated with aging in mice (22). Whether nerve terminal degeneration occurs in humans in the same fashion as it does in the laboratory rodent has not as yet been reported.

Muscle Energetics

In comparisons between young and elderly human subjects using 31P nuclear magnetic resonance (NMR) scanning, no differences were observed in

TABLE 2. *Summary of research studies related to the effect of aging on muscle fiber characteristics*

Study	Age (years)	Muscle	Fiber characteristics Fiber number	Fiber size	FT/ST area ratio	Fiber composition
HUMAN:						
Aniansson et al. 1986	73–83	Biceps Vastus l.	-----	11% mean decrease 14% decrease in IIa area 25% decrease in IIb area	15% decrease	N.S.
Clarkson et al. 1979	20–30 55–73	Vastus l.	-----	-----	44% decrease	N.S.
Larsson et al. 1979	11–70	Vastus l.	No change	42% decrease in II fibers	25% decrease	4.5% decrease in II fibers
Lexell et al. 1983	30–72	Vastus l.	24% decrease	18% decrease in gross size N.S. in mean fiber size	Decrease	-----
ANIMAL:						
Caccia et al.[a] 1979	3–4 mo 18–19 mo 30 mo	EDL Soleus	-----	25% decrease in EDL to middle age; slight increase from middle to old age	-----	Increase in ST fibers, EDL
Eddinger et al. 1985	3 mo 8–10 mo 27–28 mo	EDL Soleus	----- -----	No change in CSA	-----	10.8% increase in Type I 70% decrease in IIa between 3 to 30 months.
Hooper 1981	26 wk 70 wk	Biceps b. Tibialis a.	18% decrease 16.3% decrease 37% (BB), 18% (TA) decrease in fiber length	15% decrease 19% decrease	12.8% increase 5% increase	-----

[a]Utilized female subjects.

the muscular concentrations of ATP, PC, Pi, and pH (23). Therefore, the ability of the muscle to respond to the immediate energy requirements of daily life remains similar in the aged.

The enzyme levels of both anaerobic and aerobic enzymes in older subjects are comparable to those of young subjects in terms of activities per gram of muscle weight (12–14). This supports the earlier findings of Farrar et al. (24) that the decrease in oxidative metabolism found in aged rats is due to a decrease in mitochondrial protein with age, rather than a decrease in enzyme activity per amount of muscle protein.

When taken into account, all of the preceding changes suggest that the alterations in muscle with aging are quantitative, not qualitative, in that, for surviving fibers, the same enzymatic activity and energy-creating capacity are found per unit protein (Table 2). Therefore, by increasing muscle mass through exercise or other intervention, the older muscle should be able to operate at a functional level that is much like younger muscle. Thus, if muscle can be trained in old age, there is the possibility of increasing muscle function.

INTERVENTION STUDIES

Endurance training is widely accepted and has definitively been shown to promote resistance to fatigue through concurrent adaptations in the oxidative capacities of muscle cells and improvement in cardiorespiratory function in all age groups and both genders (12,25). The slowing of the muscle fibers and restrictions on the speed of tension development necessary for quick response, as in maintaining balance, point to the need for and advantages of strength training, in addition to endurance or aerobic training for the aging individual (13,26).

Documentation of the accompanying loss in human muscle strength with aging has emerged primarily from cross-sectional studies consisting predominantly of male subjects. Cross-sectional studies of young and old men and women indicate that the mean strength of the older female group (age 70 to 86 years) across types of contraction (knee flexion and extension) is 33 to 37% less than the mean strength of the younger female group (age 20 to 35 years) (27). Expressed in another manner, knee muscle strength of the older women was 56 to 78% of that of the younger women. In comparison, the knee muscle strength of the older men was 45 to 65% of that of the younger men, a finding that may indicate a relatively smaller decline in lean body mass with age in women than in men.

Unfortunately, cross-sectional studies assessing age-related differences in muscle strength suffer from shortcomings that may be resolved in part by longitudinal studies. In a follow-up study 7 years after the initial investigation (27a), a 10 to 22% ($p<0.05$) loss in knee extensor muscle strength was reported (12). Changes in fiber composition were not significant; however, a decrease of 14% ($p<0.02$) in the Type IIa fiber area was noted. The 10 to

TABLE 3. *Methodology of strength training studies in older men and women*

Study	Gender	Age (yrs)	Muscle group	Mode	Training Duration	Training Intensity	Training Frequency
Moritani & deVries 1980 (N=5/group)	Male	67–72 18–26	Elbow flexors	PRE	8 wk	10 reps at 2/3max	2x/day 3x/wk
Hurley et al. 1988 (N=10/group)	Male control	40–55 40–64	Upper & lower extremities	Nautilus	16 wk	8–12 RM 15–20 RM	3–4x/wk
Aniansson and Gustafsson 1981 (N=12)	Male	69–74	Knee extensors	Body weight resistance	12 wk	70% VO2max 45 mins.	3x/wk
Aniansson et al. 1984 (N=15)	Female	74–86	Knee extensors	Body weight resistance & elastic bands	10 mo	65% VO2max average	2x/wk

TABLE 4. *Findings of strength training studies in older men and women*

Study	Change in strength	Change in muscle fibers	Other
Moritani and deVries 1980	Old—26% increase in trained arm maximal strength	NC trained arm cross-sectional area. 23% increase in trained arm activation level. No change in arm efficiency of electrical activity (EEA)	
	Young—29% increase in trained arm maximal strength	9% increase in trained arm cross-sectional area 12% increase in trained arm activation level 16% decrease in EEA	
Hurley et al. 1988	50% increase in upper body strength 33% increase in lower body strength		5% decrease in LDL 10% increase in HDL 43% increase in HDL_2 8% decrease in total/HDL No change in total cholesterol or triglycerides 8–11% decrease in submaximal heart rate
Aniansson and Gustafsson 1981	9–22% increase in isometric and isokinetic strength	Increase in relative number and area of type IIa fibers Decrease in Type I fiber area No change in mean fiber area	
Aniansson et al. 1984	7–13% increase in isometric and isokinetic strength	Increase in relative number and area of Type IIa fibers	

NC, no change.

454

22% reduction in quadriceps muscle strength was greater than the 6% reduction in body cell mass (BCM), suggesting that factors other than muscle mass may account for the age-related strength changes. Furthermore, strength changes in the lower extremities (quadriceps) were reported to be greater than those of the upper extremities (biceps) (12). Finally, their data demonstrated and confirmed that the metabolic capacity of muscle is maintained in older age. Therefore, the potential for increased endurance and strength persists throughout the process of aging.

In addressing the potential changes in muscle strength of older men and women brought about by strength training, the four intervention studies (3,13,21,28) summarized in Tables 3 and 4 reflect the body of investigation in this area. In these studies, methods of assessing and quantitating muscle strength were specific to the particular mode of training utilized—one repetition maximum for the Nautilus training, isokinetic dynamometer (Cybex II) modified with strain gauge for torque measurements for body weight resistance and elastic band training, and hydraulic dynamometer and EMG instrumentation for elbow flexor training. Differences in measured changes in strength among the studies may be attributed to the muscle group analyzed (upper versus lower extremity), subject gender, genetic predisposition for the fiber type and distribution, compliance to training regimen, daily activity level, nutritional status, motivation, and emotional factors.

The ability to maintain balance through fast muscle tension development (isometric and isokinetic strength indicated by muscle activation level and Type II muscle fiber relative number and area) is a primary practical concern for the elderly. All lower extremity disabilities of strength, reflexes, gait, and balance have been shown to be significantly associated with falling (26). Therefore, strength training could be considered an appropriate method of intervention for the improvement of muscle function and reduction of risk for falls and fractures, particularly of the proximal end of the femur or femoral neck (29–31).

SUMMARY

One of the more striking characteristics of the aging process is impaired motor performance, which is demonstrated in a slowing of movements, loss of fine coordination and decrease in maximum strength. In essence, these changes have a restrictive influence on the quality of physical movement (25,27,32) as evidenced by deficiencies in motor units or neutral factors and in muscle cell morphology or fiber type distributions (12,33–35). There is a presenting trend toward a shift from a heterogeneous to a more uniform muscle fiber pattern, i.e., predominance of slow-twitch Type I muscle fibers and the age-related decline in the relative number of Type II fibers. This trend is the basis for many studies that examine methods and mechanisms by which the impending muscle fiber transformation and resultant decrease in maximum strength may be attenuated by exercise training. We have tried to present the limited information available so that the practitioner would be able to understand the methods used and the potential benefits accrued from strength training in the elderly. It is unfortunate that the literature is so devoid of good quantitative studies on older women, and we hope to encourage research in this area in the future.

REFERENCES

1. Editorial. *Lancet* 1986;2:1413.
2. Frontera WR, Meredith CN, O'Reilly KP, Knuttger HG, Evans W. *J Appl Physiol* 1988;64:1038–1044.
3. Aniansson A, Gustafsson E. *Clin Physiol* 1981;1:87–98.
4. Larsson L, Karlsson J. *Acta Physiol Scand* 1978;104:128–136.
5. Clarkson PM, Kroll W, Melchionda A. *J Gerontol* 1981;36:648–653.
6. Larsson L, Grimby G, Karlsson J. *J Appl Physiol: Respirat Environ Exerc Physiol* 1979; 46:451–456.
7. Gutmann E, Hanzlikova V. *Mech Aging Dev* 1972;1:327i–349i.
8. Sato T, Akatsuka H, Kito K, Tokoro Y, Tauchi H, Kato K. *Mech Aging Dev* 1986;34:297–304.
9. Wiswell RA, Andonian M, Merrill J. In: Bidlack WR, Clemens RA, eds. *The elderly: Nutrition, health, aging and longevity* (in press).
10. Lexell J, Henriksson-Larsen K, Winblad B, Sjostrom M. *Muscle Nerve* 1983;6:588–595.
11. Hooper A. *Gerontology* 1981;27:121–126.
12. Aniansson A, Hedberg M, Henning G-B, Grimby G. *Muscle Nerve* 1986;9:585–591.
13. Aniansson A, Ljungberg P, Rundgren A, Wetterqvist H. *Arch Gerontol Geriatr* 1984;3:229–241.
14. Grimby G, Danneskiold-Samsoe B, Hvid K, Saltin B. *Acta Physiol Scand* 1982;115: 125–134.
15. Eddinger T, Cassens R, Moss R. *Am J Physiol* 1986; 251 (Cell Physiol 20):C421–C430.
16. Eddinger T, Moss R, Cassens R. *J Histochem Cytochem* 1985;33:1033–1041.
17. Caccia M, Harris J, Johnson M. *Muscle Nerve* 1979;2:202–212.
18. Campbell M, McComas A, Petito F. *J Neurol Neurosurg Psychiatry* 1973;36:174–182.
19. Kanda K, Hashizume K, Nomoto E, Asaki S. *Neurosci Res* 1986;3:242–246.
20. Carlson K, Alston W, Feldman D. *Am J Phys Med* 1964;43:141–145.
21. Moritani T, deVries H. *J Gerontol* 1980;35:672–682.
22. Andonian MH, Fahim MA. *J Neurocytol* 1987;16:589–599.
23. Taylor D, Crowe M, Bore P, Styles P, Arnold D, Radda G. *Gerontology* 1984;30:2–7.
24. Farrar R, Martin T, Ardies C. *J Gerontol* 1981;36:642–647.
25. Suominen H, Heikkinen E, Parkatti T. *J Gerontol* 1977;32:33–37.
26. Tinetti ME, Speechley M, Ginter S. *N Engl J Med* 1988;26:1701–1707.
27. Murray MP, Duthie E, Gambert S, Sepic S, Mollinger L. *J Gerontol* 1985;40:275–280.
27a. Aniansson A, Grimby G, Hedberg M, Krotkiewski M. *Clin Physiol* 1981;1:73–86.
28. Hurley BF, Hagberg J, Goldverg A, et al. *Med Sci Sports Exerc* 1988;20:150–154.
29. Bevier WC, Wiswell RA, Pyka G, Kozak KC, Newhall KM, Marcus RA. *J Bone Min Res* 1989;4:421–432.
30. Chow R, Harrison J, Brown C, Hajek V. *Arch Phys Med Rehabil* 1986;67:231–234.
31. Pocock NA, Eisman J, Yeates J, Sambrook P, Eberi S. *J Clin Invest* 1986;78:618–621.
32. Maughan RJ, Watson J, Weir J. *J Physiol* 1983;338:37–49.
33. Grimby G. *Ann Clin Res* 1988;20:62–66.
34. Gutmann E, Hanzlikova V. *Gerontology* 1976;22:280–300.
35. Pearson MB, Bassey E, Bendall J. *Age Aging* 1985;14:49–54.

Geriatric Nutrition, edited by John E. Morley,
Zvi Glick, Laurence Z. Rubenstein.
Raven Press, Ltd., New York © 1990.

35

Interdisciplinary Teams for the Solution of Nutritional Problems

*Kenneth D. Cole and †Freddie A. Jones

*Interdisciplinary Team Training in Geriatrics (ITTG), *Geriatric Research,
Education, and Clinical Center and †Dietetics Service, VA Medical Center,
Sepulveda, California 91343 and *Department of Psychology, University of
Southern California, Los Angeles, California 90089*

Teams usually evolve from the need to integrate a broad array of information into a plan of action or a course of treatment. Even in the cockpits of modern aircraft, the once-cherished qualities of self-reliance and machismo have given way to notions of interdependence and teamwork. Because they need to incorporate a vast amount of information in making timely decisions, flight crews now undergo "cockpit resource management" training in order to work together more efficiently (1). In a similar fashion, health care once was typically administered by a sole provider, usually a physician. Now the "pilot-like" qualities of self-reliance and instant decision making necessary for the independent practice of medicine have given way to such skills as collaborating with other professionals and coordinating care. Especially in such specialties as geriatrics, the caseload is dominated by patients suffering from a multiplicity of interacting problems that require input from several disciplines. At the same time, however, elderly patients are more likely than their younger counterparts to rank continuity of care and personal attention as high priorities in receiving care (2).

In this chapter, we explore the history and function of teamwork in geriatric health care, the role of the dietitian on the team, and the structure and benefits of special nutritional support teams.

HISTORY OF TEAMWORK IN HEALTH CARE DELIVERY

The first team was the physician and patient. Early in this narrow notion of teamwork, the patient was a passive recipient of ministrations by the doctor. With more chronic diseases and conditions, which are potentially preventable by changes in lifestyle, more teamwork is needed between doctors and their patients. Lately, the team concept has been broadened to include health assistants who extend the role of the physician (3).

Surgery teams of physicians and nurses have traditionally been highly integrated and collaborative, as all professionals perform on the same patient at the same time. However, the first true interdisciplinary teams were the collaborative efforts among professionals at mission hospitals, clinics, and schools in the 1920s and 1930s, and the initial endeavors of the Montefiore Hospital in the 1940s (4,5). The Montefiore Hospital Outreach Program in New York delivered home care services through an interdisciplinary team made up of a social worker, nurse, and physician. In the 1960s the Martin Luther King Heath Care Center in the South Bronx furthered the development of the primary health care team (6). The University of Washington expanded the team concept by adding a dietitian, psychologist, medical technologist, dentist, and dental hygienist. In the 1970s interdisciplinary team development was encouraged by the provision of federal funding to support the training of both staff and trainees in team settings (5). Now treatment teams are ubiquitous in the health care industry as they function at various levels of development in many types of settings.

DEFINITION OF TEAMS

Although the terms are often used interchangeably, multidisciplinary and interdisciplinary connote different degrees of team functioning. A *multidisciplinary team* is a mix of professionals working with the same patients and usually in the same setting. *Interdisciplinary teams,* really a subset of multidisciplinary teams, take teamwork further by creating coordinated treatment plans for their patients and by negotiating common goals for themselves. These tasks are usually conducted during a team meeting when patients are discussed. Often, an added feature of an interdisciplinary team is the commitment to address the conflict that inevitably arises during teamwork.

COMPOSITION AND ORGANIZATION OF
INTERDISCIPLINARY TEAMS

The optimal time to create an interdisciplinary team is at the inception of a program or treatment unit. That is the time when careful thought can be given to the crucial issue of whom to include on the team. The key factor in establishing a team is the specific needs of the type of patients being treated (7).

There is probably no one ideal mix of professionals to include on a team. For example, a reviewer surveyed more than 200 health care teams and found almost as many discipline compositions as there were teams (8). One guideline for developing teams is the smaller, the better. With the addition of each new team member, the permutations of potential interactions—and

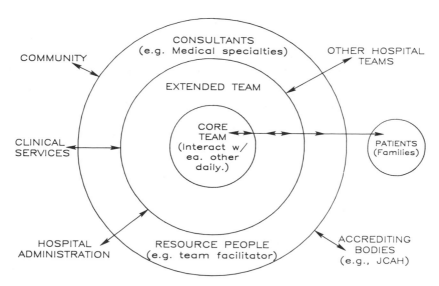

FIG. 1. A model of an interdisciplinary team in a medical center.

conflicts—among team members increase dramatically. One method to cope with the enormity of team interactions is to conceive of interdisciplinary team building as levels of inclusion, rather than any all-or-none principle. A useful division is among core members, extended members, and consultants and resource persons (Fig. 1).

Core Team Members

Core team members are the ones who work together in the same settings on the same unit every day, and they usually do not have patient responsibilities on other units. These professionals work together day in and day out, not just for the 1-hour team meeting per week. On a typical geriatric unit, these disciplines tend to be nursing, medicine, perhaps a physician assistant or nurse practitioner, social worker, and perhaps a representative of another very active discipline. Whatever the ultimate mix, this core team of professionals is responsible for developing team procedures and for deciding how to include other disciplines in the assessment and treatment of the patients.

Extended Team Members

In many geriatric settings, core team participation may be limited by personnel constraints that require staff to be assigned to multiple clinical sites. More simply, in other instances there may not be sufficient work for some disciplines to require their full-time participation in the team. Extended team members may come from such disciplines as speech pathology, audiology, psychology, optometry, pharmacy, dentistry, and dietetics. Naturally, if any of these professionals are needed and are available for core team activities, such as dietetics on a geriatric surgical unit, then they could be included. Extended team members typically interact with professionals from several teams, and they come to each unit's team meeting prepared to collaborate only on specific patients. However, usually they do not interact with the core team members in the day-to-day exigencies of patient care.

Consultants and Resource Persons

The third level of team participation is that of consultants and other resource persons. Consultants are involved only with those cases that the core team decides are necessary and appropriate. They may be invited to team meetings to discuss their findings and recommendations, or they may merely send reports. Except for issues regarding patients with whom they are working, they do not engage in team decision making (5). Resource persons are either hospital or clinic personnel specializing in team development or group communications, or they may be designated outside consultants serving to help the team with such tasks as goal clarification, role negotiation, and conflict management.

Patients

A discussion about inclusion-exclusion is not complete without consideration of patient attendance at team meetings. Their participation in team meetings may sound appealing, but as one writer pointed out, this "misplaced hospitality" is easily abused (9). Although the staff exists for the patient, their musings and conflicts do not. It is very time consuming to translate technical information into understandable terms, and in some chronic care settings the concern about discharge can frighten the patient excessively. Of course, the patient's values, resources, and goals are considered in the planning by the treatment team, but except for some specially arranged team meetings, when there is a good amount of time, patients and team meetings should be kept separate (5,9). The typical setting for such discussions is during patient rounds, with the interdisciplinary team needing to be ever mindful of all patients' concerns about privacy and confidentiality.

INTERDISCIPLINARY TEAM LEADERSHIP AND FUNCTIONING

Traditionally, the physician or the program director is the leader of the team (10). However, a persistent difficulty in team development is that often the person with the most power does not necessarily possess the greatest skill in team management (11). A number of different types of leadership may emerge as a team builds. There may be a program leader, but another person may lead the team meetings. Covert "socioemotional" leaders of the unit may emerge, despite the power being ostensibly with the team leader. In most highly functioning teams, leadership is not tightly bound to one person or discipline, but rather it resides with the team member who happens to have the most expertise for the given problem at hand.

The basis for effective team management is the delineation of team goals and negotiation of roles for each team member. Both commitment and performance are enhanced when team members periodically review their own goals (11) and partake in flexible, open communication, with shared responsibility for decisions and shared accountability for performing team tasks (10). Many interdisciplinary teams make the mistake of never creating clear-cut goals for their unit and for themselves as a team. As can happen in a marriage, conflict over basic goals can be a festering source of tension on a team for many years. With the refinement of goals, the team builds its identity and sense of purpose (12). Similarly, negotiation and clarification of roles are an integral part of team development (13).

When members on a team find themselves entrenched in goal or role conflicts, it often "feels" to them like a personality conflict. This perception makes each side's position more rigid. However, findings from social psychology indicate that, while persons initiating actions attribute the causes of their behavior to situational demands, the perceivers of such behaviors attribute their cause to stable personal dispositions (14). Known as the "fundamental error of attribution," this repeated tendency can lock team members into a stand-off for months or even years, instead of leading to fruitful exploration of the differing perceptions of team goals and personal roles from which the members are operating.

Early in the formation of the interdisciplinary team, a mechanism for making decisions and carrying out tasks should be developed. Members can become disenchanted with the team approach if initially they thought they would be consulted on all decisions, which is rarely true for practical reasons (15). In fact, many routine tasks can be handled easily by two or three members, leaving the more complicated, potentially creative decision making to the entire team (16). In general, when a task involves a simple problem of coordination, a centralized human resource network is more efficient; however, decentralized networks, such as highly functioning interdisciplinary teams, are superior in solving such complex tasks as patient management or discharge planning (17).

Group norms of interdisciplinary teams often emerge quickly without any discussion. Norms may include who is free to interrupt whom, the level of self-disclosure that is within the boundaries for the team, attendance and promptness issues, seating arrangements, and the pace of the meeting, just to name a few. Trainees and new staff generally adjust to the norms, rather than challenge them, unless they join the team at a critical developmental point.

Even with the careful use of team development principles, no group becomes an effective interdisciplinary team without going through some kind of developmental process involving four stages: forming, norming, storming, and performing (18). Teams form and readily develop tacit norms about what is appropriate behavior for the group. Eventually, certain missions, roles, and norms are challenged before the team can move on to a higher level of functioning. Teamwork is hard work; it is not just the eventual result of assembling a collection of health care professionals. Part of the initial developmental period can be used for identifying the many conflicts that will emerge. During this period strengths and weaknesses are identified and changes are attempted in order to rechannel energy going into conflict toward patient care goals. Conflict is inevitable on interdisciplinary teams, and it is not necessarily destructive. However, avoiding it or personalizing it can be devastating for a team (19,20).

CONSULTING WITH INTERDISCIPLINARY TEAMS

A team consultant or facilitator can be very useful to an interdisciplinary team, especially at the beginning stages of development or during difficult transition points (4,21,22). Consultants might look for indicators of highly functioning and poorly functioning teams. On a well-functioning team there is the freedom to voice divergent viewpoints and to question basic assumptions (23). Leadership and maintenance functions tend to be shared by all members of the team. Conversely, on a poorly functioning team, members come late or do not talk, leadership may be "locked in," and minority viewpoints can be pushed to the exclusion of other members' input. Teams may realize that decisions need to be made, yet either definitive decisions are never reached or the responsibility for follow through is not delineated.

Like a family therapist, a consultant relates to the team, but does not become enmeshed in the team's implicit system (24). First, the consultant helps the team assess itself in terms of goal development and adherence, clarity of roles, level of honest communication both within the team and with those outside the team, and the sense of identity and purpose that the team has created for itself (12). Then, by attending to the group process and behavior of team members, the consultant guides the team toward the successful negotiation of unresolved team issues.

Interactions among team members also reflect system issues and patient care problems. Sometimes, negative interactions stemming from these difficulties can pull the team apart without the team's awareness of these external forces (7). By exploring negative feelings, team members often find out the underlying reasons for another member's behavior. Team members can be encouraged to foster a problem-solving attitude about their group in which difficulties and conflicts are perceived as the norm, rather than terri-

TABLE 1. *Dietetic service nutrition profile and care plan*

S:
   FOOD
   ALLERGIES:

   FOOD
   PREFERENCES:

   PREVIOUS DIET COUNSELING:

O: DX:

   HT: _____   WT: _____   DATE _____   FRAME SIZE: _____

   IBW: _____   %IBW: _____   USUAL WT: _____   %USUAL WT: _____

   PERTINENT
   LAB VALUES:

   DIET RX:

A. DIET
   TOLERANCE: GOOD   FAIR   POOR   APPETITE: GOOD   FAIR   POOR

   SWALLOWING: GOOD   FAIR   POOR   CHEWING: GOOD   FAIR   POOR

   WT. STATUS: WITHIN IBW   _____ < IBW   _____ > IBW

   ENERGY   WT   WT   WT
   REQUIREMENTS: _____ KCAL/DAY FOR: MAINTENANCE   GAIN   LOSS

   PROTEIN REQUIREMENTS: _____ g/DAY

   DIET   NOT   LEARNING
   COUNSELING: INDICATED   INDICATED   DIFFICULTIES   REFUSE

P: RX: 1. _____ CONTINUE PRESCRIBED DIET

        2. _____ RECOMMEND DIET CHANGE TO:

        3. _____ RECOMMEND WT MONITORING

        4. _____ WILL INCORPORATE FOOD PREFERENCES WHERE POSSIBLE

        5. _____ FOLLOW UP

PT. ED: 1. _____ INFORMED OF DIET

        2. _____ NO FURTHER PLANS

        3. _____ DIET COUNSELING

SIGNATURE: DATE:

TABLE 2. *Example of an interdisciplinary care team*

MEDICAL RECORD	OVERALL TREATMENT PLAN

IMPORTANT: CHECK APPROPRIATE BOX: ☐ INITIAL
☐ CHANGE TO TREATMENT PLAN

INSTRUCTIONS: Following an assessment of the patient's problems, the initial treatment plan will be documented on this form. This plan will specify the overall diagnostic and therapeutic activities that will be undertaken in regard to each of the patient's problems and the specific staff members responsible for carrying out these activities. Specific mention will be made of plans for specialized rehabilitation services, patient education, discharge, and followup. Revisions of the treatment plan will be made on this form, if appropriate, or on additional copies of this form.

INTERDISCIPLINARY TEAM MEMBERS:	SIGNATURES		SIGNATURES
AUDIOLOGY & SPEECH THERAPY (ST)		PHYSICIAN (MD)	
COMMUNITY HEALTH NURSE (CHNC)		PHYSICIAN (MD)	
CORRECTIVE THERAPY (CT)		PSYCHIATRIC LIAISON (PSYC)	
DENTAL (DMD/DDS/RDH)		RECREATION THERAPY (RT)	
DIETETICS (RD)		REGISTERED NURSE (RN)	
LICENCED VOCATIONAL NURSE (LVN)		REGISTERED NURSE (RN)	
NURSE PRACTITIONER (NP)		SOCIAL WORKER (SW)	
NURSE SPECIALIST (CNS)			
OCCUPATIONAL THERAPY (OTR)			
PHARMACY (RPH)			
PHYSICAL THERAPY (PT)			

ble truths that should not be unleashed. Active and forthright discussion of team problems can prevent emotions from smoldering and being played out in unproductive ways toward other members or patients (3).

THE ROLE OF DIETITIANS ON AN INTERDISCIPLINARY TEAM

In the health care setting the dietitian's major goal is to ensure a high quality of life for every patient. The dietitian is responsible for helping prevent malnutrition, nutritional deficiencies, and diet-related diseases by identifying these problems and recommending appropriate and timely interven-

TABLE 2. *Continued*

DISCHARGE PLAN	The plan of care has been reviewed with Patient/Family. Signature _____ Date _____		
INTERDISCIPLINARY TREATMENT PLAN	PERSON RESPONSIBLE	EVALUATION DATE	PROGRESS NOTE—DATED
PROBLEM: Unplanned weight loss of 20% ideal body weight in the past three months. GOAL: To increase weight status by ½ to 1 pound per week until patient reaches his ideal body weight. PLAN:		Monthly	
1. Psychiatric consult to rule out psychological causes for weight loss.	Psyc.		
2. MD exam to rule out physical causes for weight loss.	MD		
3. Oral exam to determine any chewing problems.	DMD		
4. Provide food preferences.	RD		
5. Provide supplemental feedings if indicated and monitor acceptance.	RD/RN/MD		
6. Calorie count × 3 days to determine current intake.	RD		
7. Weekly weights and evaluation.	RD/RN		
8. Increase socialization at meal time (group dining).	SW/RN/OT		
9. Monthly lab tests.	MD		
Signature/Title-Practitioner	Signature/Initial of Approving Physician		Date

tions. The dietitian promotes optimal health through sound nutrition and provides nutrition education to patients to increase their level of independence in making appropriate food choices. The dietitian may even act as a patient advocate when necessary, to ensure adequate nutritional care and patient satisfaction. Maximizing food choices and catering to individual food preferences can greatly increase the quality of a patient's life.

As an interdisciplinary team member, the clinical dietitian is responsible for identifying patient problems that may require nutritional intervention. Nutrition-related problems are often discovered by conducting detailed nutritional assessments, which involve reviewing information about the patient, such as laboratory and anthropometric data; noting use of medications that may affect food intake; interviewing the patient for his diet history; and visually inspecting the patient's physical appearance. The development of a patient care plan (Table 1) becomes the framework for nutritional intervention.

In the interdisciplinary team meeting, the dietitian takes the leadership role in identifying the nutrition-related problems and ensuring that appropriate disciplines are involved in their resolution. For example, the dietitian may identify unplanned weight loss that is more than 20% of ideal body weight as a patient's major problem. The interdisciplinary team members would identify the goals for the patient's treatment plan, the person(s) responsible for implementing the plan, and the evaluation time frame to monitor progress (Table 2). The achievement of the stated goal depends on the cooperation of each team member.

The dietitian also plays a role in facilitating other disciplines' treatment goals as the effectiveness of their plans is threatened when nutritional status is compromised. Healing can be delayed; the potential for pneumonia, congestive heart failure, decubitis ulcers, and oral cavity and gum disease can be increased; the response to physical and occupational therapy can be diminished; and even self-esteem can be threatened by nutritional deficits. Everyone on the interdisciplinary team may feel comfortable making statements about food and diet, but the dietitian is the professional with the expertise to place diet history and nutritional status into a meaningful context.

NUTRITION SUPPORT TEAMS

Over the last decade we have witnessed the emergence of nutrition support teams (25). In 1978 a British report outlined the key elements of a fully functioning nutrition support team that is comprised of a core team of a physician and nurse specialist. In this early formulation of a nutrition support team, the authors remarked that the active support of a patient's care plan by a carefully organized team is essential (26). A more recent review of nutrition support teams identifies the members as follows: the physician as the team leader, the nurse who is in charge of the subclavian catheter, a pharmacologist and perhaps a second staff pharmacist who mixes the solutions, and the specialty dietitian who conducts a complete nutritional assessment, calculates the nutritional needs, and recommends the enteral feedings (27). The main goal of the nutrition support team is ensuring quality in the provision of both parenteral and enteral nutrition. Depending on the needs of specific patients, this core team also may utilize the services of physical therapy, psychology, or a lab technician.

Similar to other interdisciplinary teams, a nutrition support team has responsibilities to its patients, itself as a team, and to the community in which it is functioning. A nutrition support team has three basic functions. The first is performing direct service, such as conducting nutritional assessments of patients who are malnourished or at high risk; prescribing, preparing, and adjusting parenteral and enteral nutritional solutions; and preventing or identifying early complications associated with nutritional support. Nutrition support teams also have a record-keeping function as well—monitoring and evaluating patients' nutritional support systems with protocols (27) and collecting data on complications and patient outcomes. Third, most nutrition support teams have an education and research role as well. Teams educate other health professionals about nutrition support and conduct research, both to improve the technical quality of nutritional support and to increase its cost effectiveness.

Most nutrition support functions are not perceived as independent components, but rather as a comprehensive pattern or structure. Even though each clinician is involved in a different process, all need to have the same overarching goals, a common core of knowledge, and a set of highly developed team skills. These can be taught most effectively through an integrated team training approach, rather than segmented instruction (28). Smooth functioning within the team, although often achieved in excellent teams, is not adequate in itself and may be mistaken wrongly for evidence that the team is delivering viable services (29,30).

Although studies are difficult to design, some preliminary data indicate that nutrition support teams can lead to improved patient outcomes. An early study found a complication rate of 33% for nonteam patients compared to 3.7% for nutrition support team patients. The authors recommended the development of a protocol for administration of total parenteral nutrition (TPN) to reduce complications (31). Another group investigated total parenteral nutrition by breaking down complications into three categories: mechanical, metabolic, and septic. This group sequentially followed 28 patients with only consultative TPN team services and then 29 patients with a more involved team that spent more time with patient monitoring and verifying adherence to TPN infection control guidelines. Although mechanical and metabolic complications were clearly reduced in the patients treated by the more involved team, their incidence was still excessive, provoking the authors to suggest additional responsibilities and activities for the TPN team both to reduce complications and to improve therapy (32).

Exploring the utility of nutrition support teams in enteral nutrition, researchers have documented the efficacy of teams in reducing the number of abnormalities and optimizing nutrition delivery compared to nonteams (33,34). The teams were made up of general surgery residents, nurses, pharmacists, and a clinical dietitian. The investigators remarked on the need for close patient monitoring, proper intervention for complications, expertise, and compulsive attention to detail, all activities that require a great deal of time. It is noteworthy that, although team patients were monitored by one of the authors of the study, the physicians of the nonteam patients did not know that the studies were being conducted. Moreover, there was no random assignment of patients to conditions, but rather it appears that any patients that were referred to the nutrition team were compared to all others during a specified span of time.

Given the nature of these experimental designs, it is no wonder that teams were shown to be more effective than traditional approaches. There have been few true empirical investigations of team-delivered health care (35,36).

Although there are many inherent difficulties in comparing team-delivered care to more traditional approaches, this is a research area where investigative strides could and should occur. Multiple-site trials of teams of the same size and discipline composition could be undertaken. In more elegant studies, patients could be randomly assigned or matched on specified characteristics. The extent of team development and expertise would be difficult to hold constant across sites, but at least measures of team satisfaction and functioning could be covaried with other outcome data.

Yet, teams serve functions in addition to treatment. Especially in teaching hospitals, interdisciplinary teams have provided an important component of training for professionals who plan to practice in geriatric specialties. Teams also can play a strong role in attracting young trainees to the field. A complete evaluation of what interdisciplinary teams accomplish in health care settings will include not only carefully conceptualized and conducted patient outcome studies but also thoughtful investigation into the impact of interdisciplinary collaboration on recruitment and training.

REFERENCES

1. Foushee HC. *Am Psychol* 1984;39:885–893.
2. Fletcher RH, O'Malley MS, Earp J, et al. *Med Care* 1983;21:234–242.
3. Gosselin JY. *Can Ment Health* 1983;31:23.
4. Baldwin DC, Tsukuda RAW. In: Cassell CK, Walsh JR, eds. *Geriatric medicine, vol II, Fundamentals of geriatric care.* New York: Springer-Verlag, 1984.
5. Campbell LJ, Cole KD. *Clin Geriatr Med* 1987;3:99–110.
6. Wise H. *Making health teams work.* Cambridge, MA: Ballinger, 1974.
7. Nason F. *Soc Work Health Care* 1983;9:25–45.
8. Kane RA. *Interprofessional teamwork.* Manpower monograph, no. 8, Syracuse University School of Social Work, Syracuse, NY, 1975.
9. Kane RA. *Health Soc Work* 1982;7:2–4.
10. Lowe JI, Kerranen M. *Soc Work Health Care* 1978;3:323–330.
11. Goren S, Ottaway R. *J Nurs Admin* 1985;15:9–16.
12. Logan RL, McKendry M. *NZ Med J* 1982;95:883–884.
13. Halstead LS, Rintala DH, Kanellos M, et al. *Arch Phys Med Rehabil* 1986;67:357–361.
14. Jones EE, Nisbett RE. *The actor and the observer: Divergent perceptions of the causes of behavior.* Morristown, NJ: General Learning Press, 1971.
15. Charatan FB, Foley CJ, Libow LS. In: Andres R, Bierman EL, Hazzard WR, eds. *Principles of geriatric medicine.* New York: McGraw-Hill, 1985;
16. Cole KD, Campbell LJ. *Phys Occup Ther Geriatr* 1986;4:69–74.
17. Shaw ME. In: Berkowitz L, ed. *Advances in experimental social psychology,* vol I. New York: Academic Press, 1964.
18. Tuckman B. *Psychol Bull* 1965;63:384–399.
19. Vogt MT, Ducanis AJ. *J Allied Health* 1977;Winter:23–30.
20. Margolis H, Fiorelli JS. *J Rehabil* 1984;50:13–17.
21. Pearson PH. *Devel Med Child Neurol* 1983;25:390–395.
22. von Schilling K. *Int Nurs Rev* 1982;29:93–96.
23. Saint-Yves IFM. *Roy Soc Health J* 1982;102:232–233.
24. De Shazer S, Molnar A. *Fam Proc* 1984;23:481–486.

25. Blackburn GL, Bristrian BR, Maini BS. *JPEN* 1977;1:11–22.
26. Powell-Tuck J, Farwell JA, Nielsen T. *Lancet* 1978;2:825–828.
27. Lyman B, Pendleton S, Pemberton LB. QRB, 1987;232–240.
28. Agriesti-Johnson C, Dwyer K, Steinbaugh M. *JPEN* 1988;12:130–134.
29. Barnard D. *Soc Sci Med* 1987;25:741–746.
30. Purtillo RB. *Arch Phys Med Rehabil* 1988:69.
31. Nehme A. *JAMA* 1980;243:1906–1908.
32. Dalton MJ, Schepers G, Gee JP, Alberts CC, Eckhauser FE, Kirking DM. *JPEN* 1984;8:146–152.
33. Brown RO, Carlson SD, Gowan GSM Jr, Powers DA, Luther RW. *JPEN* 1987;11:52–56.
34. Powers DA, Brown RO, George SM Jr, et al. *JPEN* 1986;10:635–638.
35. Bloom BS, Soper KA. *J Am Geriatr Soc* 1980;28:451–455.
36. Halstead LS. *Arch Phys Med Rehabil* 1976;57:507–511.

Geriatric Nutrition, edited by John E. Morley,
Zvi Glick, Laurence Z. Rubenstein.
Raven Press, Ltd., New York © 1990.

36

Choices About Food and Water: The Emerging Ethical and Legal Standard of Care

Steven H. Miles and Gregory P. Gramelspacher

*Center for Clinical Medical Ethics, Pritzker School of Medicine, University of
Chicago, Chicago, Illinois 60637*

Geriatricians often confront the difficult and troubling decision of whether
to continue providing food and water to seriously and chronically ill patients. How should a clinician counsel a family whose demented loved one,
in the final stages of a progressive disease, no longer takes enough food to
sustain his life? Should a feeding tube be placed in a 65-year-old woman who
is comatose after a cardiac arrest? Once in place, may it be removed? Who
should decide? The moral challenge of these decisions is as stark as food is
elemental.

This chapter examines the ethical and legal issues raised by the possibility
of forgoing nourishment. First, we describe the emerging legal and ethical
consensus that the medically supervised provision of food and water is a
life-sustaining medical treatment. Then, we examine the implications of this
conclusion for clinical decision making, both for the competent patient and
the incompetent patient. Finally, we use specific clinical examples to clarify
two complicated aspects of the food and water debate: treatment of comatose patients and palliative care of demented patients.

AN EMERGING VIEW: NUTRITION AS A MEDICAL TREATMENT

A current understanding of clinicians' responsibilities for decisions about
food and water begins with the increasingly accepted, although still controversial, proposal that the medically supervised provision of food and water
is a medical treatment. As a treatment, the medical provision of food and
water is the result of a clinical decision-making process that, as with other
treatment choices, is to be made according to sound medical judgment and

the patient's interests and preference. This section explores the origin of and debate over this premise.

The premise that the medical provision of food and water is a life-sustaining medical treatment is of recent origin. Clinical decisions to withhold feeding came to public attention 5 years after the New Jersey Supreme Court authorized removing a respirator from Karen Ann Quinlan in 1976. The initial food and fluid cases involved congenitally conjoined infants in Illinois, an infant with Down's syndrome and a tracheoesophageal fistula in Indiana, and a California man (Clarence Herbert) who was comatose after suffering a perioperative respiratory arrest (1–4). Much of the public debate has focused on whether forgoing feeding is actually killing or is allowing a profoundly ill person to die of his underlying disease. In 1983, a seminal report from the President's Commission for the Study of Ethical Problems in Medicine and Biomedical and Behavioral Research (5) stated explicitly that "special feeding procedures" were a "life-sustaining treatment" that might be foregone in some circumstances. However, the Commission only briefly touched on the clinical implications of this view for the care of comatose and dying patients. The Commission's view was used in California's Herbert decision, which concluded that an evaluation of the benefits and burdens of feeding from the patient's perspective was the proper foundation for a clinical decision to stop feeding (6).

In the mid-1980s, feeding as a medical treatment was extensively debated in the medical, ethics, and legal literature. Lynn and Childress (2), in a cogent and influential early review, argued that, as with other medical treatments, food and water might be properly forgone when (a) feeding is futile in the sense of being technically impossible or because death is imminent in any case; (b) it is of no benefit to the patient (as with permanently comatose and thus insensate patients); or (c) it is disproportionately burdensome in the patient's perspective. The last two criteria refer to persons for whom the palliative or life-extending benefits of feeding are more than offset, in the patient's view, by burdens caused by the procedures or consequences of medically supervised feeding. These burdens could include the need to restrain patients to enable feeding, shortness of breath that might be increased in dying patients who are "normally" hydrated (4,7–9), or the burdens of continued existence in a profoundly disabled state in which the patient finds life-prolonging care to be unacceptable.

Public policy has generally endorsed the elective nature of clinical feeding. Living Will laws or Durable Powers of Attorney for Health Care in at least 22 states specifically accept the discontinuation of food and water (10) (Table 1). Major health professional societies—the American Medical Association (11), the American Geriatrics Society (12), the American Academy of Neurology (13), the American Nursing Association (14), and the American Dietetic Association (15)—have stated, with various nuances, that the provision of food and water is elective, as are other life-prolonging medical treatments.

TABLE 1. *Food and water in Living Will laws*

States where discontinuation of nutrition and hydration is permitted within Living Will laws			
Alabama	Alaska	Arkansas	California
Delaware	D of C	Idaho	Illinois
Kansas	Louisiana	Minnesota	Mississippi
Montana	Nevada	New Mexico	North Carolina
Oregon	Tennessee	Texas	Vermont
Virginia	Washington		

States where discontinuation of nutrition and hydration is not permitted within Living Will laws			
Colorado[a]	Connecticut	Florida[a]	Georgia
Maine[a]	Missouri		

States where discontinuation of nutrition and hydration is not addressed within Living Will laws			
Arizona	Hawaii	Indiana	Iowa
Maryland	New Hampshire	Oklahoma	South Carolina
Utah	West Virginia	Wyoming	

From Society for the Right to Die, ref. 32, and updated literature. Statutes have specific language that should be consulted.
[a]Court decisions in these states have overturned or amended this restriction.

State courts and one federal court also support the premise that food and water are elective forms of medical treatment (1,4,6,16–18) (Table 2). Courts have overturned legislation in three of six states that prohibited the termination of food and water in Living Will laws (Table 1).

In 1988, two state supreme courts disallowed the removal of feeding tubes (19,20) (Table 2). In the O'Connor decision, New York's highest court did not reject the view that food and water are elective, but did set a very high standard for concluding that such decisions represent the patient's explicit preferences. In the Cruzan decision, Missouri's Supreme Court ruled that food was obligatory given the strong state interest in preserving life and absent an explicit and fully informed directive from a patient that it should be withdrawn.

The decisions in Missouri and New York reflect the views of those who reject the premise that food and water may be withheld or withdrawn in a manner similar to other life-sustaining medical treatments. Derr (21), Siegler and Weisbard (22) and others (23) distinguish decisions to withhold food from decisions to withhold other medical therapies in several ways. First, forgoing food ensures death in any person, regardless of their health or the accuracy of the assessment of their condition. Thus, intent to kill (and perhaps euthanasia) is inherent in decisions to withhold food (24). Second, permitting health care providers to terminate feedings will induce fear into our most dependent and vulnerable patients. Third, termination of feeding, as a death-inducing act, undermines the moral foundation of the health profession. Fourth, feeding has a unique cultural significance that other treatments

TABLE 2. *Selected state court decisions on termination of feeding*

California: *Barber v. Superior Court,* 147 Cal. App. 3d 1006, 195 Cal. Rptr. 484 (Ct. App. 1983).
   Bouvia v. Superior Court (Glenchur), 179 Cal. App. 3d 1127, 225 Cal. Rptr. 297 (Ct. App. 1986), *review denied* (Cal. June 5, 1986).
Colorado: *In re Rodas,* No. 86PR139 (Colo. Dist. Ct. Mesa County Jan. 22, 1987, as modified, April 3, 1987) (Buss, Jr.).
Florida: *Corbett v. D'Alessandro,* 487 So. 2d 368 (Fla. Dist. Ct. App.), *review denied,* 492 So. 2d 1331 (Fla. 1986).
Maine: *In re Gardner,* 534 A.2d 947 (Me. 1987).
Massachusetts: *Brophy v. New England Sinai Hospital, Inc.,* 398 Mass. 417, 497 N.E. 2d 626 (1986).
Michigan: *In re Culham,* No. 87-340537-AZ (Mich. Cir. Ct. Oakland County, December 15, 1987) (Breck, J.).
Missouri: *Cruzan v. Harmon,* No. CV384-9P (Mo. Cir. Ct. Jasper County July 27, 1988) (Teel, J.), *reversed,* No. 70813 (Mo. Sup. Ct. Nov. 16, 1988).
New Jersey: *In re Conroy,* 98 N.J. 321, 486 A.2d 1209 (1985).
   In re Raquenna, 213 N.J. Super. 475, 517 A.2d 886 (Super. Ct. Ch. Div.), *aff'd,* 213 N.J. Super. 443, 517 A.2d 869 (Super. Ct. App. Div. 1986) (per curiam).
   In re Jobes, 108 N.J. 394, 529 A.2d 434 (1987).
   In re Peter, 108 N.J. 365, 529 A.2d 419 (1987).
New York: *In re Application of Brooks* (Leguerrier) (N.Y. Sup. Ct. Albany County June 10, 1987) (Conway, J.).
   Delio v. Westchester County Medical Center, 129 A.D.2d 1, 516 N.Y.S.2d. 677 (App. Div. 2d Dept 1987).
   In the Matter of Mary O'Conner, Westchester County Medical Center v. Helen Hall, No. 312 (N.Y. Ct. App. Oct. 14, 1988).
North Dakota: *In re Bayer,* No. 4131 (N.D. Burleigh County Ct. Feb. 5, 11, and Dec. 11, 1987) (Riskedahl, J.).
Pennsylvania: *In re Jane Doe,* 16 Philia. 229 (Pa. Ct. Com. Pl. 1987).
Rhode Island: *Gray v. Romeo,* 697 F. Supp. 580 (D.R.I. 1988).
Texas: *Newman v. William Beaumont Army Medical Center,* NO. EP-86-CA-276 (W. D. Tex. Oct. 30, 1986) (Hudspeth, J.).
Virginia: *Haselton [sic] v. Powhatan Nursing Home, Inc.,* 6 Va. Cir. Ct. Op. 414 (Aspen 1987) (Va. Cir. Ct. Fairfax County 1986), (Sept. 2, 1986) (Fortkort, J.), *appeal denied,* Record No. 860814 (Va. Sept. 2, 1986).
Washington: *In re Guardianship of Grant,* 109 Wash. 2d 545, 747 P.2d 445 (1987).

[a]U.S. Federal Court decision.

do not have (1,25). Because of this cultural meaning, food and fluids are basic forms of caring that engage communitarian understandings of compassion that are not adequately weighed in the mechanistic, individualistic balancing of benefits and burdens (26).

Those who hold that public policy should equate feeding with other treatments center their rebuttal on a communitarian perspective on food and water on patient autonomy and on the difference between killing and allowing to die. They believe that the symbolic significance of feeding should be evaluated on an individual basis according to the patient's own preferences, values, and interests (2,16). They argue that the public supports the right to decline artificial nourishment, suggesting that the fear of being sustained by technology outweighs the fear that health providers will wrongly terminate patient's lives. The distinction between killing and allowing to die is crucial to those who believe that feeding can be an unduly burdensome treatment, especially for those who fear that forgoing feeding suggests tacit support for direct medical killing (27,28). The lethal effect of withholding nourishment is justified as an unintended secondary result of a primary decision to reject further treatment (19).

There is a certain irony to this debate. Modern clinical ethics, which matured in its examination of decisions to forgo the most complex medical technology, now labors with the simple, yet profound psychology of feeding. The legal and ethical boundaries that circumscribe decisions about nutrition are less clear than those for more elaborate technologies, such as respirators, dialysis, or resuscitation. Even so, recent reviews (1,3,29) accept that food and water are elective therapies. These authors emphasize, however, that the symbolic significance of feeding and the lethality of stopping this therapy call for the most careful decision-making processes.

CLINICAL DECISION MAKING ABOUT FOOD AND WATER

This section examines clinical decision making about the continuation of feeding and hydration. It begins with a strong presumption in favor of the provision of food and water. Meals are a routine event in health care facilities. Feeding prolongs life, promotes healing and health, and palliates hunger and thirst. To set aside this presumption requires a documented, deliberate, and consultative review of the patient's medical condition, preferences, and interests that accommodates dissenting moral views by individual members of the health care team.

Patients' values and preferences should determine the kind of medically indicated therapy that they receive. The ethical principle of autonomy is affirmed by the common law doctrine of informed consent and a constitutionally derived respect for privacy (5). It applies to decision making about food and water (18,29,30). Sometimes, clinicians or families can directly know a patient's preference about medically supervised food and water. Many patients with advanced malignancies or other chronic conditions can discuss whether they will accept enteral feeding should they become too ill to ingest what is needed to sustain life or promote health (8). Such persons should be consulted before or soon after invasive methods of feeding are initiated. These patients can also discuss their preferences with regard to other life-sustaining treatments (CPR, ventilators) and about future clinical events that would change their treatment objectives. For example, a patient who is receiving chemotherapy might agree to enteral feeding to determine if the cancer would respond to therapy, providing that the physician promised to withdraw the feeding tube if the medical condition deteriorated so that the patient could no longer recognize family members.

In some situations, patients who are not directly confronted with a proposal for medically supervised feeding will express future preferences.

However, experience suggests that few persons specifically state their preferences about feeding, even if they have strong views about other life-sustaining treatments. Some Living Wills enable patients to express preferences about the provision of food and water in the event of future incompetence. Durable Powers of Attorney for Health Care can specifically empower a proxy to make decisions on a patient's behalf with regard to food and water, although such documents would ordinarily be interpreted as so empowering the proxy even without an explicit detail.

Clinicians should be cautious about incorporating such directives into decisions to withhold feeding. For example, where a healthy person might have strong speculative opinions about the unacceptability of treatment after a medical catastrophe, the same person might accept a lower quality of life than he or she had anticipated after adapting to a chronic, debilitating condition.

Many patients are unable to express their preferences because of coma, dementia, delirium, or communication disorders. Patients who are transiently incompetent should be supported, until they are able to participate in decision making. Patients with terminal illnesses who become incompetent after a long period of anorexia, during which they declined invasive feeding support, should be allowed to die. For noncomatose persons, the possibility that a patient experiences hunger or thirst is usually decisive in favor of providing food and water. These decisions are most difficult to make for persons with advanced degenerative dementias (17,30). Some of these persons have had eating apraxias or dysphagias that necessitated medically supervised feeding or enteral intubation earlier in their course. The evaluation of whether this support should be continued is very controversial.

The evaluation of forgoing feeding for patients without decisional capacity should engage, as proxies, families or close friends who are intimately knowledgeable of the patient's preferences, rather than the health care provider. There are several approaches to decision making (29,31). One approach—"substituted judgment"—asks those who are familiar with a patient to imagine what the patient would decide by taking into account what is known of the patient's background, values, previous attitudes to medical care, prognosis, and sensation of medical care. The "best interests" and "proportionate benefits and burdens" standards do not detail the pretense of recreating a patient's own view, but require the proxy to evaluate treatment in light of the patient's needs, rather than from the perspective of the costs or social worth of the patient (17). The views of family members that feeding is a form of care, not a treatment, may deserve respect (32), although they should not override a patient's clearly articulated preference.

Health care providers should be prepared to conduct a deliberative, consultative, and documented review of decisions to forgo food and water (29,30,31,33). The medical facts should be reviewed. For decisionally capable patients, this might include a psychiatric evaluation. Clinicians should evaluate whether family members are motivated by good intentions (see Jobes decision, Table 2). Decisions about feeding should not be swayed by misconceptions about the feeding process, by remediable deficiencies in the palliation of suffering or maintenance of dignity and independence, or by depression or transient discouragement. Local requirements for legal guardians (or ombudsmen) should be respected and may be properly appealed if their participation is deemed inappropriate, as sometimes happens. Ethics committees or consultants can help ensure that such decisions meet current standards of ethical professional practice. Given the extensive professional consensus on this issue, courts or public guardians should not be routinely engaged in these decisions unless their involvement is specifically mandated by law.

Clinicians should make a written record of the participants and their roles in the decision-making process and specify the rationale for the conclusion that consent for feeding has been withdrawn. In addition, clinicians should record positive treatment goals, including plans to address palliative goals. Health care facility policies can define the procedures for such a decision-making process (33).

Although patients may direct whether they receive a treatment, they may not oblige health care providers to violate their own deeply held moral positions. In "shared decision making," the physician informs the patient of possible outcomes and recommended courses, the patient makes a treatment choice, and the provider agrees to honor it as the therapeutic relationship continues (31,34). Once it has been determined that consent to continue feeding has been withdrawn, nurses and physicians who conscientiously object to this decision should be allowed to excuse themselves from the patient's care (29). Legal cases have been divided on whether nursing homes or hospitals can require, as a matter of policy, the transfer of patients for whom feeding is to be discontinued (33).

DIFFICULT CLINICAL CASES

The two clinical examples below illustrate when the appropriateness of providing enteral tube feedings may be questioned. One involves feeding to reduce prognostic uncertainty in comatose persons; the other addresses feeding in the palliative care of a demented and terminally ill patient.

Temporary Feeding to Reduce Prognostic Uncertainty

A 65-year-old woman is comatose 3 days after suffering a cardiac arrest during a cholecystectomy. She is being weaned from a respirator. The physician recommends enteral tube feedings to provide her nutrition. Her husband and daughter cite repeated conversations in which the patient said that she would not want to be kept alive if she became unable to care for herself or recognize her family.

The outcome of anoxic coma is variable. Some patients recover substantial cognitive or physical ability, whereas others remain in a persistent vegetative state in which they can be sustained for years with nutritional support and attentive nursing care. The prognosis for functional recovery by comatose individuals often cannot be determined for several weeks or months (13). Thus, a full prognostic evaluation often requires the aggressive use of nutritional and medical support for weeks to months.

In this situation, food and water might be initiated conditionally as part of a trial of therapy to determine if the patient will recover to a condition where he or she would desire sustained support (13,29). Such a trial is analogous to the empiric use of an antibiotic to determine if it can promote recovery from an incompletely diagnosed infectious process. Such trials offer several advantages. Families might be more willing to accept a course of aggressive life support if a re-evaluation of its continued appropriateness is promised as prognostic information became available. Furthermore, the promised re-evaluation sets a helpful context for a future discussion of therapeutic goals, which can be comforting as the final decision to discontinue food and water is made. Clinicians who make such proposals must be available to see that the promised re-evaluation of the treatment plan occurs. Feeding does not have a palliative role in the treatment of persons in a persistent vegetative state as they are believed to be insensate of pain, hunger, or thirst (13).

Feeding the Terminally Ill

An 85-year-old man with late confusional stage Alzheimer's disease has a prostate cancer with multiple axial metastases and is being cared for in the nursing home. The cancer has progressed despite hormonal therapy. Two persons are needed to transfer him from a bed to a chair, and he is unable to participate in rehabilitation. His arms have not been restrained. Nursing aides have fed him by spoon, but he has been consistently rejecting their efforts. The nutritionist notes in the nursing home record: "Calorie Count: 400 calories per day. Assessment: Inadequate. PLAN: Inform physician that tube feedings are needed."

This unfortunate situation calls for a comprehensive and individualized re-evaluation of the patient's medical condition, anorexia, treatment preferences, and treatment plan objectives. The foundation for treatment decisions rests on the choice of treatment objectives (35). If the overriding treatment objective is palliation, rather than prolonging life, the extent to which enteral feeding (by any method) is palliative should be assessed (29,30). Anorexia, assuming that the patient is capable of expressing hunger or thirst, might signify that nourishment is not palliative. In such a case tube feedings might cause rather than relieve suffering, particularly if the patient had to be restrained during the feedings. Little is known about the physical pain of not feeding such patients (4,7,9,36). If the patient is felt to be in the terminal phase of his cancer, nourishment might be futile in that it could not sustain life. In this situation, it is possible that the insistent provision of physiologic amounts of nourishment might increase his suffering (7,9,28) and thus should not be undertaken. Careful documentation should address the nutritionist's conclusion as the decision not to intubate the patient is set in the context of other palliative treatment goals.

CONCLUSION

The debate over medical nourishment reveals the way that medical technologies are instruments of care. The strong presumption in favor of providing nourishment rests on a deep sense of duties owed to the most vulnerable among us. These decisions cannot be resolved by a simple calculation of physiologic needs. Ethical clinical decision making rests on the belief that a patient is a person whose life is precious, whose mortality is a tragic fact, and whose values must be respected.

REFERENCES

1. Curran WJ. *N Engl J Med* 1985;313:940–942.
2. Lynn J, Childress JF. *Hastings Cent Rep* 1983;13:17–21.
3. Lynn J, ed. *By no extraordinary means*. Bloomington, IN: Indiana University Press, 1986.
4. Office of Technology Assessment. *Life-sustaining technologies and the elderly*. Washington, DC: US Government Printing Office, 1988.
5. President's Commission for the Study of Ethical Problems in Medicine and Biomedical and Behavioral Research. *Deciding to forego life-sustaining treatment: Ethical, medical, and legal issues in treatment decisions*. Washington, DC: US Government Printing Office. 1983.
6. Lo B. *Ann Intern Med* 1984;104:248–251.
7. Campbell-Taylor I, Fisher HR. *J Am Geriatr Soc* 1988;35:1100–1103.
8. Schmitz P, O'Brien M. In: Lynn J, ed. *By no extraordinary means*. Bloomington, IN: Indiana University Press, 1986:29–38.
9. Zerwekh JV. *Nursing* 1983;13:47–51.
10. Society for the Right to Die. *Handbook of living will laws*. New York: Society for the Right to Die, 1987.
11. American Medical Association. *Current opinions of the Council on Ethical and Judicial Affairs. Withholding or withdrawing life-prolonging medical treatment*. Chicago: AMA. 1986.
12. American Geriatrics Society. *J Am Geriatr Soc* 1984;32:915–921.
13. American Academy of Neurology. *Neurology* 1989;39:125–126.
14. Fry ST. *Nurs Outlook* 1988;36:122–123, 148–150.
15. American Dietetic Association. *J Am Dietet Assoc* 1987;87:78–85.
16. Annas GJ. *Hastings Cent Rep* 1986;16:26–28.
17. Lo B, Dornbrand L. *Ann Intern Med* 1986;104:869–873.
18. Steinbrook R, Lo B. *N Engl J Med* 1988;318:286–290.
19. Annas GJ. *Hastings Cent Rep* 1989;19:29–31.
20. Annas GJ. *Hastings Cent Rep* 1988;18:31–33.

21. Derr PG. *Hastings Cent Rep* 1986;16:28–30.
22. Siegler M, Weisbard AJ. *Arch Intern Med* 1985;145:129–131.
23. Rosner F. *NY State J Med* 1987;87(11):591–593.
24. Bopp J. *Issues Law Med* 1988;4:3–52.
25. Callahan D. *Hastings Cent Rep* 1983;13:22.
26. Meilander G. *Hastings Cent Rep* 1984;14:11–13.
27. May WE, Barry R, Griese O, Grisez G, et al. *Issues Law Med* 1987;3:203–217.
28. Schaffner KF. *Crit Care Med* 1988;16:1063–1068.
29. Hastings Center. *Guidelines on the termination of life-sustaining treatment and the care of the dying.* Briarcliff Manor, NY: The Hastings Center, 1987.
30. Watts DT, Cassel CK. *J Am Geriatr Soc* 1984;32:237–242.
31. President's Commission for the Study of Ethical Problems in Medicine and Biomedical and Behavioral Research. *Making health care decisions.* Washington, DC: US Government Printing Office, 1982.
32. Miles SH. *Theoret Med* 1987;8:293–302.
33. Miles SH, Gomez C. *Protocols for elective use of life-sustaining treatments.* New York: Springer Publishing Co, 1989.
34. Siegler M. *Bull NY Acad Med* 1981;57:56–69.
35. Volicer L, Rheaume Y, Brown J, Fabiszewski K, Brady R. *JAMA* 1986;256:2210–2213.
36. Printz LA. *Geriatrics* 1988;43:84–88.

Subject Index

A

Accident, cause of mortality, 4
Acetylcholine, Alzheimer's disease, 424
Acetylsalicylic acid, nutritional implication, 386
Acrodermatitis enteropathica, zinc deficiency, 162
Activity level, children, measurement, 427
Acute illness, incidence, 5
Adipose tissue
  anthropometric, 295
  brown, 32
  feeding control mechanism, 36
Adiposity, mortality, relative risk, 299
Advertisement, health fraud, 403
Aging
  albumin synthesis, 249–250
  demographics, 1–3
    developed nations, 2
  epidemiology, 3–8
  food restriction, 24
  gallstone disease, 251–253
  hepatocyte domains, 244
  hepatocyte organelle, 241–244
  ligand processing, hepatocyte, 248–249
  liver, 241
  liver cell, 240–241
    turnover, 244–245
  liver function, 247–248
  mono-oxygenase system, 250–251
  nonparenchymal cell, hepatic, 245–247
  reduction in activity, 31
Aging theory
  cellular-based, 12–16
  molecular theory, 11–18
  organ-system based, 12
  population-based
    type I, 11
    type II, 11–12
Albumin
  level depressed in hypozincemia, 167
  malnutrition indication, 81–82
  serum level, 105–106
Albumin synthesis, aging process, 249–250
Alcohol
  abuse in elderly, 390
  consumption, hypertension treatment, 290
  drug-food interaction, 390–391
Alpha-glucosidase inhibitor, diabetes management, 265–266
Alzheimer's disease, dietary choline intake, 424
American Diabetes Association, dietary recommendation, 46, 263
Amino acid supplement, 401
  drug interaction, 393
  health fraud, 405–406
p-Aminobenzoic acid, health fraud, 406
Amitriptyline, nutritional implication, 386
Anabolic androgen, weight maintenance, 311
Anemia
  cause, 62
  etiology, 187–188
  incidence
    hospitalized elderly, 187
    institutionalized elderly, 187
  nutritional, 183–192
  prevalence, 186–187
Anorexia, 106. See also Anorexia of aging
  diuretic medication, 320
  elderly, cause, 319
  stress, 189
  zinc deficiency, 161–165
Anorexia of aging, 106–110
  causes, 107–110
    pathophysiologic, 108
    physiologic, 107–108
    psychologic, 108–109
    social, 107
  definition, 107

Anoxic coma, feeding to determine
    prognosis, 477–478
Antacid, phosphorus absorption
    decrease, 64
Anthropometrics, 76–80
    adipose tissue mass, 295
    nutritional assessment, 78–80, 112
    upper arm, 79–80
Antiarrhythmic agent, drug-food
    interaction, 373–379
Anticoagulant medication, drug-food
    interaction, 379
Antihypertensive therapy
    medication adverse effect,
        incidence, 290
    nonpharmacologic, 282–290
    nutritional intervention, 281–292
Antineoplaston, cancer quackery,
    412
Antioxidant, longevity effect, free
    radical scavenger, 404–405
Antioxidant enzyme supplement,
    health fraud, 405
Antiparkinson agent, drug-food
    interaction, 385–389
Apathy, starvation, 419
Apoptosis, 241
Arm muscle circumference, protein
    status indication, 79
Arsenic, human requirement, 171
Arthritis, fraudulent remedy, 409–410
Artificial sweetener, diabetic diet,
    265
Ascorbic acid. *See* Vitamin C
Asialoorosomucoid, biliary secretion,
    effect of aging, 249
Aspiration, nutrient formula, 355–356
Atherogenesis, 270
    dietary component interaction
        regulation, 272
Atherosclerosis
    development, multicausal, 269
    selenium deficiency, 177–178
    vitamin B_6 deficiency, 277
Atrophic gastritis
    elderly, prevalence, 232
    physiologic consequence, 232
    vitamin B_{12} bioavailability limited,
        233
Atrophy, muscle fiber, aging-related,
    449
Attention deficit disorder, food effect,
    427–428

Autistic children, food related
    behavior, 428
Autoimmunity retardation, nutritional
    manipulation, 23
Autonomy, ethical principle, food
    withholding, 475

B

B cell, differentiation pathway, 219
Bacterial overgrowth, gut, 253
Baldness, health fraud, 407
Basal metabolic rate, 29–30
    aging reduction, 30
    metabolic origin, 29
Behavior, dietary influence, 429
Behavioral modification, weight
    reduction, 303–304
Behavioral problem, nutritional
    therapy, 419
Beriberi, 131
Beta-adrenergic blocking agent, drug-
    food interaction, 373
Bile acid, homostatistical regulation,
    252
Biliary cirrhosis, primary, 254
Biliary lipid composition, effect of
    age, 252
Biochemical index, nutritional
    assessment, 80–85
    prognostic power, 85
Bioelectrical impedance, fat-lean
    tissue proportion
    determination, 75–76
Biotin
    assessment, 140
    deficiency, 140
    function, 140
    risk factors, 140
    toxicity, 140
Bisacodyl, nutritional implication, 382
Blood modifier, drug-food interaction,
    372–380
Blood parameter, nutritional
    assessment, 81–82
Blood pressure
    calcium intake relation, 286–287
    dietary fat, 288–289
    dietary sodium intake effect, 284
    increase with aging, 281
    magnesium supplementation, 288
    orthostatic change, 282

potassium intake decreasing, 285
sodium-sensitive, 91
Body circumference measurement, 295
Body composition
  age-associated change, 28
  assessment, 75–76
  body impedance measurement, 295
  change, 74–75
Body fat
  aging increase, 44
    total, 75
  assessment technique, 294–295
  distribution
    body circumference
      measurement, 295
    health risk assessment, 293
    triceps skinfold thickness, 79
Body impedance measurement, body
  composition, 295
Body water, total
  decline with age, 75, 193–194
  measurement, 295
Body weight
  ideal, 78
  longitudinal change, 297
Bone mass
  calcium intake effect, current, 153
  calcium supplementation, 154
Bone matrix, calcium deposition,
  quantification, 63
Bone remodeling, dynamic process,
  149
Boron, function, 171–172
Brain damage, malnutrition, 420
Breakfast consumption, school
  performance, 425
Breast cancer, incidence, 308
Bronchodilator, drug-food interaction,
  389
Brown adipose tissue, diet-induced
  thermogenesis, 32
Butylated hyroxytoluene, health
  fraud, 405

C

Cachexia, pharmacologic intervention,
  311–312
Calcitriol level, decreased in elderly,
  155
Calcium
  atrophic gastritis, 233–234

calcium intake necessary, 63
  low-sodium diet effect, 153
  medication effect, 153
  negative, elderly, 150
bioavailability, 233–234
blood-pressure-lowering effect,
  286–287
bone matrix deposition,
  quantification, 63
dietary intake, 149–150
  bone mass effect, 153
  North American decrease, 283
  North American deficiency, 287
  survey data, 150
hypertensive sensitivity,
  biochemical parameter,
  286–287
increased need at menopause onset,
  63
increased requirement in older
  adult, 150–153
intestinal absorption, 154
  adaptive response, 155
  diminished, 157
  osteoporotic patient, 56
metabolism, hypertension
  abnormality, 286–287
recommended daily allowance,
  62–63
United States, 149
Calcium supplement
  bone mass, 154
  magnesium absorption interference,
  64
Caloric deprivation, thymic involution
  delay, life span determination,
  211–212
Caloric restriction
  animal study, 404
  growth period, cell-mediated
    immunity suppression, 212
  immunologic consequence, animal
    research, 211–212
  reference diet, 212
Calories
  diabetes diet, 262–266
  recommended daily allowance,
  43–44
Cancer. *See also* Specific type
  incidence increase with age,
  307–308
  malnutrition, 309
  mortality rate, 4

Cancer (*contd*)
  prevalence, dietary modulation,
    94–95
  selenium deficiency, 177
Cancer cachexia
  definition, 309
  lipid metabolism, 310–311
  pathophysiology, 309–311
Cancer quackery, 410–412
Carbohydrate
  American Diabetes Association
    recommendation, 264
  complex, dietary increase, 45
  glucose response, glycemic index,
    264–265
  recommended daily allowance,
    45–46
Cardiac cachexia, 315–323
  description, 316
  diagnostic criteria, 321
  digitalis, 319–320
  digoxin, 319–320
  Hippocrates' description, 316
  management, 321–322
  pathogenesis, 316–320
  prevalence, 315
Cardiac disease, malnutrition
    association, prevalence, 319
Cardiomyopathy, selenium deficiency,
    177
Cardiovascular disease
  nutrition, 269–279
    epidemiologic study, 273–275
  United States prevalence, 269
Cardiovascular drug
  drug-food interaction, 372–380
  nutritional concern, 375–378
Cardiovascular system, age-related
    change, 270
Care plan, dietetic service, 463
Caries, elderly, 226
Carotenoid, dietary intake, decreased
    cancer risk, 55
Catheter, indwelling, 360
Cell-mediated immune dysfunction,
    nutritional intervention,
    mechanistic approach, 219–220
Cell-mediated immunity
  depressed, micronutrient deficiency,
    210
  nutritional modulation, 209–218
Cellular change, immune response
    effect, 204–206

Cellular hypoxia, biochemical
    consequence, cardiac cachexia
    genesis, 317
Cellular milieu, immune response
    effect, 204
Central feeding drive, decrease,
    neurotransmitter effect, 109
Central nervous system medication,
    nutritional concerns, 386–388
Chemophobia, food supply, 400
Chiropractice, health fraud, 413,
    415
Chlorpropamide, hyponatremia,
    200–201
Cholecystokinin
  gallbladder muscle sensitivity, 236
  memory retention, 426
Cholesterol
  bile acid conversion, enzyme, 253
  biliary, secretion, 252
  dietary
    physiologic compensation,
      270–271
    serum cholesterol level setting,
      47–48
    serum cholesterol relation, 271
  dietary reduction, controversy,
    275–278
  hepatic, synthesis, 252
  immunosuppressive effect, 213
  life expectancy, 276–277
  low, prognostic significance, 329
  mortality unaffected by reduction,
    93
  plasma level
    dietary intake uncorrelated,
      270–271
    increase with age, 48–49, 274
  serum level
    dietary component interaction
      regulation, 272
    seasonal variation, 272
    vanadium deficiency, 179
Cholesterol-heart disease relation
  Framingham Heart Study, 49
  Pooling Project, 49
Cholesterol-lowering agent, drug-food
    interaction, 379–380
Cholestyramine, nutritional
    implication, 374
Choline supplement, brain
    acetylcholine level unrelated,
    424

Chromatin
  age-related change, 16
  thermal stability, increase, 16
  transcribability, reduction with
    aging, 16
Chromium
  glucose homeostasis, 172
  recommended daily allowance, 173
Chromium deficiency, manifestation,
    173
Chronic medical problem
  nutrition-related, diet therapy,
    338–341
  prevalence, 5
  quackery, 399
Cimetidine
  drug-food interaction, 381
  nutritional implication, 382
Cirrhosis, biliary, primary, 254
Clinical feeding, elective nature,
    public policy, 472–473
Cobalamin. *See* Vitamin B_{12}
Cobalt, function, 173
Collagen metabolism, wound healing,
    365
Collagen synthesis, thiamine
  deficiency, 367
Colon cancer, incidence, 308
Colon detoxification, 406
Compliance
  diet regimen, 394
  drug regimen, 394
Congestive heart failure
  fat absorption, 318
  functional impairment, 315
  hypoalbuminemia, 317–318
  malnutrition, diagnostic work-up,
    316
  nitrogen balance, 318
Constipation, fiber effect, 51
Consultant, interdisciplinary team, 460
Copper
  deficiency, clinical syndrome,
    173–174
  function, 173
  serum level, 66
    increase with aging, 174
Core team member, interdisciplinary
  team, 459
Coronary heart disease
  Coronary Primary Prevention Trial,
    274
  death rate, age-adjusted, 277–278

dietary change effect, 23
  lipid hypothesis, 47
  mortality, 50
  Multiple Risk Factor Intervention
    Trial, 274
  risk factor, 50
Coronary Primary Prevention Trial,
    274
Counseling, drug-food interaction,
    393–394
Creatinine excretion, malnourishment
    effect, 81
Creatinine height index
  aging effect, 80
  formula, 81
Criminal behavior, nutrition effect,
    426

D
Dark adaptation, impaired, zinc
    therapy, 163
Death rate, age-specific, definition, 20
Decision making
  clinical, feeding, 475–477
  food withholding
    best interests, 476
    proportionate benefits and
      burdens, 476
    substituted judgment, 476
Deficiency
  biotin, 140
  folic acid, 137–138
  niacin, 139
  pantothenic acid, 141
  vitamin A, 123–124
  vitamin B_1, 131
  vitamin B_2, 132
  vitamin B_6, 133–134
  vitamin B_{12}, 135–136
  vitamin C, 142–143
  vitamin D, 126–127
  vitamin E, 128–129
  vitamin K, 129–130
Degenerative disease, life expectancy
    effect, 21
Degradation system, impairment, age-
    associated, 248
7-Dehydrocholesterol, epidermal
    concentration, age-dependent
    decline, 156
Delayed hypersensitivity skin testing,
    immune status indication, 83

Dementia
  folate deficiency, 138
  malnutrition, 7
  malnutrition risk, 109
  tryptophan, 423–424
Demographics, aging, 1–3
Dental amalgam filling, mercury-
    containing, safety, 413
Dentition
  health fraud, 412–413
  nursing home food acceptability, 338
Depression
  nutrient intake effect, 108
  vitamin B_6, 420
Diabetes
  dietary change, 46
  elderly, nutrition effect, 259–268
  non-insulin-dependent, dietary
      treatment, 261–262
  pathogenesis, nutritional factor, 262
  prevalence, increase with advancing
      age, 259
  screening, 98
  Type II, caloric restriction, 263
Diabetic diet, nursing home resident,
    340
Diagnostic practice, fraudulent, 408
Diarrhea
  enteral-feeding-associated, 356
    hypoproteinemia association, 357
  zinc deficiency, 166
Diet
  calorie restriction, elderly, 303
  compliance, 394
  diabetes, 262–266
    calories, 262–266
  high-monounsaturated-fat, 263
  very low-fat, controversial, 275
Diet-induced thermogenesis, 31–32
  brown adipose tissue, 32
Diet therapy, cancer quackery, 411
Dietary calcium, hypertension
    treatment, 286–287
Dietary fat
  blood pressure, 288–289
  intake reduction, 44
Dietary fiber. *See also* Insoluble fiber;
    Soluble fiber
  calcium chelation, 152
  definition, 51
  diabetic diet, 265
  intake, 52

Dietary intake
  nursing home resident, 337
  serum cholesterol level, 48
Dietary phosphorus
  deficiency, 64
  hypertension treatment, 288
Dietary recommendation, American
    Diabetes Association, 263
Dietary supplementation,
    immunopotentiation, 217–218
Dietetic service
  care plan, 463
  nutrition profile, 463
Dietitian, interdisciplinary team,
    464–466
Digitalis, cardiac cachexia, 319–320
Digitalis glycoside, drug-food
    interaction, 372
Digoxin
  cardiac cachexia, 319–320
  nutritional implication, 374
1,25-Dihydroxyvitamin D, plasma
    level, decrease with aging, 157
Disability
  elderly, disease as cause, 239–240
  old-old, 239
  prevalence, 5
Diuretic
  anorexia, 320
  drug-food/food-drug interaction,
      372–373
  electrolyte imbalance, 319
  elevated zinc excretion, 443
  hyponatremia, 200
Diverticular disease, fiber effect,
    51–52
Dopamine, feeding control, 34–35
Drug
  compliance, 394
  disposition capacity, age-related
      decline, 239
  nutrient bioavailability, 97–98
  obesity therapy, 304
  reduced, elimination, 247
  usage by elderly, 371
Drug-food interaction
  alcohol, 390–391
  antiarrhythmic agent, 373–379
  anticoagulant medication, 379
  antiparkinson agent, 385–389
  beta-adrenergic blocking agent, 373
  blood modifier, 372–380

bronchodilator, 389
cardiovascular drug, 372–380
cause, 371–372
cholesterol-lowering agent, 379–380
cimetidine, 381
counseling, 393–394
digitalis glycoside, 372
diuretic medication, 372–373
food supplement, 391–393
gastric medication, 380–381
laxative, 380–381
lithium, 385
monamine oxidase inhibitor, 389
musculoskeletal agent, 381–384
psychotherapeutic medication,
    384–389
quinidine, 379
respiratory tract agent, 389
vasodilator, 373–379
Durable Power of Attorney for Health
    Care, food withholding, 476

E
Effector cell dysfunction, zinc
    deficiency, 217
Elderly
anemia, chronic stress causing, 188
developing nations, 2–3
drug usage, 371
health care services, 8–9
health status, variable, 3
independent community, nutrition
    survey, 327
nutritional assessment, 73–87
nutritional change, 218
nutritional requirements, 41–72
old-old
    disability, 239
    segment increase, 2
undernutrition, confounding
    problems, 38
United States
    demography, 325–328
    increase, 41
Electrolyte imbalance, diuretic
    therapy, 319
Electromyographic value, change with
    aging, 450
Endocrine disorder, obesity, 298–299
Endothelial cell, hepatic sinusoid, 246
Endurance training, 452

Enema, colon detoxification, 406
Energy allowance, current
    recommended daily allowance,
    43
Energy balance
age-associated change, 27–28
control mechanism, influence of
    aging, 27–38
physical activity, 31
Energy intake
age-related change, 32–38
age-related reduction, 33
control, 32–38
    central mechanism, 32–35
    peripheral mechanism, 35–38
Energy output
age-related change, 28–32
age-related reduction, 33
basal metabolic rate, 29–30
control, 28–32
decrease with age, 298
diet-induced thermogenesis, 31–32
physical activity, 31
resting activity, 298
thermic effect of meals, 30–31
Enteral feeding
advantage over parenteral therapy,
    346
appropriateness, 477–479
complication, 353–357
contraindication, 343–346
gastrointestinal complication,
    356–357
indication, 343–346
method, 350–353
nutrient delivery
    mode, 353
    route, 351–353
    schedule, 353
    site, 350–351
nutrition support team, utility, 467
pleural-pulmonary complication,
    355–356
septic-metabolic complication, 355
solution choice, 346–350
Enteral feeding formula
commonly available, 344–345
cost, 350
disease-specific, 347–348
modular
    carbohydrate module, 349
    fat module, 348

Enteral feeding formula, modular (*contd*)
protein module, 349
selection, 346–350
solution osmolarity, 350
trace mineral requirement, 347
water component, 347
Enteral feeding tube
mechanical complication, 354
patient intolerance, 354
Enzyme, hepatic, age-related change, 248
Epidemiology, aging, 3–8
Epidermal growth factor
biliary excretion, reduction with age, 249
transcellular pathway, 249
Epithelialization, wound healing, 366
Error catastrophy theory of Orgel, 13
Erythrocyte glutathione reductase activation coefficient, riboflavin status evaluation, 58
Erythrocyte transketolase activation coefficient, 57
Erythropoiesis
cell production, 184
group housing, age-related change, 186
normal, 183–188
effect of age, 185–186
progenitor cell, 183
red cell production regulation, 185
Esophageal function, change with aging, 231–232
Essential fatty acids, recommended daily allowance, 47
Ethics, nourishment withholding, 471–480
Exercise
benefit, 447
bone mass increase, 152
life span prolongation, 96
weight reduction, 303
Extended team member, interdisciplinary team, 459–460

F

Faith healing, cancer quackery, 411
Fat
absorption, 318
American Diabetes Association guideline, 266

body, function, 293
dietary intake, 44, 47–50, 288–289
distribution, age-related change, 297
Fat-lean tissue proportion determination, bioelectrical impedance, 75–76
Fat-storing cell, hepatic
aging process, 246
function, 246
Federal Trade Commission, health fraud, 414
Feeding
central control, 33
central control mechanism
anatomic center, 32–34
autonomic center, 32–34
neurochemical mechanism, 34–35
memory retention, 425–426
peripheral control mechanism, sensual factor, 35
temporal, prognostic uncertainty reduction, 477–478
terminally ill, 478–479
thermic effect, 30–31
Feeding drive, opiate-based, decreased, 35
Feeding termination, state court decisions, 474
Feeding tube, 112–113
removal, legal issue, 473–475
Feingold diet, hyperactivity, 427–428
Fish, dietary increase, 94
Fish oil
antihypertensive action, mechanism, 289
diabetes diet, 266
dietary increase, 94
memory enhancement, mice, 435–440
memory retention, dose effect, 438
Fluid, decreased consumption, cause, 66–67
Fluid loss, increase in elderly, 67
Fluidity, plasma membrane, hepatocyte, 241–242
Fluoride, function, 174
Fluoride deficiency, osteoporosis, 174
Folate, recommended daily allowance, 59
Folic acid
assessment, 137
deficiency, 137–138
function, 136

risk factors, 137
toxicity, 138
Food
    medical provision, life-sustaining
        medical treatment, 472
    nonnutritive substance, 430–431
Food and Drug Administration, health
    fraud, 414
Food deprivation, basal metabolic rate
    reduction, 30
Food plan, model, nursing home, 335
Food restriction
    antiaging action, mechanism, 24
    life expectancy increase, 22, 24
    rodent longevity, 23–24
Food service, nursing home
    evaluation, 335
    federal guidelines on standards,
        334–335
    management, 334–335
Food supplement, drug interaction,
    391–393
Food supply
    chemophobia, 400
    fear, 399–402
    nutritional quality, 400–402
Food withholding, decision review,
    476–477
Framingham study
    body mass index, mortality relation,
        300–301
    cholesterol-heart disease relation, 49
    egg intake, serum cholesterol level
        uncorrelated, 271
    serum cholesterol level, 273
Fraud. *See* Health fraud
Free radical scavenger, life extension,
    97
Free radical theory, 13
Fructose, diabetic diet, 265
Functional impairment, older
    population, prevalence, 5–6
Furosemide, nutritional implication,
    374

G
Gallbladder, change with aging, 236
Gallstone disease, aging process,
    251–253
Garlic
    antibiotic effect, 408
    antithrombitic effect, 408

Gastric emptying time, delayed in
    elderly, 232
Gastric medication
    drug-food interaction, 380–381
    nutritional concern, 382–383
Gastrointestinal disease, elderly,
    prevalence, 236
Gastrointestinal hormone, food intake
    effect, 38
Gastrointestinal tract
    change with aging, 231–236
    functional capacity, enteral feeding,
        348–349
Gene expression, aging change, 17
Genomic expression, aging effect, 14
Genotype, determinant of fat
    disposition, 298
Geriatric assessment and treatment
    program, multidimensional, 8–9
Gerovital, 406–407
Glomerular filtration rate, age-related
    decline, 284
Glomerular sclerosis, age increase, 22
Glucocorticoid, food intake effect, 37
Gluconeogenesis inhibition, hydrazine
    sulfate, 311
Glucose, parenteral nutrition formula,
    358
Glucose homeostasis, chromium, 172
Glucose production, whole body,
    increase with cancer, 310
Glucose response, carbohydrate,
    glycemic index, 264–265
Glucose tolerance
    age-related change, carbohydrate
        intake modification, 260–261
    decreased, role of dietary
        carbohydrates, 260
    effect of aging, 260
    impaired, age-related, 259
Glycemic index, 264–265
Glycocolic breath test, 235
Golgi apparatus, hepatocyte, volume
    density, 243
Gonadal steroid, food intake effect,
    37
Group housing, erythropoiesis, age-
    related change, 186
Growth fraction, liver, effect of aging,
    245
Growth hormone
    food intake stimulation, 36
    protein-energy malnutrition, 113

Growth retardation, zinc deficiency, 166
Gum disease. *See* Periodontitis
Gustation, 228
Gut, bacterial overgrowth, 253

H

Handicapped elderly, food intake improvement, utensil modification, 99–101
Headache, diet relation, 429–430
Health association, 414–415
Health care services
  teamwork, 457–458
  use by elderly, 8–9
    poor nutritional status, 41
Health food, 399–400
Health food industry, misinformation, 400
Health fraud, 399–416
  advertisement, 403
  chiropractice, 413, 415
  cost, 397–398
  dentition, 412–413
  Federal Trade Commission, 414
  Food and Drug Administration, 414
  package label, 403
  U.S. Postal Service, 414
  vitamin E, 405
Health status survey, older population, 6
Heat stroke, 67
Height, decrease in elderly, 76
Hematologic parameter, effect of aging, 186
Hematologic test, nutritional assessment, 82
Hemoglobin, changes of aging, 62
Hepatocyte
  effect of aging, 240
  life span, 240
  lipid level, 240
  volume, effect of aging, 240–241
Hepatocyte domains, aging process, 244
Hepatocyte organelle, aging process, 241–244
Herbal remedy, efficacy, 407
Hip fracture, vitamin D deficiency, 92
Honolulu Heart Study, serum cholesterol level, 273
Hospital Prognostic Index, 85

House Subcommittee on Health and Long-Term Health Care, health fraud investigation, 397
Hydralazine, nutritional implication, 374
Hydrazine sulfate, gluconeogenesis inhibition, 311
Hydrodensitometry, body fat calculation, 294
Hydroxylation, vitamin D, 126
25-Hydroxyvitamin D, plasma level, vitamin D status assessment, 156
Hyperactivity
  elimination diet, 428
  Feingold diet, 427–428
  sucrose intake, 428
Hypercholesterolemia
  cardiac effect, elderly resistance, 277
  coronary heart disease mortality, 47
  cut-off point, 273–274
Hyperglycemia, chromium replacement, 172
Hypernatremia, cause, 201
Hypertension, 90–91
  calcium intake effect, 91
  elderly, type, 281–282
  excess weight contribution, 91
  nonpharmacologic therapy, compliance in elderly, 290
  sodium restriction, 65
  systolic, prevalence, 181
Hypertension treatment
  alcohol consumption, 290
  dietary calcium, 286–287
  dietary phosphorus, 288
  potassium supplementation, 285–286
  sodium restriction, 283–285
  weight reduction, 289–290
Hypoosmolarity, 200
Hypoalbuminemia, 74
  congestive heart failure, 317–318
Hypoalbuminemic malnutrition, definition, 105
Hypogonadism, zinc deficiency, 163
Hypomagnesemia, 64
Hyponatremia
  chlorpropamide, 200–201
  diuretic, 200
  drug-induced, 200
  elderly, prevalence, 199
Hypophagia, nursing home, cause, 329

Hypophosphatemia, 64
Hypothalamus, lateral area, lesion, 33
Hypovitaminosis D, 158–159
Hypozincemia, skin lesion, zinc
    supplementation, 162

I

Ibuprofen, nutritional implication, 387
Ideal body weight, elderly, 78
Immobilization, negative calcium
    balance, 151
Immune cell, cellular milieu, change,
    204
Immune dysfunction
    age-associated, nutritional
        intervention, 203–223
    cell-mediated, nutritional
        intervention, 219–220
    selenium deficiency, 178
Immune function
    impaired, zinc deficiency, 165
    lipid modulation, 212–213
Immune response, T-cell-dependent,
    2-mercaptoethanol
    enhancement, 217
Immune system, deterioration, aging
    process, 12
Immune system parameter, nutritional
    assessment, 83–84
Immune therapy, cancer quackery, 412
Immunity, cell-mediated, thymus-
    dependent, 203
Immunodeficiency, zinc deficiency
    animal research, 216–217
    human research, 215–217
Immunodepression, malnutrition, 209
Immunoglobulin A, biliary secretion,
    effect of aging, 249
Immunohematopoietic function,
    malnourished subject, 191
Immunologic change, T-cell-
    dependent, senescence,
    203–206
Immunopotentiation
    dietary supplementation, 217–218
    nutritional supplementation,
        217–218
    zinc supplementation, 217–218
Impotence
    cause, 442
    zinc status, 441–446

Inactivity, functional loss acceleration,
    447
Indwelling venous catheter,
    complication, 360
Infection
    catabolic effect, 330
    cause of death, 4
    nursing home population,
        prevalence, 330
Inflammation, cytokine release, serum
    zinc depression, 167
Inflammatory injury response, wound
    healing, 364
Insoluble fiber, dietary source, 51
Insulin
    cancer cachexia treatment, 311–312
    food intake stimulation, 36–37
Insulin receptor, responsiveness loss,
    46
Interdisciplinary team
    composition, 458–460
    consultant, 460
    core team member, 459
    decision making, 461
    definition, 458
    developmental process, 462
    dietitian, 464–466
    example, 464–465
    extended team member, 459–460
    functioning, 460–462
    group norms, 461
    leadership, 460–462
    medical center, model, 459
    member interaction, 462
    nutritional problem solution,
        457–469
    organization, 458–460
    patient, 460
    resource person, 460
    team consultant, 462
    team goal delineation, 461
Interleukin-1, T cell activation, 220
Intubation, gastrointestinal tract,
    351–353
Iodine, function, 174
Iron
    bioavailability, 62
    recommended daily allowance,
        61–62
Iron cycle, 185
Iron deficiency
    learning deficit, 425
    wound healing, 368

Israel Ischemic Heart Disease Study,
    serum cholesterol level, 273

J

Jargon, quackery, 399

K

Kupffer cell
    aging process, 246–247
    endocytosis activity, effect of aging,
        246
    function, 245–246

L

Laboratory parameter
    normal range, elderly, 111–112
    nutritional assessment, 111
Lactase, deficiency, 45–46
Lactose intolerance, elderly,
        prevalence, 234
Laxative, drug-food interaction,
        380–381
Lean body mass
    decrease with age, 44, 74
    water content, disease effect, 193
Learning, nutrition effect, 425–426
Learning deficit, iron deficiency, 425
Lecithin, human bile, 252
Legal standard of care, nourishment
        withholding, 471–480
Levodopa, nutritional implication, 387
Life expectancy
    average, 3
    cholesterol level, 276–277
    definition, 19
    protein restriction effect, 22
    sex differential, 1–2
    United States, increase, 3, 89
Life Extension, 403–404
Life extension
    antioxidant, 97
    dietary restriction, 96
    free radical scavenger, 97
Life span of species
    definition, 19
    nutrition, 23–25
    rate of aging relation, 21
Ligand, extrahepatic, hepatic
        processing, 248–249

Lipid, dietary, immunoregulatory
        aspect, 212–213
Lipid hypothesis, coronary heart
        disease, 47
Lipid intake, cell-mediated immunity
        effect, 215
Lipid level
    hepatocyte, 240
    serum, dietary cholesterol
        unrelated, 273
Lipid metabolism, cancer cachexia,
        310–311
Lipid reduction, mortality unaffected,
        93
Lipid Research Coronary Prevention
        study, 50
Lipoprotein, immunoregulatory
        property, 214–215
Lipoprotein lipase, 312
Lithium
    drug-food interaction, 385
    function, 175
    nutritional implication, 387
Live-cell therapy, cancer quackery,
        412
Liver
    aging effect, 239–258
    aging process, 241
    cell aging process, 240–241
    cell turnover, aging process,
        244–245
    endothelial cell
        aging process, 246–247
        function, 246
    feeding control mechanism, 36
    function, aging process, 247–248
    growth fraction, effect of aging, 245
Liver disease
    drug-induced, aging process effect,
        253–254
    specific, aging process, 254
Living Will, food withholding, 476
Living Will law, 472–473
Longevity
    aging relation, 20–21
    disease relation, 20–21
    expression, 19–20
    measurement, 19–20
    nutrition, 19–25
    nutritional enhancement,
        misinformation, 404–406
    United States, 278

Lymphocyte
  function
    aging effect, 83–84
    protein-calorie malnutrition
      effect, 83–84
    total count, immune status
      indication, 83
Lysine-arginine regimen, thymulin
  elevation, 217
Lysosome, hepatocyte, volume
  density, 244

M

Macular degeneration, zinc
  supplementation, 164
Magnesium
  hypertension relation, 288
  recommended daily allowance, 64
Malnutrition
  brain damage, 420
  cancer, 309
  cause, 338
  congestive heart failure, diagnostic
    work-up, 316
  dementia, 7
  functional impairment associated, 6
  immunodepression, 209
  institutionalized elderly, 218
  mixed, 74
  nursing home
    epidemiology, 325–332
    incidence, 336
  protein-energy, 73–74
  risk factor
    physical impairment, 7–8
    prevalence, 6
Manganese, function, 175
Marasmus, 73–74
  definition, 105
  mixed marasmic stated, 74
Mastication
  denture wearer, 227
  function, 227
  quantitation, 227
Matol, Km, FDA regulation, 407–408
Maximum Lifespan
  calorie restriction, animal data, 404
  health food promotion, 403–404
Media, health claims, 403–404
Medical trade association, 415

Medical treatment, nutrition, 471–475
Medium chain triglyceride, enteral
  feeding, 348–349
Megavitamin, cancer quackery, 411
Megestrol acetate
  mechanism of action, 311
  weight gain, 310
Memory
  cholecystokinin, 426
  feeding, 425–426
  fish oil, dose effect, 438
  menhaden oil, 435–440
  retention test, mice, 436
Menhaden oil, memory enhancement,
  435–440
Menopause, negative calcium balance,
  150–151
Mental status
  altered, zinc deficiency, 165–166
  food ingestion alteration, 429
2-Mercaptoethanol, T cell immune
  response enhancement, 217
Mercury, dental filling, health fraud,
  413
Messenger ribonucleic acid level, age-
  related change, 15
Metabolic arthritis therapy, quackery,
  409
Metabolic therapy, cancer quackery,
  411
Metropolitan Life Insurance Weight
  Tables of 1983, 76
Microsome, hepatic, effect of aging,
  251
Midarm circumference, skeletal
  muscle estimation, 79
Migraine headache
  foods implicated, 430
  tyramine, 430
Milk, human, high-cholesterol-
  containing, 276
Mineral
  estimated safe and adequate daily
    intake, 61–66
  recommended daily allowance,
    61–66
  supplementation, 66
Mineral oil, nutritional implication,
  382
Minnesota Coronary Survey,
  cardiovascular disease, diet
  unrelated, 275

Mitochondria
  hepatocyte, volume density, 243
  protein level, effect of aging,
    243–244
Mitochondrial membrane, hepatic,
    cholesterol/phospholipid molar
    ratio, 241–242
Mitochondrial molecule, turnover
    rate, 243
Molybdenum, function, 175
Monamine oxidase inhibitor, drug-
    food interaction, 389
Mono-oxygenase enzyme, Class 2
    reaction, 251
Mono-oxygenase system, aging
    process, 250–251
Monoamine, feeding control, 34–35
Morbidity
  nutritional intervention effect, 89–90
  older population, 5–6
Mortality, adiposity, relative risk, 299
Mortality rate, protein-calorie
    undernutrition, nursing home,
    328–329
Mortality ratio, weight index, 301
Motor nerve, change with aging, 450
Mouth, change with aging, 231
Multidisciplinary team, definition, 458
Multiple Risk Factor Intervention
    Trial, coronary heart disease,
    274
Muscle
  fiber-specific change with aging,
    449–450, 451
  physiologic change with aging,
    448–452
Muscle energetics, 450–452
Muscle mass, training to increase, 452
Muscle size, gross, internal decrease
    with aging, 449
Muscle strength
  component, 448
  intervention study, 452–455
  loss with aging, 452
Muscle tension development, fast,
    balance maintenance, 455
Musculoskeletal agent, drug-food
    interaction, 381–384

N

National Health and Nutrition
    Examination Survey, weight, 77

Natriuretic inefficiency, effect of
    aging, 284–285
Nephropathy, food restriction
    influence, 22
Nerve terminal morphology, change
    with aging, 450
Neural functioning, zinc deficiency,
    420
Neurologic change, nutritional
    deficiency, 420
Neuropeptide, feeding control, 35
Neurotransmitter
  anorexia of dementia related, 109
  anorexia of depression related, 108
  nutrient precursor, 422–425
Niacin
  assessment, 139
  deficiency, 139
  function, 138
  gram dose, elevated cholesterol
    treatment, 402
  recommended daily allowance,
    58–59
  risk factors, 139
  toxicity, 140
Nickel, function, 175–176
Nicotinic acid. See Niacin
Night vision, impaired, zinc therapy,
    163
Nitrogen, jejunal absorption,
    hypoproteinemic patient, 318
Nitrogen balance
  congestive heart failure, 318
  protein intake effect, 45
Nitrogen balancing assessment,
    urinary urea nitrogen, 80–81
Nonnutritive substance, 430–431
Nonparenchymal cell, hepatic, aging
    process, 245–247
Norepinephrine, feeding control,
    34–35
Nursing home
  diet liberalization benefits, 341
  food service
    evaluation, 335
    federal guidelines on standards,
      334–335
    fiscal constraint, 335
    management, 334–335
  hypophagia, cause, 329
  malnutrition, epidemiology, 325–332
  model food plan, 335
  nutrient standard, 335

nutrition management, 333–342
population, 333
protein-calorie undernutrition
 intervention, 330
 prevalence, 325
Nursing home resident
 dentition status, decrease in food
  acceptability, 338
 diabetic, glycemic control, 340
 dietary intake, 337
 fat-modified diet, 340
 malnutrition, incidence, 336
 nutritional assessment
  anthropometric data, 337
  laboratory test, 337–338
  nutritional status, 336–338
   chronic condition affecting, 334
  therapeutic diet, need assessment,
   339
 weight loss, 338
Nutrient, estimated safe and adequate
 daily intake, 43
Nutrient bioavailability, drug
 treatment, 97–98
Nutrient deficiency, low-fat, low-
 cholesterol diet, 275
Nutrient requirement, enteral
 nutrition, 346–347
Nutrition
 cardiovascular disease, 269–279
 disease process influence, life
  expectancy effect, 21–23
 life span of species, 23–25
 longevity, 19–25
 medical treatment, 471–475
 oral function effect, 227–228
 oral pathology effect, 226–227
Nutrition intake, psychological
 condition affecting, 7
Nutrition management, nursing home,
 333–342
Nutrition profile, dietetic service, 463
Nutrition support team, 466–468
 enteral nutrition, utility, 467
Nutritional assessment, 110–112
 anthropometry, 78–80
 biochemical index, 80–85
  prognostic power, 85
 blood parameter, 81–82
 elderly, 73–87
 hematologic test, 82
 nursing home resident
  anthropometric data, 337

laboratory test, 337–338
pressure sore, 369
serum standards, 82
standard parameters, 336
Nutritional change, old age, 218
Nutritional deficiency, neurologic
 change, 420
Nutritional intake, measurement,
 118–119
Nutritional intervention, cell-mediated
 immune dysfunction,
 mechanistic approach, 219–220
Nutritional manipulation,
 autoimmunity retardation, 23
Nutritional misinformation, 399–416
Nutritional quality, food supply,
 400–402
Nutritional requirements, elderly,
 41–72
Nutritional risk factor, elderly
 population, prevalence, 6–8
Nutritional status
 disease susceptibility modulation,
  218
 healthy elderly, survey, 326–327
 institutionalized elderly, 327–328
 nursing home elderly, survey,
  327–328
 nursing home resident, 336–338
Nutritional supplement
 immunopotentiation, 217–218
 promotion, 401
Nutritional support, recent advances,
 343
Nutritional therapy, behavioral
 problem, 419

O

Obesity, 293–306
 age-related, pathogenesis, 298–299
 complication, 300
 definition, 293
 drug therapy, elderly, 304
 endocrine disorder, 298–299
 functional impairment, 302–303
 health hazards, 299–303
 hypertension association, 301
 management, 303–305
 megestrol acetate treatment, 310
 morbid, increased risk of death, 301
 mortality rate, 299
 nursing home admission, 305

Obesity (*contd*)
  prevalence
    America, 295–296
    Austria, 296
    Sweden, 296
  sleep-disordered breathing, 302
  spousal attitude, 304
  surgical treatment, 305
Older population
  cause of death, 3–5
  health status survey, 6
  morbidity, 5–6
  physician utilization, 8
Omega-3 fatty acid, diabetes diet, 266
Oral cavity
  age-related change, 225–226
  nutritional status effect, 225
Oral disease, prevalence, geriatric
    population, 225
Oral mucosa, atrophy, 225
Osmoreceptor sensitivity, increased by
    aging, 196
Osmoregulation, elderly, 195–197
Osteomalacia, 126
  early diagnosis, 158–159
  incidence, United States, 158
  severity, 158
  vitamin D status, 55–56
Osteopenia, 92
  age-related, vitamin D related, 155
  prevalence with age, 127
Osteoporosis, 127
  fluoride deficiency, 174
  postmenopausal women, 62–63
  vitamin D status, 55–56
Overweight. *See* Obesity

P

Package label, health fraud, 403
Pancreas
  change with aging, 234
  pancreatic failure, dietary factor,
    261
Pantothenic acid
  assessment, 141
  deficiency, 141
  function, 141
  risk factors, 141
  toxicity, 141
Paraventricular nucleus lesion, energy
    intake effect, 33

Parenteral nutrition formula
  glucose, 358
  lipid component, 358
Parenteral nutritional support
  complications, 467
  general principles, 357–359
  indication, 357
  limitations to use, 359–360
  monitoring, 359
  patient care, 359
  protein component, 357–358
  route of administration, 359
Patient
  interdisciplinary team, 460
  medical treatment preference,
    475–476
Patient history, nutritional assessment,
    111
Pepper, Claude, 397
Peptide chain elongation, alteration,
    15
Percutaneous endoscopic gastrostomy,
    351, 365
Periodontitis, elderly, 226–227
Peripheral hormone, feeding control,
    36–38
Peripheral neuropathy, pyridoxine
    supplementation, 391
Phenelzine, nutritional implications,
    388
Phenolphthalein, nutritional
    implication, 382
Phosphorus
  dietary
    calcium balance, 152
    deficiency, 64
    hypertension treatment,
      288
    intestinal absorption, age-related
      decrease, 288
Phylloquinone. *See* Vitamin K
Physical activity, 31
Physical examination, nutritional
    assessment, 111
Physical working capacity, aging
    decline, 31
Physician, quackery, 415
Physiologic aging, research, 240
Physiologic stress, protein
    requirement increase, 45
Plaque-forming-cell response,
    spleen, zinc deficiency
    reduction, 216

Plasma glucose concentration,
     fluctuation, alcohol-drug
     interaction, 390
Plasma volume, age-related
     expansion, 185
Polyunsaturated fatty acid
     dietary intake, lipid composition
          alteration, 214
     dietary saturation,
          immunosuppressive activity
          correlation, 213
     omega-3
          blood pressure reduction, 289
          memory enhancement study,
               435–440
Polyunsaturated/saturated fat ratio,
     serum cholesterol
     effect, 48
Pooling Project, cholesterol-heart
     disease relation, 49
Popular publication, health claims,
     403–404
Potassium, dietary intake, 65
Potassium adaptation, effect of aging,
     285–286
Potassium supplementation
     hypertension treatment, 285–286
     natriuretic effect, 285
Pressure sore
     nutritional assessment, 369
     nutritional factors
          healing, 364
          management, 368–369
          pathogenesis, 363–364
          prevalence, 363
          risk factor, nutrition, 363–364
Prevention
     nutrition intervention, life
          expectancy unchanged, 89
     nutrition role, 89–104
     primary
          cancer, 94
          cholesterol, 92–93
          exercise, 96
          fish, 94
          fish oil, 94
          hypertension, 90–91
          life extension, 96–97
          osteopenia, 92
     secondary, 97–100
     tertiary
          exercise therapy, 101
          nutritional therapy, 101

Prognosis
     cholesterol level, 85
     serum albumin concentration, 85
     total lymphocyte count, 85
Prognostic Nutritional Index, 85
Propranolol, nutritional implication,
     376
Prostaglandin, increased synthesis,
          increased precursor intake, 214
Prostate cancer, incidence, 308
Protein
     diabetic diet, 266
     dietary intake, calcium balance,
          152
     recommended daily allowance,
          44–45
Protein-calorie malnutrition
     animal research, 210
     assessment, multidisciplinary
          approach, 114
     definition, 189
     hematologic manifestation, 188–191
     hospitalized elderly, incidence, 188
     human research, 209–210
     immunologic change, 189
     multifaceted complex syndrome,
          210
     treatment, 112–113
          multidisciplinary approach, 114
Protein-calorie undernutrition, nursing
          home
     cause, 329–330
     intervention, 330
     mortality rate, 328–329
     prevalence, 325, 328–329
Protein-energy malnutrition
     classification, Bistrian, 105
     early detection, 98
     growth hormone therapy, 113
     nutritional rehabilitation,
          hematologic effect, 190
     primary prevention programs, 98
Protein metabolism, impaired, 166
     zinc deficiency, 166
Protein status indication, arm muscle
     circumference, 79
Protein supplement, 401
Protein synthesis
     age-related change, 13–15
     age-related decline, 14
     biochemical process, 14
Proxisome, hepatocyte, volume
     density, 244

Pseudohypertension syndrome,
    sclerotic change causing,
    281–282
Psychiatric medication, appetite
    alteration, 429
Psychotherapeutic medication, drug-
    food interaction, 384–389
Psyllium hydrophilic mucilloid,
    nutritional implication, 382
Pyridoxal phosphate, biochemical
    deficiency, 58
Pyridoxine. See Vitamin B6
Pyridoxine supplementation,
    peripheral neuropathy, 391

Q
Quackery
    arthritis remedy, 409–410
    chronic medical problem, 399
    definition, 398
    jargon, 399
    physician, 415
    vulnerability of elderly, 398–399
Quinidine
    drug-food interaction, 379
    nutritional implication, 376

R
Recommended daily allowance, 42–43
    calcium, 62–63
    calories, 43–44
    carbohydrate, 45–46
    chromium, 173
    definition, 119
    folate, 59
    iron, 61–62
    magnesium, 64
    mineral, 61–66
    national variation, 119
    niacin, 58–59
    nursing home diet inadequate, 335
    protein, 44–45
    vitamin A, 54–55
    vitamin B2, 57
    vitamin B6, 58
    vitamin B12, 59–60
    vitamin C, 60
    vitamin D, 55
    vitamin E, 56
    vitamin intake, elderly, 118
    vitamin K, 57

Regulatory cell, imbalance, aging, 205
Renal anatomy, change with age, 195
Renal collecting tubule, vasopressin
    responsiveness, 196–197
Renal function, water metabolism,
    194–195
Reserve capacity, reduction, aging
    process, 185
Resource person, interdisciplinary
    team, 460
Respiratory tract agent, drug-food
    interaction, 389
Resting metabolic rate, decrease, lean
    body tissue loss, 43
Retention test
    memory, mice, 436
    menhaden oil performance
        improvement, 439
Retinal function, role of zinc, 163–164
Retinol. See Vitamin A
Riboflavin. See Vitamin B2
Ribonucleic acid synthesis, age-related
    change, 15
Rodaquin, cancer quackery, 412
Rodent longevity, food restriction,
    23–24
Rough endoplasmic reticulum,
    hepatocyte, volume density,
    242–243

S
Salivation, function, 228
Salt regulation, renin secretion
    impairment, 198
Salt restriction, dietary, hypertension
    treatment, 283–285
Satiety system, peripheral, nutrient
    intake regulation, 109
Schilling test, cobalamin deficiency,
    136
School performance, breakfast
    consumption, 425
Selenium
    age effects on level, 176
    deficiency
        atherosclerotic cardiovascular
            disease, 177–178
        carcinogenesis, 177
        cardiomyopathy, 177
        drug metabolism effect, 176
        hepatic effect, 176
        immune dysfunction, 178

function, 176
soil concentration, 176
toxicity, 178
Self-medication, 406–408
Senile dementia, tryptophan level,
423–424
Sense, 35
food intake effect, 35
Serotonin
appetite regulation, 423
feeding control, 34–35
tryptophan feeding, 422–423
Sex differential, life expectancy, 1–2
Sexual function, zinc status, 441–446
Silicon, function, 178
Skeletal muscle estimation, midarm
circumference, 79
Skin lesion, hypozincemia, zinc
supplementation, 162
Skinfold measurement, age-related
change, 297
Sleep-disordered breathing, obesity,
302
Small intestine
change with aging, 234–236
feeding control mechanism, 36
Smooth endoplasmic reticulum
hepatic, reduction with aging,
250–251
hepatocyte, volume density,
242–243
Sodium
delayed response, elderly, 198
dietary intake, 65
Sodium restriction
hypertension treatment, 283–285
nursing home resident, 339
Soluble fiber
dietary source, 51
glucose absorption slowing, 52
plasma cholesterol decrease, 52
Somatic mutation theory, 13
Spironolactone, nutritional
implication, 377
Starvation, apathy, 419
Stomach
change with aging, 232–234
feeding control mechanism, 36
Stomach cancer, incidence, 308
Strength training study, older
population
findings, 454
method, 453

Stress, anorexia, 189
Stromal cell, plastic-adhering, aging
effect, 208
Sucrose
diabetic diet, 265
hyperactivity, 428
Survival curve
longevity data expression, 19–20
rat, food restriction, 24

T
T cell
activation, interleukin-1, 220
differentiation, stage-specific, 209
differentiation pathway, 219
dysfunction, effect of age, 203–206
interaction, 219
B cell, 219
nucleus
functional change, 206
morphologic alteration with age,
206
qualitative change with age, 205–206
quantitative change with age, 205
6-thioguanine-resistant, age-related
increase, 206
T-maze footshock avoidance training,
retention, menhaden oil effect,
437–439
Taste
elderly, 228
impaired, zinc supplementation,
164–165
Teamwork, health care delivery,
457–458
Tecumseh Study, serum cholesterol
level, 273
Tension production, effect of aging,
448
Testosterone level, zinc excretion
relationship, 444–445
Thermic effect of meals, 30–31
adaptive component, 30
obligatory component, 30
Thiamine. *See* Vitamin B₁
Thiazide diuretic
calcium supplement interaction, 391
nutritional implication, 377
Thirst-neurohypophyseal-arginine
vasopressin, antidiuretic
hormone-renal feedback loop,
195

Thirst perception, alteration with aging, 198–199
Thymic graft, involuting, T cell generation, 207–208
Thymic peptide, hormonal activity, 207
Thymosin alpha-1, epithelial cell containing, 207
Thymus
  age-related change, 206–209
  involution, age-related, 207
Thyroid hormone
  basal metabolic rate governance, 29
  food intake effect, 37
Tissue repair, schematic representation, 352
Tocopherol. *See* Vitamin E
Tooth, age-related change, 226
Tooth loss
  food selection alteration, 228
  masticatory ability decline, 227
Toxicity
  biotin, 140
  folic acid, 138
  niacin, 140
  pantothenic acid, 141
  selenium, 178
  vitamin A, 124
  vitamin B_1, 131
  vitamin B_2, 132
  vitamin B_6, 134
  vitamin B_{12}, 136
  vitamin C, 143–144
  vitamin D, 127
  vitamin E, 129
  vitamin K, 130
Trace element
  aging effect, 171–179
  function, 171–179
  interaction, 179
  recommended daily dose, 347
Transcobalamin II, vitamin B_{12} plasma carrier, 60
Transferrin, malnutrition indication, 82
Triceps skinfold thickness, body fat estimation, 79
Tricyclic antidepressant, drug-food interaction, 384–389
Triglyceride, medium chain, 348–349
Tryptophan
  drug interaction, 393
  senile dementia, 423–424
    serotonin concentration increase, 422
    sleep enhancement, 423
Tube feeding, complication, 113
Tumor necrosis factor/cachectin
  cachexia mediation, 311
  cancer cachexia treatment, 312
Tumorex, cancer quackery, 412
Tyramine, migraine headache, 430

U

Undernutrition, confounding problems, 38
Upper arm, anthropometry, 79–80
Urinary creatinine excretion, lean body mass indication, 81
Urinary diluting capacity, 197
Urinary urea nitrogen, nitrogen balancing assessment, 80–81
U.S. Dietary Guidelines, dietary recommendation, 46
U.S. Postal Service, health fraud, 414

V

Vanadium
  deficiency, cholesterol level, 179
  human intake, 179
Vasodilator, drug-food interaction, 373–379
Vasopressin
  end-organ resistance, molecular basis, 196–197
  plasma concentration, upright posture increase, 197
  secretion, osmoregulation, 196
  secretory capacity, unimpaired by aging, 195–196
Ventromedial nucleus lesion, energy intake effect, 33
Violent behavior, specialized diet, 426
Vitamin
  definition, 117
  recommended daily allowance, 52, 117–118
  source, 121
Vitamin A
  assessment, 123
  deficiency, 123–124
  elderly intake, 54–55
  function, 122–123

intestinal uptake, increase with age, 235
plasma level, liver storage, 55
recommended daily allowance, 54–55
risk factors, 123–124
toxicity, 124, 402
wound healing, 367
Vitamin B₁
  absorption, alcohol decrease, 57
  assessment, 130
  deficiency, 131
    collagen synthesis, 367
  dietary intake, 57
  function, 130
  recommended daily allowance, 57
  risk factors, 130–131
  toxicity, 131
Vitamin B₂
  assessment, 132
  deficiency, 57, 132
  dietary intake, 57
  function, 132
  recommended daily allowance, 57
  risk factors, 132
  toxicity, 132
Vitamin B₆
  assessment, 133
  deficiency, 133–134
    atherosclerosis, 277
  depression, 420
  function, 133
  increased requirement with age, 58
  recommended daily allowance, 58
  risk factors, 133
  toxicity, 134
Vitamin B₁₂
  assessment, 134
  atrophic gastritis limiting, 233
  calcium bioavailability limited, 233–234
  deficiency, 135–136
    Schilling test, 136
  function, 134
  recommended daily allowance, 59–60
  risk factors, 135
  serum level, decline with age, 60
  toxicity, 136
Vitamin C
  assessment, 142
  deficiency, 142–143
  function, 141–142

megadose, 401–402
plasma level, sex variation, 60
recommended daily allowance, 60
risk factors, 142
serum level, smokers vs. nonsmokers, 402
toxicity, 143–144
wound healing, 367
Vitamin D, 156–158
  absorption, age-related defect, 157
  assessment, 125
  deficiency, 126–127
    elderly, 158–159
    hip fracture pathogenesis, 92
  endogenous synthesis, 126
  function, 125
  hydroxylation, 126
  malabsorption with aging, 236
  metabolism, age-related change, 155
  recommended daily allowance, 55
  risk factors, 126
  sun exposure, 55
  supplemental, 56
  total body store, 156
  toxicity, 127
Vitamin deficiency. *See also* Specific type
  cause
    elderly, 120
    general population, 120
  developmental stages, 119
  dietary pattern causing, 52
  manifestation in elderly, 122
  supplementation effect, 53–54
Vitamin disorder, elderly, 117–147
Vitamin E
  assessment, 128
  blood level, 56
  deficiency, 128–129
  function, 128
  health fraud, 405
  recommended daily allowance, 56
  risk factors, 128
  toxicity, 129
  wound healing, 367–368
Vitamin K
  assessment, 129
  deficiency, 129–130
  dietary intake, 56–57
  function, 129
  recommended daily allowance, 57
  risk factors, 129
  toxicity, 130

Vitamin/mineral supplement
  elderly consumption, 53
  nutritional status effect, 53–54
Vitamin requirement, advanced age,
  61
Vitamin supplement
  oral anticoagulant interaction, 391
  patient instruction, 144
Volume regulation, elderly, 198

W
Warfarin
  nutritional implication, 378
  vitamin supplement interaction, 391
Water
  free clearance, decreased, 200
  impaired access to, 199
Water homeostasis, fluid access
    impairment, 199
Water metabolism, 193–202
  clinical syndrome, 199–201
  disordered, cause, 194
  renal function, 194–195
  systemic modifier, 198–199
Weight
  age-associated change, 28
  Metropolitan Life Insurance Tables
    of 1983, 76
  National Health and Nutrition
    Examination Survey, 77
Weight index, mortality ratio, 301
Weight loss
  duration, 78
  exercise program, 303
  hypertension treatment, 289–290
  nursing home resident, 338
  nutritional risk indication, 77–78
  serum albumin level maintained,
    105–106
  technique in elderly, 305
Weight maintenance, anabolic
    androgen, 311
Wernicke's syndrome, 131
Wound contraction, 365–366
Wound healing
  age-related change, 366
  biology, 364–366
  carbohydrate function, 367
  collagen metabolism, 365
  epithelialization, 366

fat function, 367
impaired, zinc deficiency, 166
inflammatory response to injury,
  364
iron deficiency, 368
mineral function, 368
nutritional requirements, 366–368
protein function, 367
schematic representation, 352
vitamin A, 367
vitamin C, 367
vitamin E, 367–368
zinc deficiency, 368

X
Xerostomia, elderly, 228
D-Xylose, urinary excretion decline
    with age, 235

Z
Zinc
  depressed, elderly, 161
  dietary intake, 65
  excretion, diuretic elevation,
    444–445
  function, 161
  sexual function, 441–446
Zinc deficiency
  acrodermatitis enteropathica, 162
  anorexia, 161–165
  delayed sexual maturation, 444
  diabetes pathogenesis, 262
  diarrhea, 166
  effector cell dysfunction, 217
  growth period, effect, 216
  growth retardation, 166
  hypogonadism, 163
  immunodeficiency
    animal research, 216–217
    human research, 215–217
  impotence, 441–446
  manifestation, 162
  mechanism, multifactorial, 167
  neural functioning, 420
  prevalence, 215
  protein-calorie malnutrition, 215
  wound healing, 368

Zinc metabolism
  altered, clinical implication, 162–166
  elderly, 161–169
Zinc supplementation
  complication, 167

immune function effect, 165
immunopotentiation, 217–218
macular degeneration, 164
recommended dose, 168
response, 162

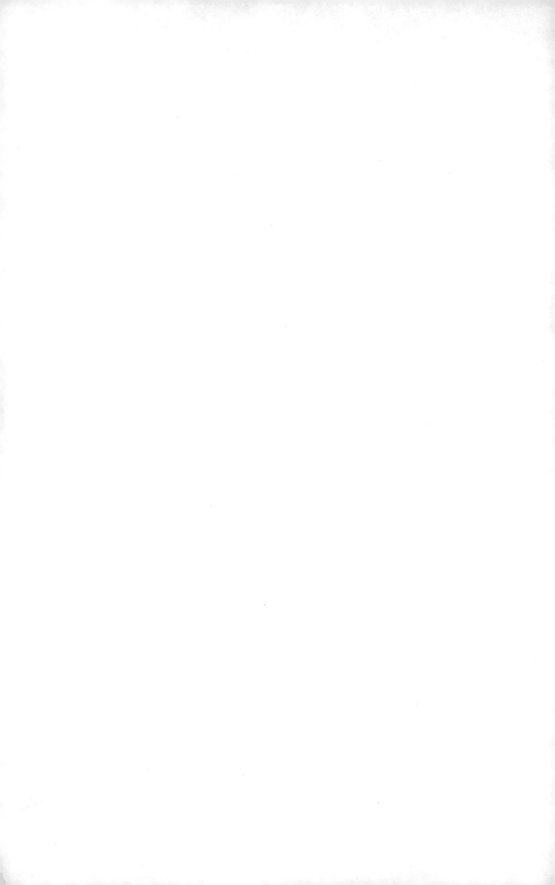